MW01675353

Clinical Rheumatology

Clinical Rheumatology

Edited by Mary Kellar

AMERICAN
MEDICAL PUBLISHERS
www.americanmedicalpublishers.com

American Medical Publishers,
41 Flatbush Avenue,
1st Floor, New York,
NY 11217, USA

Visit us on the World Wide Web at:
www.americanmedicalpublishers.com

© American Medical Publishers, 2022

This book contains information obtained from authentic and highly regarded sources. Copyright for all individual chapters remain with the respective authors as indicated. All chapters are published with permission under the Creative Commons Attribution License or equivalent. A wide variety of references are listed. Permission and sources are indicated; for detailed attributions, please refer to the permissions page and list of contributors. Reasonable efforts have been made to publish reliable data and information, but the authors, editors and publisher cannot assume any responsibility for the validity of all materials or the consequences of their use.

ISBN: 978-1-63927-474-1

Trademark Notice: Registered trademark of products or corporate names are used only for explanation and identification without intent to infringe.

Cataloging-in-Publication Data

Clinical rheumatology / edited by Mary Kellar.
p. cm.
Includes bibliographical references and index.
ISBN 978-1-63927-474-1
1. Rheumatology. 2. Rheumatism--Treatment. I. Kellar, Mary.
RC927 .C55 2022
616.723--dc23

Table of Contents

Preface

This book was inspired by the evolution of our times; to answer the curiosity of inquisitive minds. Many developments have occurred across the globe in the recent past which has transformed the progress in the field.

Rheumatology is a field of medicine that is concerned with the diagnosis and management of rheumatic diseases. The immune-mediated disorders of the musculoskeletal system, vasculitides, autoimmune diseases and heritable connective tissue disorders are under the scope of this field. These encompass degenerative arthropathies, systemic conditions and connective tissue diseases, inflammatory arthropathies, and soft tissue rheumatism. The diagnosis of a rheumatic disease may be based on multiple joint inspection, musculoskeletal examination, Schober's test, ultrasounds, X-rays, and the chemical pathology and cytopathology of the fluid aspirated from affected joints. Rheumatic diseases are generally treated with NSAIDs, analgesics, steroids, monoclonal antibodies and disease-modifying anti-rheumatic drugs. Rheumasurgical interventions may be directed at the prevention of disease progression or may be correctional interventions. This book includes some of the vital pieces of work being conducted across the world, on various topics related to rheumatology. It strives to provide a fair idea about this discipline and to help develop a better understanding of the latest advances within this field. It is appropriate for students seeking detailed information in this area as well as for experts.

This book was developed from a mere concept to drafts to chapters and finally compiled together as a complete text to benefit the readers across all nations. To ensure the quality of the content we instilled two significant steps in our procedure. The first was to appoint an editorial team that would verify the data and statistics provided in the book and also select the most appropriate and valuable contributions from the plentiful contributions we received from authors worldwide. The next step was to appoint an expert of the topic as the Editor-in-Chief, who would head the project and finally make the necessary amendments and modifications to make the text reader-friendly. I was then commissioned to examine all the material to present the topics in the most comprehensible and productive format.

I would like to take this opportunity to thank all the contributing authors who were supportive enough to contribute their time and knowledge to this project. I also wish to convey my regards to my family who have been extremely supportive during the entire project.

Editor

1

Comorbidity in gout at the time of first diagnosis: sex differences that may have implications for dosing of urate lowering therapy

Panagiota Drivelegka[1*], Valgerdur Sigurdardottir[1,2], Anna Svärd[2], Lennart T. H. Jacobsson[1] and Mats Dehlin[1]

Abstract

Background: The aim of this study is to examine the occurrence of comorbidities at the time of first diagnosis of gout compared with matched population controls, overall and by sex, as well as to examine the crude and age-standardized prevalence of these comorbidities in men and women with gout at first diagnosis.

Methods: A population-based study used data from Swedish national and regional registers, including 14,113 gout patients aged ≥ 20 years, with a first recorded diagnosis of gout between 1 January 2006 and 31 December 2012, and 65,782 population controls, matched by age, sex and county. Prevalence ratios (95% confidence intervals) comparing gout cases and controls were calculated, overall and by sex. Crude and age-standardized prevalence (95% confidence interval) of all comorbidities in gout patients were calculated, to show differences between sexes, taking also the higher age at diagnosis in women into account.

Results: All examined comorbidities were 1.2–2.5-fold more common in gout patients at diagnosis than in population controls in both sexes. Women with gout were on average 6 years older than men at first gout diagnosis and most comorbidities, including obesity and diuretic use, were or tended to be more frequent in women than in men. When standardizing for age, women had a higher prevalence of thromboembolism (6.6% vs 5.2%) and chronic obstructive pulmonary disease (3.1% vs 2.4%). Men, on the other hand, had a higher prevalence of coronary heart disease (9.4% vs 6.4%), atrial fibrillation (9.0% vs 6.0%), congestive heart failure (7.7% vs 6.6%) and stroke (4.1% vs 3.3%).

Conclusions: The occurrence of most comorbidities was significantly increased at first diagnosis of gout in both sexes. Women were older at diagnosis and had higher occurrence of most comorbidities, including obesity and diuretic use, factors that increase serum urate, and this needs to be taken into account when starting and optimizing urate lowering therapy. These sex differences were attenuated when standardizing for age and the occurrence of cardiovascular diseases was actually higher in men.

Keywords: Gout, Comorbidity, Epidemiology, Gender, Urate lowering treatment

* Correspondence: panagiota.drivelegka@vgregion.se
[1]Department of Rheumatology and Inflammation Research, Sahlgrenska Academy, University of Gothenburg, Grona Straket 12, Sahlgrenska University Hospital, 413 45 Gothenburg, Sweden
Full list of author information is available at the end of the article

Background

Gout is the most common form of inflammatory arthritis and is caused by deposition of monosodium urate (MSU) crystals in peripheral joints and surrounding tissues as a result of chronic elevation of serum urate (SU) levels. The incidence and prevalence of gout are increasing in many parts of the world and the prevalence is > 1% in North America and Europe [1].

Gout has been linked with an increased occurrence of several comorbidities, which all may influence the overall effect on quality of life and increased mortality [2–4]. Some of these comorbidities, such as use of diuretics [5, 6], renal disease [7–14], obesity [15, 16], transplantation [17–20], psoriasis [21, 22] and alcohol overconsumption [23, 24], have also been suggested to increase SU levels and hence be part of the causal pathway for developing hyperuricemia and clinical gout. Epidemiological studies examining the relationship between gout and risk for cardiovascular diseases (CVD) overall and in men and women separately report conflicting findings, with a significant association reported by some studies [3, 4, 25, 26], but not others [27–29]. There is only limited evidence for positive associations with cerebrovascular disease [30–33] or peripheral vascular disease (PVD) [34, 35].

Current clinical guidelines and management pathways endorsed by the European League against Rheumatism [36], American College of Rheumatology [37] and British Society for Rheumatology [38] agree on the importance of assessing comorbidities before deciding to initiate treatment of gout with urate lowering therapy (ULT). In addition, there are also results supporting the need for higher doses of ULT if patients have comorbid conditions, such as renal disease, use of diuretics or obesity [39]. This effect of decreased eGFR and diuretic use is probably explained by their ability to increase SU levels and not by any effect on the dose–response relationship between given allopurinol dose and change in urate levels [40].

It is well known that several comorbidities occur more commonly in patients with gout compared to the general population [20, 41–43], although there are relatively few population representative studies from Europe [43]. Furthermore, the timing of comorbidity occurrence relative to gout diagnosis has not always been addressed. In particular, there are very few studies examining the prevalence of comorbidities in patients with gout by sex [44–47] and none of them have presented results at the time of gout diagnosis. If such differences between sexes were found, they could indicate that pathological pathways differ in importance in men and women. In addition, such differences could be of importance to take into consideration when initiating and dosing ULT [39].

Using healthcare register data in the Western Swedish Health Care Region (VEGA) to identify cases and population registers to identify matched controls, and linking these groups to several national registers, this study aimed to: examine the occurrence of several comorbidities at the time of first diagnosis of gout compared with matched controls, overall and by sex; and examine the crude and age-standardized prevalence of these comorbidities in men and women with gout at first diagnosis.

Methods

Study design

We conducted a population-based and register-based case–control study using register data from 1 January 2000 through 31 December 2012 comparing patients at the time of first gout diagnosis to matched general population controls.

Ethical approval for the study was granted from the Ethical Review Board of Gothenburg, Sweden. Informed consent from the patients was not needed as the study only involved quality register linkage and no actual handling of patients.

Setting

According to Statistics Sweden, in 2016 the population of Sweden was 9,995,153 and in Västra Götaland, a county in the western part of Sweden, where the study was conducted, the population was 1,671,783 (http://www.scb.se/hitta-statistik/statistik-efter-amne/befolkning/befolkningens-sammansattning/befolkningsstatistik/).

Swedish health care is public and tax funded. Health and demographic information on all inhabitants is recorded in a series of different healthcare registers. Linkage of data from these registers is possible using the 10-digit personal identification number automatically assigned to all Swedish residents [48].

Data sources

The Western Swedish Health Care Region (VEGA) was used to identify cases with gout. This register contains information back to 2000 about all healthcare contacts at inpatient and outpatient specialty clinics, as well as at primary care clinics, and includes the date of visit and diagnoses given by the treating physician according to the Swedish version of the International Statistical Classification of Diseases (ICD). Since 1997, the 10th version of ICD (ICD-10) is used in Sweden. The vast majority of patients with gout are treated by general practitioners.

The Swedish Prescribed Drug Register (PDR) (http://www.socialstyrelsen.se/register/halsodataregister/lakemedelsregistret) contains information about all prescribed drugs dispensed by Swedish pharmacies since July 2005.

This register was used to determine the exposure of patients and controls to treatment with diuretics within 6 months prior to first diagnosis of gout, as well as to support the obesity and hypertension diagnoses. The Anatomical Therapeutic Chemical Classification System (ATC codes) was used to identify the medical treatments (Additional file 1: Table S1).

Demographic data were obtained from Statistics Sweden (http://www.scb.se/en/), which holds data on immigration, emigration and residency. Data on education level were retrieved from the Longitudinal Integration Database for Health Insurance and Labor Market Studies (LISA), which is administered by Statistics Sweden and holds annual registers on all individuals 16 years of age and older.

Vital status on 31 December 2012 was determined via the Cause-of-death Register (https://www.socialstyrelsen.se/register/dodsorsaksregistret), which provides information on the date and cause(s) of death for all residents since 1961.

Study populations

We identified all patients who attended any inpatient, outpatient or primary care clinic between 1 January 2000 and 31 December 2012. In this study we included all patients who had received their first ICD-coded diagnosis corresponding to gout (Additional file 1: Table S1) between 1 January 2006 and 31 December 2012. This time period was chosen in order to be able to link our data to the PDR and to be able to define these cases as incident. Cases with a diagnosis of gout before that period, cases receiving ULT before gout diagnosis and cases aged < 20 years were excluded (Fig. 1). Up to five general population comparators, alive and without gout by the time of the index patients' first gout diagnosis were identified for each gout patient and matched by year of birth, sex and county from the population register held by Statistics Sweden.

Comorbidities and medication of interest

We classified comorbidities into two diagnostic categories: comorbidities which have been 'suggested to increase the SU level' and consequently increase the risk for clinical gout (psoriasis, transplantation, renal disease, use of diuretics, obesity and alcoholism); and 'other comorbidities', such as diabetes, hypertension, coronary heart disease (CHD), congestive heart failure (CHF), atrial fibrillation (AF), stroke, thromboembolism, PVD and chronic obstructive pulmonary disease (COPD), in which the causal relationship to urate levels and clinical gout is not clear. With the exceptions of hypertension and obesity (based on both ICD codes and/or ever previously dispensed prescription of antihypertensive or anti-obesity drugs respectively according to ATC codes in the PDR), comorbidities were defined as the presence of at least one visit to a physician in primary or specialized care with a corresponding ICD-coded diagnosis (Additional file 1: Table S1). Treatment with diuretics (including thiazide, loop and thiazide-related diuretics) was defined as having dispensed a prescription of these agents within 6 months prior to first diagnosis of gout.

Comparison by sex

We compared demographic characteristics and pattern of comorbidities separately in men and women, with their respective controls.

Statistical analysis

Data are expressed as mean ± SD for continuous variables and number and percentages for categorical variables. The prevalence of a specific comorbidity was calculated by dividing the number of subjects diagnosed with that comorbidity prior to the date of first gout diagnosis of the index patient as numerator (for both cases and controls) by the total number of patients with gout or controls as denominator. Prevalence ratios (PRs) and 95% confidence intervals (CIs) were used to estimate the association between gout and each coexisting medical condition. In a sensitivity analysis, only cases with two or more visits with an ICD-coded diagnosis of gout [49] were included and compared with their matched controls. In the sex--stratified analyses we compared both the crude and standardized prevalence for each comorbidity. Standardization was done by the indirect method, with the Swedish census population in 2012 as the standard population. Nonoverlapping 95% CIs were considered statistically significant for all comparisons. All analyses were conducted using SAS software, version 9.3 (SAS Institute Inc. Cary, NC, USA).

Results

Population

A total of 14,113 individuals who received their first ICD-coded gout diagnosis between 1 January 2006 and 31 December 2012 were identified and matched to 65,782 general population comparator subjects (Fig. 1). There were 4600 women and 9513 men matched to 22,052 and 43,730 controls, respectively (Table 1). Women were approximately 6 years older than men at the time of gout diagnosis and had lower education level (Table 1).

Prevalence of comorbidities in the study population

Comorbidities suggested to increase SU level

At the time of gout diagnosis, 59.1% of gout cases had at least one comorbidity of this category, which was 2.1-

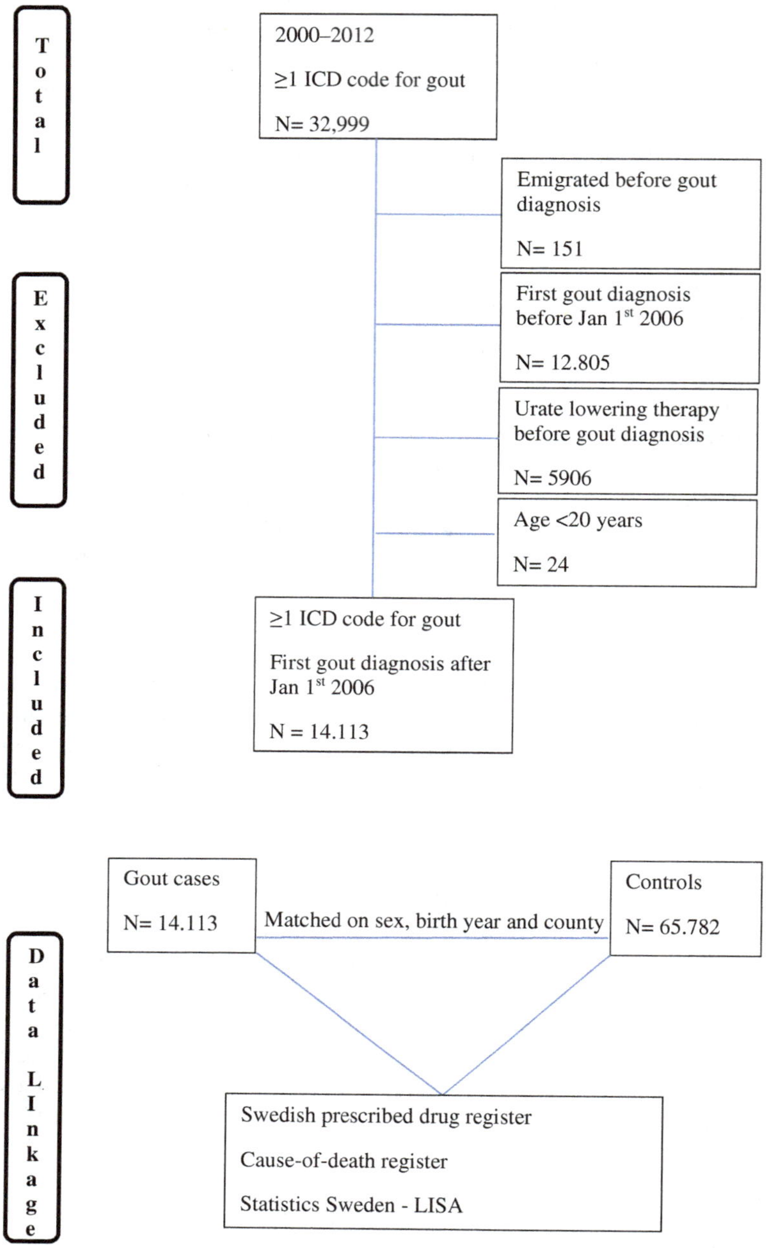

Fig. 1 Study design. ICD International Statistical Classification of Diseases, LISA Longitudinal Integration Database for Health Insurance and Labor Market Studies

fold higher than in controls (27.7%) (Table 1). Exposure to diuretics (43.7%), renal disease (11.8%) and obesity (10.4%) were the most frequent of these comorbidities in gout patients and were 2.3–2.7-fold more common in gout patients at diagnosis vs matched controls (Table 1). The proportions of individuals having undergone organ transplantation and those having diagnosed alcoholism and to a lesser extent psoriasis were also more common in gout patients compared to controls (Table 1).

Other comorbidities

At the time of gout diagnosis, the overall proportion of patients having at least one comorbidity of this category was 71.8% in comparison to 51.3% of the controls (Table 1). All cardiovascular diseases were both common and highly associated with gout at the time of gout diagnosis (Table 1), with hypertension being the most frequent in both gout patients (67.0%) and controls (44.3%) (Table 1).

Table 1 Demographic characteristics of the study population and prevalence (95% CI) of comorbidities in gout cases at the time of first diagnosis and statistical comparisons between all gout patients and controls

	Gout cases			Controls			PR (95% CI) (total gout cases – total controls)	*p* value (total gout cases – total controls)
	Men (*N* = 9513)	Women (*N* = 4600)	Total (*N* = 14,113)	Men (*N* = 43,730)	Women (*N* = 22,052)	Total (*N* = 65,782)		
Age at diagnosis (years), mean (SD)	65.3 (14.9)	71.1 (15.1)	67.2 (15.2)	64.4 (14.6)	70.7 (15.0)	66.5 (15.0)		
Level of education, *N* (%)								
≤ 9 years	3560 (37.4)	2169 (47.2)		15,531 (35.5)	9419 (42.7)			
10–12 years	4047 (42.6)	1655 (36.0)		17,349 (39.7)	7699 (34.9)			
> 12 years	1766 (18.6)	690 (15.0)		10,254 (23.5)	4509 (20.5)			
Comorbidities, total (%)	74.4	81.2	76.6	52.8	61.3	55.7		
Comorbidities suggested to increase SU level (%)	52.2	62.8	59.1	25.7	31.7	27.7		
Psoriasis, PR (95% CI)	3.6 (3.3–4.0)	4.0 (3.4–4.6)	3.7 (3.4–4.1)	2.7 (2.5–2.8)	2.8 (2.6–3.0)	2.7 (2.6–2.8)	1.4 (1.3–1.5)	< 0.001
Organ transplantation, PR (95% CI)	1.1 (0.9–1.3)	1.2 (0.9–1.5)	1.1 (1.0–1.3)	0.4 (0.3–0.5)	0.5 (0.4–0.5)	0.4 (0.4–0.5)	2.8 (2.3–3.4)	< 0.001
Renal disease, PR (95% CI)	12.2 (11.5–12.9)	11.1 (10.1–12.1)	11.8 (11.3–12.4)	5.1 (4.9–5.3)	3.4 (3.2–3.6)	4.5 (4.4–4.7)	2.6 (2.5–2.8)	< 0.001
Use of diuretics, PR (95% CI)	39.1 (37.8–40.4)	53.4 (51.3–55.5)	43.7 (42.7–44.8)	15.8 (15.5–16.2)	24.3 (23.6–25.0)	18.7 (18.4–19.0)	2.3 (2.3–2.4)	< 0.001
Obesity, PR (95% CI)	9.5 (8.9–10.1)	12.2 (11.2–13.2)	10.4 (10.0–11.0)	3.5 (3.3–3.7)	4.8 (4.5–5.1)	3.9 (3.8–4.1)	2.6 (2.5–2.8)	< 0.001
Alcoholism	5.1 (4.6–5.5)	1.8 (1.5–2.2)	4.0 (3.7–4.3)	2.9 (2.7–3.1)	0.9 (0.8–1.1)	2.2 (2.1–2.3)	1.8 (1.6–2.0)	< 0.001
Other comorbidities (%)	69.3	76.9	71.8	48.4	57.3	51.3		
Diabetes, PR (95% CI)	14.9 (14.1–15.7)	18.3 (17.1–19.6)	16.0 (15.4–16.7)	9.5 (9.2–9.8)	8.6 (8.2–9.0)	9.2 (9.0–9.4)	1.7 (1.7–1.8)	< 0.001
Hypertension, PR (95% CI)	64.5 (62.9–66.1)	72.3 (69.9–74.8)	67.0 (65.7–68.4)	41.4 (40.8–42.0)	50.2 (49.3–51.1)	44.3 (43.8–44.9)	1.5 (1.5–1.6)	< 0.001
Coronary heart disease, PR (95% CI)	19.5 (18.6–20.4)	18.2 (17.0–19.5)	19.1 (18.4–19.8)	13.7 (13.3–14.0)	11.8 (11.4–12.3)	13.0 (12.8–13.3)	1.5 (1.4–1.5)	< 0.001
Congestive heart failure, PR (95% CI)	16.2 (16.1–17.8)	21.4 (20.1–22.8)	18.4 (17.7–19.1)	6.5 (6.3–6.8)	7.7 (7.3–8.1)	6.9 (6.7–7.1)	2.7 (2.5–2.8)	< 0.001
Atrial fibrillation, PR (95% CI)	18.6 (17.7–19.5)	19.0 (17.8–20.3)	18.7 (18.0–19.5)	7.5 (7.3–7.8)	7.7 (7.3–8.1)	7.6 (7.4–7.8)	2.5 (2.4–2.6)	< 0.001
Stroke, PR (95% CI)	8.3 (7.7–8.9)	9.4 (8.6–10.3)	8.7 (8.2–9.2)	6.9 (6.6–7.1)	7.9 (7.5–8.3)	7.2 (7.0–7.4)	1.2 (1.1–1.3)	< 0.001
Thromboembolism, PR (95% CI)	9.7 (9.1–10.4)	13.6 (12.6–14.7)	11.0 (10.5–11.6)	5.4 (5.2–5.6)	7.3 (7.0–7.7)	6.0 (5.8–6.2)	1.8 (1.7–1.9)	< 0.001
Peripheral vascular disease, PR (95% CI)	4.5 (4.1–5.0)	5.5 (4.8–6.2)	4.8 (4.5–5.2)	2.2 (2.0–2.3)	2.6 (2.4–2.8)	2.3 (2.2–2.4)	2.1 (1.9–2.3)	< 0.001
Chronic obstructive pulmonary disease, PR (95% CI)	4.9 (4.5–5.4)	6.5 (5.8–7.3)	5.5 (5.1–5.9)	2.3 (2.1–2.4)	3.2 (3.0–3.4)	2.6 (2.5–2.7)	2.1 (1.9–2.3)	< 0.001

CI confidence interval, *PR* prevalence ratio, *SD* standard deviation, *SU* serum urate

Comparison by sex

Crude prevalence At the time of first gout diagnosis, all comorbidities were more frequent in cases compared to controls both overall and stratified by sex (Table 1).

All comorbidities, except for alcoholism, renal disease and CHD, had higher point prevalence in women compared to men, with nonoverlapping 95% CIs for use of diuretics (53.4% vs 39.1%), obesity (12.2% vs 9.5%), diabetes (18.3% vs 14.9%), hypertension (72.3% vs 64.5%), CHF (21.4% vs 16.2%), thromboembolism (13.6% vs 9.7%) and COPD (6.5% vs 4.9%). In men, only diagnosed alcoholism (5.1% vs 1.8%) was significantly more common.

Age-standardized prevalence The higher age of women at diagnosis (71.1 years compared to 65.3 years in men) was taken into account in two separate analyses.

First, the PRs for comorbidities were calculated by sex for each comorbidity (Fig. 2) compared to age-matched controls. The pattern of PRs was overall similar for men and women, although there were slightly higher PRs (nonoverlapping 95% CIs) for men for diagnosed hypertension and use of diuretics, and for women with regard to diagnosed renal disease and diabetes compared to the opposite sex (Fig. 2).

Second, we compared the age-standardized prevalence of comorbidities in men and women with gout (Table 2). In these analyses, comorbidities suggested to increase SU levels did not differ substantially (overlapping 95% CIs) and were numerically similar in men and women, with the exception of a slightly higher prevalence (but overlapping 95% CIs) for diagnosed obesity and use of diuretics in women.

On the other hand, the age-standardized prevalence for other comorbidities such as CHD, CHF and AF was significantly higher in men (nonoverlapping 95% CIs) compared to that for women, whereas the age-standardized prevalence for thromboembolism and COPD was significantly higher in women (nonoverlapping 95% CIs).

Sensitivity analyses

To assess the robustness of the results we also calculated the prevalence of the various comorbidities, defining gout by a stricter definition of having had two or more visits to a physician with gout over time. The prevalence of comorbidities when using the stricter case definition was overall similar to that in the main analyses (Additional file 2: Table S2).

Discussion

In this large, population-based study of patients with gout, recruited from both primary and specialized health care, we found that both comorbidities suggested to increase SU level and other comorbidities were more common in gout cases vs population-based controls, both overall and for men and women separately. All

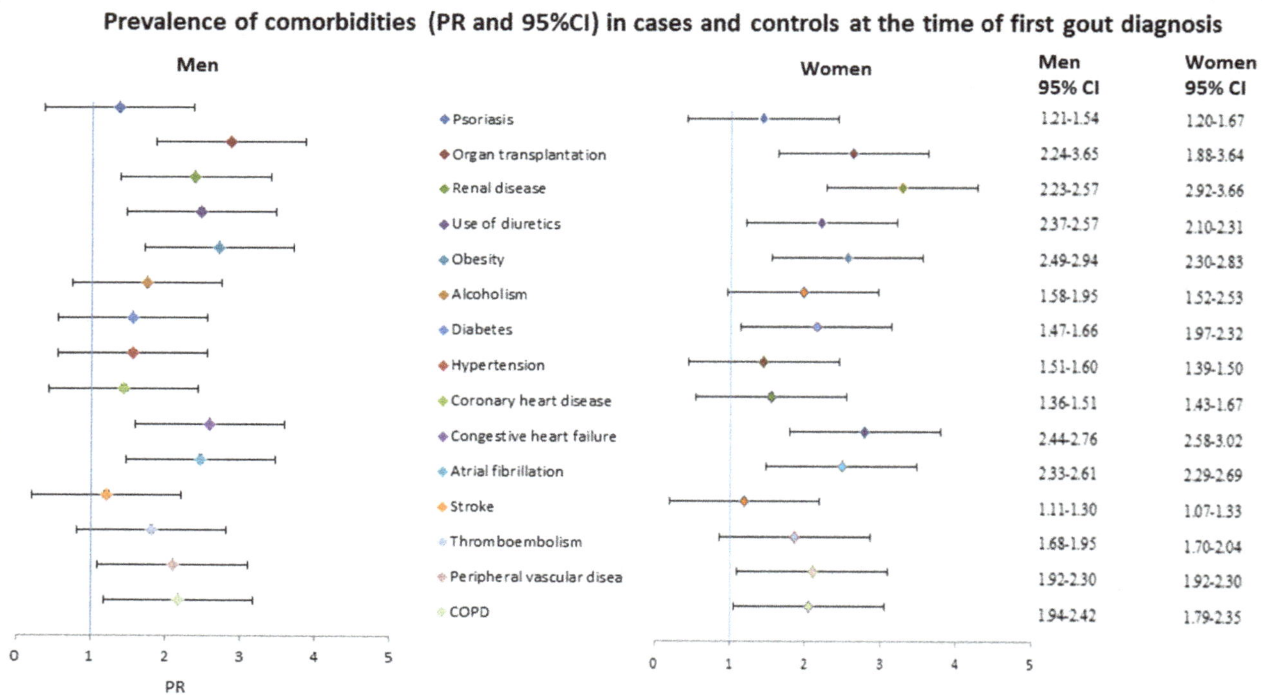

Fig. 2 Prevalence rates (95% CIs) of comorbidities in cases and controls for men and women at first gout diagnosis. CI confidence interval, COPD chronic obstructive pulmonary disease, PR prevalence ratio

Table 2 Age-standardized prevalence (95% CI) of comorbidities in men and women with gout at the time of first diagnosis

	Gout cases (N = 14,113)			
	Men (N = 9513), prevalence (%)	95% CI	Women (N = 4600), prevalence (%)	95% CI
Comorbidities suggested to increase SU level				
Psoriasis	3.7	2.8–4.5	3.3	2.6–4.1
Organ transplantation	1.3	0.8–1.8	1.8	0.9–2.6
Renal disease	8.2	7.4–9.0	8.3	6.8–9.8
Use of diuretics	21.9	20.9–22.8	24.1	22.7–25.6
Obesity	10.2	8.9–11.6	12.5	10.8–14.3
Alcoholism	5.5	4.7–6.3	3.5	2.1–4.8
Other comorbidities				
Diabetes	8.7	8.1–9.3	9.9	8.9–10.9
Hypertension	40.1	38.6–41.6	39.4	36.9–41.9
Coronary heart disease	9.4	9.0–9.9	6.4	5.8–7.0
Congestive heart failure	7.7	7.3–8.1	6.6	6.0–7.1
Atrial fibrillation	9.0	8.4–9.5	6.0	5.4–6.5
Stroke	4.1	3.7–4.5	3.3	2.8–3.7
Thromboembolism	5.2	4.8–5.6	6.6	5.8–7.5
Peripheral vascular disease	2.1	1.9–2.3	2.1	1.7–2.5
COPD	2.4	2.1–2.6	3.1	2.6–3.5

CI confidence interval, *COPD* chronic obstructive pulmonary disease, *SU* serum urate

comorbidities, except for alcoholism, were or tended to be more frequent in women than in men at the time of first gout diagnosis. When standardizing for age, these sex differences were attenuated, and diagnoses of CVD were actually more prevalent in men. Since gout may be diagnosed several years after the first attack [50], both hyperuricemia and gout may have been present for a considerable time before and a causal relation to CVD or other comorbidities is not possible to deduce from the present study. Regarding occurrence of comorbidities suggested to increase SU level, there were only minor sex differences after age standardization, which suggests large similarities in the pathophysiologic pathways leading to gout in men and women.

The prevalence of some comorbidities in our study, such as hypertension, CHF, diabetes, PVD and renal disease, was higher than that in the study by Kuo et al. [43], despite the fact that both studies are register based, include a large group of patients and report occurrence of comorbidities at the time of first gout diagnosis. The prevalence of psoriasis, however, was almost the same in both studies. Possible explanations, apart from the different geographical setting, could be that the mean age of gout patients in our study was 5 years higher and that our study had a slightly higher proportion of women (32.6% vs 27.5%), who were found to have higher occurrence of associated comorbidities than men.

Other studies that have examined sex differences in occurrence of comorbidities by sex differ to some extent from ours. One previous study on established gout by Harrold et al. from 2017 [44] showed, in line with the present study, that women had higher prevalence of obesity, hypertension and diabetes mellitus and were more likely to take diuretics compared to men, although this study was based on a smaller sample of patients identified from an American network of rheumatologists. In another previous American study [45] based on 6133 patients diagnosed with gout as part of their health insurance plans, all evaluated comorbidities (obesity was not included) were more frequent in women with gout compared to men. On the other hand, these studies showed that women had higher prevalence of kidney disease compared to men, which is not confirmed in our study. One possible explanation could be that our study is conducted at the time of first diagnosis of gout, whereas the previous studies examined prevalent gout, and that the mean age of our male patients was 5 and 7 years higher respectively than in the two previous studies. There is also one small clinical study by De Souza et al. [47] based on only 58 patients that showed no differences in the occurrence of comorbidities between women and men, which could be explained by the small sample size of the study. We have also shown that thromboembolism and COPD were more frequent in women with gout compared to men. The association between these comorbidities and gout has not been studied before. The higher prevalence in women might suggest some differences in pathophysiologic pathways or risk profile between men and women, but it is not possible to study the underlying mechanisms in the present study.

Regarding CVD, we found a higher occurrence in men compared to women, when adjusting for age. Current literature on risk for cardiovascular events in men and women with gout reports conflicting results. In line with the present study that showed higher prevalence of CHD and CHF in men, when we standardized for age, Krishnan et al. [26] showed that men with hyperuricemia had an increased risk for myocardial infarction in a controlled trial examining the efficacy of risk reduction in men at high risk for vascular events. Results from the Framingham study [25] showed an increased risk for CHD and angina in men with gout, but not in women, independently of other cardiovascular risk factors. Choi and Curhan [4] showed in a large prospective study that men with gout had higher overall mortality compared to men without gout. In contrast, De Vera et al. [51] in a population-based cohort showed higher risk for myocardial infarction in women compared to men, and Clarson et al. [34] in a population representative cohort in the UK showed that female patients with gout were at greater risk for any vascular event compared to men with gout. These discrepancies could be explained by differences between studies in study design, sample size and selection of the study population. Regarding potential explanatory mechanisms for higher frequency of CVD in men, we showed that other conventional risk factors for CVD, such as obesity, hypertension or diabetes, were not higher in men, although smoking and dyslipidemia could not be taken into account due to lack of data.

A previous study by Wright et al. [39] showed that obesity, use of diuretics and, to a lesser extent, renal disease had a significant influence on plasma urate concentrations and allopurinol daily maintenance dose. According to this study, dose requirements to achieve treatment goals for SU were found to increase by 2-fold to over 3-fold with increasing total body weight and were 1.25–2 times higher in those taking diuretics, whereas renal function had a relatively modest impact on the required allopurinol dose. Another study [40] suggests that the effect of decreased eGFR and diuretic use is explained by their ability to increase SU levels and not by any effect on the dose–response relationship between the given allopurinol dose and the change in urate levels. Considering that women in our study and previous studies [44] have a trend toward a higher prevalence of obesity and use of diuretics, factors that increase urate levels in serum, these comorbidities should be considered when initiating and adjusting ULT in women.

Some possible limitations should be acknowledged. The identification of gout patients was based on ICD codes, which may have led to some misclassification bias. However, according to a previous validation study [49], a more strict definition of gout requiring one or more visits with an ICD-coded gout diagnosis by a rheumatologist or two or more visits in primary care was found to have a high positive predictive value for fulfilling the various classification criteria for gout. The comorbidity pattern of gout cases in the present study was very similar to the comorbidity pattern of those fulfilling the stricter case definition (Additional file 2: Table S2), suggesting similar validity for both case definitions. Regarding definition of comorbidities, the validity of ICD codes in the Swedish national patient registry is generally very high [48], although not all diagnoses used in this study have been validated. There is, thus, a possible risk for underestimation of some comorbidities, in particular obesity and alcoholism, when ICD codes are used for definitions. However, there is no reason to believe that such underestimation would be of different magnitude in cases compared to controls and in women compared to men. Smoking, which is a major risk factor for CVD, could not be taken into account because of a lack of data. Finally, the study was performed in the western part of Sweden, which may hamper generalizability. However, according to previous reports, the sociodemographic distribution and healthcare seeking in this region are very similar to Sweden as a whole [52, 53].

This study has also several strengths. First, it is a population-based study, including all gout cases in the region, which reduces the risk of selection bias. Second, patients were identified from both primary and specialized health care, which covers all of the different phenotypes of gout, from mild to severe disease. Third, several unrelated independent data sources were used. For instance, case identification and information regarding medication or education level were retrieved from completely independent sources. Fourth, the study includes a large number of subjects with gout and controls, which generates statistically robust estimates for the occurrence of the various comorbidities.

Conclusions

This large, population-based study shows that all patients with gout have higher occurrence of many comorbid conditions at the time of first diagnosis, compared to matched controls from the general population. The majority of these comorbidities are more common in women than in men with gout. In particular, the higher occurrence of diuretic use and obesity in women may need to be taken into account when initiating ULT.

Abbreviations

AF: Atrial fibrillation; ATC: Anatomical Therapeutic Chemical Classification System; CHD: Coronary heart disease; CHF: Congestive heart failure; CI: Confidence interval; COPD: Chronic obstructive pulmonary disease CVD: Cardiovascular disease; eGFR: Estimated glomerular filtration rate; ICD: International Statistical Classification of Diseases; LISA: Longitudinal Integration Database for Health Insurance and Labor Market Studies; MSU: Monosodium urate; PDR: Swedish Prescribed Drug Register; PR: Prevalence ratio; PVD: Peripheral vascular disease; SD: Standard deviation; SU: Serum urate; ULT: Urate lowering therapy; VEGA: Western Swedish Health Care Region

Funding

This study was supported by grants from The University of Gothenburg and The Swedish Rheumatism Association.

Authors' contributions

All authors were involved in the conception and design of the study. LTHJ and MD contributed to the acquisition of the data. All authors contributed to analysis and interpretation of the data and take responsibility for the integrity of the data and the accuracy of the analyses. All authors participated in the drafting of the manuscript or revised it critically for intellectual content. All authors approved the final version to be published.

Competing interests

The authors declare that they have no competing interests.

Author details

[1]Department of Rheumatology and Inflammation Research, Sahlgrenska Academy, University of Gothenburg, Grona Straket 12, Sahlgrenska University Hospital, 413 45 Gothenburg, Sweden. [2]Centre of Clinical Research Dalarna, Falun, Sweden.

References

1. Kuo CF, Grainge MJ, Zhang W, Doherty M. Global epidemiology of gout: prevalence, incidence and risk factors. Nat Rev Rheumatol. 2015; 11(11):649–62.
2. Kuo CF, Yu KH, See LC, Chou IJ, Tseng WY, Chang HC, et al. Elevated risk of mortality among gout patients: a comparison with the national population in Taiwan. Joint Bone Spine. 2011;78(6):577–80.
3. Kuo CF, See LC, Luo SF, Ko YS, Lin YS, Hwang JS, et al. Gout: an independent risk factor for all-cause and cardiovascular mortality. Rheumatology (Oxford). 2010;49(1):141–6.
4. Choi HK, Curhan G. Independent impact of gout on mortality and risk for coronary heart disease. Circulation. 2007;116(8):894–900.
5. Hueskes BA, Roovers EA, Mantel-Teeuwisse AK, Janssens HJ, van de Lisdonk EH, Janssen M. Use of diuretics and the risk of gouty arthritis: a systematic review. Semin Arthritis Rheum. 2012;41(6):879–89.
6. Bruderer S, Bodmer M, Jick SS, Meier CR. Use of diuretics and risk of incident gout: a population-based case-control study. Arthritis Rheumatol. 2014;66(1):185–96.
7. Roughley MJ, Belcher J, Mallen CD, Roddy E. Gout and risk of chronic kidney disease and nephrolithiasis: meta-analysis of observational studies. Arthritis Res Ther. 2015;17:90.
8. Fathallah-Shaykh SA, Cramer MT. Uric acid and the kidney. Pediatr Nephrol. 2014;29(6):999–1008.
9. Juraschek SP, Kovell LC, Miller ER 3rd, Gelber AC. Association of kidney disease with prevalent gout in the United States in 1988-1994 and 2007-2010. Semin Arthritis Rheum. 2013;42(6):551–61.
10. Prasad Sah OS, Qing YX. Associations between hyperuricemia and chronic kidney disease: a review. Nephrourol Mon. 2015;7(3):e27233.
11. Avram Z, Krishnan E. Hyperuricaemia—where nephrology meets rheumatology. Rheumatology (Oxford). 2008;47(7):960–4.
12. Yu KH, Kuo CF, Luo SF, See LC, Chou IJ, Chang HC, et al. Risk of end-stage renal disease associated with gout: a nationwide population study. Arthritis Res Ther. 2012;14(2):R83.
13. Feig DI. Serum uric acid and the risk of hypertension and chronic kidney disease. Curr Opin Rheumatol. 2014;26(2):176–85.
14. Johnson RJ, Nakagawa T, Jalal D, Sanchez-Lozada LG, Kang DH, Ritz E. Uric acid and chronic kidney disease: which is chasing which? Nephrol Dial Transplant. 2013;28(9):2221–8.
15. Haslam DW, James WP. Obesity. Lancet. 2005;366(9492):1197–209.
16. Gheita TA, El-Fishawy HS, Nasrallah MM, Hussein H. Insulin resistance and metabolic syndrome in primary gout: relation to punched-out erosions. Int J Rheum Dis. 2012;15(6):521–5.
17. Clive DM. Renal transplant-associated hyperuricemia and gout. J Am Soc Nephrol. 2000;11(5):974–9.
18. Neal DA, Tom BD, Gimson AE, Gibbs P, Alexander GJ. Hyperuricemia, gout, and renal function after liver transplantation. Transplantation. 2001;72(10):1689–91.
19. Schwab P, Lipton S, Kerr GS. Rheumatologic sequelae and challenges in organ transplantation. Best Pract Res Clin Rheumatol. 2010;24(3):329–40.
20. Stamp L, Ha L, Searle M, O'Donnell J, Frampton C, Chapman P. Gout in renal transplant recipients. Nephrology (Carlton). 2006;11(4):367–71.
21. Merola JF, Wu S, Han J, Choi HK, Qureshi AA. Psoriasis, psoriatic arthritis and risk of gout in US men and women. Ann Rheum Dis. 2015;74(8):1495–500.
22. Kwon HH, Kwon IH, Choi JW, Youn JI. Cross-sectional study on the correlation of serum uric acid with disease severity in Korean patients with psoriasis. Clin Exp Dermatol. 2011;36(5):473–8.
23. Choi HK, Atkinson K, Karlson EW, Willett W, Curhan G. Alcohol intake and risk of incident gout in men: a prospective study. Lancet. 2004;363(9417): 1277–81.
24. Tu HP, Tung YC, Tsai WC, Lin GT, Ko YC, Lee SS. Alcohol-related diseases and alcohol dependence syndrome is associated with increased gout risk: a nationwide population-based cohort study. Joint Bone Spine. 2017;84(2):189–96.
25. Abbott RD, Brand FN, Kannel WB, Castelli WP. Gout and coronary heart disease: the Framingham Study. J Clin Epidemiol. 1988;41(3):237–42.
26. Krishnan E, Baker JF, Furst DE, Schumacher HR. Gout and the risk of acute myocardial infarction. Arthritis Rheum. 2006;54(8):2688–96.
27. Gelber AC, Klag MJ, Mead LA, Thomas J, Thomas DJ, Pearson TA, et al. Gout and risk for subsequent coronary heart disease. The Meharry-Hopkins Study. Arch Intern Med. 1997;157(13):1436–40.
28. Janssens HJ, van de Lisdonk EH, Bor H, van den Hoogen HJ, Janssen M. Gout, just a nasty event or a cardiovascular signal? A study from primary care. Fam Pract. 2003;20(4):413–6.
29. Teng GG, Ang LW, Saag KG, Yu MC, Yuan JM, Koh WP. Mortality due to coronary heart disease and kidney disease among middle-aged and elderly men and women with gout in the Singapore Chinese Health Study. Ann Rheum Dis. 2012;71(6):924–8.
30. Seminog OO, Goldacre MJ. Gout as a risk factor for myocardial infarction and stroke in England: evidence from record linkage studies. Rheumatology (Oxford). 2013;52(12):2251–9.
31. Chen JH, Chuang SY, Chen HJ, Yeh WT, Pan WH. Serum uric acid level as an independent risk factor for all-cause, cardiovascular, and ischemic stroke mortality: a Chinese cohort study. Arthritis Rheum. 2009;61(2):225–32.
32. Bos MJ, Koudstaal PJ, Hofman A, Witteman JC, Breteler MM. Uric acid is a risk factor for myocardial infarction and stroke: the Rotterdam study. Stroke. 2006;37(6):1503–7.
33. Hozawa A, Folsom AR, Ibrahim H, Nieto FJ, Rosamond WD, Shahar E. Serum uric acid and risk of ischemic stroke: the ARIC Study. Atherosclerosis. 2006; 187(2):401–7.
34. Clarson LE, Hider SL, Belcher J, Heneghan C, Roddy E, Mallen CD. Increased risk of vascular disease associated with gout: a retrospective, matched cohort study in the UK clinical practice research datalink. Ann Rheum Dis. 2015;74(4):642–7.

35. Baker JF, Schumacher HR, Krishnan E. Serum uric acid level and risk for peripheral arterial disease: analysis of data from the multiple risk factor intervention trial. Angiology. 2007;58(4):450–7.
36. Zhang W, Doherty M, Bardin T, Pascual E, Barskova V, Conaghan P, et al. EULAR evidence based recommendations for gout. Part II: Management. Report of a task force of the EULAR Standing Committee for International Clinical Studies Including Therapeutics (ESCISIT). Ann Rheum Dis. 2006; 65(10):1312–24.
37. Khanna D, Fitzgerald JD, Khanna PP, Bae S, Singh MK, Neogi T, et al. 2012 American College of Rheumatology guidelines for management of gout. Part 1: systematic nonpharmacologic and pharmacologic therapeutic approaches to hyperuricemia. Arthritis Care Res (Hoboken). 2012;64(10):1431–46.
38. Jordan KM, Cameron JS, Snaith M, Zhang W, Doherty M, Seckl J, et al. British Society for Rheumatology and British Health Professionals in Rheumatology guideline for the management of gout. Rheumatology (Oxford). 2007;46(8):1372–4.
39. Wright DF, Duffull SB, Merriman TR, Dalbeth N, Barclay ML, Stamp LK. Predicting allopurinol response in patients with gout. Br J Clin Pharmacol. 2016;81(2):277–89.
40. Kannangara DRW, Graham GG, Wright DFB, Stocker SL, Portek I, Pile KD, et al. Individualising the dose of allopurinol in patients with gout. Br J Clin Pharmacol. 2017;83(9):2015–26.
41. Zhu Y, Pandya BJ, Choi HK. Comorbidities of gout and hyperuricemia in the US general population: NHANES 2007-2008. Am J Med. 2012;125(7): 679–87. e1
42. Primatesta P, Plana E, Rothenbacher D. Gout treatment and comorbidities: a retrospective cohort study in a large US managed care population. BMC Musculoskelet Disord. 2011;12:103.
43. Kuo CF, Grainge MJ, Mallen C, Zhang W, Doherty M. Comorbidities in patients with gout prior to and following diagnosis: case-control study. Ann Rheum Dis. 2016;75(1):210–7.
44. Harrold LR, Etzel CJ, Gibofsky A, Kremer JM, Pillinger MH, Saag KG, et al. Sex differences in gout characteristics: tailoring care for women and men. BMC Musculoskelet Disord. 2017;18(1):108.
45. Harrold LR, Yood RA, Mikuls TR, Andrade SE, Davis J, Fuller J, et al. Sex differences in gout epidemiology: evaluation and treatment. Ann Rheum Dis. 2006;65(10):1368–72.
46. Yu TF. Some unusual features of gouty arthritis in females. Semin Arthritis Rheum. 1977;6(3):247–55.
47. De Souza A, Fernandes V, Ferrari AJ. Female gout: clinical and laboratory features. J Rheumatol. 2005;32(11):2186–8.
48. Ludvigsson JF, Otterblad-Olausson P, Pettersson BU, Ekbom A. The Swedish personal identity number: possibilities and pitfalls in healthcare and medical research. Eur J Epidemiol. 2009;24(11):659–67.
49. Dehlin M, Stasinopoulou K, Jacobsson L. Validity of gout diagnosis in Swedish primary and secondary care—a validation study. BMC Musculoskelet Disord. 2015;16:149.
50. Andres M, Bernal JA, Sivera F, Quilis N, Carmona L, Vela P, et al. Cardiovascular risk of patients with gout seen at rheumatology clinics following a structured assessment. Ann Rheum Dis. 2017;76(7):1263–8.
51. De Vera MA, Rahman MM, Bhole V, Kopec JA, Choi HK. Independent impact of gout on the risk of acute myocardial infarction among elderly women: a population-based study. Ann Rheum Dis. 2010;69(6):1162–4.
52. Ministry of Health and Social Affairs SGO. Updated high-cost protection—outpatient care and medication. 2013. ISBN 978-91-7555-111-1.
53. Statistiska C. Folkmängden efter region, civilstånd, ålder och kön. År 1968–2017. http://www.statistikdatabasen.scb.se/pxweb/en/ssd/START__BE__BE0101__BE0101A/BefolkningNy/?rxid=313a85a4-865b-47db-8892-54b5d5dff618. 2012.

2

In-vivo monitoring of anti-folate therapy in arthritic rats using [^{18}F]fluoro-PEG-folate and positron emission tomography

Durga M. S. H. Chandrupatla[1], Gerrit Jansen[1], Ricardo Vos[2], Mariska Verlaan[2], Qingshou Chen[3], Philip S. Low[3], Albert D. Windhorst[2], Adriaan A. Lammertsma[2], Conny J. van der Laken[1] and Carla F. M. Molthoff[2*]

Abstract

Background: Folate receptor β (FRβ) is involved in facilitating cellular uptake of folates and anti-folates (such as methotrexate (MTX)). In rheumatoid arthritis, FRβ is expressed on synovial macrophages and recently has been explored as a biomarker for imaging in arthritic rats using the folate-based positron emission tomography (PET) tracer [^{18}F]fluoro-PEG-folate. The purpose of this study was to examine whether this folate tracer can also be used to monitor therapeutic efficacy of MTX in arthritic rats.

Methods: Arthritic rats received either no treatment or MTX therapy (1 mg/kg, either 2× or 4×). Healthy rats did not receive any arthritic induction or therapy. [^{18}F]fluoro-PEG-folate PET-CT scans (60 min) were performed before and after MTX therapy. Following PET, the ex-vivo tissue distribution of radioactivity was determined in excised knees and multiple tissues. Synovial macrophage infiltration in knee sections was quantified by immunohistochemistry using ED1 and ED2 antibodies.

Results: PET scans clearly visualized increased uptake of [^{18}F]fluoro-PEG-folate in arthritic knees compared with contralateral knees. Significantly lower standard uptake values (1.5-fold, $p < 0.01$) were observed in arthritic knees of both MTX-treated groups after therapy, approximating the levels seen in healthy rats. Consistently, ex-vivo tissue distribution demonstrated a 2–4-fold lower tracer uptake in the arthritic knee of 2× and 4× MTX-treated rats, respectively, compared with control rats. These results were corroborated with significantly reduced (2–4-fold, $p < 0.01$) ED1-positive and ED2-positive synovial macrophages in arthritic knees of the MTX-treated rats compared with those of the control rats.

Conclusion: This study in arthritic rats underscores the potential and usefulness of [^{18}F]fluoro-PEG-folate PET as a therapeutic monitoring tool of MTX therapy and potentially other anti-folate treatment of arthritis.

Keywords: [^{18}F]fluoro-PEG-folate, Folate receptor β, Methotrexate, Rheumatoid arthritis, Macrophages

Background

Methotrexate (MTX) is the anchor drug in rheumatoid arthritis (RA) therapy, either as a single agent or in combination with disease-modifying anti-rheumatic drugs and biological agents [1–4]. Membrane transport via carrier-mediated and receptor-mediated routes is the first regulatory step in the mechanism of action of MTX in immunological target cells [5–7]. Notably, in RA (synovial) macrophages, the folate receptor β (FRβ) has been recognized as a major transport route for MTX, next to the reduced folate carrier [8, 9]. FRβ expression is confined to cells of the myeloid lineage [10, 11] as opposed to the α-isoform of FR (FRα), which is selectively expressed in specific types of cancer (ovary, breast) [12–14]. Given the high binding affinity (low nanomolar Kd) of FR for folic acid, this receptor has been exploited for therapeutic targeting with folate-conjugated drugs [15, 16] as well as imaging of FRα-positive tumours and activated FRβ-positive macrophages in RA [17–19]. FRs harbour several

* Correspondence: cfm.molthoff@vumc.nl
[2]Department of Radiology & Nuclear Medicine, VU University Medical Center, De Boelelaan 1117, 1081 HV Amsterdam, The Netherlands
Full list of author information is available at the end of the article

interesting properties for targeting with folate-based positron emission tomography (PET) tracers; for example, easy accessibility as an extracellular GPI-anchored membrane protein, high binding affinities for folates, and specific expression on activated macrophages in inflammatory diseases, allowing receptor targeting for imaging with folate-based PET tracers [9, 10].

In humans, macrophages have been identified as a sensitive biomarker for therapy monitoring, regardless of the choice of treatment [20]. Moreover, RA remission has been positively correlated with lower numbers of synovial macrophages [21]. These findings, however, were obtained by invasive histological studies. Clearly, non-invasive imaging of macrophages may be an attractive alternative approach to detect and monitor synovial activity in body tissues [22]. Animal models of arthritis can serve as a pre-clinical step to explore macrophage expression through novel imaging modalities. Beyond successful application of single-photon imaging agents—for example, EC20, a ^{99m}Tc-labelled folate [23–25]—to image arthritis, recently a folate-based PET tracer, [^{18}F]fluoro-PEG-folate, has been synthesized [26]. Such a tracer could potentially employ the higher sensitivity of PET and its ability to quantify uptake, which is essential for intervention studies. The potential of [^{18}F]fluoro-PEG-folate for imaging macrophages has been demonstrated in an arthritic animal model [26]. However, the potential of [^{18}F]fluoro-PEG-folate to monitor the efficacy of therapeutic interventions, in particular using anti-folates, such as MTX, has not been explored.

In the present study, the potential of [^{18}F]fluoro-PEG-folate as a macrophage-targeted PET agent for monitoring MTX therapy efficacy in arthritic rats was examined.

Methods

Animals

Wistar rats (male, 150–200 g; Charles River International Inc, Sulzfeld, Germany) were provided with standard food (16% protein rodent diet; Harlan Laboratories Inc., Madison, WI, USA) and water ad libitum. Rats were housed in groups of three to six in conventional cages and kept in a room with a 12-hour light/dark cycle, and constant room temperature (20 °C) and humidity level (50%). Animal experiments were performed in accordance with the European Community Council Directive 2010/63/EU for laboratory animal care and the Dutch Law on animal experimentation. The experimental protocol was validated and approved by the local committee on animal experimentation of the VU University Medical Center (DEC PET13-07).

Arthritic induction and therapeutic interventions

Wistar rats received 4× intra-articular (i.a.) mBSA injections, 4 or 5 days apart, in the arthritic knee as described previously [27]. This model had resemblance to human arthritis because after immunization and an i.a. mBSA injection in one knee, arthritis develops within a week as manifested by an increased knee thickness and synovial macrophage infiltration in the arthritic vs contralateral knee. This adds another major advantage to this model because the contralateral knee serves as an internal control over the arthritic knee. Additionally, by applying successive intra-articular mBSA injections after the first i.a. mBSA injection, a prolonged chronic phase of arthritis is maintained allowing assessments of therapeutic interventions. MTX (VU University Medical Center's pharmacy, the Netherlands) was administered (1 mg/kg) intraperitoneally (i.p.) once at days 22, 24, 29 and 33 (after the first i.a. injection) for the 4 × -MTX group ($n = 4$ rats) or once 3 days before (day 31) and once 3 days after (day 37) the fourth i.a. injections (2 × -MTX group, $n = 4$). Control rats (untreated control group, $n = 4$ rats) received phosphate-buffered saline (PBS) i.p. once at days 22, 24, 29 and 33 (after the first i.a injection). Healthy rats did not undergo arthritis induction or receive any treatment. At the end of therapy (~day 40), all rats were sacrificed and tissues were excised for further processing. Figure 1 summarizes the schedule of arthritis induction, therapeutic interventions and various analyses.

[^{18}F]fluoro-PEG-folate synthesis and PET-CT

[^{18}F]fluoro-PEG-folate was synthesized as described previously [26], with a radiochemical purity > 97% and mean specific activity of 31.4 ± 5.5 GBq/μmol. Rats were anaesthetized using inhalation anaesthetics (isoflurane 2–2.5% and oxygen 0.45 volume %). The tail vein was cannulated with a poly-urethane 3-French cannula. During PET-CT (Mediso nanoPET-CT, Budapest, Hungary) rats were placed in an integrated heating bed while monitoring respiratory function. A computed tomography (CT) scan was performed for 5 min, followed by tracer administration (10.5 ± 1.1 MBq) at the start of a dynamic PET scan of 60 min. PET data were normalized, and corrected for scatter, randomization, attenuation, decay and dead time. List-mode PET data were re-binned in 19 successive frames (4 × 5, 4 × 10, 2 × 30, 3 × 60, 2 × 300, 3 × 600 and 1 × 900 s), which were reconstructed using an iterative 3D Poisson ordered-subsets expectation-maximization algorithm with four iterations and six subsets. Resulting images had a matrix size of 170 × 170 × 157 voxels, each with a dimension of 0.6 × 0.6 × 0.6 mm^3.

PET data analysis

Images were analysed using AMIDE software (A Medical Image Data Examiner, version 0.9.2) [28]. CT and PET images were superimposed for drawing regions of interest (ROI). Fixed-size ellipsoidal-shaped ROIs (dimensions:

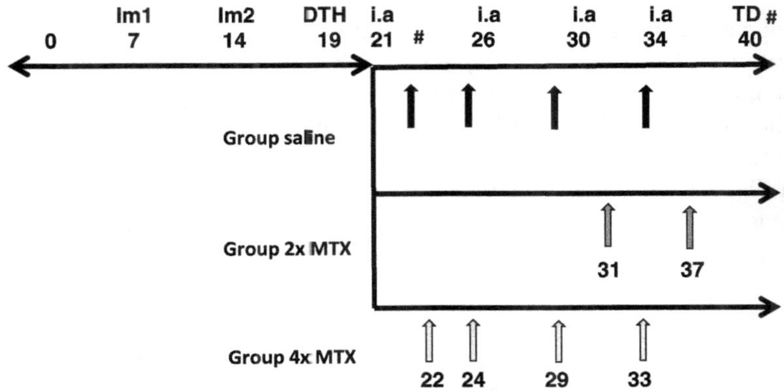

Fig. 1 Timeline depicting the induction of arthritis in rats and thereupon methotrexate (*MTX*) interventions. On day 7 and day 14 the first and second immunization (*Im1* and *Im2*) was administered, on day 19 the delayed type hypersensitivity (*DTH*) test and thereupon four intra-articular (*i.a.*) injections were administered. Upon arthritic induction the rats were administered saline (*black arrows*) or 2× MTX (*dark grey arrows*) or 4× MTX (*light grey arrows*). PET-CT (*#*) was performed before (day 22) and after (day 40) MTX therapy. At the end of the study (day 40), ex-vivo tissue distribution (*TD*) was performed. Healthy rats did not receive any arthritic induction or MTX treatment and were sacrificed on day 40

$7 \times 4 \times 7$ mm^3) were drawn manually over the area of both arthritic and contralateral knees in the last frame. Next, ROIs were projected onto the dynamic image sequence and time–activity curves (TACs) were generated. TACs were expressed as standardized uptake values (SUV); that is, mean ROI radioactivity concentration normalized to injected dose and body weight.

Ex-vivo tissue distribution studies

All rats were sacrificed (60 min after tracer administration) and knees, blood and various internal organs were excised, rinsed, dipped dry, weighed and the amount of radioactivity determined using an LKB 1282 Compugamma CS gamma counter (LKB, Wallac, Turku, Finland). Results were expressed as percentage of the injected dose per gram of tissue (%ID/g) [27].

Histopathology and immunohistochemistry

Both knees were dissected in toto and fixed for 7 days at 4 °C in 10% freshly made paraformaldehyde in PBS with 2% sucrose (pH 7.3) prior to decalcification in osteosoft (101728; Merck, Darmstadt, Germany) for ~2.5 weeks at room temperature. Thereafter, knees were embedded in paraffin. Sections of 5 μm were cut through the centre of the joint in a longitudinal direction and stained with haematoxylin and eosin to assess the degree of inflammation in synovial tissue. Staining for macrophages was performed as described previously [27]. Briefly, after antigen retrieval, sections were incubated with the specific mouse anti-rat monoclonal antibodies ED1, homologous to human CD68, and ED2, homologous to human CD163, or isotype control antibody for 1 hour at RT. All antibodies were obtained from Hycult (Plymouth Meeting, PA, USA). The detection EnVision™ kit (K4063 dual-link-HRP rabbit/mouse; DAKO, Glostrup, UK) was used according to the instructions of the manufacturer with 3,3′-diaminobenzidine tetrahydrochloride (DAB; DAKO) containing 0.01% H_2O_2. Subsequently, sections were counterstained with haematoxylin, dehydrated and mounted. Images were captured using a Leica 4000B microscope and Leica digital camera DC500 (Microsystems B.V. Rijswijk, the Netherlands).

All stained slides were blinded and counted by two independent observers, guided by an experienced pathologist, for ED1-positive and ED2-positive synovial macrophages. For this purpose, knee sections were divided into four quadrants (Q1–Q4), each representing the joint capsule with synovial tissue lining on either side of the proximal and distal side of the bone. Under the microscope (Leica, Amsterdam, the Netherlands) at 400× magnification, in each quadrant two to three areas were evaluated for macrophages in the lining and sub-lining (1–10 layers) of the synovium. The average number of macrophages per area from all four quadrants were combined and presented as total number of ED1 or ED2 macrophages (± standard deviation (SD)).

Statistical analysis

Statistical analysis was performed using SPSS (version 15) for Windows (SPSS Inc., Chicago, IL, USA). The Wilcoxon signed-rank (exact) test was used to determine differences in paired observations, such as uptake of [^{18}F]fluoro-PEG-folate in arthritic versus contralateral knees. Mann–Whitney (exact) tests were performed to analyse differences in [^{18}F]fluoro-PEG-folate uptake in groups (i.e. arthritic versus normal and control knees). $p < 0.05$ was considered statistically significant. All results are represented as mean ± SD.

Results

Arthritis induction and therapeutic interventions

Arthritis induction in rats (see Fig. 1 for timeline) was associated with macroscopic thickening of the arthritic knee compared with the contralateral knee (data not shown). Therapeutic interventions with MTX at the time points depicted in Fig. 1 were not associated with any adverse effects or visible effects on knees and no significant changes in body weight were observed.

[^{18}F]fluoro-PEG-folate PET studies in untreated and MTX-treated arthritic rats

At baseline, [^{18}F]fluoro-PEG-folate PET scans (Fig. 2a–c) clearly visualized high uptake in the arthritic knee of control rats, which decreased in both the 2 × -MTX and 4 × -MTX groups. Before treatment, [^{18}F]fluoro-PEG-folate SUV in the arthritic knee (1.01 ± 0.07) was significantly ($p < 0.01$) higher than in the contralateral knee (0.67 ± 0.04) (Fig. 2a, d). After MTX treatment, both the 2 × -MTX (0.67 ± 0.11) (Fig. 2b) and 4 × -MTX (0.70 ± 0.10) groups (Fig. 2c) showed a significantly ($p < 0.01$) 1.5-fold lower uptake of [^{18}F]fluoro-PEG-folate compared with untreated arthritic rats. In fact, SUV values in the arthritic knee of both 2 × -MTX and 4 × -MTX rats (Fig. 2e, f) were comparable with the level of uptake in knees of healthy rats (0.67 ± 0.07) (data not shown).

Ex-vivo tissue distribution studies

Before treatment, control rats showed a significantly 1.5-fold ($p < 0.05$) higher uptake (expressed as %ID/g) of [^{18}F]fluoro-PEG-folate in arthritic knees (0.22 ± 0.04) compared with contralateral knees (0.14 ± 0.04). After MTX treatment, [^{18}F]fluoro-PEG-folate uptake in arthritic knees was significantly 2-fold ($p < 0.05$) lower in the 2 × -MTX group (0.11 ± 0.01) and 4-fold ($p < 0.01$) lower in the 4 × -MTX group (0.06 ± 0.03) compared with untreated arthritic rats (Fig. 3).

Uptake of [^{18}F]fluoro-PEG-folate in plasma did not differ between control vs 2 × -MTX and 4 × -MTX rats (0.010 ± 0.006 vs 0.009 ± 0.001 and 0.009 ± 0.001, respectively) (Table 1). MTX treatment, however, did

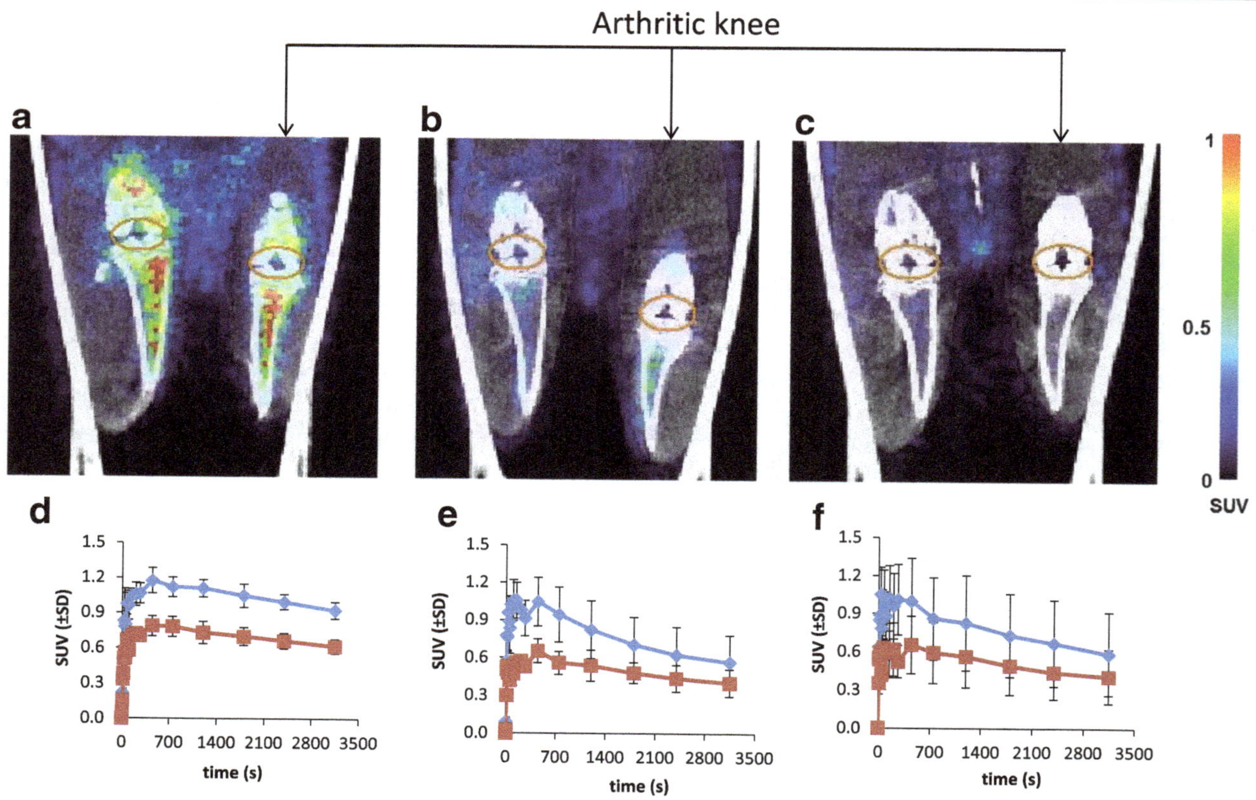

Fig. 2 Representative coronal PET-CT scans of [^{18}F]fluoro-PEG-folate in control and arthritic rats. **a** Control (before therapy, day 22); **b** 2× MTX and **c** 4× MTX (after therapy, day 40). *Orange ellipsoid*: ROI drawn around the synovium of the knee joint. Arthritic (*right*) and contralateral knees (*left*) depicted on each image. Standardized uptake value (*SUV*) scale bar from minimum 0 to maximum 1, represent the uptake of the tracer. TACs of [^{18}F]fluoro-PEG-folate uptake are expressed as SUV (±SD) in arthritic and contralateral knees of the control group (**d**), 2 × -MTX group (**e**) and 4 × -MTX group (**f**)

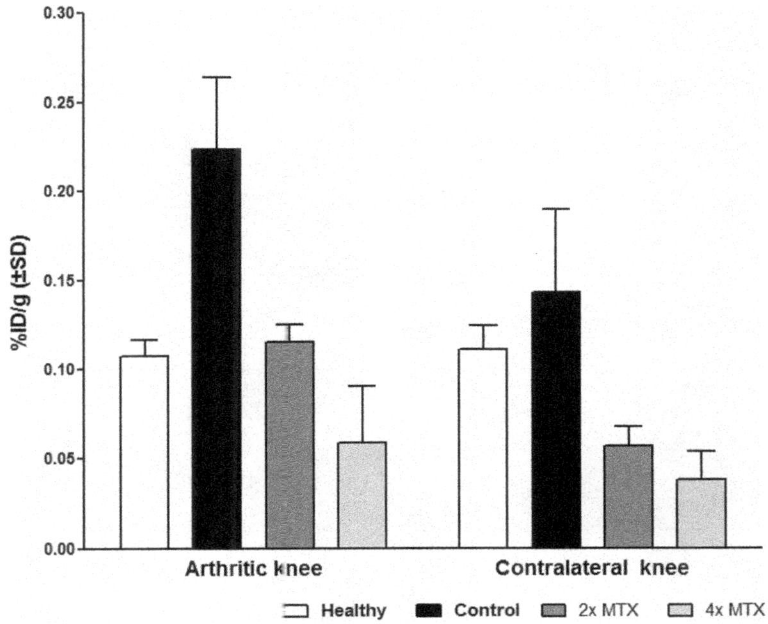

Fig. 3 Ex-vivo tissue distribution of [^{18}F]fluoro-PEG-folate in arthritic and contralateral knees of healthy (*white bars*), control rats (*black bars*) and 2 × -MTX (*dark grey*) and 4 × -MTX (*light grey*) rats at 60 min post tracer injection. Results expressed as mean percentage injected dose per gram (*%ID/g*). *Error bars* indicate SD. *MTX* methotrexate

reduce [^{18}F]fluoro-PEG-folate uptake in high macrophage resident organs, as illustrated in Table 1 for the control group vs both 2 × -MTX and 4 × -MTX groups in the liver, heart, spleen, lung and bone. In the kidney and intestine, MTX treatment had no major impact on tracer uptake in control, 2 × -MTX and 4 × -MTX rats (Table 1).

Immunohistochemistry of synovial macrophages

To examine whether the lower [^{18}F]fluoro-PEG-folate uptake in arthritic knees after MTX treatment was due to reduced infiltration of synovial macrophages, ED1-positive and ED2-positive macrophages in synovial tissue were quantified. Microscopically, synovial tissue of arthritic rats showed cellular influx of ED1$^+$ and ED2$^+$ macrophages (Fig. 4a–l), the latter of which were significantly ($p < 0.01$) more abundant: 3-fold (42 ± 9 vs 15 ± 4) and 2-fold (36 ± 8 vs 13 ± 3), respectively, in the arthritic and contralateral knees (Figs. 4a vs d, g vs j and 5). Both the 2 × -MTX and 4 × -MTX treatment groups of arthritic rats showed a marked and significant reduction of ED1$^+$ and ED2$^+$ synovial macrophages in the arthritic knees compared with the untreated counterparts (Fig. 4). Quantification showed a 4-fold and 3-fold ($p < 0.01$) reduction in ED1$^+$ synovial macrophages after 2 × -MTX and 4 × -MTX treatments (Fig. 5a), respectively. For ED2$^+$ the reduction was 3-fold ($p < 0.01$) for both groups (Fig. 5b). Notably, MTX treatment reduced ED1$^+$ and ED2$^+$ synovial macrophages in arthritic knees to levels observed in contralateral knees (Fig. 5).

Table 1 Ex-vivo tissue distribution of [^{18}F]fluoro-PEG-folate in various tissues of healthy control, 2 × -MTX and 4 × -MTX rats at 60 min post tracer injection

Tissue	Healthy rats	Control rats	2 × -MTX group	4 × -MTX group
Bone	0.103 ± 0.040	0.134 ± 0.022	0.064 ± 0.011	0.032 ± 0.016
Plasma	0.013 ± 0.007	0.010 ± 0.006	0.009 ± 0.002	0.010 ± 0.001
Blood	0.007 ± 0.009	0.007 ± 0.001	0.005 ± 0.002	0.006 ± 0.001
Lung	0.051 ± 0.019	0.074 ± 0.024	0.025 ± 0.016	0.024 ± 0.005
Heart	0.045 ± 0.015	0.080 ± 0.028	0.034 ± 0.004	0.022 ± 0.006
Liver	0.081 ± 0.049	0.106 ± 0.041	0.053 ± 0.006	0.042 ± 0.01
Spleen	0.393 ± 0.131	0.551 ± 0.218	0.132 ± 0.027	0.062 ± 0.034
Kidney	3.106 ± 0.317	2.077 ± 0.895	3.386 ± 0.186	3.098 ± 0.612
Skin	0.116 ± 0.017	0.138 ± 0.025	0.090 ± 0.012	0.063 ± 0.027

Results expressed as mean percentage injected dose per gram (%ID/g) ± standard deviation
MTX methotrexate

Discussion

The present study, using [^{18}F]fluoro-PEG-folate, investigated the feasibility of non-invasively monitoring efficacy of anti-folate therapeutic interventions in RA. Lower accumulation of [^{18}F]fluoro-PEG-folate in arthritic knees corroborated with decreased numbers of active macrophages in MTX-treated rats compared with the untreated rats. This was illustrated for MTX, because this is the golden standard in clinically active RA treatment [1, 3, 4].

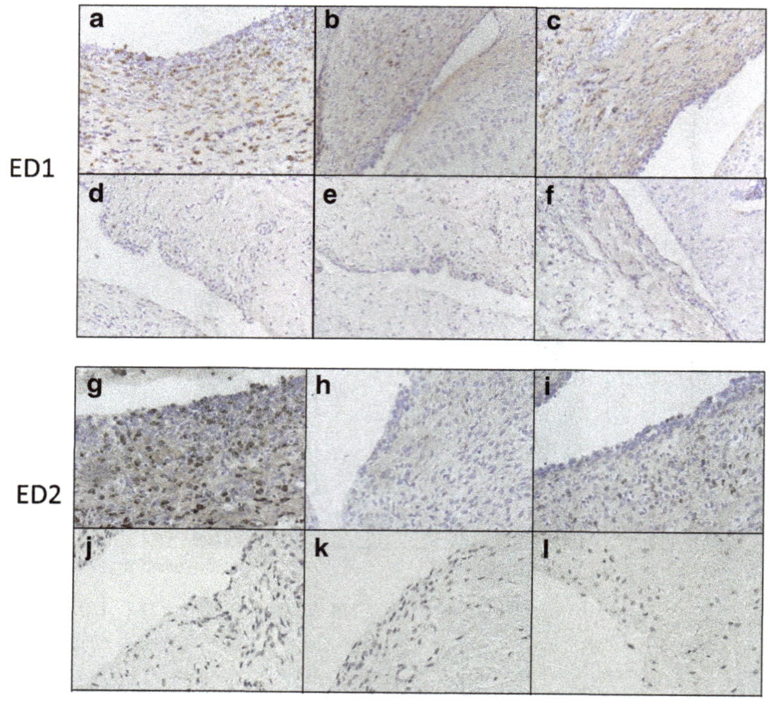

Fig. 4 Representative images of ED1$^+$ and ED2$^+$ synovial macrophages in knee sections of control and MTX-treated rats. **a**, **b**, **c** Images represent ED1$^+$ synovial macrophages in the arthritic knee of control, 2 × -MTX and 4 × -MTX rats, respectively. **d**, **e**, **f** ED1$^+$ synovial macrophages in the contralateral knee of control, 2 × -MTX and 4 × -MTX rats, respectively. **g**, **h**, **i** images of ED2$^+$ synovial macrophages in the arthritic knee of control and 2 × -MTX and 4 × -MTX rats, respectively. **j**, **k**, **l** ED2$^+$ synovial macrophages in the contralateral knee of control, 2 × -MTX and 4 × -MTX rats, respectively. All images captured at 200x magnification

Folate receptor expression on activated macrophages has been exploited for imaging and therapeutic monitoring of arthritis with various folate PET tracers including 4-[^{18}F]fluorophenylfolate and [^{68}Ga]-DOTA-folate [29]. These PET tracers showed a significantly improved specificity over a general inflammation tracer [^{18}F]-FDG, which relates to increased glucose metabolism in, for example, activated macrophages. In the present study, we made use of a pegylated folate tracer, [^{18}F]fluoro-PEG-folate, which harbours improved plasma pharmacokinetic properties over other folate tracers. In a side-by-side comparison in a rat model for RA [27], [^{18}F]fluoro-PEG-folate demonstrated a 1.5× improved target to background ratio compared with the mitochondrial translocator protein

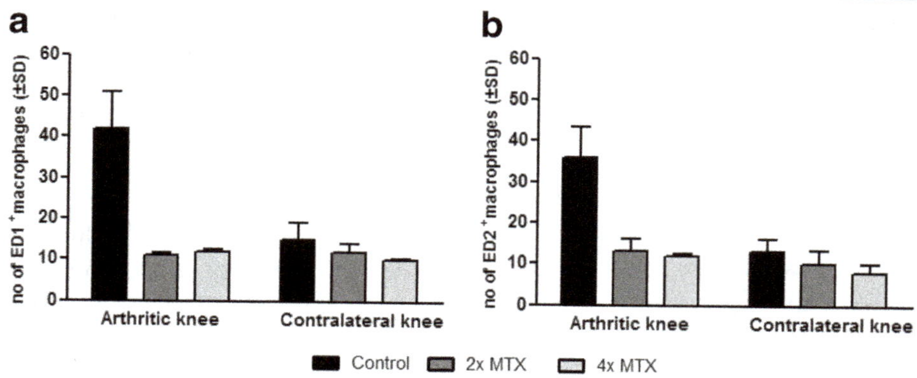

Fig. 5 Quantification of ED1$^+$ and ED2$^+$ synovial macrophages in knee sections of control and treated rats. **a** ED1$^+$ synovial macrophages, 6 days after the third boost, of control rats (*black bars*) and 2 × -MTX (*dark grey*) and 4 × -MTX (*light grey*) rats. **b** ED2$^+$ synovial macrophages, 6 days after the third boost, of control rats (*black bars*) and 2 × -MTX (*dark grey*) and 4 × -MTX (*light grey*) rats. Values represent mean number of macrophages counted in predefined areas of the synovium. *Error bars* indicate SD. *MTX* methotrexate, *SD* standard deviation

targeted macrophage tracer (R)-[^{11}C]PK11195 [26]. Moreover, [^{18}F]fluoro-PEG-folate also displayed promising PET imaging potential [26], which was taken a step further in the present study for monitoring therapeutic interventions, such as MTX therapy.

[^{18}F]fluoro-PEG-folate PET combined with a CT has advantage over the previous reported [^{18}F]fluoro-PEG-folate PET study [26], because the region of interest (ROI) around the synovium can be depicted more precisely. [^{18}F]fluoro-PEG-folate showed a marked reduction in tracer uptake in arthritic knees of the rats following two different MTX treatment regimens. It is unlikely that reduced tracer uptake in the MTX-treated rats is due to direct competition of the radiolabelled tracer with MTX for FRβ for various reasons: PET scans were acquired in the last week after the last MTX dose and, based on MTX pharmacokinetics [30] at that time, residual plasma levels will be <10 nM; the binding affinity of FRβ for [^{18}F]fluoro-PEG-folate outweighs the binding affinity for MTX by at least 100-fold; and also the binding affinity of the natural circulating plasma folate (i.e. 5-methyltetrahydrofolate) is 3-fold higher than the tracer [9, 26], and thus competitive effects are not anticipated. In addition, immunohistochemical analysis of the arthritic joints showed a significant reduction of macrophages in synovial tissue which was in line with reduced joint uptake of the folate tracer. Consistent with our PET results, Kelderhouse et al. [31] also demonstrated a markedly lower accumulation of the SPECT folate targeted imaging agent [^{99m}Tc]-EC20 in a collagen-induced arthritis (CIA) model upon administration of anti-rheumatic drugs. In the same CIA model, OTL0038, a novel folate-conjugated near-infrared dye, also showed low accumulation following anti-rheumatic therapies [32]. Together, whereas SPECT and optical imaging each has proven value with folate-based imaging agents, PET folate harbours advantages over SPECT (low-resolution and low-sensitivity images) [26] and optical imaging (no deep tissue imaging) [32]. Although costs of PET are relatively high at this moment, it is anticipated that with the widespread application of PET technology worldwide, costs will come down in the near future as also happened in the past decennia for the other imaging techniques such as CT and MRI.

Previously, apart from prominent arthritis induction in the arthritic knee, signs of systemic inflammation were also observed [27], reflected by tracer uptake in macrophage-rich organs, especially the liver and spleen. Ex-vivo tissue distribution data indicated that MTX therapy also had systemic effects by reducing [^{18}F]fluoro-PEG-folate uptake in these organs as well as in the contralateral knee. Independent of MTX therapy, the increased accumulation of [^{18}F]fluoro-PEG-folate in kidneys and intestinal tissue could be attributed to tracer clearance and/or high expression of FRα on kidney proximal tubule cells [15, 17] and intestinal tissue [33] to which receptor the folate tracer also binds.

Immunohistochemical analyses indicated that markedly reduced numbers of macrophages in the synovium of MTX-treated arthritic rats accounted for reduced [^{18}F]fluoro-PEG-folate tracer uptake. Interestingly, reduction in macrophages upon MTX treatment involved both ED1-positive and ED2-positive macrophages—although CD68 (and possibly its rat homologue ED1 used in the present study) is not an absolute marker for macrophages because its expression has also been demonstrated on fibroblasts. To extend on this point, an experienced pathologist examined the (arthritic) knee sections for morphological assessment of cellularity and immunohistochemical staining of ED1$^+$ cells. ED1$^+$ synovial fibroblasts were identified but morphologically discerned from macrophages and were not taken into account for macrophage scoring assessments. Moreover, from the perspective of macrophage polarization, we also examined numbers of ED2$^+$ macrophages (the rat homologue of human CD163, so-called 'M2', 'anti-inflammatory macrophages') in synovial tissue before and after therapy. Notably, studies by Puig-Kroger et al. [34] showed that FRβ is differentially expressed on M2 macrophages upon ex-vivo skewing of monocytes with macrophage-colony stimulating factor. However, studies by Tsuneyoshi et al. [35] in human RA synovial tissue demonstrated mixed patterns of FRβ expression on 'M1' ('pro-inflammatory') and M2 macrophages. In this context it is also important to note that M2 macrophages in an RA environment with complex IgG autoantibodies and/or ACPA antibodies are triggered to produce pro-inflammatory cytokines [36, 37]. Thus, MTX targeting with respect to polarization of macrophages and the role of FRβ therein warrant further investigations. Given the fact that beyond MTX several other second-generation anti-folates have been developed which have demonstrated potential pre-clinical anti-arthritic activity [7, 9, 38–40], [^{18}F]fluoro-PEG-folate PET imaging may be useful for monitoring their efficacy.

Conclusion

The present study demonstrates the feasibility of in-vivo monitoring of MTX therapy in arthritic rats using [^{18}F]fluoro-PEG-folate PET, paving the way for its future use in human clinical RA.

Abbreviations

FDG: FluoroDeoxyGlucose; FRβ: Folate receptor beta; i.a.: Intra-articular; ID/g: Injected dose/gram; M-CSF: Macrophage-colony stimulating factor; MTX: Methotrexate; PEG: Polyethylene glycol; PET-CT: Positron emission tomography–computer tomography; RA: Rheumatoid arthritis; ROI: Region of interest; SD: Standard deviation; SUV: Standardized uptake value

Acknowledgements
The authors gratefully acknowledge Dr H. Niessen for histopathological help, Marjon Al and Inge de Greeuw for expert technical assistance with in-vivo and ex-vivo studies, Elise Mantel for technical support with macrophage quantification, Eline Elshof for technical support with animal experiments, Rolph van Kooij for synthesis of [^{18}F]fluoro-PEG-folate and Martien Mooijer for tracer planning.

Funding
This study was supported by the Center for Translational Molecular Medicine (CTMM; project—TRACER), VU University Medical Center—Cancer Center Amsterdam (CCA—PV13/87) and the Dutch Arthritis Association (Reumafonds NRF 09-01-404).

Authors' contributions
DMSHC contributed to the acquisition, analysis and interpretation of the data and drafted the manuscript. RV and MV were involved in the animal studies and acquisition of PET-CT scans. CFMM, GJ and CJvdL were involved in the design of the study, contributed to the interpretation of the data and critically revised the manuscript. ADW coordinated the development of the PET tracer and made contributions to the manuscript. AAL contributed to the data analysis of the PET scans and editing of the manuscript. PSL and QC made contributions to PET tracer precursor synthesis and revision of the manuscript. All authors read and approved the final manuscript.

Competing interests
PSL is a stockholder from Endocyte Inc. The other authors declare that they have no competing interests.

Author details
[1]Amsterdam Rheumatology and Immunology Center, VU University Medical Center, De Boelelaan 1117, 1081 HV Amsterdam, The Netherlands. [2]Department of Radiology & Nuclear Medicine, VU University Medical Center, De Boelelaan 1117, 1081 HV Amsterdam, The Netherlands. [3]Department of Chemistry, Purdue University, 720 Clinic Drive, West Lafayette, IN 47907-2084, USA.

References

1. Kremer JM, Lawrence DA, Hamilton R, McInnes IB. Long-term study of the impact of methotrexate on serum cytokines and lymphocyte subsets in patients with active rheumatoid arthritis: correlation with pharmacokinetic measures. RMD Open. 2016;2(1):e000287.
2. Swierkot J, Szechinski J. Methotrexate in rheumatoid arthritis. Pharmacol Rep. 2006;58(4):473–92.
3. Hazlewood GS, Barnabe C, Tomlinson G, Marshall D, Devoe D, Bombardier C. Methotrexate monotherapy and methotrexate combination therapy with traditional and biologic disease modifying antirheumatic drugs for rheumatoid arthritis: abridged Cochrane systematic review and network meta-analysis. BMJ. 2016;353:i1777.
4. Bergstra SA, Allaart CF, Stijnen T, Landewe R. Meta-regression of a dose-response relationship of methotrexate in mono- and combination therapy in DMARD naive early rheumatoid arthritis patients. Arthritis Care Res. 2016. doi:10.1002/acr.23164 [Epub ahead of print].
5. Jansen G, Peters GJ. Novel insights in folate receptors and transporters: implications for disease and treatment of immune diseases and cancer. Pteridines. 2015;26(2):41–53.
6. Zhao R, Matherly LH, Goldman ID. Membrane transporters and folate homeostasis: intestinal absorption and transport into systemic compartments and tissues. Expert Rev Mol Med. 2009;11:e4.
7. Blits M, Jansen G, Assaraf YG, van de Wiel MA, Lems WF, Nurmohamed MT, van Schaardenburg D, Voskuyl AE, Wolbink GJ, Vosslamber S, et al. Methotrexate normalizes up-regulated folate pathway genes in rheumatoid arthritis. Arthritis Rheum. 2013;65(11):2791–802.
8. Nakashima-Matsushita N, Homma T, Yu S, Matsuda T, Sunahara N, Nakamura T, Tsukano M, Ratnam M, Matsuyama T. Selective expression of folate receptor beta and its possible role in methotrexate transport in synovial macrophages from patients with rheumatoid arthritis. Arthritis Rheum. 1999;42(8):1609–16.
9. van der Heijden JW, Oerlemans R, Dijkmans BA, Qi H, van der Laken CJ, Lems WF, Jackman AL, Kraan MC, Tak PP, Ratnam M, et al. Folate receptor beta as a potential delivery route for novel folate antagonists to macrophages in the synovial tissue of rheumatoid arthritis patients. Arthritis Rheum. 2009;60(1):12–21.
10. Elnakat H, Ratnam M. Distribution, functionality and gene regulation of folate receptor isoforms: implications in targeted therapy. Adv Drug Deliv Rev. 2004;56(8):1067–84.
11. Feng Y, Shen J, Streaker ED, Lockwood M, Zhu Z, Low PS, Dimitrov DS. A folate receptor beta-specific human monoclonal antibody recognizes activated macrophage of rheumatoid patients and mediates antibody-dependent cell-mediated cytotoxicity. Arthritis Res Ther. 2011;13(2):R59.
12. Boogerd LS, Boonstra MC, Beck AJ, Charehbili A, Hoogstins CE, Prevoo HA, Singhal S, Low PS, van de Velde CJ, Vahrmeijer AL. Concordance of folate receptor-alpha expression between biopsy, primary tumor and metastasis in breast cancer and lung cancer patients. Oncotarget. 2016;7(14):17442–54.
13. O'Shannessy DJ, Somers EB, Maltzman J, Smale R, Fu YS. Folate receptor alpha (FRA) expression in breast cancer: identification of a new molecular subtype and association with triple negative disease. Springerplus. 2012;1:22.
14. van Dam GM, Themelis G, Crane LM, Harlaar NJ, Pleijhuis RG, Kelder W, Sarantopoulos A, de Jong JS, Arts HJ, van der Zee AG, et al. Intraoperative tumor-specific fluorescence imaging in ovarian cancer by folate receptor-alpha targeting: first in-human results. Nat Med. 2011;17(10):1315–9.
15. Low PS, Henne WA, Doorneweerd DD. Discovery and development of folic-acid-based receptor targeting for imaging and therapy of cancer and inflammatory diseases. Acc Chem Res. 2008;41(1):120–9.
16. Assaraf YG, Leamon CP, Reddy JA. The folate receptor as a rational therapeutic target for personalized cancer treatment. Drug Resist Updat. 2014;17(4-6):89–95.
17. Muller C, Schibli R. Prospects in folate receptor-targeted radionuclide therapy. Front Oncol. 2013;3:249.
18. Nagai T, Kyo A, Hasui K, Takao S, Matsuyama T. Efficacy of an immunotoxin to folate receptor beta in the intra-articular treatment of antigen-induced arthritis. Arthritis Res Ther. 2012;14(3):R106.
19. Lu Y, Stinnette TW, Westrick E, Klein PJ, Gehrke MA, Cross VA, Vlahov IR, Low PS, Leamon CP. Treatment of experimental adjuvant arthritis with a novel folate receptor-targeted folic acid-aminopterin conjugate. Arthritis Res Ther. 2011;13(2):R56.
20. Haringman JJ, Gerlag DM, Zwinderman AH, Smeets TJ, Kraan MC, Baeten D, McInnes IB, Bresnihan B, Tak PP. Synovial tissue macrophages: a sensitive biomarker for response to treatment in patients with rheumatoid arthritis. Ann Rheum Dis. 2005;64(6):834–8.
21. Smith MD, Kraan MC, Slavotinek J, Au V, Weedon H, Parker A, Coleman M, Roberts-Thomson PJ, Ahern MJ. Treatment-induced remission in rheumatoid arthritis patients is characterized by a reduction in macrophage content of synovial biopsies. Rheumatology. 2001;40(4):367–74.
22. Gent YY, Ahmadi N, Voskuyl AE, Hoetjes N, van Kuijk C, Britsemmer K, Turkstra F, Boers M, Hoekstra OS, van der Laken CJ. Detection of subclinical synovitis with macrophage targeting and positron emission tomography in patients with rheumatoid arthritis without clinical arthritis. J Rheumatol. 2014;41(11):2145–52.
23. Leamon CP, Parker MA, Vlahov IR, Xu LC, Reddy JA, Vetzel M, Douglas N. Synthesis and biological evaluation of EC20: a new folate-derived, (99m)Tc-based radiopharmaceutical. Bioconjug Chem. 2002;13(6):1200–10.
24. Henne WA, Rothenbuhler R, Ayala-Lopez W, Xia W, Varghese B, Low PS. Imaging sites of infection using a 99mTc-labeled folate conjugate targeted to folate receptor positive macrophages. Mol Pharm. 2012;9(5):1435–40.
25. Matteson EL, Lowe VJ, Prendergast FG, Crowson CS, Moder KG, Morgenstern DE, Messmann RA, Low PS. Assessment of disease activity in rheumatoid arthritis using a novel folate targeted radiopharmaceutical Folatescan. Clin Exp Rheumatol. 2009;27(2):253–9.
26. Gent YY, Weijers K, Molthoff CF, Windhorst AD, Huisman MC, Smith DE, Kularatne SA, Jansen G, Low PS, Lammertsma AA, et al. Evaluation of the novel folate receptor ligand [18F]fluoro-PEG-folate for macrophage targeting in a rat model of arthritis. Arthritis Res Ther. 2013;15(2):R37.
27. Chandrupatla DM, Weijers K, Gent YY, de Greeuw I, Lammertsma AA, Jansen G, van der Laken CJ, Molthoff CF. Sustained macrophage infiltration upon multiple intra-articular injections: an improved rat model of rheumatoid arthritis for PET guided therapy evaluation. Biomed Res Int. 2015;2015:509295.

28. Loening AM, Gambhir SS. AMIDE: a free software tool for multimodality medical image analysis. Mol Imaging. 2003;2(3):131–7.
29. Kularatne SA, Belanger MJ, Meng X, Connolly BM, Vanko A, Suresch DL, Guenther I, Wang S. Low PS, McQuade P, et al. Comparative analysis of folate derived PET imaging agents with [(18)F]-2-fluoro-2-deoxy-d-glucose using a rodent inflammatory paw model. Mol Pharm. 2013;10(8):3103–11.
30. Hoekstra M, Haagsma C, Neef C, Proost J, Knuif A, van de Laar M. Bioavailability of higher dose methotrexate comparing oral and subcutaneous administration in patients with rheumatoid arthritis. J Rheumatol. 2004;31(4):645–8.
31. Kelderhouse LE, Robins MT, Rosenbalm KE, Hoylman EK, Mahalingam S, Low PS. Prediction of response to therapy for autoimmune/inflammatory diseases using an activated macrophage-targeted radioimaging agent. Mol Pharm. 2015;12(10):3547–55.
32. Kelderhouse LE, Mahalingam S, Low PS. Predicting response to therapy for autoimmune and inflammatory diseases using a folate receptor-targeted near-infrared fluorescent imaging agent. Mol Imaging Biol. 2016;18(2):201–8.
33. Parker N, Turk MJ, Westrick E, Lewis JD, Low PS, Leamon CP. Folate receptor expression in carcinomas and normal tissues determined by a quantitative radioligand binding assay. Anal Biochem. 2005;338(2):284–93.
34. Puig-Kroger A, Sierra-Filardi E, Dominguez-Soto A, Samaniego R, Corcuera MT, Gomez-Aguado F, Ratnam M, Sanchez-Mateos P, Corbi AL. Folate receptor beta is expressed by tumor-associated macrophages and constitutes a marker for M2 anti-inflammatory/regulatory macrophages. Cancer Res. 2009;69(24):9395–403.
35. Tsuneyoshi Y, Tanaka M, Nagai T, Sunahara N, Matsuda T, Sonoda T, Ijiri K, Komiya S, Matsuyama T. Functional folate receptor beta-expressing macrophages in osteoarthritis synovium and their M1/M2 expression profiles. Scand J Rheumatol. 2012;41(2):132–40.
36. Vogelpoel LT, Hansen IS, Rispens T, Muller FJ, van Capel TM, Turina MC, Vos JB, Baeten DL, Kapsenberg ML, de Jong EC, et al. Fc gamma receptor-TLR cross-talk elicits pro-inflammatory cytokine production by human M2 macrophages. Nat Commun. 2014;5:5444.
37. Clavel C, Ceccato L, Anquetil F, Serre G, Sebbag M. Among human macrophages polarised to different phenotypes, the M-CSF-oriented cells present the highest pro-inflammatory response to the rheumatoid arthritis-specific immune complexes containing ACPA. Ann Rheum Dis. 2016;75(12):2184–91.
38. van der Heijden JW, Assaraf YG, Gerards AH, Oerlemans R, Lems WF, Scheper RJ, Dijkmans BA, Jansen G. Methotrexate analogues display enhanced inhibition of TNF-alpha production in whole blood from RA patients. Scand J Rheumatol. 2014;43(1):9–16.
39. Nagayoshi R, Nakamura M, Ijiri K, Yoshida H, Komiya S, Matsuyama T. LY309887, antifolate via the folate receptor suppresses murine type II collagen-induced arthritis. Clin Exp Rheumatol. 2003;21(6):719–25
40. Castaneda O, Nair MG. Controlled trial of methotrexate versus CH-1504 in the treatment of rheumatoid arthritis. J Rheumatol. 2006;33(5):862–4.

3

Decrease in bone mineral density during three months after diagnosis of early rheumatoid arthritis measured by digital X-ray radiogrammetry predicts radiographic joint damage after one year

Michael Ziegelasch[1*], Kristina Forslind[2,3], Thomas Skogh[1], Katrine Riklund[4], Alf Kastbom[1] and Ewa Berglin[5]

Abstract

Background: Periarticular osteopenia is an early sign of incipient joint injury in rheumatoid arthritis (RA), but cannot be accurately quantified using conventional radiography. Digital X-ray radiogrammetry (DXR) is a computerized technique to estimate bone mineral density (BMD) from hand radiographs. The aim of this study was to evaluate whether decrease in BMD of the hands (BMD loss), as determined by DXR 3 months after diagnosis, predicts radiographic joint damage after 1 and 2 years in patients with early RA.

Methods: Patients (n = 176) with early RA (<12 months after onset of symptoms) from three different Swedish rheumatology centers were consecutively included in the study, and 167 of these patients were included in the analysis. Medication was given in accordance with Swedish guidelines, and the patients were followed for 2 years. Rheumatoid factor and antibodies to cyclic citrullinated peptides (anti-CCP) were measured at baseline, and 28-joint Disease Activity Score (DAS28) was assessed at each visit. Radiographs of the hands and feet were obtained at baseline, 3 months (hands only) and 1 and 2 years. Baseline and 1-year and 2-year radiographs were evaluated by the Larsen score. Radiographic progression was defined as a difference in Larsen score above the smallest detectable change. DXR-BMD was measured at baseline and after 3 months. BMD loss was defined as moderate when the decrease in BMD was between 0.25 and 2.5 mg/cm^2/month and as severe when the decrease was greater than 2.5 mg/cm^2/month. Multivariate regression was applied to test the association between DXR-BMD loss and radiographic damage, including adjustments for possible confounders.

Results: DXR-BMD loss during the initial 3 months occurred in 59% of the patients (44% moderate, 15% severe): 32 patients (19%) had radiographic progression at 1 year and 45 (35%) at 2 years. In multiple regression analyses, the magnitude of DXR-BMD loss was significantly associated with increase in Larsen score between baseline and 1 year ($p = 0.033$, adjusted R-squared = 0.069).

Conclusion: DXR-BMD loss during the initial 3 months independently predicted radiographic joint damage at 1 year in patients with early RA. Thus, DXR-BMD may be a useful tool to detect ongoing joint damage and thereby to improve individualization of therapy in early RA.

Keywords: Digital X-ray radiogrammetry, Bone mineral density, Disease progression, Early rheumatoid arthritis

* Correspondence: michael.ziegelasch@regionostergotland.se
[1]Department of Rheumatology, Department of Clinical and Experimental Medicine, Linköping University, Linköping, Sweden
Full list of author information is available at the end of the article

Background

Early stages of rheumatoid arthritis (RA) are characterized by gradually developing joint swelling, stiffness and pain, and the patients often have a history of several months of symptoms when first presenting to the rheumatologist. Periarticular bone loss may already be present at this stage, representing an early radiologic manifestation visible on plain radiographs [1, 2]. The disease course in RA shows considerable inter-individual variation, ranging from mild and self-limiting to severe erosive disease, sometimes with extra-articular manifestations. Early treatment with disease-modifying anti-rheumatic drugs (DMARDs) is known to improve disease outcome [3–5], and may limit disease-associated bone loss [6]. However, further improved individual prediction of the disease course and outcome remains an important issue in order to optimize anti-rheumatic therapy.

Digital X-ray radiogrammetry (DXR) is a technique that uses computerized analyses of standard hand radiographs to estimate peripheral bone mineral density (BMD) of the three middle metacarpal bones (DXR-BMD) [7, 8]. DXR-BMD loss has repeatedly been shown to predict radiographic joint progression in early RA [9–14]. However, the majority of previous DXR-BMD studies have been based on 12-month change, and by that time, conventional X-ray assessments of joint damage are at least as informative about disease progression [9, 11–14]. A Dutch study addressing DXR-BMD change after 4 months, reported an independent association between DXR-BMD loss and subsequent radiographic damage [10]. This study was part of a clinical trial with selected patients, and the treatment regimens were slightly different from standard care in Sweden. Therefore, we wished to investigate whether 3-month change in DXR-BMD predicts radiographic joint damage after 1 and 2 years in "real-world" patients with recent-onset RA.

Methods

Patients

Patients (n = 176) with early RA (64% women, symptom duration < 12 months), fulfilling the inclusion criteria (see subsequent text) and giving their informed consent, were consecutively included from three Swedish regions (one in Northern and two in Southern Sweden) in 2008–2014 and were followed for 2 years. All patients fulfilled the 2010 American College of Rheumatology (ACR)/European League Against Rheumatism (EULAR) [15] and/or the 1987 ACR [16] classification criteria. Pharmacotherapy was prescribed as found appropriate by the treating rheumatologist, according to Swedish guidelines. Baseline characteristics are detailed in Table 1.

At baseline, 83% of patients were prescribed oral prednisolone, 49% received osteoporosis prophylaxis with low-dose calcium phosphate and vitamin D, and 6% with bisphosphonates. 91% received conventional synthetic DMARDs (csDMARD) (88% methotrexate, 2.4% other csDMARDs and 0.6% combination therapy). One patient (0.6%) was started on a tumor necrosis factor (TNF) inhibitor at baseline. During the follow-up period 14.4% received biologic therapy (bDMARDs) as displayed in Table 2.

Radiographic assessment and digital X-ray radiogrammetry (DXR)

Radiographs (posterior-anterior projection) of the hands, wrists and forefeet were performed at baseline, 3 months (hands only) and 1 and 2 years. The baseline and 1-year and 2-year radiographs were read in chronological order and evaluated according to the Larsen score [17] by one investigator at each center (MZ, KF and EB). The scoring system included 32 areas; metacarpal-phalangeal joints II – V, all proximal interphalangeal joints, the wrists divided into four areas and the metatarsophalangeal joints II–V. Each joint and joint area was graded 0–5. The maximum total score was 160. The smallest detectable change (SDC) was calculated for the three readers individually (EB, 2; KF, 1; MZ, 3) according to the method of Bruynesteyn [18]. Radiographic progression was defined as a difference in Larsen score above the SDC of the corresponding reader. The intra-rater and inter-rater reliability of the readers was assessed by calculating the intraclass correlation coefficient (ICC). The ICC was 0.903.

BMD was estimated on hand radiographs of the second, third and fourth metacarpal bones using DXR (the online Pronosco X-posure System, SECTRA, Linköping, Sweden), a computerized version of the traditional technique of radiogrammetry measuring cortical bone thickness [8, 19]. DXR-BMD was assessed at inclusion and after 3 months. The mean value of both hands was used in all analyses. DXR-BMD values are given in mg/cm^2. DXR-BMD loss was categorized either as a moderate decrease in DXR-BMD (≥ 0.25 but < 2.5 mg/cm^2 per month) or a severe decrease (≥ 2.5 mg/cm^2 per month), as defined by the provider (Sectra) [20]. To ensure consistent image acquisition, the images for each patient were always taken in a frontal position of the hands using the same X-ray machine. The images were sent unprocessed to Sectra for DXR analysis.

Clinical and laboratory assessments

The erythrocyte sedimentation rate (ESR, mm/1 h) and C-reactive protein (CRP, mg/L) were determined at baseline and after 3, 6, 12 and 24 months. At the same time points, the 28-joint Disease Activity Score (DAS28) was calculated by the patient's regular physician [21]. Therapy response was determined according to EULAR response criteria [22]. Functional status was evaluated

Table 1 Baseline characteristics by radiographic progression at 1 year and bone mineral density loss after 3 months

	Total	Radiographic progression			BMD loss		
		No	Yes	*p* value	No	Yes	*p* value
Age	58 (14.5)	57.9 (14.4)	60.3 (14.7)	0.41	55.7 (15.5)	60.3 (13.4)	*0.042*
Women, *n* (%)	107 (64)	84/135 (62.2)	23/32 (71.9)	0.41	38/69 (55.1)	69/98 (70.4)	0.05
Symptom duration (months)	6 (3.7)	5.5 (3.3)	6.4 (5.0)	0.35	6 (3.2)	5.5 (3.9)	0.31
Anti-CCP2 positive, *n* (%)	107 (64)	88/135 (65.2)	19/32 (59.4)	0.54	42/69 (60.8)	65/98 (66.3)	0.51
RF positive, *n* (%)	103 (63)	83/131 (63.4)	20/32 (62.5)	1.0	40/68 (58.8)	63/95 (66.3)	0.41
ESR (mm/h)	29 (21.4)	27.3 (21.1)	35.4 (21.8)	0.055	25.4 (18.2)	31.3 (23.2)	0.066
CRP (mg/ml)	22 (24.4)	21.6 (25.0)	24.7 (22.2)	0.51	18.2 (23)	25 (25.1)	0.074
DAS 28	4.86 (1.30)	4.79 (1.3)	5.12 (1.4)	0.21	4.57 (1.27)	5.06 (1.29)	*0.023*
HAQ	0.94 (0.60)	0.91 (0.59)	1.08 (0.59)	0.15	0.86 (0.55)	1 (0.62)	0.16
Larsen total	4.1 (4.9)	3.57 (4.63)	6.25 (5.46)	*0.005*	3.16 ((4.23)	4.73 (5.24)	*0.034*
DXR-BMD	579.5 (86.1)	584.7 (84.2)	558.0 (91.7)	0.115	600.6 (84.2)	564.8 (84.7)	*0.008*
DXR-BMD loss	0.68 (1.81)	−0.52 (1.65)	−1.37 (2.31)	0.058	0.83 (1.05)	−1.74 (1.45)	*< 0.001*

Values are mean (SD) unless otherwise stated
Abbreviations: *CCP* cyclic citrullinated peptides, *RF* rheumatoid factor, *ESR* erythrocyte sedimentation rate, *CRP* C-reactive protein, *DAS28* Disease Activity Score, *HAQ* Health Assessment Questionnaire, *DXR-BMD* bone mineral density measured by digital X-ray radiogrammetry
p values in italics are statistically significant

using the Swedish version of the Stanford Health Assessment Questionnaire (HAQ) [23]. Rheumatoid factor (RF) and antibodies to cyclic citrullinated peptides (anti-CCP2) were analyzed in baseline serum samples at the clinical immunology units of the local hospitals.

Statistics

Statistical calculations were performed using SPSS software (version 23, IBM Corporation, Armonk, USA). Linear regression analyses were used to explore the effect of DXR-BMD alone, and in combination with various clinical and laboratory variables, chosen with respect to clinical assumptions, for associations with change in Larsen score after 1 and 2 years. After testing each variable in a simple regression analysis with change in Larsen score at 1 and 2 years as the dependent variable, multiple regression analyses were performed including variables with $p < 0.2$. Radiographic progression was defined as a difference in Larsen score above the SDC between baseline and 1 and 2 years, respectively. Thus, for example, radiographs assessed by KF with a difference > 1 between the two time points were graded as the actual difference, otherwise as 0. As sensitivity analyses, we also performed linear regression with the same variables, but with absolute changes in Larsen, i.e. not considering the SDC. In addition, logistic regression analysis was performed, in which radiographic progression was defined as change in Larsen score greater than SDC. The Pearson chi^2 test or Fisher's exact test were used for categorical variables, and the independent samples t test was used for continuous variables. All p values are two-sided, and p values less than 0.05 were considered statistically significant.

Table 2 Treatment characteristics

Treatment	Number (percentage) of patients
csDMARDs/biologics started at baseline, *n* (%)	152 (91.0)
- MTX, *n* (%)	147 (88.0)
- Other csDMARDs, *n* (%)	4 (2.4)
- csDMARD triple therapy, *n* (%)	1 (0.6)
Anti-TNF at baseline, *n* (%)	1 (0.6)
Anti-TNF ever, *n* (%)	18 (10.8)
Other bDMARDs	6 (3.6)
Oral glucocorticoids, *n* (%)	138 (82.6)
Calcium supplements, *n* (%)[a]	79 (49.1)
Bisphosphonates, *n* (%)[b]	7 (6.0)

Abbreviations: *MTX* methotrexte, *cDMARDs* conventional disease modifying anti-rheumatic drugs, *TNF* tumor necrosis factor, *bDMARDs* biologic disease modifying anti-rheumatic drugs
[a]Data available for 161 patients
[b]Data available for 124 patients

Results

In total, 176 patients without previous DMARD exposure were included in the study. Table 1 shows the patient characteristics and Table 2 the anti-rheumatic therapy including glucocorticoids (GC), and treatments that influence BMD, initiated at baseline. There were no significant differences in these background characteristics between the participating sites (data not shown). Nine patients were lost because of missing radiographs at 3 months. Thus, the evaluation included 167 patients with radiographs at baseline, 3 months and 1 year

(Helsingborg, n = 38; Linköping, n = 65; Umeå, n = 64). Of the 167 patients, 129 also underwent radiography at 2 years (Fig. 1). Compared with the patients with 2-year radiographs available, patients without 2-year radiographs had lower mean Larsen score at baseline (2.1 (SD = 3.17) vs 4. 7 (SD = 5.17); $p < 0.001$) and at 1 year (2.6 (SD = 3.34) vs 5.8 (SD = 5.66); $p < 0.001$), and were to a lesser extent RF positive (48.6% vs 67.5%; $p = 0.037$). Other baseline characteristics, as detailed in Tables 1 and 2 did not significantly differ from those in patients with radiographs available at 2 years.

At 3 months, 105 (63%) patients had low disease activity (DAS28 ≤ 3.2) and 80 (48%) had reached EULAR remission (DAS28 ≤ 2.6): 46 (28%) of the patients had moderate and 6 (4%) high disease activity (DAS28 > 5.2). DAS28 values from the 3-month visits were missing for 10 (6%) patients. After 1 year, 108 (65%) of the patients had low disease activity, 36 (22%) patients had moderate and 7 (4%) high disease activity: 88 (53%) of the patients had reached EULAR remission. DAS28 values from the 1-year visit were missing in 16 patients (10%).

The mean age of the male patients (n = 60) at baseline was 61 years (SD = 14.5) and the mean age of the female

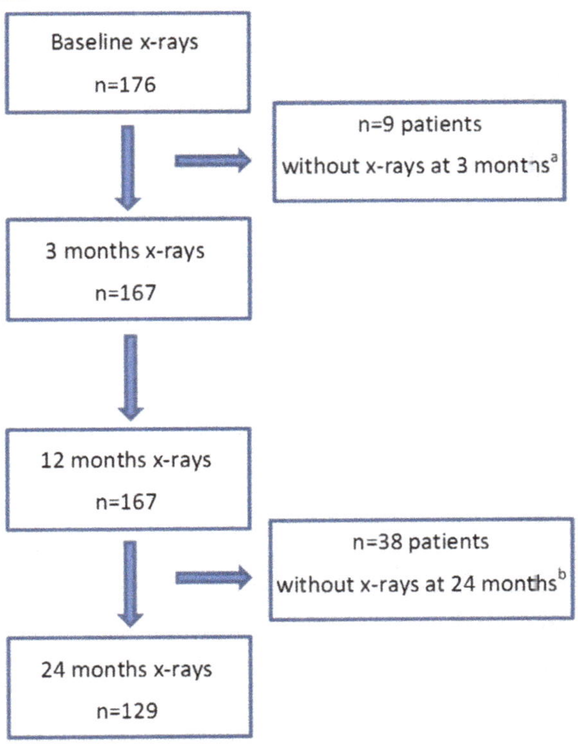

Fig. 1 Availability of radiographs at baseline and follow up. There were 176 patients included in the study. [a]Nine patients were lost because of missing radiographs at 3 months, and thus, the evaluation included 167 patients with radiographs at baseline, 3 months and 1 year. [b]Of the 167 patients included in the evaluation, 129 also underwent radiography at 2 years

patients (n = 107) was 57 years (SD = 14.3). Comparing our DXR-BMD values with a Danish reference cohort of healthy individuals [24], 92 patients (55.1%) in our cohort had bone loss in the hand exceeding the age-related bone loss in the hand among the Danish controls.

Of the 167 patients, 32 (19%) had radiographic progression at 1 year and 45 of 129 patients (35%) had radiographic progression at 2 years. The change in DXR-BMD over 3 months showed BMD loss in 98 patients (59%). The DXR-BMD loss was moderate in 73/167 patients (44%) and severe in 25/167 patients (15%). Radiographic joint damage was significantly different across the three categories of DXR-BMD loss at baseline and at 1 year ($p = 0.039$ and $p = 0.024$, respectively) and there was a trend towards statistical significance after 2 years ($p = 0.056$) (Table 3). Categorizing DXR-BMD loss according to the age-related reference material presented by Ornbjerg et al. [24] yielded very similar results (data not shown).

Patients with change in Larsen score greater than the SDC after 1 year had significantly higher Larsen scores (mean) at baseline (3.6 vs 6.2; $p = 0.005$). Compared with patients without DXR-BMD loss, patients with DXR-BMD loss after 3 months were significantly older (60.3 years vs 55.7; $p = 0.042$), had significantly higher baseline DAS28 (5.1 vs 4.6; $p = 0.023$) and significantly higher Larsen scores at baseline (4.7 vs 3.2; $p = 0.034$). Also, the proportion of women was significantly higher (70.4% vs 55.1%; $p = 0.05$) among patients with BMD loss (Table 2). There was no significant difference in the DXR value at baseline in the anti-CCP2-positive compared with the anti-CCP-negative patients (576 vs 587 mg/cm^2; $p = 0.426$).

Simple regression analyses with change in Larsen score greater than the SDC at 1 year as the dependent variable were performed, including the following covariates: age, sex, oral corticosteroid treatment, DXR-BMD loss/month, baseline DAS28, CRP, ESR, Larsen score, anti-CCP2 status, and RF status. Also, DAS28 > 2.6 at 3 months (yes/no) was included. Covariates with a p value < 0.2 in these analyses were included in a multiple regression model (Table 4). This model, adjusting for sex and baseline values of ESR, DAS28, Larsen score and anti-CCP2 status, showed a significant association between 3-month BMD loss and increase in Larsen score above the SDC after 1 year ($p = 0.033$, adjusted R-squared = 0.069) (Table 4). No significant association was observed between early bone loss and increase in the Larsen score above the SDC at 2 years ($p = 0.604$). When using the same covariates but with change in Larsen score without considering the SDC as the dependent variable, DXR-BMD loss was significantly associated with the 1-year Larsen score ($p = 0.048$), but not the Larsen score at 2 years ($p = 0.491$). In logistic regression analysis, there was no significant association between

Table 3 Mean Larsen scores and 3-month bone mineral density loss in early rheumatoid arthritis

	Mean (SD) Larsen score			p value
	No BMD loss	Moderate BMD loss	Severe BMD loss	
Baseline (SD)	3.2 (4,23)	4.3 (4.81)	6.0 (6.28)	0.039
1 year (SD)	4.0 (4.68)	5.3 (5.45)	7.3 (6.38)	0.024
2 years (SD)	5.4 (5.1)	6.9 (5.6)	8.8 (6.04)	0.056

BMD bone mineral density

DXR-BMD loss and 1-year radiographic progression defined as a change in Larsen score above the SDC ($p = 0.158$). Treatment with bisphosphonates, calcium and vitamin D did not influence the DXR-BMD loss (data not shown).

When analyzing only patients without erosions at baseline (n = 123), using the same multivariate model (adjusted for the same variables but not for the Larsen score at baseline), 3-month DXR-BMD loss remained associated with radiographic progression after 1 year ($p = 0.021$, R-squared = 0.07). Also, when analyzing the 1-year outcome among the 129 patients with 2-year radiographs available, the association between DXR-BMD loss and radiographic progression remained statistically significant ($p = 0.039$, adjusted R-squared = 0.08).

Discussion

To our knowledge, this is the first study addressing the predictive value of 3-month DXR-BMD in patients with recent-onset RA compared with radiography and clinical data. In clinical practice, evaluation of prescribed DMARDs is commonly performed 3 months after initiation. At this occasion, particularly in early disease, additional information on the patient's radiographic prognosis would be highly valuable in order to optimize therapy decisions. In this study, we found DXR-BMD loss during the first 3 months to independently predict radiographic joint damage at 1 year and the 1-year progression from baseline.

Our results on metacarpal bone loss among patients with early RA are in line with previous reports [9–14]. The shortest interval of DXR-BMD assessments among previous studies was 3 months in the study from Bøyesen et al. [25], addressing 3-month change in DXR-BMD as a predictive factor for erosive progression identified on magnetic resonance imaging (MRI) in patients with early RA. In the 53 patients completing that study there was only a trend towards higher MRI synovitis score and 3-month DXR BMD loss in patients developing MRI erosions, and no significant changes. Wevers-de Boer and coworkers [10] presented 4-month data with similar findings on the 1-year radiographic outcome as in the current study. Thus, early DXR-BMD assessments seem to be of clinical value, in order to optimize early institution of anti-rheumatic pharmacotherapy and thereby diminish the risk of future disability [4, 26–30]. However, we found no predictive value of DXR-BMD loss in relation to the 2-year radiographic outcome. This was somewhat

Table 4 Regression analyses with change in Larsen score between baseline and 12 months as dependent variable

	Simple regression			Multiple regression		
Variable	Adjusted R-square	β-coeff	p value	Adjusted R-square	β-coeff	p value
DXR decrease (mg/cm²/month)[a]	0.049	−0.235	0.002	0.069	−0.181	0.033
DAS28[b]	0.015	0.148	0.070		0.028	0.767
Larsen score[b]	0.017	0.153	0.049		0.068	0.404
Age[b]	0.001	0.082	0.291			
Gender	0.007	0.114	0.143		0.071	0.381
anti-CCP2 status[b]	0.010	−0.125	0.107		−0.128	0.114
RF[b]	−0.001	−0.069	0.385			
Corticosteroid treatment	−0.002	0.042	0.417			
Disease duration (months)[b]	−0.006	0.026	0.739			
CRP (mg/L)[b]	−0.004	0.045	0.566			
ESR (mm/h)[b]	0.024	0.173	0.025		0.133	0.165
DAS28 > 2.6 at 3 months	−0.002	0.065	0.422			

Abbreviations: *DXR* digital X-ray radiogrammetry, *DAS28* Disease Activity Score in 28 joints, *CCP* cyclic citrullinated peptides, *RF* rheumatoid factor, *CRP* C-reactive protein, *ESR* erythrocyte sedimentation rate, *BMD* bone mineral density

[a]Decrease in DXR-BMD between baseline and 3 months

[b]Baseline value

surprising, since existing radiographic damage often predicts radiographic progression. One possible explanation for the disparate 1-year and 2-year findings in our study could be that potent instituted pharmacotherapy attenuated radiographic differences over time. Also, missing data from 2-year radiographs (n = 38) need to be considered, but the association between DXR-BMD loss and radiographic damage at 1 year remained statistically significant, also after excluding the 38 patients without 2-year radiographs. Thus, difference in statistical power appears to be an unlikely explanation for the discordance between 1-year and 2-year data. A previous study by Forslind et al. [9] showed that patients with early RA, who were on prednisolone 7.5 mg per day in addition to conventional DMARDS, had significantly less DXR-BMD loss as compared with patients with RA who were not receiving corticosteroids. This finding was attributed to the anti-inflammatory effect of prednisolone, hampering osteopenia induced by inflammation. Although not primarily designed to address this, our study did not identify a significant impact of oral corticosteroid on BMD loss or radiographic progression. Similarly, treatment with bisphosphonates, calcium and vitamin D did not significantly impact BMD loss.

In our study we did not observe a significant difference in the DXR value at baseline in the anti-CCP2-positive compared with the anti-CCP-negative patients. This fact is contrary to the findings in other studies [31–33] in which BMD loss was significantly more widespread in anti-CCP-positive patients. Different methods for estimating BMD loss (comparative micro computed tomography (micro-CT) analysis and dual-energy X-ray absorptiometry) may influence the differing results. Also, it needs to be pointed out that our study was not primarily designed to address the influence of anti-CCP on BMD loss.

Whenever a patient with RA presents with erosions at the time of diagnosis, an aggressive disease course is assumed, and treatment is chosen accordingly. Thus, information on the radiographic prognosis is even more important in the large category of patients without evidence of erosive disease at diagnosis. Interestingly, we found that 3-month DXR-BMD loss also predicted 1-year radiographic damage in this subgroup of patients. However, the comparative value of DXR-BMD compared with other imaging modalities needs to be assessed.

Limitations of this study are the missing 2-year radiographs in 38 patients (23%), and the fact that the baseline Larsen score and RF status differed between patients with radiographs available at 2 years and those without. Nevertheless, analyzing the 129 patients with all radiographs available up to 2 years did not substantially alter the findings.

Conclusion

In this real-world study of patients with early RA, we found that DXR-BMD loss during the initial 3 months independently predicted radiologic damage at 1 year. However, DXR-BMD loss predicts only a minor part of the variation in radiographic damage, and an association was not established after 2 years of disease. Future studies should compare the value of DXR-BMD with other imaging modalities.

Abbreviations

ACR: American College of Rheumatology; bDMARD: Biologic disease modifying anti-rheumatic drug; BMD: Bone mineral density; CCP: Cyclic citrullinated peptides; csDMARD: Conventional synthetic disease modifying anti-rheumatic drug; CRP: C-reactive protein; DAS: Disease Activity Score; DAS28: DAS with 28 joints; DXR: Digital X-ray radiogrammetry; DXR-BMD: Bone mineral density measured by digital X-ray radiogrammetry; ESR: Erythrocyte sedimentation rate; EULAR: European League Against Rheumatism; GC: Glucocorticoid; HAQ: Health Assessment Questionnaire; ICC: Intraclass correlation coefficient; MRI: Magnetic resonance imaging; MTX: Methotrexate; RA: Rheumatoid arthritis; RF: Rheumatoid factor; SDC: Smallest detectable change; TNF: Tumor necrosis factor

Acknowledgements

This work was financially supported by the Swedish Rheumatism Association, the Norrbacka-Eugenia foundation, the King Gustav V 80-year Foundation, the Swedish Medical Society, ALF Grants from Region Östergötland, the Linköping University Hospital Research Fund and the Foundation for Assistance to Disabled People in Skane (Stiftelsen för Bistånd åt Rörelsehindrade i Skåne).

Funding

Not applicable.

Authors' contributions

KF, AK, TS, EB and MZ designed the study and participated in patient enrollment and characterization. MZ, KF and EB scored radiographs. MZ and EB analyzed the data. All authors contributed to the interpretation of data, drafting the article and revising it critically. All authors approved the final version of the manuscript.

Competing interests

The authors declare that they have no competing interests.

Author details

[1]Department of Rheumatology, Department of Clinical and Experimental Medicine, Linköping University, Linköping, Sweden. [2]Section of Rheumatology, Department of Medicine, Helsingborg Hospital, Helsingborg, Sweden. [3]Department of Clinical Sciences, Section of Rheumatology, Lund University, Helsingborg, Sweden. [4]Department of Diagnostic radiology, Umeå university Hospital, Umeå, Sweden. [5]Department of Public Health and Clinical Medicine/Rheumatology, Umeå university Hospital, Umeå, Sweden.

References

1. Brook A, Corbett M. Radiographic changes in early rheumatoid disease. Ann Rheum Dis. 1977;36(1):71–3.
2. Grassi W, et al. The clinical features of rheumatoid arthritis. Eur J Radiol. 1998;27 Suppl 1:S18–24.

3. Darawankul B, et al. The good EULAR response at the first year is strongly predictive of clinical remission in rheumatoid arthritis: results from the TARAC cohort. Clin Rheumatol. 2015;34(1):43–9.
4. Markusse IM, et al. Long-term outcomes of patients with recent-onset rheumatoid arthritis after 10 years of tight controlled treatment: a randomized trial. Ann Intern Med. 2016;164(8):523–31.
5. Schneider M, Kruger K. Rheumatoid arthritis–early diagnosis and disease management. Dtsch Arztebl Int. 2013;110(27-28):477–84.
6. Dolan AL, et al. Does active treatment of rheumatoid arthritis limit disease-associated bone loss? Rheumatology (Oxford). 2002;41(9):1047–51.
7. Jorgensen JT, et al. Digital X-ray radiogrammetry: a new appendicular bone densitometric method with high precision. Clin Physiol. 2000;20(5):330–5.
8. Rosholm A, et al. Estimation of bone mineral density by digital X-ray radiogrammetry: theoretical background and clinical testing. Osteoporos Int. 2001;12(11):961–9.
9. Forslind K, et al. Hand bone loss measured by digital X-ray radiogrammetry is a predictor of joint damage in early rheumatoid arthritis. Scand J Rheumatol. 2009;38(6):431–8.
10. Wevers-de Boer KV, et al. Four-month metacarpal bone mineral density loss predicts radiological joint damage progression after 1 year in patients with early rheumatoid arthritis: exploratory analyses from the IMPROVED study. Ann Rheum Dis. 2015;74(2):341–6.
11. Guler-Yuksel M, et al. Changes in hand and generalised bone mineral density in patients with recent-onset rheumatoid arthritis. Ann Rheum Dis. 2009;68(3):330–6.
12. Hoff M, et al. Cortical hand bone loss after 1 year in early rheumatoid arthritis predicts radiographic hand joint damage at 5-year and 10-year follow-up. Ann Rheum Dis. 2009;68(3):324–9.
13. Rezaei H, et al. Evaluation of hand bone loss by digital X-ray radiogrammetry as a complement to clinical and radiographic assessment in early rheumatoid arthritis: results from the SWEFOT trial. BMC Musculoskelet Disord. 2013;14:79.
14. Forslind K, et al. Does digital X-ray radiogrammetry have a role in identifying patients at increased risk for joint destruction in early rheumatoid arthritis? Arthritis Res Ther. 2012;14(5):R219.
15. Aletaha D, et al. 2010 Rheumatoid arthritis classification criteria: an American College of Rheumatology/European League Against Rheumatism collaborative initiative. Arthritis Rheum. 2010;62(9):2569–81.
16. Arnett FC, et al. The American Rheumatism Association 1987 revised criteria for the classification of rheumatoid arthritis. Arthritis Rheum. 1988;31(3):315–24.
17. Larsen A. How to apply Larsen score in evaluating radiographs of rheumatoid arthritis in long-term studies. J Rheumatol. 1995;22(10):1974–5.
18. Bruynesteyn K, et al. Deciding on progression of joint damage in paired films of individual patients: smallest detectable difference or change. Ann Rheum Dis. 2005;64(2):179–82.
19. Barnett E, Nordin BE. The radiological diagnosis of osteoporosis: a new approach. Clin Radiol. 1960;11:166–74.
20. de Rooy DP, et al. Loss of metacarpal bone density predicts RA development in recent-onset arthritis. Rheumatology (Oxford). 2012;51(6): 1037–41.
21. Prevoo ML, et al. Modified disease activity scores that include twenty-eight-joint counts. Development and validation in a prospective longitudinal study of patients with rheumatoid arthritis. Arthritis Rheum. 1995;38(1):44–8.
22. van Gestel AM, Haagsma CJ, van Riel PL. Validation of rheumatoid arthritis improvement criteria that include simplified joint counts. Arthritis Rheum. 1998;41(10):1845–50.
23. Ekdahl C, et al. Assessing disability in patients with rheumatoid arthritis. Use of a Swedish version of the Stanford Health Assessment Questionnaire. Scand J Rheumatol. 1988;17(4):263–71.
24. Ornbjerg LM, et al. Establishment of age- and sex-adjusted reference data for hand bone mass and investigation of hand bone loss in patients with rheumatoid arthritis treated in clinical practice: an observational study from the DANBIO registry and the Copenhagen Osteoarthritis Study. Arthritis Res Ther. 2016;18:53.
25. Boyesen P, et al. Prediction of MRI erosive progression: a comparison of modern imaging modalities in early rheumatoid arthritis patients. Ann Rheum Dis. 2011;70(1):176–9.
26. Goekoop-Ruiterman YP, et al. Clinical and radiographic outcomes of four different treatment strategies in patients with early rheumatoid arthritis (the BeSt study): A randomized, controlled trial. Arthritis Rheum. 2008;58(2 Suppl):S126–35.
27. Breedveld F. The value of early intervention in RA – a window of opportunity. Clin Rheumatol. 2011;30 Suppl 1:S33–9.
28. Ahlstrand I, et al. Pain and activity limitations in women and men with contemporary treated early RA compared to 10 years ago: the Swedish TIRA project. Scand J Rheumatol. 2015;44(4):259–64.
29. Kudo-Tanaka E, et al. Early therapeutic intervention with methotrexate prevents the development of rheumatoid arthritis in patients with recent-onset undifferentiated arthritis: A prospective cohort study. Mod Rheumatol. 2015;25(6):831–6.
30. Kyburz D, Finckh A. The importance of early treatment for the prognosis of rheumatoid arthritis. Swiss Med Wkly. 2013;143:w13865.
31. Kleyer A, et al. Bone loss before the clinical onset of rheumatoid arthritis in subjects with anticitrullinated protein antibodies. Ann Rheum Dis. 2014; 73(5):854–60.
32. Bugatti S, et al. Anti-citrullinated protein antibodies and high levels of rheumatoid factor are associated with systemic bone loss in patients with early untreated rheumatoid arthritis. Arthritis Res Ther. 2016;18(1):226.
33. Orsolini G, et al. Titer-dependent effect of anti-citrullinated protein antibodies on systemic bone mass in rheumatoid arthritis patients. Calcif Tissue Int. 2017;101(1):17–23.

4

Patient-reported outcomes of baricitinib in patients with rheumatoid arthritis and no or limited prior disease-modifying antirheumatic drug treatment

Michael Schiff[1*], Tsutomu Takeuchi[2], Roy Fleischmann[3], Carol L. Gaich[4], Amy M. DeLozier[4], Douglas Schlichting[4], Wen-Ling Kuo[4], Ji-Eon Won[5], Tara Carmack[4], Terence Rooney[4], Patrick Durez[6,7], Saeed Shaikh[8], Rodolfo Pardo Hidalgo[9], Ronald van Vollenhoven[10] and Cristiano A. F. Zerbini[11]

Abstract

Background: This study evaluates patient-reported outcomes (PROs) in a double-blind, phase III study of baricitinib as monotherapy or combined with methotrexate (MTX) in patients with active rheumatoid arthritis (RA) with no or minimal prior conventional synthetic disease-modifying antirheumatic drugs (DMARDs) and naïve to biological DMARDs.

Methods: Patients were randomized 4:3:4 to MTX administered once weekly ($N = 210$), baricitinib monotherapy (4 mg once daily (QD), $N = 159$), or combination of baricitinib (4 mg QD) and MTX (baricitinib + MTX, $N = 215$). PROs included the Patient's Global Assessment of Disease Activity (PtGA), patient's assessment of pain, Health Assessment Questionnaire-Disability Index (HAQ-DI), Functional Assessment of Chronic Illness Therapy-Fatigue (FACIT-F), duration of morning joint stiffness (MJS), worst joint pain, worst tiredness, Work Productivity and Activity Impairment-Rheumatoid Arthritis (WPAI-RA), Short Form 36 version 2, Acute (SF-36); and EuroQol 5-Dimensions (EQ-5D) Health State Profile. Comparisons were assessed with analysis of covariance (ANCOVA) and logistic regression models.

Results: Compared to MTX, patients in both baricitinib groups reported greater improvement ($p \leq 0.01$) in HAQ-DI, PtGA, pain, fatigue, worst join pain, SF-36 physical component score, and EQ-5D at weeks 24 and 52. For the SF-36 mental component score, patients in both baricitinib groups reported statistically significant improvements ($p \leq 0.01$) at week 52 compared to MTX-treated patients. Statistically significant improvements ($p \leq 0.05$) were observed with the WPAI-RA for the baricitinib groups vs. MTX at week 24 and for the WPAI-RA daily activity and work productivity measures for baricitinib + MTX at week 52.

Conclusions: In this study, baricitinib alone or in combination with MTX, when used as initial therapy, resulted in significant improvement compared to MTX in the majority of the pre-specified PRO measures.

Keywords: Baricitinib, PRO, JAK inhibitor, RA, Rheumatoid, tsDMARD, Health-related quality of life, health status indicators, HAQ-DI

* Correspondence: michael.schiff@me.com
[1]University of Colorado School of Medicine, Denver, CO 80045, USA
Full list of author information is available at the end of the article

Background

Patients with rheumatoid arthritis (RA) experience progressive and significant restrictions in daily living and frequently report pain, fatigue, sleep disturbances, and functional impairment in work and leisure-time physical activities [1–3]. Patient-reported symptoms are generally present early in the disease, and, when present, can be a significant burden on patients' quality of life. The American College of Rheumatology (ACR) established a core set of measures to assess disease activity in clinical trials, which includes several patient-reported outcomes (PROs) associated with RA [4]. Additional PROs for use in clinical trials have been suggested by Outcome Measures in Rheumatology Clinical Trials (OMERACT) [5]. The ACR and the European League Against Rheumatism (EULAR) have recognized PROs as important factors in the assessment of patient disease activity and have recommended the evaluation of PROs in daily clinical practice when considering response to therapy [6, 7]. Regulatory authorities have recommended that PROs be used as additional measures of effectiveness in clinical trials of RA [8].

Treatment recommendations for RA highlight the importance of early diagnosis and of intensive treatment strategies, with the target of remission or lowest possible disease activity [9]. The treatment regimen for RA suggested by the ACR and EULAR includes initial conventional synthetic disease-modifying anti-rheumatic drugs (csDMARDs), especially methotrexate (MTX); if not effective, combining csDMARDs with biological DMARDs (bDMARDs), or oral targeted synthetic DMARDs (tsDMARDs) that target the intracellular Janus kinase (JAK) pathways, are recommended [6, 7]. This early intensive disease management has been shown to mitigate joint damage and inflammation, to avoid disability from RA, and to improve patient health-related quality of life [10–13].

It has been advocated that the treatment of RA should be a shared decision-making process between the patient and the physician [9]. Together, they must address questions of significance to the patients, including the potential improvement of PROs [9]. A relevant question to both patients and physicians is whether bDMARDs or tsDMARDs require co-administration of methotrexate (MTX), which itself is associated with potential adverse effects that may affect patient function (fatigue, nausea, etc.) [14, 15].

Baricitinib is a selective JAK1 and JAK2 inhibitor that was recently approved for the treatment of moderately to severely active RA in adults in the European Union and is under development for RA in other regions. Baricitinib interferes with pathways that are believed to be important in the pathogenesis of RA. RA-BEGIN was a phase III study (NCT01711359) conducted in patients with active RA who were naïve to csDMARDs (no or limited exposure to MTX) or bDMARDs. Baricitinib alone or in combination with MTX demonstrated superior clinical efficacy with acceptable safety compared to MTX as the initial therapy for patients with active RA [1]. In the present analysis of the RA-BEGIN study, we report the effects of baricitinib, administered as monotherapy or in combination with MTX compared to MTX monotherapy, on the PRO measures.

Methods

Patients

Full details regarding the primary efficacy and safety outcomes of this study have been reported previously [1]. In summary, patients were ≥ 18 years old with moderately to severely active RA (≥6/68 tender and ≥ 6/66 swollen joints; high-sensitivity C-reactive protein ≥ 3.6 mg/L (upper limit of normal 3.0 mg/L); seropositive for rheumatoid factor or anti-citrullinated peptide antibodies) and naïve (or had no more than three prior doses of MTX) to DMARDs.

Study protocol and oversight

RA-BEGIN was a randomized, 52-week, double-blind, active comparator-controlled study conducted in 18 countries. Patients were randomized 4:3:4 to receive oral MTX monotherapy (administered orally once weekly), baricitinib monotherapy (4 mg once daily (QD)), or the combination of baricitinib (4 mg QD) and MTX (baricitinib + MTX). Methotrexate was initiated at 10 mg/week and, if tolerated, increased to 20 mg/week by week 8. A lower dose of MTX was available for patients in whom a lower dose was clinically indicated or required by national guidelines (initial dose of 7.5 mg and a maximum dose of 12.5 mg). Rescue treatment (baricitinib + MTX) was available, beginning at week 24, for those patients whose tender and swollen joint counts did not improve by ≥ 20% from baseline. The study was conducted in accordance with ethical principles of the Declaration of Helsinki and Good Clinical Practice guidelines and was approved by each center's institutional review board or ethics committee. All patients provided written informed consent.

Patient-reported outcomes

Pre-specified secondary PROs were included in the study. The Patient's Global Assessment of Disease Activity (PtGA) and the patient's assessment of pain were evaluated using visual analog scales (VAS) of 0–100 mm. Physical function was assessed by the Health Assessment Questionnaire-Disability Index (HAQ-DI) [2, 3]; scores range from 0 to 3, with lower scores reflecting better physical function and less disability. An HAQ-DI score of ≤ 0.25 is considered the normative value and an improvement of ≥ 0.22 has been shown to be the minimum clinically important difference (MCID) [16, 17]. Fatigue was assessed by the Functional Assessment of Chronic Illness Therapy-Fatigue (FACIT-F) scale; scores range from 0 to 52, with higher scores representing less fatigue; in this study a value of 3.56 was used for the MCID [18–20]. Duration of morning joint stiffness (MJS) was reported by the patient as the length of time in minutes that MJS lasted on the day prior to each study visit. The patients' assessments of the worst joint pain and the worst tiredness over the past 24 hours were measured using novel Worst Joint Pain and Worst Tiredness Numeric Rating Scales (NRS). Scores for both the NRSs range from 0 (no joint pain/tiredness) to 10 ("as bad as you can imagine").

Health-related quality of life (HRQOL) was evaluated using the Medical Outcomes Study (MOS) Short Form-36 (SF-36; version 2, Acute) [21, 22], which assesses eight domains scored from 0 to 100 that can be aggregated into physical and mental component scores (PCS, MCS) and compared to values from normal individuals. An MCID change of 5 was used to assess the clinical relevance of changes in SF-36 component scores [23, 24]. The EuroQol 5-Dimensions (EQ-5D) Health State Profile was also used to assess HRQOL. The EQ-5D consists of two components: a descriptive system of the respondent's health and a rating of their current state (0 – 100 mm VAS) [25]. The UK and US scoring algorithms provide an index score using the UK or US population weighting normalized to that population [25–27].

The Work Productivity and Activity Impairment-Rheumatoid Arthritis (WPAI-RA) instrument was used to measure overall work productivity and impairment of regular activities during the past 7 days. Scores are calculated as impairment percentages [28], with higher percentages indicating greater work and activity impairment and less productivity.

The PROs were assessed at baseline, week 1, week 2, week 4, and every 4 weeks thereafter to week 24; after week 24 they were assessed at weeks 32, 40, and 52; with the exception of the FACIT-F, which was assessed at baseline, week 1, week 4 and then followed the same schedule as the other PROs and the SF-36, EQ-5D, and WPAI-RA, which were assessed at baseline and week 4 and then followed the same schedule as the other PROs.

Statistical analysis

Randomized patients were included in the analyses under a modified intention-to-treat principle (mITT analysis set), which included all patients treated with ≥ 1 dose of study drug. Treatment comparisons for categorical and continuous measures were performed using logistic regression and analysis of covariance (ANCOVA), respectively, with baseline value (for continuous measures only), treatment, geographical region, and presence of baseline joint erosions (yes/no) in the model. The Fisher exact test was used for categorical data when sample size requirements for the logistic regression model were not met (< 5 responders in any category for any factor). Differences in the duration of MJS were assessed with the Wilcoxon rank sum test. Any duration of MJS lasting > 12 hours was truncated to 720 minutes for the purpose of this analysis.

Patients who were rescued or discontinued from the study or study treatment were thereafter defined as non-responders (non-responder imputation (NRI)) for all categorical data. These patients also had their last observations before rescue or discontinuation (modified last observation carried forward (mLOCF)) used for analyses of continuous data. The WPAI-RA analyses were censored after rescue or study discontinuation without imputation applied.

Results

Patients

A total of 588 patients were randomized and 584 patients received treatment; 210 initially received MTX, 159 baricitinib monotherapy, and 215 baricitinib + MTX. Patient demographics and disposition have been described by Fleischmann et al. [1]. Briefly, baseline demographics and clinical characteristics were similar among treatment groups (Table 1) [1]. The median disease duration was 0.2 years and more than 90% of patients were DMARD-naïve. The mean MTX dose achieved was 17.7 mg per week in both the MTX and combination groups; approximately 23% of patients received the lower MTX dose regimen. The mean doses prescribed in the full-dose/low-dose groups were 19.6 mg/12.1 mg in the MTX monotherapy group and 19.2 mg/12 mg in the baricitinib + MTX group, respectively, at week 24. Patients had active disease, impaired physical function, moderate levels of pain and tiredness/fatigue, a median duration of MJS of 60–90 minutes, and reduced HRQOL (Table 1) at baseline.

PROs

In the RA-BEGIN study, although MTX monotherapy was an effective therapy in many patients, statistically significant improvements in PROs were seen at week 24 across the majority of measures and were maintained through week 52 for both the baricitinib monotherapy and baricitinib + MTX groups compared to MTX. For some measures, statistically significant improvements were seen as early as week 1.

HAQ-DI, PtGA, and patient's assessment of pain

As reported by Fleischmann et al. [1] for HAQ-DI, PtGA and patient's assessment of pain, improvements in both the baricitinib monotherapy and baricitinib + MTX groups were evident as early as week 1 compared to MTX. Significant improvements in physical function, PtGA and patient's assessment of pain were maintained through week 24 to week 52 (Table 2).

The percentages of patients with improvement in HAQ-DI scores that exceeded the MCID (≥ 0.22) with MTX, baricitinib monotherapy, and baricitinib + MTX,

Table 1 Patient characteristics, disease activity, and patient-reported outcomes at baseline*

Parameter[a]	MTX (*N* = 210)	Baricitinib 4 mg (*N* = 159)	Baricitinib 4 mg + MTX (*N* = 215)
Age, years	50.5 (13)	50.9 (13)	48.5 (14)
Female, *n* (%)	148 (70)	121 (76)	156 (73)
Duration of RA, years	1.3 (4.0)	1.9 (4.7)	1.3 (2.7)
Duration of RA, years, median	0.2	0.2	0.2
Concomitant corticosteroid use, *n* (%)	76 (36)	47 (30)	83 (39)
Number of previous cDMARDs used, *n* (%)			
0	190 (90)	146 (92)	197 (92)
1	20 (10)	13 (8)	18 (8)
2	0	0	0
Ever used DMARD (≤ 3 doses of MTX permitted), *n* (%)	20 (10)	13 (8)	18 (8)
Disease activity			
Swollen joint count, of 66	16 (11)	16 (9)	16 (10)
Tender joint count, of 68	27 (15)	26 (14)	28 (15)
DAS28-hsCRP	5.9 (1.0)	5.9 (1.0)	5.9 (0.9)
DAS28-ESR	6.6 (1.0)	6.6 (1.1)	6.6 (1.0)
Simplified Disease Activity Index	42 (14)	43 (14)	43 (13)
Clinical Disease Activity Index	39 (13)	40 (13)	40 (13)
Patient-reported outcomes			
HAQ-DI (0–3)	1.7 (0.7)	1.6 (0.7)	1.6 (0.7)
PtGA VAS (0–100)	66 (24)	65 (22)	63 (24)
Patient's assessment of pain, VAS (0–100)	65 (24)	64 (22)	63 (23)
Fatigue (FACIT-F; 0–52)	27 (11)	28 (11)	28 (11)
Median (IQR) duration of morning joint stiffness, minutes	90 (30, 180)	60 (30, 180)	90 (30, 180)
Worst Joint Pain NRS (0–10)	7 (2)	7 (2)	7 (2)
Worst Tiredness NRS (0–10)	6 (2)	6 (3)	6 (2)
QoL (SF-36; 0–100)			
PCS	32 (8)	33 (8)	32 (9)
MCS	47 (12)	45 (13)	47 (13)
EQ-5D			
Health State Index Score, UK algorithm (-0.594,1)	0.473 (0.256)	0.485 (0.255)	0.489 (0.251)
Self-perceived health score VAS (0–100)	51 (23)	50 (23)	51 (23)

Score ranges for individual patient-reported outcomes measures are indicated in brackets. Lower scores indicate better outcomes for HAQ-DI, PtGA, patient's assessment of pain, Worst Joint Pain, Worst Tiredness. Higher scores indicate better outcomes for FACIT-F, SF-36 and EQ-5D

EQ-5D European Quality of Life-5 Dimensions, *FACIT-F* Functional Assessment of Chronic Illness Therapy–Fatigue, *HAQ-DI* Health Assessment Questionnaire-Disability Index, *IQR* interquartile range, *MCS* Mental Component Score, *MTX* methotrexate, *NRS* numeric rating scale, *PCS* Physical Component Score, *PtGA* Patient's Global Assessment of Disease Activity, *QoL* quality of life, *RA* rheumatoid arthritis, *SF-36* Short Form-36, *UK* United Kingdom, *VAS* visual analog scale

[a]Data are presented as mean (standard deviation) unless stated otherwise

*Further details can be found in Fleischmann et al. 2017 [1]

respectively, were 70%, 81%, and 79% ($p \leq 0.05$ for both baricitinib groups vs. MTX) at week 24 and were 57%, 68%, and 72% ($p \leq 0.05$ for baricitinib monotherapy vs. MTX; $p \leq 0.001$ for baricitinib + MTX vs. MTX) at week 52. The percentage of patients who achieved the normative value of ≤ 0.25 at week 24 for MTX, baricitinib monotherapy, and baricitinib + MTX, respectively, were 21%, 33%, and 34% ($p \leq 0.05$ for the baricitinib monotherapy vs. MTX; $p \leq 0.01$ for baricitinib + MTX vs. MTX) and were 18%, 29%, and 34% ($p \leq 0.05$ for the baricitinib monotherapy vs. MTX; $p \leq 0.001$ for baricitinib + MTX vs. MTX) at week 52.

Table 2 Change from baseline at week 24 and week 52 for patient-reported outcomes

PRO measure[a] (95% CI)	Week 24			Week 52		
	MTX (*N* = 210)	Baricitinib 4 mg (*N* = 159)	Baricitinib 4 mg + MTX (*N* = 215)	MTX (*N* = 210)	Baricitinib 4 mg (*N* = 159)	Baricitinib 4 mg + MTX (*N* = 215)
Physical Function (HAQ-DI)	− 0.74 (− 0.83, − 0.66)	− 1.04 (− 1.14, − 0.95)***	− 1.03 (− 1.11, − 0.95)***	− 0.71 (− 0.79, − 0.62)	− 0.99 (− 1.08, − 0.89)***	− 1.06 (− 1.14, − 0.97)***
Patient's Global Assessment of Disease Activity (PtGA)	− 31 (− 34, − 27)	− 41 (− 45, − 38)***	− 40 (− 43, − 37)***	− 29 (− 32, − 26)	− 40 (− 44, − 37)***	− 43 (− 46, − 39)***
Patient's assessment of pain	− 30 (− 33, − 27)	− 41 (− 45 − 37)***	− 41 (− 44, − 38)***	− 31 (− 34, − 27)	− 40 (− 44, − 37)***	− 43 (− 47, − 40)***
FACIT-F	8.9 (7.6, 10.1)	13.3 (11.8, 14.7)***	12.2 (11.0, 13.5)***	8.9 (7.6, 10.2)	11.7 (10.2, 13.1)**	12.6 (11.4, 13.9)***
MJS Duration, median change from baseline	− 35.0 (− 55.0, − 25.0)	− 50.0 (− 60.0, − 30.0)	− 59.0 (− 85.0, − 40.0)**	− 40.0 (− 55.0, − 30.0)	− 55.0 (− 60.0, − 40.0)	− 60.0 (− 80.0, − 50.0)**
Worst Joint Pain NRS	− 2.8 (− 3.2, − 2.5)	− 4.0 (− 4.3, − 3.6) ***	− 4.0 (− 4.3, − 3.7)***	− 3.0 (− 3.4, − 2.7)	− 3.9 (− 4.3, − 3.6)***	− 4.1 (− 4.4, − 3.8)***
Worst Tiredness NRS	− 2.1 (− 2.5, − 1.8)	− 3.1 (− 3.5, − 2.7)***	− 3.0 (− 3.3, − 2.7)***	− 2.2 (− 2.5, − 1.8)	− 3.0 (− 3.4, − 2.6)**	− 2.9 (− 3.3, − 2.6)**
EuroQol-5 Dimensions (EQ-5D)						
Health State Index Score, UK algorithm	0.200 (0.173, 0.227)	0.288 (0.257, 0.318)***	0.288 (0.261, 0.315)***	0.191 (0.161, 0.221)	0.272 (0.239, 0.306)***	0.273 (0.244, 0.303)***
US algorithm	0.138 (0.119, 0.158)	0.199 (0.177, 0.221) ***	0.199 (0.179, 0.218) ***	0.133 (0.111, 0.154)	0.187 (0.163, 0.211)***	0.189 (0.168, 0.210)***
Self-perceived health score	15 (12, 18)	24 (20, 27)***	22 (18, 25)**	14 (11, 18)	25 (21, 28)***	25 (22, 28)***

CI confidence interval, *MJS* morning joint stiffness, *MTX* methotrexate, *NRS* numeric rating scale, *PRO* patient-reported outcomes, *RA* rheumatoid arthritis

[a]Data are presented as least-squares mean unless stated otherwise

*$p \leq 0.05$; **$p \leq 0.01$; ***$p \leq 0.001$ vs. MTX

FACIT-F, duration of MJS, worst joint pain and worst tiredness

Compared to MTX monotherapy, statistically significant improvements in the FACIT-F for both baricitinib groups were observed as early as the first assessment at week 1 ($p \leq 0.001$ for both baricitinib groups vs. MTX; Fig. 1). The duration of MJS, worst joint pain, and worst tiredness were significantly reduced in both baricitinib groups compared to MTX from week 1 (MJS duration, $p \leq 0.05$ for baricitinib monotherapy vs. MTX, $p \leq 0.001$ for baricitinib + MTX vs. MTX; worst joint pain, $p \leq 0.001$ for both baricitinib groups vs. MTX; worst tiredness, $p \leq 0.001$ for baricitinib monotherapy vs. MTX, $p \leq 0.01$ for baricitinib + MTX vs. MTX; Fig. 1). The improvements in the FACIT-F score and reductions in duration of MJS, worst joint pain, and worst tiredness were maintained to week 24 and week 52 in both baricitinib groups (Fig. 1 and Table 2). The duration of MJS was not statistically significantly different, however, in the baricitinib monotherapy group vs. the MTX group at week 24 or week 52.

The percentage of patients with improvement in the FACIT-F that exceeded the MCID at week 24 (≥ 3.56) was 65%, 75%, and 71% for MTX, baricitinib monotherapy, and baricitinib + MTX, respectively, at week 24 ($p \leq 0.05$ for baricitinib monotherapy vs. MTX; $p = 0.268$ for baricitinib + MTX vs. MTX). The percentage of patients with improvement in the FACIT-F that exceeded the MCID (≥ 3.56) was 54%, 62%, and 62%, respectively at week 52 (neither baricitinib group was statistically significantly different from the MTX group).

Health-related quality of life

Compared to MTX monotherapy, statistically significant improvements in SF-36 PCS were observed in both the baricitinib monotherapy and the baricitinib + MTX groups as early as the first assessment at week 4 (Fig. 2); these improvements were maintained during the study. For the SF-36 MCS, numeric improvements were observed at all time points in both baricitinib treatment groups compared to the MTX group and the differences were statistically significant at weeks 4, 40 and 52 ($p \leq 0.05$).

For the SF-36 PCS, at week 24, the percentage of patients who met or exceeded the MCID for MTX, baricitinib monotherapy, and baricitinib + MTX, respectively, was 62%, 71%, and 74% ($p = 0.091$ for baricitinib monotherapy vs. MTX; $p \leq 0.05$ for baricitinib + MTX vs. MTX). At week 52, the percentage of patients who met or exceeded the MCID for the SF-36 PCS was 48%, 65%, and 65%, respectively ($p \leq 0.05$ for baricitinib monotherapy vs. MTX; $p \leq 0.001$ for baricitinib + MTX vs. MTX). In contrast, for the SF-36 MCS, there were no statistically significant

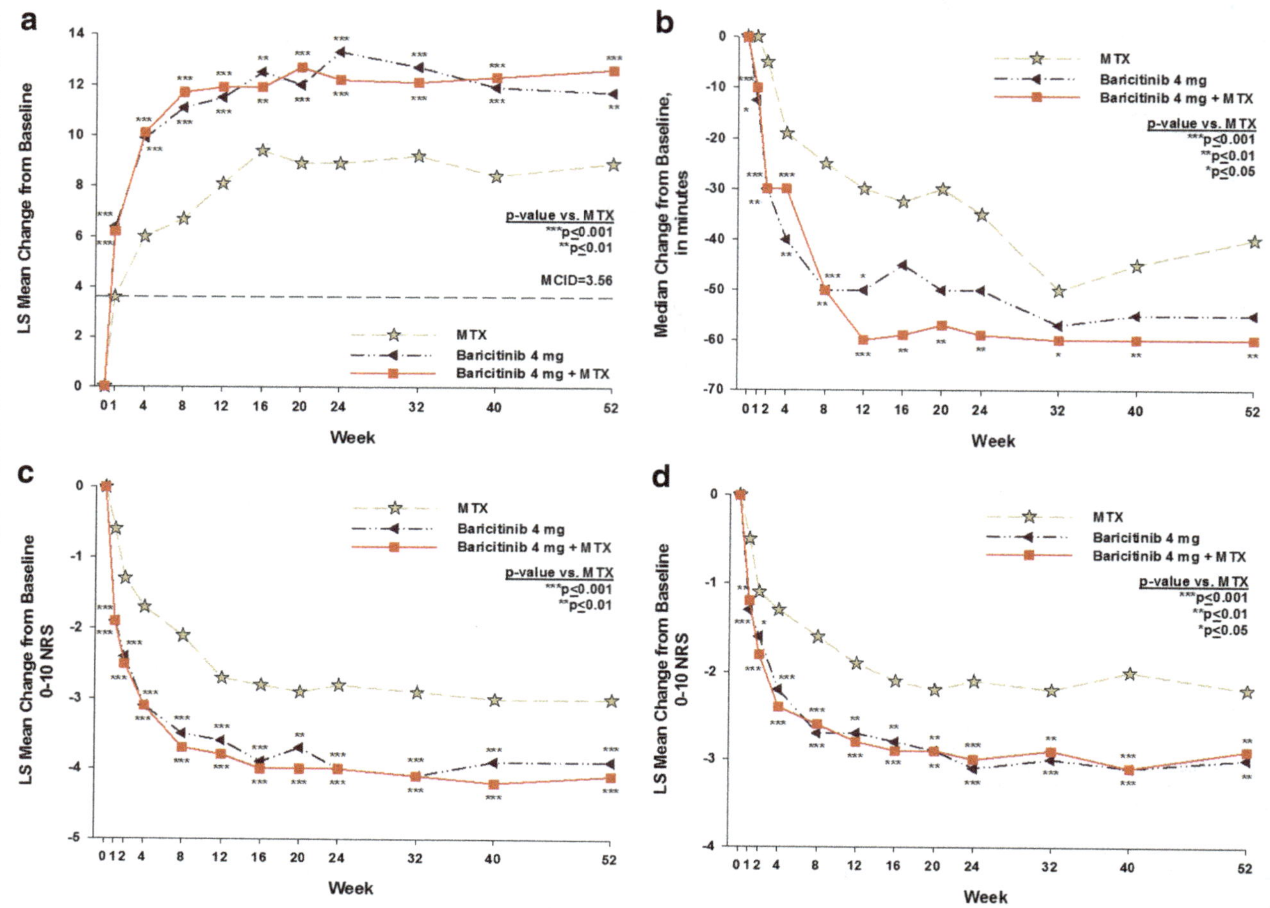

Fig. 1 Change from baseline over time for the Functional Assessment of Chronic Illness Therapy-Fatigue (FACIT-F) (**a**), morning joint stiffness duration (**b**), worst joint pain (**c**), and worst tiredness (**d**). The dashed line represents the minimum clinically important difference (MCID) in the FACIT-F (≥ 3.56 points). The question asked for morning joint stiffness duration was "Please indicate how long your morning joint stiffness lasted yesterday (duration in minutes)." The question for worst joint pain was "Please rate your joint pain by selecting the one number that describes your joint pain at its WORST in the last 24 hours (0 = no pain; 10 = pain as bad as you can imagine)." The question for worst tiredness was "Please rate your tiredness by selecting the one number that describes your WORST level of tiredness during the past 24 hours (0 = no tiredness; 10 = as bad as you can imagine)", MTX methotrexate

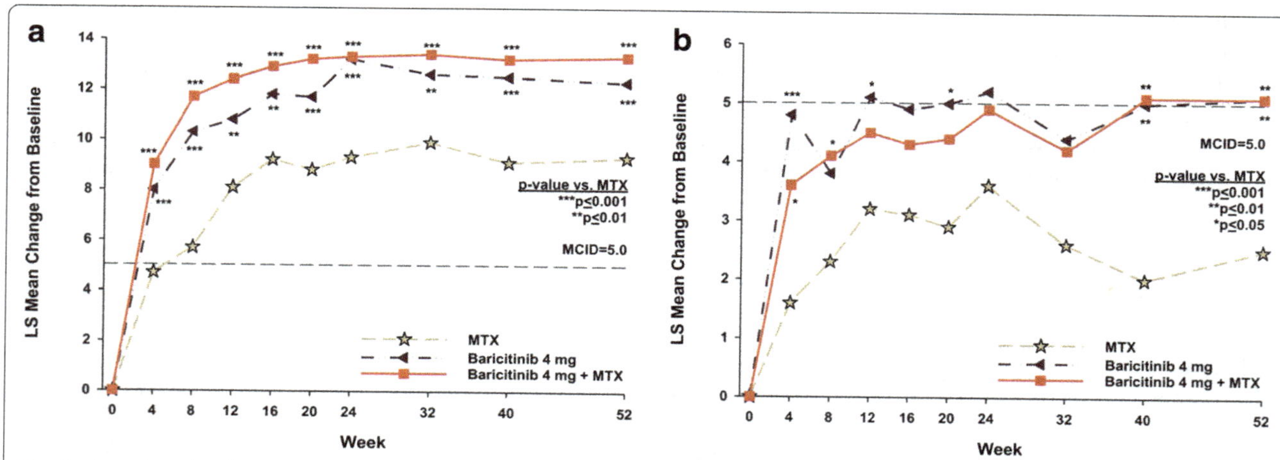

Fig. 2 Change from baseline over time in the Physical Component Score (PCS) (**a**) and Mental Component Score (MCS) (**b**) of the Short Form-36 (SF-36). The dashed line represents the minimum clinically important difference (MCID) in the SF-36 PCS (≥ 5 points) and SF-36 MCS (≥ 5 points). MTX methotrexate

differences between the baricitinib groups and the MTX group in the percentage of patients who met or exceeded the MCID.

For the EQ-5D UK index score at week 4, the first post-baseline assessment, there were statistically significant improvements in both the baricitinib monotherapy and baricitinib + MTX groups compared to MTX ($p \leq 0.001$ for both baricitinib groups vs. MTX). These differences were maintained through week 52 (Table 2). A statistically significant improvement was seen in the EQ-5D VAS in both baricitinib groups compared to the MTX group, beginning at week 4 ($p \leq 0.001$ for both baricitinib groups vs. MTX). These results were maintained through the end of the study (Table 2). Similar results were seen for the US index score (Table 2).

WPAI-RA

For the WPAI-RA assessment, patients in the baricitinib monotherapy and baricitinib + MTX groups reported improved daily activity compared to MTX monotherapy (Table 3). Among those patients employed at baseline and who maintained employment at week 24, there were statistically significant improvements in both baricitinib groups compared to the MTX group across all measures; these statistically significant improvements were only maintained at week 52 in the baricitinib + MTX group compared to the MTX group, with respect to work productivity loss ($p \leq 0.05$) (Table 4).

Discussion

The primary objective of the RA-BEGIN study was to evaluate baricitinib, an oral tsDMARD that selectively inhibits JAK1 and JAK2, as monotherapy or combined with MTX compared to MTX monotherapy in patients with active RA and no prior DMARD therapy or limited prior MTX therapy. The current analysis has focused on PROs which, in conjunction with clinical assessment measures, are a valuable and practical tool for comprehensive disease management and provide important insights into the patient's response to therapy and as such, should be utilized in the clinic [29]. Although MTX was effective in this population, particularly at later time points, the majority of the pre-specified PROs of physical function, HRQOL, PtGA, pain, fatigue, duration of MJS, tiredness, and joint pain were all statistically significantly improved to a greater extent at many or all time points in patients treated with baricitinib monotherapy and baricitinib + MTX compared to the MTX monotherapy.

The clinical relevance of these PRO improvements with baricitinib is emphasized by their consistent superiority to MTX, the oral standard of care in the treatment of RA, in contrast to simply being compared to a placebo control. The ACR guidelines and EULAR recommendations propose that MTX be the first-line DMARD treatment for DMARD-naïve patients because of its effectiveness in controlling disease activity, improving patient function and limiting radiographic progression in up to one third of patients, and having an acceptable and well-known safety profile and a low cost [1, 6, 7]. These recommendations have relied on studies in MTX-naïve patients that compared MTX to bDMARD monotherapy and indicated that MTX was as clinically effective (including PRO data) as bDMARD monotherapy [30–32]. One study, TEMPO, used a similar design to RA-BEGIN to compare etanercept either as monotherapy or in combination with MTX vs. MTX in patients with mean disease duration of over 6 years. In TEMPO, etanercept monotherapy had similar benefit to MTX monotherapy in improving PROs [33].

There are, however, a number of patients for whom MTX monotherapy is unsuitable. There is, therefore, an unmet need for alternative therapeutic choices for such patients; novel, orally administered tsDMARDs, such as baricitinib, would appear to have desirable attributes in this setting. Importantly, in RA-BEGIN, the comparable effects on PRO improvements in the baricitinib monotherapy and baricitinib + MTX groups suggest that baricitinib may be an effective monotherapy treatment.

These results from the current analysis are similar to what has been reported from studies of bDMARDs plus MTX in patients with early RA. For example, the PREMIER trial compared MTX monotherapy, adalimumab monotherapy, and adalimumab + MTX in patients with early RA

Table 3 Work Productivity and Activity Impairment Questionnaire - Rheumatoid Arthritis (WPAI-RA): impairment of regular activities among all patients at baseline and least-squares mean change from baseline at week 24 and at week 52

WPAI-RA question administered to all patients[a]	Baseline, Mean (SD)			Week 24, LSM (95% CI)			Week 52, LSM (95% CI)		
	MTX (*N* = 210)	Baricitinib 4 mg (*N* = 159)	Baricitinib 4 mg + MTX (*N* = 215)	MTX (*N* = 210)	Baricitinib 4 mg (*N* = 159)	Baricitinib 4 mg + MTX (*N* = 215)	MTX (*N* = 210)	Baricitinib 4 mg (*N* = 159)	Baricitinib 4 mg + MTX (*N* = 215)
Percent activity impairment due to RA	61 (26)	62 (25)	59 (25)	− 25 (− 29, − 22)	− 37 (− 40, − 33)***	− 33 (− 37, − 30)***	− 29 (− 32, −25)	− 35 (− 38, − 31)*	− 38 (− 42, − 35)***

CI confidence interval, *LSM* least-squares mean, *MTX* methotrexate *RA* rheumatoid arthritis
[a]Data are presented as mean (standard deviation) unless stated otherwise
*$p \leq 0.05$; ***$p \leq 0.001$ vs. MTX

Table 4 Work Productivity and Activity Impairment Questionnaire - Rheumatoid Arthritis (WPAI-RA): mean presenteeism, absenteeism, and work productivity loss at baseline and least-squares mean change from baseline at week 24 and at week 52 among patients employed at baseline and at Week 24 or Week 52

WPAI-RA questions administered to patients who were employed[a]	Baseline, Mean (SD)			Week 24, LSM (95% CI)			Week 52, LSM (95% CI)		
	MTX (*N* = 210)	Baricitinib 4 mg (*N* = 159)	Baricitinib 4 mg + MTX (*N* = 215)	MTX (*n* = 85)	Baricitinib 4 mg (*n* = 63)	Baricitinib 4 mg + MTX (*n* = 105)	MTX (*n* = 67)	Baricitinib 4 mg (*n* = 58)	Baricitinib 4 mg + MTX (*n* = 96)
Percent employed at time point[b], *n* (%)	94 (45)	67 (42)	117 (55)	80 (94)	59 (94)	94 (90)	57 (85)	55 (95)	80 (83)
Percent impairment while working due to RA (presenteeism)	49 (28)	49 (26)	50 (26)	− 20 (− 25, − 15)	− 29 (− 35, − 24)*	− 31 (− 35, − 26)**	− 26 (− 31, − 20)	− 29 (− 35, − 23)	− 31 (− 35, − 27)
Percent overall work impairment due to RA (work productivity loss)	53 (29)	51 (27)	55 (27)	− 18 (− 24, − 13)	− 29 (− 36, − 23)*	− 30 (− 35, − 25)**	− 23 (− 30, − 17)	− 30 (− 37 − 23)	− 32 (− 38, − 27)*
Percent work time missed due to RA (absenteeism)	19 (31)	14 (29)	15 (25)	− 2 (− 7, 2)	− 10 (− 15, − 5)*	− 9 (− 12, − 5)*	− 3 (− 7, 1)	− 8 (− 12, − 3)	− 8 (− 11, − 4)

CI confidence interval, *LSM* least-squares mean, *MTX* methotrexate, *RA* rheumatoid arthritis

[a]Data are presented as mean (standard deviation) or LSM (95% CI)

[b]For weeks 24 and 52, the percentage of patients employed at baseline and who continued to be employed at that time point

*$p \leq 0.05$; **$p \leq 0.01$ vs. MTX

who were naive to MTX therapy [10]. For MTX, adalimumab, and adalimumab + MTX, respectively, the baseline HAQ-DI values were 1.5, 1.6, and 1.5 with decrements of − 0.8, − 0.8 and − 1.1 at 1 year [10]. In the current RA-BEGIN analysis, at baseline, the mean baseline HAQ-DI scores for MTX, baricitinib monotherapy, and baricitinib + MTX, respectively, were 1.7, 1.6, and 1.6 with decrements of − 0.71, − 0.99 and − 1.06 at one year. Similar trends were also observed in the ORAL Start trial, which compared tofacitinib monotherapy, both 5 and 10 mg twice daily, to MTX monotherapy in MTX-naïve patients. On physical functioning, tofacitinib 5 mg and 10 mg demonstrated benefit compared to MTX as monotherapy [11].

In RA-BEGIN, trends in the PRO results were also generally similar to PRO results from other studies. The HAQ-DI results in the OPTIMA trial were similar to the HAQ-DI observations described above [34]. In the OPTIMA trial, which compared adalimumab + MTX with MTX monotherapy in patients with RA who were naïve to MTX therapy, the baseline mean HAQ-DI values were 1.61 for adalimumab + MTX and 1.60 for MTX. At week 26, the mean HAQ-DI values were 0.7 for adalimumab + MTX and 0.9 for MTX ($p < 0.001$) [34].

Similar trends were observed with the FACIT-F, which measures fatigue, a major concern for patients and an important outcome measure in RA studies [35]. Notably, as with most other PROs, it is not captured in the ACR response criteria or Disease Activity Score (DAS) response composite indices. The FACIT-F was assessed in the ORAL Start trial. At 6 months, the least-squares mean (LSM) changes from baseline for MTX, tofacitinib 5 mg, and tofacitinib 10 mg, respectively, were 6.3, 8.7, and 9.1 [11, 36]. In the current analysis, the LSM changes from baseline to 6 months for MTX, baricitinib monotherapy, and baricitinib + MTX were 8.9, 13.3, and 12.2.

For the HRQOL assessments, patients in both baricitinib treatment groups reported statistically significant improvements in the EQ-5D index scores and VAS scores and the SF-36 PCS measure compared with MTX monotherapy at 4 weeks post baseline. These results were maintained through week 52. For the SF-36 MCS measure there was no statistically significant difference in the percentage of patients who met or exceeded the MCID (≥ 5) across the treatment groups. These SF-36 MCS results are consistent with previous observations from other clinical trials [19, 20]. Of note, the baseline values for the SF-36 MCS ranged from 45 to 47 in the current analysis, which demonstrates a modest, rather than severe impairment. Patients, therefore, may have had less opportunity to improve their SF-36 MCS scores.

Work productivity and activity impairment have a significant economic impact on patients. In this trial, all three treatments were effective in improving work impairment, with earlier benefit noted in both baricitinib groups, but with comparable benefits at one year.

This study has a number of limitations. In clinical practice, in contradistinction to this study, MTX will typically be started either as monotherapy or in combination with other csDMARDs prior to the use of a bDMARD or a tsDMARD, such as baricitinib. However, the intent of this study was to compare the effectiveness of baricitinib to

MTX and given current treatment paradigms, this is best accomplished in MTX-naïve patients. Following initial escalation, the maintenance dose of MTX was limited to no more than 20 mg/week; it is conceivable that there could have been a better response with MTX if the dose could have been increased or switched to subcutaneous MTX. In addition, other initial treatment regimens, such as MTX in combination with other csDMARDs, were not evaluated. Additionally, the use of carrying forward the last observations before rescue or discontinuation assumes that the PRO values would not change over time had these events not occurred. This is an appropriate statistical method for this analysis, but the assumption is not verifiable. Last, as in most double-blind comparator trials, the inclusion and exclusion criteria limited the participation of some patients, who are routinely seen in clinical practice. This may potentially impact the generalizability of the study results.

Conclusions

We have shown that the majority of the pre-specified PRO measures in this study improved in each of the active treatment groups evaluated, but there were statistically and clinically significant improvements with either baricitinib group over MTX monotherapy, many from as early as week 1. Early improvement in PROs is an important clinical outcome. The PRO data from this trial reinforce the outcomes for other signs and symptoms observed in the RA-BEGIN study [1]. This trial demonstrates that baricitinib may either be used as monotherapy or in combination with MTX, as improvements across measures of how patients feel and function were comparable for each regimen, both appearing consistently more effective than MTX. This may be of importance to physicians and their patients for whom use of MTX is not desirable, and adds to previously published data showing that baricitinib can be an effective agent in the treatment of RA [1, 37].

Abbreviations

ACR: American College of Rheumatology; ANCOVA: Analysis of covariance; csDMARDs: Conventional synthetic disease-modifying anti-rheumatic drugs; DAS: Disease Activity Score; EQ-5D: EuroQol-5 Dimensions; EULAR: European League Against Rheumatism; FACIT-F: Functional Assessment of Chronic Illness Therapy-Fatigue; HAQ-DI: Health Assessment Questionnaire-Disability Index; HRQOL: Health-related quality of life; JAK: Janus kinase; MCID: Minimum clinically important difference; mITT: Modified intention-to-treat; MJS: Morning joint stiffness; mLOCF: Modified last observation carried forward; MTX: Methotrexate; NRI: Non-responder imputation; NRS: Numeric rating scale; OMERACT: Outcome Measures in Rheumatology; PROs: Patient-reported outcomes; PtGA: Patient's Global Assessment of Disease Activity; QD: Twice daily; RA: Rheumatoid arthritis; SF-36 MCS: Short Form-36 Mental Component Score; SF-36 PCS: Short Form-36 Physical Component Score; tsDMARDs: Targeted synthetic DMARDs; VAS: Visual analog scale; WPAI-RA: Work Productivity and Activity Impairment-Rheumatoid Arthritis

Acknowledgements

The authors would like to thank Barbara Coffey, MS, and Molly Tomlin, MS, of Eli Lilly and Company for their assistance with manuscript preparation and process support and Melanie McEwen, PhD, and Julie Sherman, of Eli Lilly and Company, for their assistance with the manuscript tables and figures.

Funding

This study and manuscript were sponsored by Eli Lilly and Company and Incyte Corporation.

Authors' contributions

MS, TT, RF, CG, DS, and TR made substantial contributions to the conception and design of the study; MS, TT, RF, SS, RPH, RvV, and CAFZ participated in the acquisition of the data; W-LK and TC analyzed the data; all authors participated in the interpretation of the data; MS, TT, RF, CG, and CAFZ have been involved in the drafting of the manuscript; all authors helped to revise the paper critically with important intellectual content; and all authors read and approved the final manuscript and have agreed to be accountable for all aspects of the work.

Competing interests

Financial Support and Disclosures: MS has received consulting fees from AbbVie, Amgen, Bristol-Myers Squibb, Eli Lilly and Company, Johnson & Johnson, Novartis, Roche, and UCB (< US$10,000 each) and speaking fees from AbbVie and Bristol-Myers Squibb (> US$10,000). TT has received consulting fees from Pfizer Japan Inc., Astra Zeneca K.K., Eli Lilly Japan K.K., Novartis Pharma K.K., Daiichi Sankyo Co., Ltd., Nipponkayaku Co., Ltd, Janssen Pharmaceutical K.K., Merck Serono Co., Ltd., Takeda Pharmaceutical Co., Ltd. (< US$10,000 each), and from Mitsubishi Tanabe Pharma Co., Astellas Pharma Inc, AbbVie GK, Bristol–Myers K.K. Asahi Kasei Medical K.K (> US$10,000 each), and speaking fees from Celtrion, Nipponkayaku Co., Ltd, Pfizer Japan Inc., UCB Japan, Diaichi Sankyo Co., Ltd., Takeda Pharmaceutical Co., Ltd., (< US$10,000 each) and from Chugai Pharmaceutical Co,. Ltd., AbbVie GK, Bristol–Myers K.K., Eisai Co., Ltd., Mitsubishi Tanabe Pharma Co., Janssen Pharmaceutical K.K., and Astellas Pharma Inc., (> US$10,000 each). RF has received consulting fees from AbbVie, Amgen, Bristol–Myers Squibb, Janssen, Eli Lilly and Company, and Sanofi-Aventis (< US$10,000 each), and consulting fees from Pfizer and UCB (> US$10,000 each). CG, AD, DS, W-LK, J-EW, TC, and TR are employees of Eli Lilly and Company and all, except TC and AD are shareholders. PD has received consulting fees from Eli Lilly and Company. SS has received consulting fees from Abbvie, Eli Lilly, Roche, and UCB. RPH has no conflicts of interest related to this manuscript. RvV has received consulting fees from AbbVie, Biotest, BMS, Celgene, Crescendo, GSK, Janssen, Lilly, Merck, Novartis, Pfizer, Roche, UCB, and Vertex and research grants from AbbVie, Amgen, BMS, GSK, Pfizer, Roche, and UCB. CAFZ has received consulting fees from Merck, Pfizer, Sanofi, and Eli Lilly and Company (< US$10,000 each).

Author details

[1]University of Colorado School of Medicine, Denver, CO 80045, USA. [2]Keio University, Tokyo, Japan. [3]Metroplex Clinical Research Center, University of Texas Southwestern Medical Center, Dallas, TX 75231, USA. [4]Eli Lilly and Company, Indianapolis, IN 46285, USA. [5]Eli Lilly and Company, Seoul, Republic of Korea. [6]Service et Pôle de Rhumatologie, Cliniques Universitaires Saint-Luc, Brussels, Belgium. [7]Institut de Recherche Expérimentale et Clinique, Université catholique de Louvain, Rheumatology, Brussels, Belgium. [8]McMaster University, Hamilton, ON, Canada. [9]CER, San Juan, Argentina. [10]Amsterdam Rheumatology and Immunology Center ARC, Amsterdam, The Netherlands. [11]Centro Paulista de Investigação Clinica, São Paulo, Brazil.

References

1. Fleischmann R, Schiff M, van der Heijde D, Ramos-Remus C, Spindler A, Stanislav M, Zerbini CAF, Gurbuz S, Dickson C, de Bono S, et al. Baricitinib, methotrexate, or combination in patients with rheumatoid arthritis and no or limited prior disease-modifying antirheumatic drug treatment. Arthritis Rheumatol. 2017;69:506–17. doi:10.1002/art.39953.

2. Bruce B, Fries JF. The Health Assessment Questionnaire (HAQ). Clin Exp Rheumatol. 2005;23:S14–8.
3. Ramey D, Fries J, Singh G. The Health Assessment Questionnaire 1995 — status and review. In: Spilker B, editor. Quality of life and pharmacoeconomics in clinical trials. 2nd ed. Philadelphia: Lippincott-Raven; 1996. p. 227–37.
4. Felson DT, Anderson JJ, Boers M, Bombardier C, Chernoff M, Fried B, et al. The American College of Rheumatology preliminary core set of disease activity measures for rheumatoid arthritis clinical trials. The Committee on Outcome Measures in Rheumatoid Arthritis Clinical Trials. Arthritis Rheum. 1993;36:729–40.
5. Kirwan JR, Newman S, Tugwell PS, Wells GA, Hewlett S, Idzera L, et al. Progress on incorporating the patient perspective in outcome assessment in rheumatology and the emergence of life impact measures at OMERACT 9. J Rheumatol. 2009;36:2071–6.
6. Singh JA, Saag KG, Bridges Jr SL, Akl EA, Bannuru RR, Sullivan MC, et al. 2015 American College of Rheumatology Guideline for the Treatment of Rheumatoid Arthritis. Arthritis Rheumatol. 2016;68:1–26.
7. Smolen JS and Landewé R. EULAR recommendations for the management of rheumatoid arthritis-2016 Update. EULAR Web site. Available at: http://www.eular.org/myUploadData/files/EULAR%20RA%20Management%20recommendations%202016%20update%20June%202016-c_2.pdf. Accessed 01 Dec 2016.
8. Food and Drug Administration. Guidance for industry: rheumatoid arthritis: developing drug products for treatment: draft guidance. May 2013. Available at http://www.fda.gov/downloads/Drugs/GuidanceComplianceRegulatoryInformation/Guidances/UCM354468.pdf. Accessed 20 June 2017.
9. Smolen JS, Breedveld FC, Burmester GR, Bykerk V, Dougados M, Emery P, et al. Treating rheumatoid arthritis to target: 2014 update of the recommendations of an international task force. Ann Rheum Dis. 2016;75:3–15.
10. Breedveld FC, Weisman MH, Kavanaugh AF, Cohen SB, Pavelka K, van Vollenhoven R, et al. The PREMIER study: a multicenter, randomized, double-blind clinical trial of combination therapy with adalimumab plus methotrexate versus methotrexate alone or adalimumab alone in patients with early, aggressive rheumatoid arthritis who had not had previous methotrexate treatment. Arthritis Rheum. 2006;54:26–37.
11. Lee EB, Fleischmann R, Hall S, Wilkinson B, Bradley JD, Gruben D, et al. Tofacitinib versus methotrexate in rheumatoid arthritis. N Engl J Med. 2014;370:2377–86.
12. Jones G, Sebba A, Gu J, Lowenstein MB, Calvo A, Gomez-Reino JJ, et al. Comparison of tocilizumab monotherapy versus methotrexate monotherapy in patients with moderate to severe rheumatoid arthritis: the AMBITION study. Ann Rheum Dis. 2010;69:88–96.
13. Emery P, Breedveld FC, Hall S, Durez P, Chang DJ, Robertson D, et al. Comparison of methotrexate monotherapy with a combination of methotrexate and etanercept in active, early, moderate to severe rheumatoid arthritis (COMET): a randomised, double-blind, parallel treatment trial. Lancet. 2008;372:375–82.
14. Nash P, Nicholls D. Perceptions of methotrexate use in rheumatoid arthritis by rheumatologists and their patients: an Australian survey study. Int J Rheum Dis. 2013;16:652–61.
15. RHEUMATREX® (methotrexate) [package insert]. Fort Lee: DAVA Pharmaceuticals, Inc; 2013. https://dailymed.nlm.nih.gov/dailymed/drugInfo.cfm?setid=2cb70aa1-f73a-41c8-9a7f-edbcf1a06efd. Accessed 5 Sept 2017.
16. Wells GA, Tugwell P, Kraag GR, Baker PR, Groh J, Redelmeier DA. Minimum important difference between patients with rheumatoid arthritis: the patient's perspective. J Rheumatol. 1993;20:557–60.
17. Krishnan E, Sokka T, Hakkinen A, Hubert H, Hannonen P. Normative values for the Health Assessment Questionnaire disability index: benchmarking disability in the general population. Arthritis Rheum. 2004;50:953–60.
18. Cella D, Yount S, Sorensen M, Chartash E, Sengupta N, Grober J. Validation of the Functional Assessment of Chronic Illness Therapy Fatigue Scale relative to other instrumentation in patients with rheumatoid arthritis. J Rheumatol. 2005;32:811–9.
19. Strand V, Burmester GR, Zerbini CA, Mebus CA, Zwillich SH, Gruben D, et al. Tofacitinib with methotrexate in third-line treatment of patients with active rheumatoid arthritis: patient-reported outcomes from a phase III trial. Arthritis Care Res (Hoboken). 2015;67:475–83.
20. Keystone E, Burmester GR, Furie R, Loveless JE, Emery P, Kremer J, et al. Improvement in patient-reported outcomes in a rituximab trial in patients with severe rheumatoid arthritis refractory to anti-tumor necrosis factor therapy. Arthritis Rheum. 2008;59:785–93.
21. Brazier JE, Harper R, Jones NM, O'Cathain A, Thomas KJ, Usherwood T, et al. Validating the SF-36 health survey questionnaire: new outcome measure for primary care. BMJ. 1992;305:160–4.
22. Ware Jr JE, Sherbourne CD. The MOS 36-item short-form health survey (SF-36). I. Conceptual framework and item selection. Med Care. 1992;30:473–83.
23. Kosinski M, Zhao SZ, Dedhiya S, Osterhaus JT, Ware Jr JE. Determining minimally important changes in generic and disease-specific health-related quality of life questionnaires in clinical trials of rheumatoid arthritis. Arthritis Rheum. 2000;43:1478–87.
24. Strand V, Singh JA. Newer biological agents in rheumatoid arthritis: impact on health-related quality of life and productivity. Drugs. 2010;70:121–45.
25. EuroQol Group. EQ-5D-5L User Guide. Version 2.1. 2015 [cited August 11, 2016]; Available from: https://euroqol.org/wp-content/uploads/2016/09/EQ-5D-5L_UserGuide_2015.pdf. Accessed 5 Sept 2017.
26. Brooks R. EuroQol: the current state of play. Health Policy. 1996;37:53–72.
27. Herdman M, Gudex C, Lloyd A, Janssen M, Kind P, Parkin D, et al. Development and preliminary testing of the new five-level version of EQ-5D (EQ-5D-5L). Qual Life Res. 2011;20:1727–36.
28. Reilly MC, Zbrozek AS, Dukes EM. The validity and reproducibility of a work productivity and activity impairment instrument. Pharmacoeconomics. 1993;4:353–65.
29. Daul P, Grisanti J. Monitoring response to therapy in rheumatoid arthritis - perspectives from the clinic. Bull NYU Hosp Jt Dis. 2009;67:236–42.
30. Emery P, Fleischmann RM, Moreland LW, Hsia EC, Strusberg I, Durez P, et al. Golimumab, a human anti-tumor necrosis factor alpha monoclonal antibody, injected subcutaneously every four weeks in methotrexate-naive patients with active rheumatoid arthritis: twenty-four-week results of a phase III, multicenter, randomized, double-blind, placebo-controlled study of golimumab before methotrexate as first-line therapy for early-onset rheumatoid arthritis. Arthritis Rheum. 2009;60:2272–83.
31. Emery P, Burmester GR, Bykerk VP, Combe BG, Furst DE, Barre E, et al. Evaluating drug-free remission with abatacept in early rheumatoid arthritis: results from the phase 3b, multicentre, randomised, active-controlled AVERT study of 24 months, with a 12-month, double-blind treatment period. Ann Rheum Dis. 2015;74:19–26.
32. Burmester GR, Rigby WF, van Vollenhoven RF, Kay J, Rubbert-Roth A, Kelman A, et al. Tocilizumab in early progressive rheumatoid arthritis: FUNCTION, a randomised controlled trial. Ann Rheum Dis. 2016;75:1081–91.
33. van der Heijde D, Klareskog L, Singh A, Tornero J, Melo-Gomes J, Codreanu C, et al. Patient reported outcomes in a trial of combination therapy with etanercept and methotrexate for rheumatoid arthritis: the TEMPO trial. Ann Rheum Dis. 2006;65:328–34.
34. Kavanaugh A, Fleischmann RM, Emery P, Kupper H, Redden L, Guerette B. Clinical, functional and radiographic consequences of achieving stable low disease activity and remission with adalimumab plus methotrexate or methotrexate alone in early rheumatoid arthritis: 26-week results from the randomised, controlled OPTIMA study. Ann Rheum Dis. 2013;72:64–71.
35. Kirwan JR, Minnock P, Adebajo A, Bresnihan B, Choy E, de Wit M, et al. Patient perspective: fatigue as a recommended patient centered outcome measure in rheumatoid arthritis. J Rheumatol. 2007;34:1174–7.
36. Alten R, Strand V, Fleischmann R, Koncz T, Zwillich S, Bradley J, et al. Effects of tofacitinib monotherapy versus methotrexate on patient-reported outcomes in the 2-year phase 3 Oral Start trial in methotrexate-naïve patients with rheumatoid arthritis [abstract]. Ann Rheum Dis. 2014;73:118–9.
37. Genovese MC, Kremer J, Zamani O, Ludivico C, Krogulec M, Xie L, et al. Baricitinib in patients with refractory rheumatoid arthritis. N Engl J Med. 2016;374:1243–52.

5

A somatization comorbidity phenotype impacts response to therapy in rheumatoid arthritis: post-hoc results from the certolizumab pegol phase 4 PREDICT trial

Jeffrey R. Curtis[1*], Christopher Herrem[2], 'Matladi N. Ndlovu[3], Cathy O'Brien[3] and Yusuf Yazici[4]

Abstract

Background: Comorbidities may contribute to disease activity and treatment response in rheumatoid arthritis (RA) patients. We defined a somatization comorbidity phenotype (SCP) and examined its influence on response to certolizumab pegol (CZP) using data from the PREDICT trial.

Methods: Patients in PREDICT were randomized to the patient-reported Routine Assessment of Patient Index Data 3 (RAPID3) or physician-based Clinical Disease Activity Index (CDAI) for treatment response assessment. Post-hoc analyses identified patients with the SCP, which included diagnosis of depression, fibromyalgia/myalgias, and/or use of medications indicated for treatment of depression, anxiety, or neuropathic pain. The effect of the SCP on RAPID3 or CDAI response at week 12 and low disease activity (LDA; Disease Activity Score in 28 joints based on erythrocyte sedimentation rate ≤ 3.2) at week 52, in week-12 responders, was analyzed using non-parametric analysis of covariance (ANCOVA).

Results: At baseline, 43% (313/733) of patients met the SCP classification. Patients with the SCP were 9% more likely to withdraw from the trial. American College of Rheumatology 20% (ACR20), ACR50, and ACR70 responses were 5–14% lower among those with the SCP, and 11% more patients reported adverse events (AEs). Patients without SCP in the CDAI arm were twice as likely to achieve LDA at week 52 compared with those with SCP (32% versus 16%). No differentiation by SCP was observed in the RAPID3 arm (pooled result 21.5%).

Conclusions: We operationalized a potentially important somatization comorbidity phenotype in a trial setting that was associated with a substantially lower likelihood of treatment response and a higher frequency of AEs. Including large numbers of patients with this phenotype in RA trials may reduce the measured clinical effectiveness of a new molecule.

Keywords: Rheumatoid arthritis, Disease activity, Patient-reported outcomes, Comorbidities, Depression, Anxiety, Fibromyalgia, RAPID3, CDAI

* Correspondence: jrcurtis@uabmc.edu
[1]Division of Clinical Immunology and Rheumatology, University of Alabama at Birmingham, FOT 802, 510 20th Street South, Birmingham, AL 35294, USA
Full list of author information is available at the end of the article

Background

Comorbidities have been shown to substantially contribute to disease activity and treatment response in rheumatoid arthritis (RA) and should therefore be considered when devising treatment strategies for patients with RA [1–4]. Anxiety and depression are more common in people with RA than in the general population [5], and depression, fatigue, and fibromyalgia have been associated with increased disease activity, reduced odds for reaching clinical remission in RA, and reduced treatment effects and quality of life [4–8]. However, the impact of these comorbidities on the magnitude of response in a clinical trial setting has not been well characterized, and an efficient approach to identifying patients with these conditions within an RA trial program has not been previously well-described.

Clinical assessment tools, such as the Disease Activity Score in 28 joints (DAS28) and Clinical Disease Activity Index (CDAI), and patient-reported outcome-only tools, such as the Routine Assessment of Patient Index Data 3 (RAPID3), have proven effective for evaluating RA disease activity and predicting treatment response to guide patient management in RA [9–11]. The presence of comorbidities may also influence treatment outcomes indirectly due to the varying definitions of the state of remission or low disease activity (LDA) across different assessment tools [12]. There is currently no universal agreement on the best measurement tool for RA disease activity, given the strengths and limitations of each [9, 12–14].

The goal of these exploratory, post-hoc analyses was to define a "somatization comorbidity phenotype" (SCP) that could classify patients with RA participating in a clinical trial who had one or more conditions (e.g. fibromyalgia) that might have contributed to chronic pain independent of RA disease activity, or who had conditions (e.g. depression) other than RA that could have influenced pain and the patient's self-management of their condition. The second aim was to evaluate whether this phenotype influenced treatment response as assessed by the CDAI and RAPID3 tools and more traditional measures (e.g. ACR response). The analysis was conducted in the Patient/Physician Reported Efficacy Determination in Clinical Practice (PREDICT) trial, among patients with moderate to severe RA initiating treatment with the anti-tumor necrosis factor (anti-TNF) agent, certolizumab pegol (CZP).

Methods

Study design

The PREDICT trial (NCT01255761) was a randomized, phase 4 trial that examined the predictability of CZP treatment success at week 52 based on treatment response at week 12, as assessed by the patient-reported RAPID3 or the mostly physician-based CDAI in patients with RA with moderate to severe, active disease. The primary hypotheses tested were whether the RAPID3 was comparable to the CDAI tool in assessing response to CZP therapy at week 12, and evaluating the positive predictive value of this classification against the RA disease state at week 52. Detailed methods and the primary results of the PREDICT study have been published previously [15].

In brief, patients aged ≥ 18 years, with a diagnosis of adult-onset RA for > 3 months' duration at baseline were eligible for this 52-week study. RA was diagnosed according to the American College of Rheumatology (ACR) 1987 classification criteria [16]. Patients were also required to have an unsatisfactory response or intolerance to ≥ 1 disease-modifying antirheumatic drug (DMARD). Patients with fibromyalgia requiring treatment were excluded from the study as per protocol. The purpose of this exclusion was to remove patients who were hypothesized to have an attenuated treatment response as measured by the two tools (i.e. RAPID3 and CDAI) used in the trial, as both contain a patient measurement component. This exclusion was similar to a general exclusion in many RA trials where investigators are requested to exclude patients who have concomitant medical conditions that might interfere with the interpretation of the study results [17–19]. The exclusion was implemented by each local site investigator; no systematic identification or exclusion at the time of randomization was enforced.

Both RAPID3 and CDAI assessments were performed on all patients throughout the study at each visit. Patients were randomized 1:1 to protocolized management based upon either the RAPID3 or CDAI, and patients remained blinded throughout the study to their randomized group. Randomization was performed through an interactive voice/web-based response system (IXRS). All patients received a loading dose of CZP (400 mg at weeks 0, 2, and 4), followed by CZP 200 mg every second week (Q2W) until week 50.

At week 12, all patients were classified as responders or non-responders according to their randomized assessment group. RAPID3 response was defined as ≤ 6 (LDA) or ≥ 20% improvement from baseline, and CDAI response was defined as ≤ 10 (LDA) or ≥ 20% improvement from baseline. These cutoffs for CDAI and RAPID3 response were established in the PREDICT study protocol prior to published reports of a minimal clinically important difference (MCID) for CDAI [20] and RAPID3 [21]. All patients who were not week-12 RAPID3 or CDAI responders, or were withdrawn prior to week 12, were classified as non-responders. The non-responders included a subset of patients who had no improvement by week 12 ("week-12 failures"; those with no RAPID3 improvement or < 1 point CDAI improvement, based on the assessment group to which they were randomized), and were withdrawn from the study and CZP treatment. All other non-responders who were not week-12 failures continued treatment with CZP 200 mg Q2W, unless they reached a high disease activity state (CDAI >22 or RAPID3 >12) [22] at two consecutive visits, at which point they were withdrawn from the study.

Somatization comorbidity phenotype

The somatization comorbidity phenotype (SCP) was defined post hoc to the trial, but a priori to conducting these analyses. Based on clinical interest and suggestions from observational data that fibromyalgia, depression, anxiety, psychological distress and similar conditions might influence RA assessment [17, 23–26], we hypothesized that patients with this phenotype might have a suboptimal treatment response in an RA clinical trial. The phenotype was operationally defined by use of concomitant medications indicated for the treatment of depression, anxiety, or neuropathic pain (i.e. selective serotonin reuptake inhibitors (SSRIs), duloxetine, venlafaxine, milnacipran, pregabalin, gabapentin, amitriptyline, tizanidine, cyclobenzaprine, methocarbamol, or metaxalone), or ongoing baseline medical diagnosis of depression, chronic pain, fibromyalgia, or myalgias (classified using the *Medical Dictionary for Regulatory Activities* (MedDRA) version 15.1 with the terms: cervical tension myalgia, generalized muscle pain; muscle pain; muscle pain hip area; myalgia; and myalgias). Information classifying patients by SCP status was taken from the medical history and concomitant medication data taken at the beginning of the study. Data on the duration of medical diagnoses were not collected, therefore there was no requirement for the use of these concomitant medications or diagnoses to be of a chronic nature. A diagnosis of insomnia and use of narcotics was not included in the SCP definition, given that RA-related symptoms might commonly affect sleep, and RA-specific pain may be treated with narcotics.

Statistical analysis

All data were analyzed post hoc and the full analysis set was used, which included all patients who had a valid baseline efficacy measurement and at least one valid post-baseline efficacy measurement. The RAPID3 and CDAI arms were stratified by SCP status. RAPID3/CDAI response at week 12 and the DAS28 (based on erythrocyte sedimentation rate (ESR)) LDA (defined as ≤ 3.2) at week 52, including 95% confidence intervals (CIs) of the difference in response rates between groups, were analyzed using non-parametric analysis of covariance (ANCOVA) [27–29], with assessment tool (RAPID3 or CDAI) or SCP status (plus SCP or minus SCP) as a factor and baseline DAS28(ESR) score, gender, age, prior anti-TNF use, and duration of RA (<2 or ≥ 2 years) as covariates. Imputation for missing data was based on non-responder imputation for dichotomous variables, and last observation carried forward (LOCF) for continuous variables.

The safety set consisted of all enrolled patients who received at least one dose of study medication, with treatment-emergent adverse events (AEs) defined as taking place at any time between the first dose and 70 days after the last dose of study drug. All AEs were classified by primary system organ class (SOC), using MedDRA version 15.1. Incidence rates (IRs) were calculated per 100 patient-years (PY), with 95% CIs. Time at risk was measured from initiation of CZP up to the occurrence of the first serious infectious event (SIE), or the total time at risk for patients without SIEs (up to 70 days after the last study dose or patient withdrawal). All statistical analyses were performed in SAS® software (SAS Institute, Cary, NC, USA), version 9.1.3 or later.

Results

Patient characteristics

The full analysis set included 733 patients, with 368 patients randomized to RAPID3 and 365 patients randomized to the CDAI arm of the study. A total of 313 patients (43% overall; RAPID3, n = 151; CDAI, n = 162) met the SCP classification criteria at study baseline. Of these, 92 patients (29.4%; RAPID3, n = 47; CDAI, n = 45) met the SCP classification due to concomitant medications only (predominantly use of central acting agents (i.e. baclofen, tizanidine, cyclobenzaprine) or SSRIs); 71 patients (22.7%; RAPID3, n = 33; CDAI, n = 38) met the phenotype due to medical diagnoses only (predominantly depression). The remaining 150 patients (47.9%; RAPID3, n = 71; CDAI, n = 79) had both concomitant medications and a medical diagnosis (e.g. SSRIs, plus a diagnosis of depression) (Fig. 1, Additional file 1: Table S1).

Baseline characteristics including CDAI, RAPID3, Patient's Global Assessment of Disease Activity (PtGADA), Multi-Dimensional Health Assessment Questionnaire (MDHAQ) Pain, and physical function scores were relatively comparable between patients with and without the phenotype (+SCP and −SCP) (Table 1). A similar proportion of +SCP patients (7.9%, 12/151 RAPID3 and 7.4%, 12/162 CDAI assessed) and −SCP patients (10.6%, 23/217 RAPID3 and 7.4%, 15/203 CDAI assessed) were withdrawn from the study by week 12 due to lack of efficacy. However, a larger proportion of +SCP patients (16.5%, 34/206) than −SCP patients (7.6%, 22/290) were withdrawn after week 12 due to lack of efficacy, a 9% difference between groups (Additional file 1: Table S2).

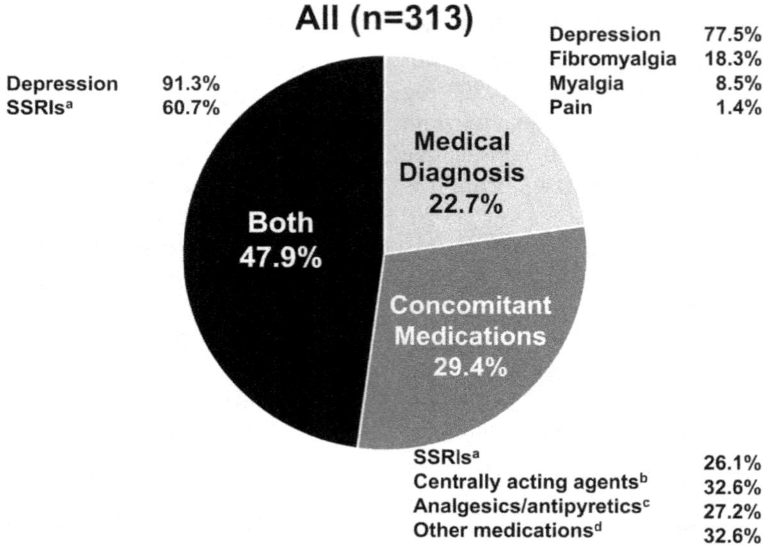

Fig. 1 Proportions of patients meeting criteria for the somatization comorbidity phenotype classification. Full analysis set. The denominator used to calculate the percentage for each category was based upon the total number of patients within the comorbidity/treatment assignment category; the sum of percentages was over 100% due to some patients taking more than one concomitant medication and/or possessing more than one medical diagnosis. [a]Defined as Anatomical Therapeutic Chemical Classification System (ATC) code N06AB. [b]Defined as ATC code M03BX. [c]Defined as ATC code N02BG. [d]Included medications in ATC codes N06AA (non-selective monoamine reuptake inhibitors), N06AX (other antidepressants), M03BA (carbamic acid esters), and M03BB (oxazol, thiazine, and triazine derivatives). SSRI selective serotonin reuptake inhibitors

Disease activity control and response at week 12

The proportion of patients classified as responders at week 12 according to RAPID3 or CDAI definitions was similar, irrespective of SCP status (+SCP 70.6%, 221/313; −SCP 70.5%, 296/420; difference in proportion 0.8% (95% CI − 5.9%, 7.4%)) (Fig. 2a). However, in the CDAI group, the likelihood of being classified as a week-12 responder was incrementally smaller for +SCP patients (73.5%, 119/162) versus −SCP patients (78.8%, 160/203) (Fig. 2a). Combining the RAPID3 and CDAI arms, fewer +SCP patients (23.3%, 73/313) than −SCP patients achieved DAS28(ESR) LDA at week 12 (29.0%, 122/420; difference in proportion − 4.9% (95% CI − 11.0%, 1.2%)) (Fig. 2b).

Disease activity control and response at week 52

At week 52, only half as many +SCP patients (16.0%, 26/162) in the CDAI assessment group achieved LDA, in comparison with the −SCP patients (32.0%, 65/203) (Fig. 2c). Similarly, only about half of the +SCP patients (21.0%, 25/119) in the CDAI assessment group who were week-12 responders achieved LDA at week 52 in comparison to the −SCP patients (40.6%, 65/160) (Fig. 2d). In contrast, this phenotype was less differentiating among patients randomized to the RAPID3 assessment arm (Fig. 2c, d). Overall, a smaller proportion of +SCP patients (19.2%, 60/313) achieved LDA at week 52 than −SCP patients (26.2%, 110/420; difference in proportion − 6.2% (95% CI − 12.2%, − 0.2%)) (Fig. 2c). Amongst the week 12 responders, fewer +SCP patients (25.3%, 56/221) achieved LDA at week 52 in comparison with the −SCP patients (36.8%, 109/296; difference in proportion − 10.6% (95% CI − 18.4%, − 2.8%−)) (Fig. 2d).

The improvement in mean DAS28(ESR) scores was consistently better in −SCP patients throughout the duration of the study. The difference according to SCP status was most apparent for patients randomized to the CDAI assessment group (Additional file 1: Figure S1). At week 52, the median DAS28(ESR) score for week-12 responders was 3.97 for the 221 +SCP patients, versus 3.37 for the 296 −SCP patients, equivalent to a 0.6-unit difference between presence and absence of the SCP. Similar trends were observed for RAPID3 and CDAI, where +SCP patients reported higher DAS28(ESR) scores (RAPID3 9.06 ± 6.19, CDAI 15.34 ± 13.07 (mean ± SD)) than −SCP patients (RAPID3 6.99 ± 6.10, CDAI 11.17 ± 11.41).

Clinical response by achievement of ACR20/50/70

Overall, approximately 5–10% fewer +SCP patients achieved ACR 20% response (ACR20), ACR50, and ACR70 throughout the study. At week 52, 44.8% (188/420), 31.7% (133/420), and 21.0% (88/420) of −SCP patients achieved ACR20, ACR50, and ACR70, respectively, versus 35.1%

Table 1 Patient baseline characteristics by SCP status[a]

	+SCP (n = 313)	−SCP (n = 420)
Mean (SD), *n* unless otherwise stated		
Randomized to assessment arm		
RAPID3, *n* (% overall)	151 (48.2)	217 (51.7)
CDAI, *n* (% overall)	162 (51.8)	203 (48.3)
DAS28(ESR)	6.34 (1.07), 306	6.27 (1.07), 411
CDAI	41.41 (13.25), 307	39.30 (13.01), 416
RAPID3	16.76 (5.31), 308	15.56 (5.73), 415
TJC	16.82 (6.81), 308	15.08 (6.74), 416
SJC	12.12 (5.65), 308	12.26 (5.66), 416
PhGADA (VAS)[b]	6.19 (1.83), 308	6.21 (1.78), 416
PtGADA (VAS)[b]	6.21 (2.23), 308	5.74 (2.35), 416
Pain MDHAQ-PN (0–10 scale)	6.83 (2.07), 308	6.33 (2.16), 415
Physical function MDHAQ-FN (converted to 0–10 scale for RAPID3)	3.73 (1.82), 308	3.49 (1.92), 416

Full analysis set of the PREDICT trial. For these baseline values, some patients (<3% overall) were excluded due to prohibited concomitant medications affecting their assessments. Those with valid assessments at subsequent study visits were not excluded from the overall study

Abbreviations: *SCP* somatization comorbidity phenotype, *ESR* erythrocyte sedimentation rate, *CDAI* Clinical Disease Activity Index, *DAS28* Disease Activity Score in 28 joints, *MDHAQ* Multidimensional Health Assessment Questionnaire, *PhGADA* Physician's Global Assessment of Disease Activity, *PtGADA* Patient's Global Assessment of Disease Activity, *RAPID3* Routine Assessment of Patient Index Data 3, *SJC* swollen joint count, *TJC* tender joint count

[a]Combining the RAPID3 and CDAI arms

[b]Visual analog scale (0–100 mm converted to cm)

(110/313), 25.2% (79/313), and 16.6% (52/313) of +SCP patients (Fig. 3a–c).

This trend was particularly noticeable in the group assessed by CDAI, with 46.8% (95/203), 34.0% (69/203), and 23.6% (48/203) of −SCP patients versus 32.7% (53/162), 22.2% (36/162), and 13.6% (22/162) of +SCP patients achieving ACR20, ACR50, and ACR70, respectively, at week 52. These results indicate an approximate 10–14% lower ACR clinical response in +SCP patients (Fig. 4a–c). Smaller differences in ACR20, ACR50, and ACR70 response rates were observed for those patients randomized to RAPID3 (Fig. 4a–c).

Safety results

The safety set comprised a total of 736 patients. Overall, the cumulative one-year incidence of treatment-emergent adverse events (TEAEs) was higher in +SCP patients (82.5%, 259/314) versus −SCP patients (71.1%, 300/422), with an incidence rate (IR) of 351.3/100 PY for +SCP patients versus 201.9/100 PY for −SCP patients. In particular, the incidence of infections and infestations was higher in +SCP patients compared to −SCP patients (108.6/100 PY versus 56.0/100 PY) (Table 2). Similarly, the IR of serious infectious events (SIEs) was also higher in +SCP patients compared with −SCP patients (5.0/100 PY versus 1.7/100 PY, a difference of 3.3/100 PY). The number of study discontinuations due to AEs was similar among +SCP and −SCP patients.

Discussion

In this large RA population with moderate to severe, active RA, we have described a method to efficiently identify a potentially important patient phenotype in a clinical trial setting that includes depression, anxiety, and chronic pain syndromes such as fibromyalgia and neuropathic pain. Patients enrolled in the PREDICT study were assigned to this phenotype based on concomitant medications and/or medical diagnosis at baseline. In total, 43% of patients met the SCP classification at study baseline, and patients with this phenotype demonstrated a substantially lower likelihood of treatment response.

In particular, the SCP that we have defined appears to be important with respect to both predicting treatment response at week 12 (23.3% of +SCP patients achieved DAS28(ESR) LDA versus 29.0% of −SCP patients) and the likelihood of achieving an LDA state after one year of treatment with CZP (25.3% of +SCP patients versus 36.8% of −SCP patients). Furthermore, +SCP patients were 5–14% less likely to achieve ACR20, ACR50, and ACR70 throughout the duration of the 52-week study. Those with the SCP were also 9% more likely to withdraw over the course of this one-year trial. Although speculative, this higher rate of withdrawal for patients with the SCP could be due to perceived lack of benefit of CZP, lower adherence, a higher rate of some AEs, or other factors.

Overall, when using CDAI as the assessment tool, patients with the SCP appeared less likely to be classified as treatment responders by week 12. Response rates appeared to be more comparable regardless of SCP status when the RAPID3 tool was used. This may reflect the fact that CDAI and the DAS28(ESR) – the primary outcome used in the PREDICT trial – are more highly correlated with each other than the RAPID3 and the DAS28(ESR) [30–32].

Our results may have implications for routine clinical care in deciding which tool to use for RA assessment, given that the RAPID3 reflects a more patient-centric and arguably more holistic assessment than the CDAI, and it is also likely to be easier to implement in busy practices [33]. Irrespective of the SCP phenotype, the primary results of the PREDICT trial showed some differences between the CDAI versus the RAPID3 in the proportion of people classified as responders at 12 weeks [15]. Ultimately, the choice of the preferred tool to assess RA disease activity and treatment response for patients both with and without the SCP phenotype must balance multiple considerations related

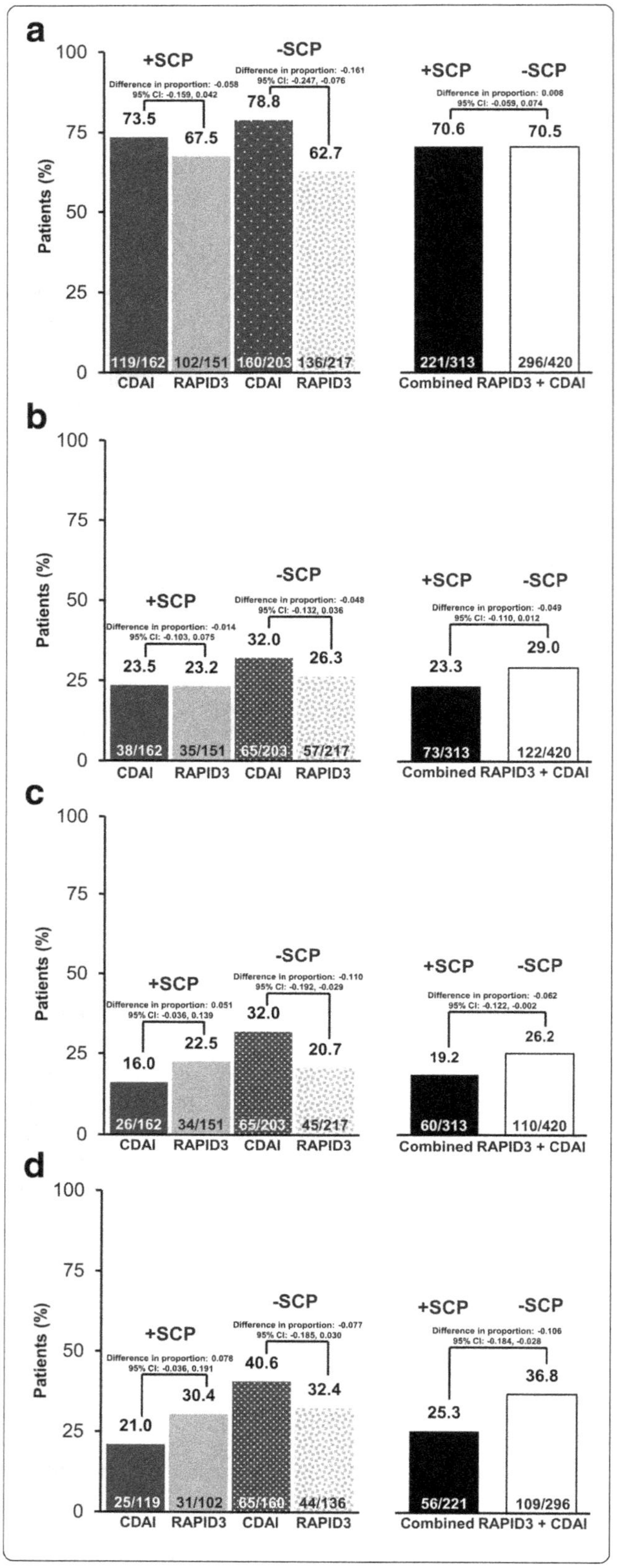

Fig. 2 Clinical response by assessment tool and presence of somatization comorbidity phenotype (SCP). **a** Proportion of Routine Assessment of Patient Index Data 3 (RAPID3) and Clinical Disease Activity Index (CDAI) responders[a] at week 12. **b** Proportion of patients assigned to RAPID3 and CDAI with Disease Activity Score in 28 joints based on erythrocyte sedimentation rate (DAS28(ESR)) low disease activity (LDA) at week 12. **c** Proportion of patients with DAS28(ESR) LDA at week 52. **d** Proportion of RAPID3 and CDAI week 12 responders[a] with DAS28(ESR) LDA at week 52. Full analysis set. LDA was defined as DAS28(ESR) ≤ 3.2. [a]RAPID3 response was defined as ≤ 6 or 20% improvement from baseline, and CDAI response was defined by ≤ 10 or 20% improvement from baseline. Missing data were handled by non-responder imputation

to performance, feasibility, and the relative importance of physician versus patient data.

The results of our study align with data from previous reports, which demonstrate that depression, anxiety, fibromyalgia, and neuropathic pain are prevalent comorbidities in patients with RA and are associated with increased disease activity, poor treatment adherence, and a reduced likelihood of achieving LDA or remission [2, 6, 7, 24, 34, 35]. Ours is among the first to quantify the impact on a large RA clinical trial patient population with active disease starting treatment with a therapeutic agent known to be effective based on the results of previous phase 3 studies. These differences extended not only to the clinical efficacy outcomes, but also to safety endpoints. The incident rate of TEAEs was higher in +SCP patients than in −SCP patients, with a notably higher rate of infectious events in the +SCP group, including SIEs. The magnitude of the difference in the rates of SIEs between +SCP and −SCP patients (3.3/100 PY) in this analysis, all of whom were receiving CZP therapy, was comparable to the difference between CZP and placebo treatment in other RA studies [36]. Depression and other patient factors have been associated with adverse events such as infections [37], cardiovascular disease [38], myocardial infarction [39], and an increased risk of mortality [40], according to past studies. This may reflect a true biologic association, as inflammatory markers such as C-reactive protein have been shown to be associated with depression [41], although these conditions may be a proxy for related factors (e.g. health-seeking behavior, perceived illness severity) that could impact the reporting of more subjective or less severe adverse events. Collectively, these findings suggest that the SCP phenotype may be a useful and easily ascertained proxy in an RA clinical trial population for factors making patients less likely to achieve a good clinical response and less likely to tolerate some RA treatments.

The limitations of these analyses included the fact that the PREDICT study only enrolled patients in the USA, and the patients with fibromyalgia symptomatic enough

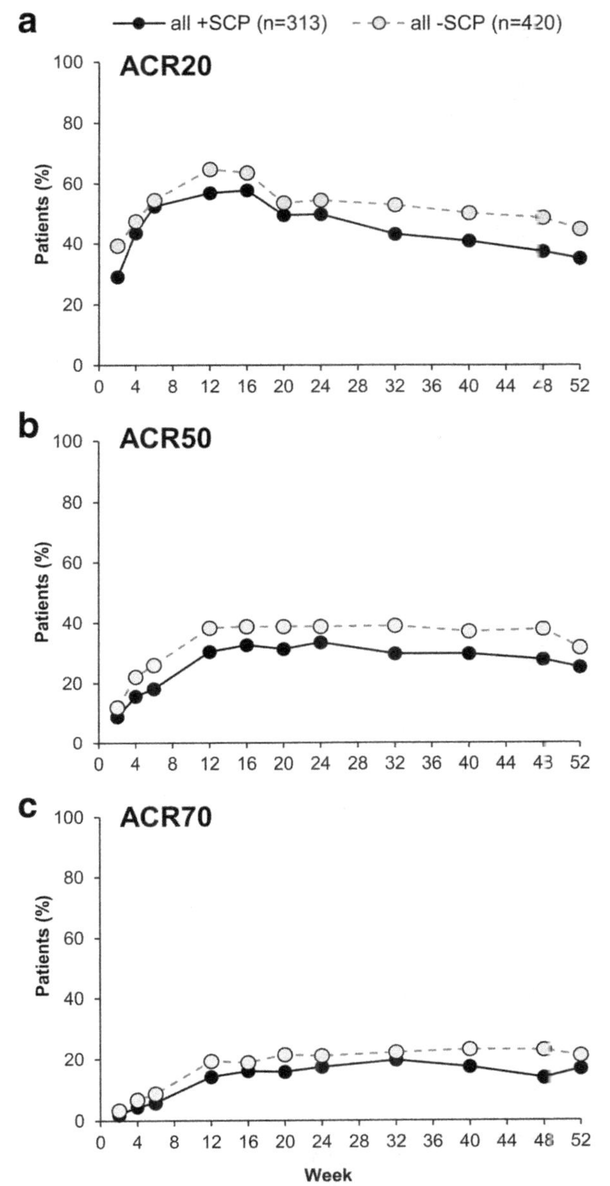

Fig. 3 American College of Rheumatology (ACR) response rates by somatization comorbidity phenotype (SCP) status. **a** ACR20. **b** ACR50. **c** ACR70. Full analysis set. Missing data were handled by non-responder imputation

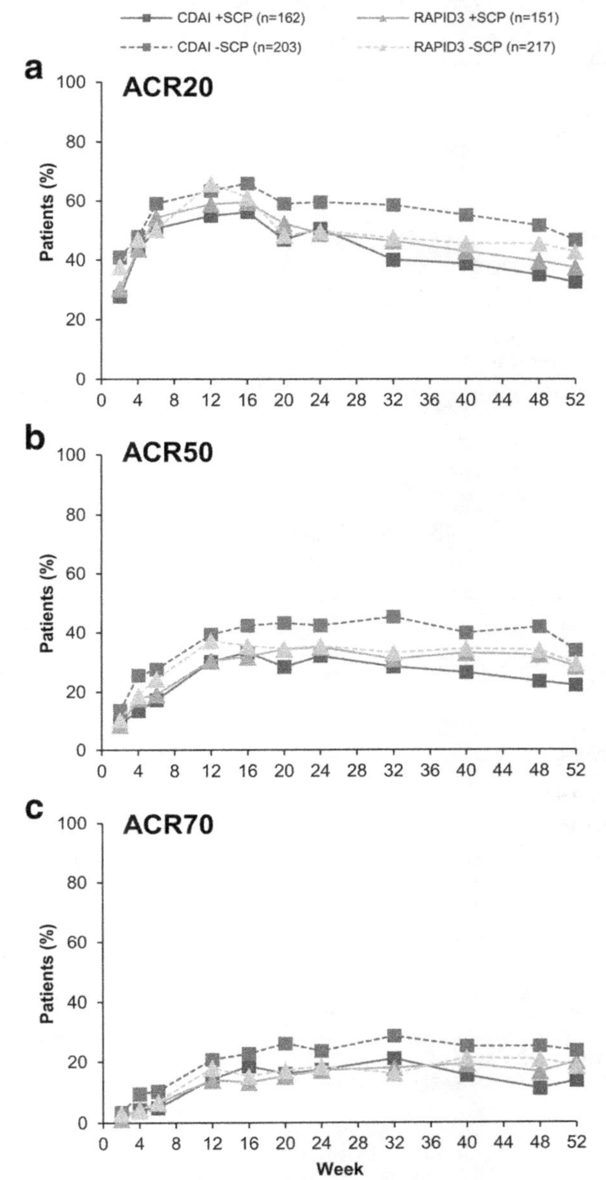

Fig. 4 American College of Rheumatology (ACR) response rates by assessment group and somatization comorbidity phenotype (SCP) status. **a** ACR20. **b** ACR50. **c** ACR70. Full analysis set. Missing data were handled by non-responder imputation

to be treated were excluded by protocol at the discretion of the local investigator, though no systematic identification or exclusion at the time of randomization was enforced. In addition, it is possible that patients with the SCP but who did not have a formal diagnosis and who were not taking any indicated medications, were misclassified. Assuming that the patients with the most severe manifestations of this condition were excluded from the study, and that some patients had not been diagnosed nor were using medication to manage their SCP, our results likely represent a conservative estimate of the effect that the SCP phenotype had on treatment response as measured by standard tools such as the achievement of DAS28(ESR) LDA and ACR response, suggesting that the impact of this phenotype in real-world settings may be even more profound. This exclusion might raise concerns about the generalizability of the study's results to the typical RA patient population seen in the USA. However, even with the exclusion in place, we note that a high proportion of patients using

Table 2 Summary of adverse events by SCP status[a]

Number (percentage), incidence ratio (95% CI)[b], unless otherwise indicated	+SCP (n = 314)	−SCP (n = 422)	All patients (n = 736)
Total time at risk (100 PY)	2.44	3.49	5.92
Any TEAEs	259 (82.5), 351.3 (309.8, 396.8)	300 (71.1), 201.9 (179.7, 226.1)	559 (76.0), 251.4 (231.0, 273.2)
TEAEs (≥5% in any SOC[c])			
Gastrointestinal disorders	65 (20.7), 31.3 (24.2, 39.9)	73 (17.3), 24.0 (18.8, 30.2)	138 (18.8), 26.9 (22.6, 31.8)
General disorders and administration site conditions	48 (15.3), 22.5 (16.6, 29.8)	53 (12.6), 17.1 (12.8, 22.3)	101 (13.7), 19.3 (15.7, 23.4)
Infections and infestations	166 (52.9), 108.6 (92.7, 126.4)	144 (34.1), 56.0 (47.2, 65.9)	310 (42.1), 75.6 (67.4, 84.5)
Injury, poisoning, and procedural complications	41 (13.1), 18.6 (13.4, 25.3)	34 (8.1), 10.2 (7.1, 14.3)	75 (10.2),13.6 (10.7, 17.0)
Investigations	39 (12.4), 17.6 (12.5, 24.1)	50 (11.8), 15.8 (11.7, 20.8)	89 (12.1), 16.5 (13.3, 20.4)
Metabolism and nutrition disorders	21 (6.7), 9.1 (5.6, 13.9)	22 (5.2), 6.6 (4.1, 9.9)	43 (5.8), 7.6 (5.5, 10.2)
Musculoskeletal and connective tissue disorders	100 (31.8), 52.5 (42.7, 63.9)	80 (19.0), 26.0 (20.6, 32.4)	180 (24.5), 36.2 (31.1, 41.8)
Nervous system disorders	59 (18.8), 28.5 (21.7, 36.8)	34 (8.1), 10.3 (7.1, 14.3)	93 (12.6), 17.3 (14.0, 21.2)
Psychiatric disorders	29 (9.2), 12.8 (8.5, 18.3)	10 (2.4), 2.9 (1.4, 5.4)	39 (5.3), 6.9 (4.9, 9.4)
Respiratory, thoracic, and mediastinal disorders	48 (15.3), 22.4 (16.5, 29.7)	48 (11.4), 14.9 (11.0, 19.8)	96 (13.0), 17.9 (14.5, 21.9)
Skin and subcutaneous tissue disorders	44 (14.0), 20.1 (14.6, 27.0)	50 (11.8), 15.5 (11.5, 20.5)	94 (12.8), 17.4 (14.0, 21.3)
Vascular disorders	26 (8.3), 11.4 (7.5, 16.8)	17 (4.0), 5.0 (2.9, 8.0)	43 (5.8), 7.6 (5.5, 10.2)
Serious TEAEs	34 (10.8), 14.8 (10.3, 20.7)	37 (8.8), 10.9 (7.7, 15.0)	71 (9.6), 12.5 (9.8, 15.8)
Serious infections and infestations	12 (3.8), 5.0 (2.6, 8.7)	6 (1.4), 1.7 (0.6, 3.8)	18 (2.4), 3.1 (1.8, 4.8)
Discontinuation due to TEAEs[d]	34 (10.8), NA	44 (10.4), NA	78 (10.6), NA
Drug-related TEAEs	80 (25.5), NA	93 (22.0), NA	173 (23.5), NA
Severe TEAEs	38 (12.1), NA	38 (9.0), NA	76 (10.3), NA
Deaths (TEAEs leading to death)	1 (0.3), NA	1 (0.2), NA	2 (0.3), NA

Safety set. *Medical Dictionary for Regulatory Activities* (MedDRA) v15.1

SCP somatization comorbidity phenotype, *TEAEs* treatment-emergent adverse events, *PY* patient-years, *NA* data not available

[a]Combining the RAPID3 and CDAI arms.

[b]n: number of subjects reporting at least one TEAE in that category, incidence rates reported per 100 patient-years

[c]System organ class

[d]There was one patient in this group reporting a TEAE of pneumonia, who did not discontinue the study drug permanently

medications indicated for depression, anxiety, neuropathic pain, and fibromyalgia were in fact enrolled in the study and had the SCP (43% of the PREDICT trial population). Moreover, in many other RA trials, study criteria commonly exclude patients with conditions deemed by the site investigator "to be symptomatic enough to interfere with the measurement of treatment response" [19, 42]. However, this exclusion criterion is highly subjective and is rarely enforced in a reproducible fashion. For this reason, RA trials can be expected to include a mix of these patients, but previously these individuals have not been easily identified without the added burden of incorporating additional, specific screening tools to classify patients as having fibromyalgia [43] or depression [44]. While these types of screening instruments could be systematically applied to an RA cohort or trial [45], the phenotype we defined has the advantage that it can be applied to data routinely captured at baseline in RA clinical trials, requiring only concomitant medications and/or diagnoses instead of a specific screening instrument, thereby minimizing participant burden for additional data collection.

These analyses have highlighted that the inclusion of large numbers of patients with the phenotype in an RA trial may appreciably affect the proportion of patients who are able to achieve an absolute disease state treatment target, such as LDA or remission. On the other hand, if new trials excluded individuals with the somatization comorbidity phenotype from a trial, this could somewhat limit the generalizability of the results and hinder comparability between trials, as the proportion of such patients in RA trials across the globe is likely to vary widely. In addition, allowing patients with the somatization comorbidity phenotype in RA studies may contribute to a ceiling effect, as patients may not demonstrate as much improvement with effective RA therapies in comparison to patients without this phenotype.

Conclusions

In the PREDICT clinical trial, 43% of patients met the "somatization comorbidity phenotype" classification criteria for diagnosis and/or use of medications indicated for depression, fibromyalgia, anxiety, or neuropathic pain. These patients were significantly more likely to withdraw from the trial and/or experience adverse events, and approximately 10–14% less likely to achieve a clinical response. These results suggest that depending on the outcome measure used (e.g. DAS28), enrolling large numbers of patients with this phenotype may affect the proportion able to achieve LDA or remission, making it advisable to consider whether to include, identify, or stratify these patients during the study design or study screening processes in future RA clinical trials.

Abbreviations

ACR: American College of Rheumatology; AE: Adverse event; ANCOVA: Analysis of covariance; CDAI: Clinical Disease Activity Index; CI: Confidence interval; CZP: Certolizumab pegol; DAS: Disease activity score; DMARD: Disease-modifying anti-rheumatic drug; ESR: Erythrocyte sedimentation rate; IR: Incidence rate; IXRS: Interactive voice/web-based response system; LDA: Low disease activity; LOCF: Last observation carried forward; MCID: Minimal clinically important difference; MDHAQ: Multi-Dimensional Health Assessment Questionnaire; MedDRA: Medical Dictionary for Regulatory Activities; NMSC: Non-melanoma skin cancer; PhGADA: Physician's Global Assessment of Disease Activity; PtGADA: Patient's Global Assessment of Disease Activity; PY: Patient years; Q2W: Every 2 weeks; RA: Rheumatoid arthritis; RAPID3: Routine Assessment of Patient Index Data 3; SCP: Somatization comorbidity phenotype; SD: Standard deviation; SIE: Serious infectious event; SJC: Swollen joint count; SOC: System organ class; SSRIs: Selective serotonin reuptake inhibitors; TEAE: Treatment-emergent adverse event; TNF: Tumor necrosis factor

Acknowledgements

We thank the patients and their caregivers in addition to the investigators and their teams who contributed to this study. The authors acknowledge Lisa Wulund, PhD, of Costello Medical Consulting Ltd (Cambridge, UK), for medical writing and editorial assistance in preparing this manuscript for publication based on the authors' input and direction. All costs associated with the development of this manuscript were funded by UCB Pharma.

Funding

UCB Pharma sponsored the study and the development of this publication. In addition to critically revising the manuscript/publication for important intellectual content, the authors approved the final version to be published. UCB Pharma performed a full review to ensure that the data presented in the publication are scientifically, technically and medically supportable, and in compliance with the intellectual property rights of UCB Pharma. Furthermore, UCB Pharma ensured that the publication complies with applicable laws, regulations, guidelines, and good industry practice.

Authors' contributions

JRC, CH, MNN, COB, and YY made substantial contributions to study conception/design, and/or acquisition/analysis/interpretation of data. JRC, CH, MNN, COB, and YY were involved in drafting of the publication, and revising it critically for important intellectual content. JRC, CH, MNN, COB, and YY gave final approval of the publication. All authors read and approved the final manuscript.

Competing interests

JRC: research grants and consulting fees from UCB Pharma, Janssen, CORRONA, Amgen, Pfizer, Bristol-Myers Squibb, Crescendo Bioscience. CH: Medical Director at Mylan, former employee of UCB Pharma. MNN: employee of UCB Pharma. COB: employee of UCB Pharma. YY: research grants from Bristol-Myers Squibb, Genentech, Celgene; consulting fees from Bristol-Myers Squibb, Celgene, Samumed.

Author details

[1]Division of Clinical Immunology and Rheumatology, University of Alabama at Birmingham, FOT 802, 510 20th Street South, Birmingham, AL 35294, USA. [2]Mylan, 1000 Mylan Blvd, Canonsburg, PA 15317, USA. [3]UCB Pharma, Allée de la Recherche 60, 1070 Brussels, Belgium. [4]NYU Hospital for Joint Diseases, New York University School of Medicine, 301 East 17th Street, New York, NY 10003, USA.

References

1. Roubille C, Richer V, Starnino T, McCourt C, McFarlane A, Fleming P, Siu S, Kraft J, Lynde C, Pope J, et al. Evidence-based recommendations for the management of comorbidities in rheumatoid arthritis, psoriasis, and psoriatic arthritis: expert opinion of the Canadian Dermatology-Rheumatology Comorbidity Initiative. J Rheumatol. 2015;42(10):1767–80.
2. Radner H, Yoshida K, Frits M, Iannaccone C, Shadick NA, Weinblatt M, Smolen JS, Solomon DH. The impact of multimorbidity status on treatment response in rheumatoid arthritis patients initiating disease-modifying anti-rheumatic drugs. Rheumatology (Oxford, England). 2015;54(11):2076–84.
3. Theis KA, Brady TJ, Helmick CG. No one dies of old age anymore: a coordinated approach to comorbidities and the rheumatic diseases. Arthritis Care Res. 2017;69(1):1–4.
4. Simoes D, Araujo FA, Severo M, Monjardino T, Cruz I, Carmona L, Lucas R. Patterns and consequences of multimorbidity in the general population: there is no chronic disease management without rheumatic disease management. Arthritis Care Res. 2017;69(1):12–20.
5. Murphy LB, Sacks JJ, Brady TJ, Hootman JM, Chapman DP. Anxiety and depression among US adults with arthritis: prevalence and correlates. Arthritis Care Res. 2012;64(7):968–76.
6. Lage-Hansen PR, Chrysidis S, Lage-Hansen M, Hougaard A, Ejstrup L, Amris K. Concomitant fibromyalgia in rheumatoid arthritis is associated with the more frequent use of biological therapy: a cross-sectional study. Scand J Rheumat. 2015;45(1):45–8.
7. Matcham F, Norton S, Scott DL, Steer S, Hotopf M. Symptoms of depression and anxiety predict treatment response and long-term physical health outcomes in rheumatoid arthritis: secondary analysis of a randomized controlled trial. Rheumatology (Oxford, England). 2016;55(2):268–78.
8. Overman CL, Kool MB, Da Silva JA, Geenen R. The prevalence of severe fatigue in rheumatic diseases: an international study. Clin Rheumatol. 2016;35(2):409–15.
9. Anderson J, Caplan L, Yazdany J, Robbins ML, Neogi T, Michaud K, Saag KG, O'Dell JR, Kazi S. Rheumatoid arthritis disease activity measures: American College of Rheumatology recommendations for use in clinical practice. Arthritis Care Res. 2012;64(5):640–7.
10. Castrejon I, Pincus T. Patient self-report outcomes to guide a treat-to-target strategy in clinical trials and usual clinical care of rheumatoid arthritis. Clin Exp Rheumatol. 2012;30(4 Suppl 73):S50–55.
11. Pincus T, Swearingen CJ, Bergman M, Yazici Y. RAPID3 (Routine Assessment of Patient Index Data 3), a rheumatoid arthritis index without formal joint counts for routine care: proposed severity categories compared to disease activity score and clinical disease activity index categories. J Rheumatol. 2008;35(11):2136–47.
12. Sokka T, Hetland ML, Makinen H, Kautiainen H, Horslev-Petersen K, Luukkainen RK, Combe B, Badsha H, Drosos AA, Devlin J, et al. Remission and rheumatoid arthritis: data on patients receiving usual care in twenty-four countries. Arthritis Rheum. 2008;58(9):2642–51.
13. Saag KG, Teng GG, Patkar NM, Anuntiyo J, Finney C, Curtis JR, Paulus HE, Mudano A, Pisu M, Elkins-Melton M, et al. American College of Rheumatology 2008 recommendations for the use of nonbiologic and biologic disease-modifying antirheumatic drugs in rheumatoid arthritis. Arthritis Rheum. 2008;59(6):762–84.
14. Smolen JS, Boers M, Abadie EC, Breedveld FC, Emery P, Bardin T, Goel N, Ethgen DJ, Avouac BP, Dere WH, et al. Recommendations for an update of

2003 European regulatory requirements for registration of drugs to be used in the treatment of RA. Curr Med Res Opin. 2011;27(2):315–25.
15. Curtis JR, Churchill M, Kivitz A, Samad A, Gauer L, Gervitz L, Koetse W, Melin J, Yazici Y. A randomized trial comparing disease activity measures to assess and predict response in rheumatoid arthritis patients initiating certolizumab pegol. Arthritis Rheumatol (Hoboken, NJ). 2015;67(12):3104–12.
16. Arnett FC, Edworthy SM, Bloch DA, McShane DJ, Fries JF, Cooper NS, Healey LA, Kaplan SR, Liang MH, Luthra HS, et al. The American Rheumatism Association 1987 revised criteria for the classification of rheumatoid arthritis. Arthritis Rheum. 1988;31(3):315–24.
17. Wolfe F, Michaud K, Busch RE, Katz RS, Rasker JJ, Shahouri SH, Shaver TS, Wang S, Walitt BT, Hauser W. Polysymptomatic distress in patients with rheumatoid arthritis: understanding disproportionate response and its spectrum. Arthritis Care Res. 2014;66(10):1465–71.
18. Pincus T, Castrejón I, Block J, Cook N. Patients with fibromyalgia in general have higher self-report questionnaire scores than patients with rheumatoid arthritis: implications for clinical trials and clinical research. Arthritis Rheumatol. 2016;68(Suppl10):54.
19. Pincus T, Yazici Y, van Vollenhoven R. Why are only 50% of courses of anti-tumor necrosis factor agents continued for only 2 years in some settings? Need for long term observations in standard care to complement clinical trials. J Rheumatol. 2006;33(12):2372–5.
20. Curtis JR, Yang S, Chen L, Pope JE, Keystone EC, Haraoui B, Boire G, Thorne JC, Tin D, Hitchon CA, et al. Determining the minimally important difference in the clinical disease activity index for improvement and worsening in early rheumatoid arthritis patients. Arthritis Care Res. 2015;67(10):1345–53.
21. Pincus T, Hines P, Bergman MJ, Yazici Y, Rosenblatt LC, MacLean R. Proposed severity and response criteria for Routine Assessment of Patient Index Data (RAPID3): results for categories of disease activity and response criteria in abatacept clinical trials. J Rheumatol. 2011;38(12):2565–71.
22. Pincus T, Yazici Y, Bergman MJ. RAPID3, an index to assess and monitor patients with rheumatoid arthritis, without formal joint counts: similar results to DAS28 and CDAI in clinical trials and clinical care. Rheum Dis Clin N Am. 2009;35(4):773–8. viii.
23. Duran J, Combe B, Niu J, Rincheval N, Gaujoux-Viala C, Felson DT. The effect on treatment response of fibromyalgic symptoms in early rheumatoid arthritis patients: results from the ESPOIR cohort. Rheumatology (Oxford, England). 2015;54(12):2166–70.
24. Inanc N, Yilmaz-Oner S, Can M, Sokka T, Direskeneli H. The role of depression, anxiety, fatigue, and fibromyalgia on the evaluation of the remission status in patients with rheumatoid arthritis. J Rheumatol. 2014; 41(9):1755–60.
25. Andersson ML, Svensson B, Bergman S. Chronic widespread pain in patients with rheumatoid arthritis and the relation between pain and disease activity measures over the first 5 years. J Rheumatol. 2013; 40(12):1977–85.
26. Ton E, Bakker MF, Verstappen SM, Ter Borg EJ, van Albada-Kuipers IA, Schenk Y, van der Veen MJ, Bijlsma JW, Jacobs JW. Utrecht Rheumatoid Arthritis Cohort Study Group. Look beyond the disease activity score of 28 joints (DAS28): tender points influence the DAS28 in patients with rheumatoid arthritis. J Rheumatol. 2012;39(1):22–7.
27. Koch GG, Tangen CM, Jung JW, Amara IA. Issues for covariance analysis of dichotomous and ordered categorical data from randomized clinical trials and non-parametric strategies for addressing them. Stat Med. 1998;17(15-16):1863–92.
28. LaVange LM, Durham TA, Koch GG. Randomization-based nonparametric methods for the analysis of multicentre trials. Stat Methods Med Res. 2005;14(3):281–301.
29. Zink RC, Koch GG. SAS® Macro NParCov Version 2, Non-parametric analysis of covariance user's guide. 2002.
30. Aletaha D, Nell VP, Stamm T, Uffmann M, Pflugbeil S, Machold K, Smolen JS. Acute phase reactants add little to composite disease activity indices for rheumatoid arthritis: validation of a clinical activity score. Arthritis Res Ther. 2005;7(4):R796–806.
31. Pincus T, Furer V, Keystone E, Yazici Y, Bergman MJ, Luijtens K. RAPID3 (Routine Assessment of Patient Index Data 3) severity categories and response criteria: Similar results to DAS28 (Disease Activity Score) and CDAI (Clinical Disease Activity Index) in the RAPID 1 (Rheumatoid Arthritis Prevention of Structural Damage) clinical trial of certolizumab pegol. Arthritis Care Res. 2011;63(8):1142–9.
32. Pincus T. Can RAPID3, an index without formal joint counts or laboratory tests, serve to guide rheumatologists in tight control of rheumatoid arthritis in usual clinical care? Bull NYU Hosp Jt Dis. 2009;67(3):254–66.
33. Berthelot J-M. RAPID3? Aptly named! Clin Exp Rheumatol. 2014;32 (Suppl 85):S80–84.
34. Wolfe F, Michaud K. Severe rheumatoid arthritis (RA), worse outcomes, comorbid illness, and sociodemographic disadvantage characterize RA patients with fibromyalgia. J Rheumatol. 2004;31(4):695–700.
35. Toms J, Soukup T, Bradna P, Hrncir Z. Disease activity composite indices in patients with rheumatoid arthritis and concomitant fibromyalgia. J Rheumatol. 2010;37(2):468. Author reply 469.
36. Bykerk VP, Cush J, Winthrop K, Calabrese L, Lortholary O, de Longueville M, van Vollenhoven R, Mariette X. Update on the safety profile of certolizumab pegol in rheumatoid arthritis: an integrated analysis from clinical trials. Ann Rheum Dis. 2015;74(1):96–103.
37. Kunutsor SK, Whitehouse MR, Blom AW, Beswick AD, Team I. Patient-related risk factors for periprosthetic joint infection after total joint arthroplasty: a systematic review and meta-analysis. PLoS One. 2016;11(3):e0150866.
38. Treharne GJ, Hale ED, Lyons AC, Booth DA, Banks MJ, Erb N, Douglas KM, Mitton DL, Kitas GD. Cardiovascular disease and psychological morbidity among rheumatoid arthritis patients. Rheumatology (Oxford, England). 2005;44(2):241–6.
39. Scherrer JF, Virgo KS, Zeringue A, Bucholz KK, Jacob T, Johnson RG, True WR, Carney RM, Freedland KE, Xian H, et al. Depression increases risk of incident myocardial infarction among Veterans Administration patients with rheumatoid arthritis. Gen Hosp Psychiatry. 2009;31(4):353–9.
40. Ang DC, Choi H, Kroenke K, Wolfe F. Comorbid depression is an independent risk factor for mortality in patients with rheumatoid arthritis. J Rheumatol. 2005;32(6):1013–9.
41. Kojima M, Kojima T, Suzuki S, Oguchi T, Oba M, Tsuchiya H, Sugiura F, Kanayama Y, Furukawa TA, Tokudome S, et al. Depression, inflammation, and pain in patients with rheumatoid arthritis. Arthritis Rheum. 2009;61(8): 1018–24.
42. Pincus T, Sokka T. Should contemporary rheumatoid arthritis clinical trials be more like standard patient care and vice versa? Ann Rheum Dis. 2004; 63(Suppl2):ii32–9.
43. Wolfe F, Clauw DJ, Fitzcharles MA, Goldenberg DL, Katz RS, Mease P, Russell AS, Russell IJ, Winfield JB, Yunus MB. The American College of Rheumatology preliminary diagnostic criteria for fibromyalgia and measurement of symptom severity. Arthritis Care Res. 2010;62(5):600–10.
44. Kroenke K, Spitzer RL, Williams JB. The PHQ-9: validity of a brief depression severity measure. J Gen Intern Med. 2001;16(9):606–13.
45. Perrot S, Peixoto M, Dieude P, Hachulla E, Avouac J, Ottaviani S, Allanore Y. Patient phenotypes in fibromyalgia comorbid with systemic sclerosis or rheumatoid arthritis: influence of diagnostic and screening tests. Screening with the FiRST questionnaire, diagnosis with the ACR 1990 and revised ACR 2010 criteria. Clin Exp Rheumatol. 2017;35 Suppl 105(3):35-42.

6

Changes in clinical disease activity are weakly linked to changes in MRI inflammation on treat-to-target escalation of therapy in rheumatoid arthritis

Fiona M. McQueen[1,5*], Peter Chapman[6], Terina Pollock[2], Dena D'Souza[1], Arier C. Lee[3], Nicola Dalbeth[4,5], Lisa Stamp[7], Karen Lindsay[5] and Anthony Doyle[2]

Abstract

Background: Rheumatoid arthritis (RA) treat-to-target (T2T) regimens often use the disease activity score (28 joints) incorporating C-reactive protein ($DAS28_{CRP}$) as an outcome measure. We compared changes in the $DAS28_{CRP}$ with changes in magnetic resonance imaging (MRI) inflammation on treatment escalation.

Methods: Eighty seropositive RA patients with active disease were enrolled. Group A ($N = 57$) escalated to another conventional disease-modifying therapy (cDMARD) combination, and Group B ($N = 23$) to anti-TNF therapy/cDMARDs. Contrast-enhanced 3T-MRI wrist scans were obtained before and 4 months after regimen change. Scan pairs were scored for inflammation (MRI(i)) and damage. Disease activity was assessed using the $DAS28_{CRP}$.

Results: Eighty patients were enrolled and 66 MRI scan pairs were available for analysis. Intra-reader reliability was high: intraclass correlation coefficient (average) 0.89 (0.56–0.97). $\Delta DAS28_{CRP}$ did not differ between groups: Group A, −0.94 (−3.30, 1.61); Group B, −1.53 (−3.59, 0.56) ($p = 0.45$). ΔMRI(i) also did not differ: Group A, 0 (−25, 10); Group B, −1 (−15, 28) ($p = 0.12$). Combining groups, ΔMRI(i) correlated weakly with $\Delta DAS28_{CRP}$ (Spearman's 0.36, $p = 0.003$). Using multiple linear regression analysis adjusting for confounders, $\Delta DAS28_{CRP}$ was associated with ΔMRI(i) ($p = 0.056$). Of the individual MRI measures, only Δtenosynovitis correlated with $\Delta DAS28_{CRP}$ (Spearman's 0.33, $p = 0.007$). ΔMRI(i) was negatively associated with the MRI erosion score at entry ($p = 0.0052$).

Conclusions: We report the first study investigating the link between changes in clinical and imaging inflammation in a real-world RA cohort escalating to conventional and biologic DMARDs. The association was significant but relatively weak, suggesting that MRI targets cannot yet be advocated as outcomes for T2T escalation.

Background

Rheumatologists routinely manage rheumatoid arthritis (RA) using a treat-to-target (T2T) regimens [1], escalating therapy in patients who fail to reach remission or a low disease activity state [2]. Management is often initiated with methotrexate alone and then escalation proceeds to combination therapy with conventional disease-modifying anti-rheumatic agents (cDMARDs) and biologic DMARDs (bDMARDs). In New Zealand, cDMARD combinations include triple therapy (methotrexate, sulphasalazine, hydroxychloroquine) and methotrexate/leflunomide, although other options are available. The New Zealand Pharmaceutical Management Agency (PHARMAC), responsible for buying and funding pharmaceuticals, has defined criteria for funding bDMARDs including a trial of three different cDMARD combinations [3]. For those with an inadequate response to cDMARDs, escalation to methotrexate/anti-tumour necrosis factor (anti-TNF) agents follows and

* Correspondence: f.mcqueen@auckland.ac.nz
[1]Department of Molecular Medicine and Pathology, Faculty of Medical and Health Sciences, The University of Auckland, Private Bag 92019, Auckland, New Zealand
[5]Department of Rheumatology, Greenlane Clinical Centre, Auckland District Health Board, 214 Green Lane West, Epsom, Auckland 1051, New Zealand
Full list of author information is available at the end of the article

subsequently other bDMARDs. Adequacy of response is usually measured by the $DAS28_{CRP}$ [4, 5].

MRI is a sensitive imaging modality that can reveal articular inflammation and joint damage [6, 7]. The OMERACT RA MRI score (RAMRIS) [8] and the Harvaardsholm tenosynovitis score [9] can quantify inflammation in a relatively reproducible manner. Studies show that MRI can detect more inflammation than physical examination. Up to 96% of asymptomatic RA patients with normal joints have MRI synovitis and 46% have MRI bone oedema/osteitis [10]. Krabben et al. [11] found MRI inflammation in 66% of non-swollen wrist joints in patients with early RA. Severe grades of bone oedema (osteitis) were common in non-swollen joints. We and others have found that osteitis is a predictor of joint erosion [12, 13]. Although MRI is more sensitive than clinical assessment for detection of joint inflammation and damage, MRI outcomes are not yet part of accepted clinical practice because of feasibility issues including cost and accessibility. It is also not clear whether using the change in MRI inflammation scores to dictate escalation of therapy would lead to better outcomes than using easily administered clinical scores such as the $DAS28_{CRP}$. While clinical trials of bDMARDs including golimumab [14] and tocilizumab [15] indicated that clinical responses were associated with improvements in MRI inflammation scores, there is little information comparing clinical and MRI responses to cDMARDs in the T2T "real-world" setting.

The aim of this study was to compare the response in clinical disease activity ($DAS28_{CRP}$) with response in MRI inflammation scores after T2T-dictated escalation of therapy in two groups of RA patients: those escalating from cDMARDs to a different cDMARD combination and those escalating to a combination that includes anti-TNF therapy.

Methods

Power calculation

Studies exploring the relation between ΔMRI synovitis scores and $\Delta DAS28_{CRP}$ [7, 16, 17] indicated a simple correlation of 0.4. Using a two-sided test at the 5% significance level with 80% power, the required total sample size would be 46 patients. Allowing for 10% dropout, the estimated sample size required was 50. For comparing MRI(i) responses between patients escalating to cDMARDs versus cDMARD/anti-TNFs, sample size was calculated based on the one-sided hypothesis that triple therapy would not be inferior to MTX/anti-TNF. We estimated that with 50 patients per group the study would have 80% power at 5% significance to establish non-inferiority, assuming a between-group difference in change from baseline to 3 months of 2 (SD = 2). Although enrolment was continued for 3 years, only 80 patients with seropositive RA were recruited from rheumatology outpatients' clinics from Auckland and Christchurch, New Zealand between 2014 and 2016. Two cohorts were recruited: Group A included patients on cDMARD therapy (either methotrexate alone or a cDMARD combination), escalating to a different cDMARD combination; and Group B included patients on a cDMARD combination who were escalating to bDMARDs including an anti-TNF agent. Patients were required to have a $DAS28_{CRP} \geq 3.2$ at the first clinical visit. Tender joint counts (28 and 68 joints) and swollen joint counts (28 and 66 joints) were performed by trained research nurses and patients filled out questionnaires to assess function. Serum was obtained for inflammatory markers and rheumatoid serology. Written informed consent was obtained from all patients. The study was approved by the Health and Disability Ethics Committees, New Zealand.

MRI scans and scoring

The dominant wrist was scanned using a 3 T scanner (Philips MR Systems Achieve 3 T; Koninklijke Philips Electronics NV, Eindhoven, the Netherlands). An eight-element Philips SENSE 3.0 T Wrist Coil 8 Channel (Invivo Corp, Gainsville, FL, USA) (receive only) was used. The dominant hand in the wrist coil fitted snugly by the patient' s side, palm to body, thumb anteriorly. The field of view included the carpus, distal radioulnar joint (dRUJ) and metacarpal (MC) bases. The following were used: turbo spin echo sequences, T1 weighted (T1w) and T2 weighted (T2w) with fat saturation (FS) using spectral adiabatic inversion recovery (SPAIR) in axial and coronal planes and proton density (PD) coronals (without FS). T1wFS axial and coronal sequences were obtained post intravenous gadolinium diethylenetriamine pentaacetic acid (GdDTPA) at standard dosage (Omniscan (Gadodiamide; 5.0 mmol/10 ml or 2.87 g/10 ml); GE Healthcare, Inc., Princeton, NJ, USA). Synovitis, osteitis and erosions were scored according to RAMRIS [8] and tenosynovitis in the flexor and extensor compartments [9]. MRI scan pairs (baseline, 4 months) were scored in known chronological order by one experienced reader (AD), blinded to clinical and X-ray data. Ten scans were selected randomly and rescored 6 months later. The intra-reader reliability was high: ICC (av) = 0.89 (99% CI 0.56–0.97).

X-rays

Plain radiographs of the hands and feet were obtained for all patients on enrolment. They were scored for damage using the Sharp van der Heijde (SvdH) score [18] by a rheumatologist (ND), blinded to clinical and MRI data.

Statistical analysis

Intra-reader reliability for MRI scores was determined using intraclass correlation coefficients (ICCs). Spearman's correlations were used to examine the association between $\Delta DAS28_{CRP}$ and ΔMRI scores. Clinical characteristics for

Groups A and B were compared using the chi-square test and median two-sample test. The effect of $\Delta DAS28_{CRP}$ and treatment group on ΔMRI(i) were analysed using multiple linear regression adjusting for age, gender, duration, anti-CCP titre and MRI erosion score at baseline. Four patients transited from Group A into Group B, providing eight scan pairs. Apart from analyses investigating baseline patient characteristics where the four patients were included only in their initial Group A, all analyses were performed including these patients in both groups and were conducted using SAS for Windows version 9.4 (SAS Institute Inc., Cary, NC, USA).

Results

A total of eighty patients were enrolled, fifty-seven in Group A (42 female, 15 male) and 23 patients in Group B (5 female, 18 male) [5, 18]. Dropout throughout the protocol is summarized in Fig. 1. One patient began adalimumab for disease control 1 month after enrolment and remained on this bDMARD for 3 months before the second MRI scan and so was switched to Group B. Full clinical and contrast-enhanced MRI data from Visit 1 (baseline) and Visit 2 (4 months) were available for 62 patients. However, 66 scan pairs were available for analysis (including eight pairs from four patients who were sequentially enrolled into Group A then Group B).

Clinical characteristics

Patients in Group A and Group B were of similar age and gender but those in Group B had a longer disease duration (Table 1). Consistent with their different places on the T2T escalation ladder, swollen and tender joint counts and disease duration (Visit 1) were lower in Group A than Group B (Table 2). The $DAS28_{CRP}$ was also lower for Group A than Group B: 4.24 vs 5.15 ($p = 0.007$). Interestingly, there was no difference between groups for MRI synovitis or tenosynovitis scores at Visit 1 but total MRI inflammation and osteitis scores were lower in Group A than Group B ($p = 0.05$ and 0.02 respectively) (Table 2). MRI erosion scores were also lower in Group A than Group B: 4 (0–50) and 9 (1–47) respectively ($p = 0.03$). The total SvdH X-ray damage score (Visit 1) was also lower in Group A than Group B: 20.5 (0–217) and 63 (0–209) respectively ($p = 0.03$).

Changes in clinical disease activity and MRI inflammation on escalation

Patients' responses were measured by $\Delta DAS28_{CRP}$. Both groups improved from Visit 1 to Visit 2 so that $\Delta DAS28_{CRP}$ for Group A was −0.94 (−3.30, 1.61) and for Group B was −1.53 (−3.59, 0.56). There was no difference between groups ($p = 0.45$). For Groups A and B, 83.3% and 87.5% respectively had a fall in the $DAS28_{CRP}$ from Visit 1 to Visit 2 indicating clinical improvement, while in 16.7% and 12.5% there was worsening. ΔMRI(i) from Visit 1 to Visit 2 varied between patients but median scores showed little change over 4 months, despite escalation of therapy, and there was no difference between groups. For Group A, ΔMRI(i) median (range) was 0 (−25, 10); for Group B, −1 (−15, 28) ($p = 0.12$). Table 3 shows how patients responded in terms of MRI inflammation (total and sub-scores) and MRI erosion score. Only a few showed MRI erosion progression (three patients (6.98%) in Group A and five patients

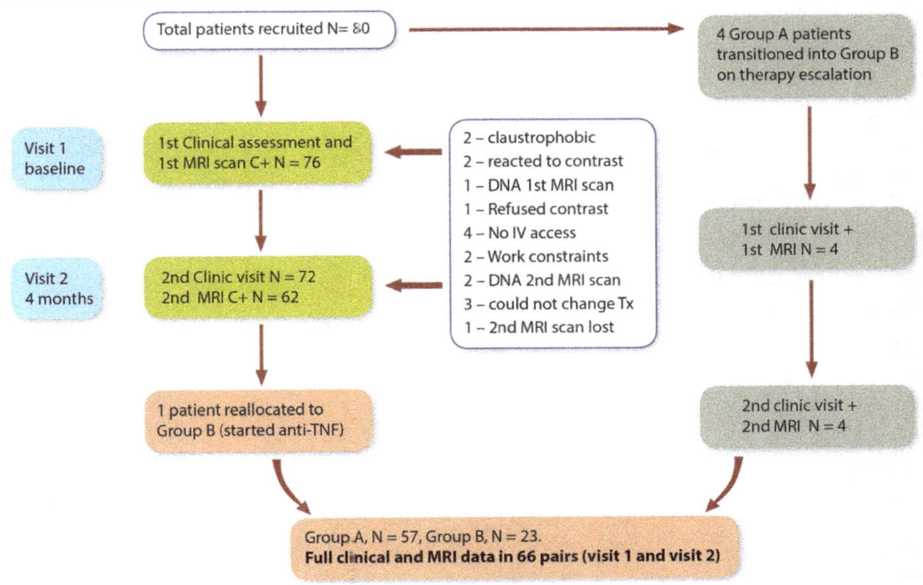

Fig. 1 Clinical and MRI data gathered as patients progressed through the study. IV intravenous, MRI magnetic resonance imaging, TNF tumour necrosis factor, Tx therapy

Table 1 Patient characteristics on enrolment

Clinical characteristic at recruitment	Total		Group A		Group B		Chi-square *p* value*
	(*N* = 80)		(*N* = 57)		(*N* = 23)		
Gender							
Female	60	75%	42	73.68%	18	78.26%	0.67
Male	20	25%	15	26.32%	5	21.74%	
Age (months)	54.5 (24, 82)		53 (24, 81)		56 (27, 82)		0.22
Disease duration (months)	36 (3, 408)		30 (3, 408)		72 (15, 240)		0.0014
On methotrexate							
Yes	70	87.5%	49	85.96%	21	91.3%	0.72
No	10	12.5%	8	14.04%	2	8.7%	

Data presented as *n* (%). Age and disease duration expressed as median (minimum, maximum) values
*Median two-sample test *p* value

Table 2 Clinical and imaging scores at Visit 1 and Visit 2 (4 months later)

	Total (*N* = 84)				Group A (*N* = 57)				Group B (*N* = 27*)				Median two-sample test *p* value
	N	Median	Minimum	Maximum	*N*	Median	Minimum	Maximum	*N*	Median	Minimum	Maximum	
Clinical scores at Visit 1													
Tender 28 joints	84	11	1	28	57	10	1	28	27	14	1	28	0.050
Swollen 28 joints	84	4	0	20	57	4	0	11	27	6	0	20	0.097
HAQ	84	1.06	0	2.5	57	0.88	0	2.13	27	1.38	0.13	2.5	0.037
$DAS28_{CRP}$	84	4.5	3.24	6.64	57	4.24	3.24	6.04	27	5.15	3.36	6.64	0.003
MRI scores at Visit 1													
Synovitis	77	3	0	9	51	3	0	9	26	4	0	9	0.102
Tendonitis	77	3	0	15	51	3	0	15	26	3	0	15	0.931
Osteitis	77	2	0	34	51	2	0	34	26	3	0	24	0.021
Erosion	76	5	0	50	50	4	0	50	26	9	1	47	0.030
Total inflammation	77	9	0	45	51	8	0	45	26	13	1	36	0.050
X-ray scores at Visit 1													
Erosions	62	13	0	130	42	5.5	0	112	20	33.5	0	130	0.001
Total SvdH score	62	35.5	0	217	42	20.5	0	217	20	63	0	209	0.031
Clinical scores at Visit 2													
Tender 28 joints	72	6	0	28	48	5	0	28	24	7	0	24	0.399
Swollen 28 joints	72	1	0	20	48	1	0	20	24	0.5	0	9	0.337
HAQ	72	0.63	0	2.13	48	0.5	0	2	24	0.75	0	2.13	0.155
$DAS28_{CRP}$	72	3.47	1.42	6.64	48	3.28	1.42	6.64	24	3.66	1.42	5.49	0.047
MRI scores at Visit 2													
Synovitis	66	3	0	9	42	3	0	9	24	3	0	8	0.851
Tendonitis	66	2.5	0	15	42	2	0	15	24	3	0	12	0.612
Osteitis	68	2	0	34	44	2	0	32	24	3.5	0	34	0.102
Erosion	67	6	0	50	43	4	0	50	24	9.5	1	47	0.009
Total inflammation	66	9	1	53	42	9	1	43	24	9	1	53	1.000

*Includes the four patients who transitioned from Group A to Group B on escalation of therapy (see text)
$DAS28_{CRP}$ disease activity score (28 joints) incorporating C-reactive protein, *MRI* magnetic resonance imaging, *SvdH* Sharp van der Heijde, *HAQ* Health assessment questionnaire

Table 3 Direction of change for MRI scores from Visit 1 to Visit 2

	Group A		Group B		Total
	n	%	*n*	%	
Change in MRI(i)					
Decrease	16	38.1	13	54.17	29
Increase	16	38.1	3	12.5	19
No change	10	23.81	8	33.33	18
Total	42		24		66
Change in MRI osteitis					
Decrease	15	34.09	8	33.33	23
Increase	9	20.45	6	25	15
No change	20	45.45	10	41.67	30
Total	44		24		68
Change in MRI synovitis					
Decrease	15	35.71	11	45.83	26
Increase	9	21.43	1	4.17	10
No change	18	42.86	12	50	30
Total	42		24		66
Change in MRI tenosynovitis					
Decrease	12	28.57	9	37.5	21
Increase	10	23.81	5	20.83	15
No change	20	47.62	10	41.67	30
Total	42		24		66
Change in MRI erosion					
Increase	3	6.98	5	20.83	8
No change	40	93.02	19	79.17	59
Total	43		24		67

MRI magnetic resonance imaging, *MRI(i)* total MRI inflammation score at the wrist (sum of synovitis, osteitis and tendonitis scores)

(20.83%) in Group B). The majority had no change in MRI erosion scores (93.0% and 79.17% respectively).

Combining groups, there was a weak positive correlation between ΔMRI(i) and $\Delta DAS28_{CRP}$ (Spearman's 0.36, $p = 0.003$). Only ΔMRI tenosynovitis correlated with $\Delta DAS28_{CRP}$ (Spearman's 0.33, $p = 0.007$); MRI sub-scores for Δosteitis, Δsynovitis and Δerosions did not (Table 4). Multiple linear regression analysis was used to assess the effect of group and $\Delta DAS28_{CRP}$ on ΔMRI(i) adjusting for age, gender, duration, anti-CCP titre and MRI erosion score at Visit 1. $\Delta DAS28_{CRP}$ was associated with ΔMRI(i) so that for every unit increase in $\Delta DAS28_{CRP}$ there was a 1.77-U increase in ΔMRI(i) ($p =$ 0.056). Findings are summarized in Fig. 2.

Change in MRI score did not differ between groups

There was no difference between groups for ΔMRI(i) although the point estimate of the fall in score was numerically greater for Group A (−3.68 (95% CI −6.16 to − 1.20)) than Group B (−0.84 (95% CI −4.27 to 2.60), $p = 0.18$). We did note an outlier in Group B in whom there was a significant fall in the $DAS28_{CRP}$ (from 5.15 (V1) to 3.31 (V2)) despite a marked rise in MRI inflammation scores (from 25 to 53). Data for this patient were excluded in a sensitivity analysis but the difference between groups remained non-significant ($p = 0.27$).

Table 4 Correlations between $\Delta DAS28_{CRP}$ and ΔMRI scores

Change in MRI scores (over 4 months)	Number of observations	Spearman correlation coefficients	*p* value
Δtotal MRI(i)	66*	0.36	0.003
Δosteitis	68	0.12	0.33
Δsynovitis	66	0.21	0.09
Δtendonitis	66	0.33	0.007
Δerosion	67	−0.02	0.87

*Sixty-six scan pairs available, includes eight pairs from the four patients who transitioned from Group A to Group B

$DAS28_{CRP}$ disease activity score (28 joints) incorporating C-reactive protein, *MRI* magnetic resonance imaging, *MRI(i)* total MRI inflammation score at the wrist (sum of synovitis, osteitis and tendonitis scores)

MRI erosion score at V1 was associated with change in MRI(i)

The MRI erosion score (V1) was negatively associated with ΔMRI(i) (parameter estimate −0.28; $p = 0.0052$), so those with higher MRI erosion scores at V1 had a greater fall in MRI(i) from V1 to V2. For every 1-U increase in the V1 erosion score, the MRI(i) score would be estimated to fall from V1 to V2 by 0.28 U. The X-ray erosion score (V1) was not associated with ΔMRI(i) ($p = 0.79$).

Discussion

This is the first real-world study to investigate the link between changes in clinical disease activity and imaging (MRI) joint inflammation, in a cohort of RA patients undergoing escalation of therapy according to T2T principles. In this setting, the clinical target is most often a low disease activity state or complete remission ($DAS28_{CRP} \leq 1.9$). It has been suggested that more stringent imaging targets should be used so that patients are treated aggressively, aiming to reach a state where there is no imaging evidence of inflammation at all [19]. MRI scanning can inform about inflammation affecting different tissues including synovium (synovitis), bone (osteitis) and tendon sheaths/tendons (tenosynovitis). We found a significant but relatively weak association between change in clinical disease activity as measured by the $DAS28_{CRP}$ over the 4-month period after escalation of therapy, and change in the total MRI inflammation score. The only MRI sub-score separately associated with $\Delta DAS28_{CRP}$ was the ΔMRI tendonitis score, although there was a trend towards an association with

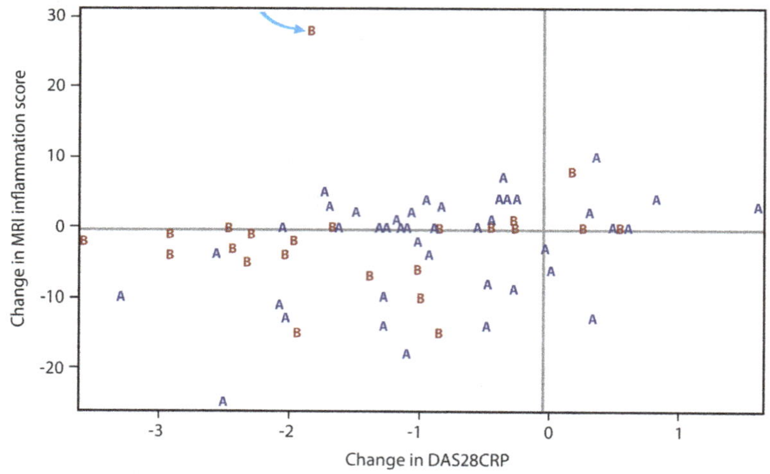

Fig. 2 Change in MRI inflammation score (over 4 months) plotted against change in $DAS28_{CRP}$ for each individual patient (labelled A or B according to group). Arrow points to an outlier in Group B (see text). $DAS28_{CRP}$ disease activity score (28 joints) incorporating C-reactive protein, MRI magnetic resonance imaging

the ΔMRI synovitis score. These findings are consistent with observations by Krabben et al. [11], who found in their analysis of 1790 joints in 179 patients that synovitis and tenosynovitis on MRI were independently associated with clinical swelling. In that study, MRI inflammation was most often observed at the wrist, validating our choice of site for MRI scanning.

Although we did observe an association between change in clinical disease activity and change in MRI inflammation scores, it was obvious from inspection of the data that many individual patients improved clinically over the 4 months after treatment escalation, with only minor changes in their MRI inflammation scores. In some instances MRI inflammation worsened despite clinical improvement. Could this be due to the much greater sensitivity of MRI for detecting joint inflammation? Clinicians are familiar with high-grade clinical joint inflammation manifesting as Virchow's triad of redness, swelling and tenderness, while lesser degrees may only be detectable as pain on movement. MRI can detect inflammation below the clinical threshold by revealing thickened synovium and tenosynovium, which often enhance post contrast, reflecting increased vascularity. However, if MRI inflammation simply represents the low end of the inflammatory spectrum, one might expect a closer correlation between clinical and imaging observations than we have found. A ceiling effect for MRI inflammation scores could be part of the explanation. Thus, a severely inflamed wrist joint might achieve a very high MRI inflammation score, which remains high even when joint swelling and tenderness have subsided. A period of 4 months might also have been insufficient time for MRI(i) to fall in some patients [20]. Another explanation for the relative disparity between changes in clinical and MRI scores is that they capture slightly different information. Clinical disease activity scores incorporate (through joint tenderness) an assessment of pain and this is missing from the MRI inflammation score. The MRI inflammation score incorporates osteitis, which is not directly detectable clinically. Additionally, low-grade synovitis may occur in normal individuals, especially older people [21], and this could contribute to background "noise" within the MRI inflammation score. In this study we have used the $DAS28_{CRP}$ as a "gold standard" against which changes in MRI inflammation were compared, but this measure has its own shortcomings and in some studies the physician global assessment is a better predictor of clinical decision-making [22].

Another possible explanation for the relatively poor correlation between change in MRI inflammation scores and change in the $DAS28_{CRP}$ might be that MRI scans in this study imaged one region only, the dominant wrist, while the $DAS28_{CRP}$ reflected disease activity at 28 joints. We were able to retrieve joint count data and found evidence for tenderness and/or swelling at the scanned wrist in 71.2% of patients at Visit 1 and 47% at Visit 2. Thus, the wrist was quite frequently involved. How well do MRI scans of the wrist reflect, or in other words act as a surrogate marker for, overall rheumatoid disease activity? The evidence for this is indirect. In an early study by McQueen et al. [12], MRI wrist bone oedema (osteitis) scores were predictive of radiographic erosion progression at the hands and feet 6 years later. In 2014, Baker et al. [20] reported a very similar result for MRI osteitis and synovitis from one hand (wrist and MCPs), which were again highly predictive of radiographic progression in the joints of the hands and feet 1 and 2 years later. In 2017, Glinatsi et al. [23] published a post-hoc analysis of clinical trial data from the CIMESTRA/OPERA cohorts and concluded that MRI-assessed inflammation at the wrist (rather than at the MCP joints) was the most important parameter reflecting physical function, pain and global assessment of disease activity in early RA. Thus, although MRI scanning of one joint area may potentially suffer from "sampling error", there is evidence that the wrist is a particularly informative region.

One of the aims of the study was to compare MRI parameters between patients escalating from one cDMARD combination to another cDMARD combination (Group A) and patients escalating to anti-TNF therapy/cDMARDs (Group B). Group B patients, who were further up the T2T escalation ladder, differed from Group A patients in that they had higher scores for MRI erosion and osteitis at their first visit. Interestingly, there were no differences between groups in terms of synovitis or tendonitis. This is consistent with the known association between MRI osteitis and erosion progression in RA [12, 13], and emphasizes that bone inflammation (osteitis) may be qualitatively and prognostically different from soft tissue joint inflammation (synovitis and tenosynovitis). Molenaar et al. [24] observed that clinically relevant damage progression can occur in patients in prolonged remission. Thus, MRI may have an important role in the detection of osteitis and prediction of damage progression; a role that cannot be duplicated by clinical assessment alone. Very few of our patients demonstrated MRI erosion progression over 4 months but longer follow-up would be required to determine whether those with clinically normal joints but high levels of osteitis had a worse erosive outcome. We did not find evidence for a greater reduction in MRI inflammation scores in those receiving anti-TNF therapy than those on cDMARDs. Although Groups A and B cannot be directly compared because of differences in disease duration, this supports the observations of O'Dell et al. [25] who showed equivalent clinical improvement in patients treated with triple therapy and those receiving anti-TNF/methotrexate therapy. Our findings also go some way towards validating the NZ PHARMAC escalation protocol that requires patients to have first tried cDMARD therapy before escalating to more costly bDMARD options.

What are the implications of our findings for the treating clinician? T2T regimens using clinical targets have been profoundly effective in limiting the progression of joint damage and disability in RA patients on cDMARD and bDMARD regimens [26]. If the goal posts are shifted to more stringent imaging targets, what is the evidence for better outcomes? The OMERACT group have studied this by looking for evidence of a "safe level" of MRI inflammation below which damage progression did not to occur, using MRI data from several RA clinical trial cohorts [27]. Gandjbakhch et al. identified an "acceptable MRI inflammatory activity state" as a RAMRIS synovitis score below 6. In these individuals, radiographic progression rarely occurred. As yet there is no evidence that clinical or functional outcomes are better in such patients. Our study has indicated considerable disparity between clinical disease activity and MRI joint inflammation, and has emphasized that the goal of complete imaging resolution of inflammation is far off in the majority of real-world patients. Is it appropriate to treat these individuals more aggressively? Issues of feasibility, cost and patient acceptability mean that clinical goals are probably to be preferred over MRI goals at least in the short term. Whether ultrasound can step into the gap remains an open question [28]. Both the ARCTIC [29] and the TaSER [30] studies have recently investigated whether ultrasound imaging can improve patient outcomes if used by clinicians to inform decision-making. Both studies concluded that an ultrasound-driven T2T strategy was not associated with significantly better clinical or imaging outcomes than a DAS28-driven strategy. Further large prospective studies of this type are now needed for MRI scanning.

Our study has a number of limitations. Firstly, the study was observational. It was not possible to stipulate what disease-suppressing therapies could be given and the associations we observed could have been influenced by individual DMARDs. We considered stratifying patients according to therapy but there were many combinations of cDMARDs used and groups would have been too small for useful comparison. However, we did establish that a similar proportion of Group A and Group B patients were taking methotrexate at their first visit. Secondly, although we found no difference between groups in clinical or MRI responses to therapy, this comparison was flawed by insufficient statistical power and also by the fact that the groups differed in terms of disease duration and radiographic erosions at baseline [31]. Despite extending enrolment by a year we did not reach the numbers required to satisfy the original power calculation. Nevertheless, our comparative clinical and MRI data do shed light on what is actually happening in terms of joint inflammation in rheumatoid patients undergoing escalation of therapy in routine rheumatology practice, and should be of help to clinicians working towards the aim of improving quality of life in their patients.

Conclusions

Full clinical and MRI data were available at two time points, before and 4 months after a change of therapy, in 66 out of 80 RA patients undergoing real-world T2T escalation. There was no or minimal change in the median MRI inflammation score over 4 months, despite clinical improvement. There was no difference in the MRI inflammation response between those escalating to a different cDMARD regimen and those escalating to a cDMARD/anti-TNF regimen. For the entire group there was a significant correlation between the change in the

$DAS28_{CRP}$ and the change in the MRI inflammation score (Spearman's 0.36, $p = 0.003$), but this was relatively weak. These results suggest that MRI outcomes should not be adopted to direct T2T escalation as clinically driven strategies are already successful in improving patient outcomes. A randomized controlled trial comparing MRI-driven and DAS-driven strategies is needed.

Abbreviations

3T-MRI: 3-Tesla magnetic resonance imaging; Anti-CCP: Anti-cyclic citrullinated peptide antibodies; bDMARD: Biological disease-modifying therapy; cDMARD: Conventional disease-modifying therapy; CRP: C-reactive protein; $DAS28_{CRP}$: Disease activity score (28 joints) incorporating CRP; dRUJ: Distal radioulnar joint; FS: Fat saturation; GdDTPA: Gadolinium diethylenetriamine pentaacetic acid; ICC (av): Intraclass correlation coefficient (average); MC: Metacarpal; MRI(i): Total MRI inflammation score at the wrist (sum of synovitis, osteitis and tendonitis scores); MTX/anti-TNF: Methotrexate combined with anti-tumour necrosis therapy; OMERACT: Outcome Measures in Rheumatology; PD: Proton density; PHARMAC: Pharmaceutical Management Agency (New Zealand); RA: Rheumatoid arthritis; RAMRIS: Rheumatoid Arthritis Magnetic Resonance Imaging Score; SAS: Statistical Analysis System; SPAIR: Spectral adiabatic inversion recovery; SvdH: Sharp van der Heijde; T1w: T1 weighted; T2T: Treat to target; T2w: T2 weighted; V1: Visit one; V2: Visit two; $\Delta DAS28_{CRP}$: Change in the $DAS28_{CRP}$; ΔMRI(i): Change in the total MRI inflammation score (wrist)

Acknowledgements

The authors thank all patients who participated in this study. They thank Mrs Megan Johnston, Ms Niamh Fanning and Clinical Nurse Specialist Jan Ipenburg for their assistance with patient recruitment for the Christchurch centre. The authors also thank the staff of Specialist Radiology and MRI Greenlane (SRG, Auckland), especially Mrs Desiree Mulders, charge radiographer, for their technical expertise with MRI scanning and documentation. They thank the staff of Hagley Radiology, Christchurch, for their technical expertise in performing MRI scans. The authors thank Dr Quentin Reeves (radiologist SRG) for his assistance in developing the MRI scan protocol used in the study.

Funding

The study was supported by the Auckland Medical Research Foundation (grant reference 1114001), Arthritis New Zealand (R234) and Lotteries Health NZ (3707583).

Disclosures

FMM has no disclosures. ND reports personal fees from Abbvie, outside the submitted work. The remaining authors have no disclosures.

Authors' contributions

FMM created and designed the project, supervised collection, analysis and interpretation of the data and wrote the manuscript. PC contributed to the study design, patient enrolment, data collection and analysis plus review of the manuscript. TP contributed to MRI data management and analysis and review of the manuscript. DD supervised patient recruitment and data collection and management. AL advised on initial study design and power calculation, performed statistical analysis and advised on manuscript presentation. ND advised on study design, scored X-ray images and contributed to manuscript submission. LS assisted in patient recruitment, data collection and review and advised on analysis. KL participated in the initial study design, oversaw review by the regulatory authorities and reviewed the manuscript. AD participated in study creation, read all MRI scans and formatted MRI scan data and reviewed the manuscript. Approval of the final version of the manuscript was obtained from all co-authors.

Authors' information

Not applicable.

Competing interests

The authors declare that they have no competing interests.

Author details

[1]Department of Molecular Medicine and Pathology, Faculty of Medical and Health Sciences, The University of Auckland, Private Bag 92019, Auckland, New Zealand. [2]Department of Radiology, Auckland City Hospital, 2 Park Rd, Grafton, Auckland 1023, New Zealand. [3]Section of Epidemiology & Biostatistics, School of Population Health (Tamaki Campus), University of Auckland, Auckland 1142, New Zealand. [4]Bone & Joint Research Group, Department of Medicine, The University of Auckland, Private Bag 92019, Auckland, New Zealand. [5]Department of Rheumatology, Greenlane Clinical Centre, Auckland District Health Board, 214 Green Lane West, Epsom, Auckland 1051, New Zealand. [6]Department of Rheumatology, Immunology & Allergy, Christchurch Hospital, PO Box 4710, Christchurch 8140, New Zealand. [7]Department of Medicine, University of Otago, PO Box 4345, Christchurch 8140, New Zealand.

References

1. Grigor C, Capell H, Stirling A, McMahon AD, Lock P, Vallance R, et al. Effect of a treatment strategy of tight control for rheumatoid arthritis (the TICORA study): a single-blind randomised controlled trial. Lancet. 2004;364(9430):263–9.
2. Smolen JS, Landewe R, Bijlsma J, Burmester G, Chatzidionysiou K, Dougados M, et al. EULAR recommendations for the management of rheumatoid arthritis with synthetic and biological disease-modifying antirheumatic drugs: 2016 update. Annals of the Rheumatic Diseases. 2017;76(6):960–77.
3. Pharmac. Decision relating to the funding of TNF inhibitors (Humira and Enbrel) and gabapentin (Neurontin) 2015 [updated 19 June 201720.6.17]. Available from: https://www.pharmac.govt.nz/news/notification-2015-09-09-tnf-inhibitors/.
4. van Riel PLCM, Fransen J. DAS28: a useful instrument to monitor infliximab treatment in patients with rheumatoid arthritis. Arthritis Research and Therapy. 2005;7(5):189–90.
5. Prevoo ML, Van 't Hof MA, Kuper HH, van Leeuwen MA, van de Putte LB, van Riel PL. Modified disease activity scores that include twenty-eight-joint counts. Development and validation in a prospective longitudinal study of patients with rheumatoid arthritis.[see comment]. Arthritis & Rheumatism. 1995;38(1):44–8.
6. McQueen FM, Ostergaard M. Established rheumatoid arthritis - new imaging modalities. Baillieres Best Pract Res Clin Rheumatol. 2007;21(5):841–56.
7. McQueen FM, McHaffie A, Clarke A, Lee AC, Reeves Q, Curteis B, et al. MRI osteitis predicts cartilage damage at the wrist in RA: a three-year prospective 3T MRI study examining cartilage damage. Arthritis Research and Therapy. 2014;16:R33.
8. Ostergaard M, Peterfy C, Conaghan P, McQueen F, Bird P, Ejbjerg B, et al. OMERACT Rheumatoid Arthritis Magnetic Resonance Imaging Studies. Core set of MRI acquisitions, joint pathology definitions, and the OMERACT RA-MRI scoring system. J Rheumatol. 2003;30(6):1385–6.
9. Haavardsholm EA, Ostergaard M, Ejbjerg BJ, Kvan NP, Kvien TK. Introduction of a novel magnetic resonance imaging tenosynovitis score for rheumatoid arthritis: reliability in a multireader longitudinal study. Annals of the Rheumatic Diseases. 2007;66(9):1216–20.
10. Brown AK, Quinn MA, Karim Z, Conaghan PG, Peterfy CG, Hensor E, et al. Presence of significant synovitis in rheumatoid arthritis patients with disease-modifying antirheumatic drug-induced clinical remission: evidence from an imaging study may explain structural progression. Arthritis. Rheumatism. 2006;54(12):3761–73.
11. Krabben A, Stomp W, Huizinga TW, van der Heijde D, Bloem JL, Reijnierse M, et al. Concordance between inflammation at physical examination and on MRI in patients with early arthritis. Annals of the Rheumatic Diseases. 2015;74(3):506–12.
12. McQueen F, Benton N, Perry D, Crabbe J, Robinson E. Bone Edema Scored on Magnetic Resonance Imaging Scans of the Dominant Carpus at Presentation Predicts Radiographic Joint Damage of the Hands and Feet Six Years Later in Patients with Rheumatoid Arthritis. Arthritis Rheum. 2003; 48(7):1814–27.
13. Hetland ML, Ejbjerg B, Horslev-Petersen K, Jacobsen S, Vestergaard A, Jurik AG, et al. MRI bone oedema is the strongest predictor of subsequent radiographic progression in early rheumatoid arthritis. Results from a 2-year

randomised controlled trial (CIMESTRA). Annals of the Rheumatic Diseases. 2009;68(3):384–90.
14. Ostergaard M, Emery P, Conaghan PG, Fleischmann R, Hsia EC, Xu W, et al. Significant improvement in synovitis, osteitis, and bone erosion following golimumab and methotrexate combination therapy as compared with methotrexate alone: a magnetic resonance imaging study of 318 methotrexate-naive rheumatoid arthritis patients. Arthritis. Rheumatism. 2011;63(12):3712–22.
15. Conaghan PG, Peterfy C, Olech E, Kaine J, Ridley D, Dicarlo J, et al. The effects of tocilizumab on osteitis, synovitis and erosion progression in rheumatoid arthritis: results from the ACT-RAY MRI substudy. Annals of the Rheumatic Diseases. 2014;73(5):810–6.
16. Emery P, van der Heijde D, Ostergaard M, Conaghan PG, Genovese MC, Keystone EC, et al. Exploratory analyses of the association of MRI with clinical, laboratory and radiographic findings in patients with rheumatoid arthritis. Annals of the Rheumatic Diseases. 2011;70(12):2126–30.
17. McQueen FM, Clarke A, McHaffie A, Reeves Q, Williams M, Robinson E, et al. Assessment of cartilage loss at the wrist in rheumatoid arthritis using a new MRI scoring system. Annals of the Rheumatic Diseases. 2010;69:1971–5.
18. van der Heijde DM, van Riel PL, Nuver-Zwart IH, Gribnau FW. vad de Putte LB. Effects of hydroxychloroquine and sulphasalazine on progression of joint damage in rheumatoid arthritis. Lancet. 1989;1(8646):1036–8.
19. Porter D, Dale J, Sattar N. How low to aim in rheumatoid arthritis? Learning from other disciplines. Annals of the Rheumatic Diseases. 2014;73(3):480–2.
20. Baker JF, Ostergaard M, Emery P, Hsia EC, Lu J, Baker DG, et al. Early MRI measures independently predict 1-year and 2-year radiographic progression in rheumatoid arthritis: secondary analysis from a large clinical trial. Annals of the Rheumatic Diseases. 2014;73(11):1968–74.
21. Nieuwenhuis WP, Mangnus L, van Steenbergen HW, Newsum EC, Huizinga TW, Reijnierse M, et al. Older age is associated with more MRI-detected inflammation in hand and foot joints. Rheumatology (Oxford). 2016;55(12): 2212–9.
22. Lindsay K, Ibrahim G, Sokoll K, Tripathi M, Melsom RD, PS H. The composite DAS Score is impractical to use in daily practice: evidence that physicians use the objective component of the DAS in decision making. Journal of clinical rheumatology. 2009;15(5):223–5.
23. Glinatsi D, Baker JF, Hetland ML, Horslev-Petersen K, Ejbjerg BJ, Stengaard-Pedersen K, et al. Magnetic resonance imaging assessed inflammation in the wrist is associated with patient-reported physical impairment, global assessment of disease activity and pain in early rheumatoid arthritis: longitudinal results from two randomised controlled trials. Annals of the Rheumatic Diseases. 2017;76(10):1707–15.
24. Molenaar ET, Voskuyl AE, Dinant HJ, Bezemer PD, Boers M, Dijkmans BA. Progression of radiologic damage in patients with rheumatoid arthritis in clinical remission. Arthritis & Rheumatism. 2004;50(1):36–42.
25. O'Dell JR, Mikuls TR, Taylor TH, Ahluwalia V, Brophy M, Warren SR, et al. Therapies for active rheumatoid arthritis after methotrexate failure. N Engl J Med. 2013;369(4):307–18.
26. Steunebrink LM, Vonkeman HE, ten Klooster PM, Hoekstra M, van Riel PL, van de Laar MA. Recently diagnosed rheumatoid arthritis patients benefit from a treat-to-target strategy: results from the DREAM registry. Clin Rheumatol. 2016;35(3):609–15.
27. Gandjbakhch F, Haavardsholm EA, Conaghan PG, Ejbjerg B, Foltz V, Brown AK, et al. Determining a magnetic resonance imaging inflammatory activity acceptable state without subsequent radiographic progression in rheumatoid arthritis: results from a followup MRI study of 254 patients in clinical remission or low disease activity. J Rheumatol. 2014;41(2):398–406.
28. Mandl P, Kurucz R, Niedermayer D, Balint PV, Smolen JS. Contributions of ultrasound beyond clinical data in assessing inflammatory disease activity in rheumatoid arthritis: current insights and future prospects. Rheumatology (Oxford). 2014;53(12):2136–42.
29. Haavardsholm EA, Aga AB, Olsen IC, Lillegraven S, Hammer HB, Uhlig T, et al. Ultrasound in management of rheumatoid arthritis: ARCTIC randomised controlled strategy trial. Bmj. 2016;i4205:354.
30. Dale J, Stirling A, Zhang R, Purves D, Foley J, Sambrook M, et al. Targeting ultrasound remission in early rheumatoid arthritis: the results of the TaSER study, a randomised clinical trial. Annals of the Rheumatic Diseases. 2016; 75(6):1043–50.
31. Hyrich KL, Watson KD, Silman AJ, Symmons DP. British Society for Rheumatology Biologics R. Predictors of response to anti-TNF-alpha therapy among patients with rheumatoid arthritis: results from the British Society for Rheumatology Biologics Register. Rheumatology (Oxford). 2006;45(12):1558–65.

7

Predictors of remission with etanercept-methotrexate induction therapy and loss of remission with etanercept maintenance, reduction, or withdrawal in moderately active rheumatoid arthritis: results of the PRESERVE trial

Josef S. Smolen[1,2*], Annette Szumski[3], Andrew S. Koenig[4], Thomas V. Jones[4] and Lisa Marshall[4]

Abstract

Background: The aim was to analyze characteristics that predict remission induction and subsequent loss of remission in patients with moderately active rheumatoid arthritis (RA) who received full-dose combination etanercept plus methotrexate induction therapy followed by reduced-dose etanercept or etanercept withdrawal.

Methods: Patients with Disease Activity Score based on 28-joint count (DAS28) >3.2 and ≤5.1 received open-label etanercept 50 mg once weekly (QW) plus methotrexate for 36 weeks. Those who achieved DAS28 low disease activity by 36 weeks were randomized to double-blind treatment with etanercept 50 mg or 25 mg QW plus methotrexate or placebo plus methotrexate for 52 weeks. All analyses were adjusted for the continuous baseline variables of their respective remission outcomes.

Results: Younger age, body mass index (BMI) <30 kg/m^2, and lower Health Assessment Questionnaire (HAQ) score at baseline were significant predictors of week-36 remission ($P < 0.05$) based on DAS28, Simplified Disease Activity Index (SDAI), and Clinical Disease Activity Index (CDAI). Baseline DAS28, SDAI, and CDAI were significantly predictive of all three remission endpoints ($P < 0.05$). For all three treatments, the strongest predictors of loss of DAS28 remission included failure to achieve sustained remission (DAS28 < 2.6 at weeks 12, 20, 28, and 36) with induction therapy, higher DAS28/SDAI/CDAI at randomization and at 1 month, increase in DAS28/SDAI/CDAI at 1 month, and increase in DAS28/CDAI/SDAI components and patient-reported outcomes (PROs) at 1 month. With the exception of not achieving sustained remission, very similar significant predictors were observed for loss of SDAI and CDAI remission.

(Continued on next page)

* Correspondence: Josef.Smolen@wienkav.at
[1]Division of Rheumatology, Department of Medicine 3, Medical University of Vienna, Waehringer Guertel 18-20, 1090 Vienna, Austria
[2]Hietzing Hospital, Vienna, Austria
Full list of author information is available at the end of the article

(Continued from previous page)

Conclusion: These findings suggest that patients with moderately active RA who are younger and have lower BMI, lower HAQ, and lower disease activity at baseline are most likely to achieve remission when receiving combination etanercept and methotrexate induction therapy. In addition, patients who fail to achieve sustained remission with induction therapy and those with worse disease activity and PROs at early time points after initiating maintenance therapy with a full-dose or reduced-dose etanercept-methotrexate regimen or methotrexate monotherapy are most likely to lose remission across all treatment arms. These findings may help guide clinicians' decision-making as they treat patients to remission and beyond.

Keywords: Rheumatoid arthritis, Treatment, Remission, Low disease activity, Etanercept, Methotrexate

Background

Clinical remission is a critical treatment target in all patients with rheumatoid arthritis (RA), regardless of the level of their disease activity [1]. In the clinical practice setting, a large proportion of patients have moderately active RA [2, 3], which is associated with an elevated risk of joint destruction and functional disability [4, 5]. Although treatment with biologics such as tumor necrosis factor (TNF) inhibitors is effective in inducing and maintaining remission in patients with RA, the determining factors associated with remission induction with biologic therapy, and remission maintenance after such therapy is reduced or discontinued, have not yet been well-studied. However, this information would be important to clinicians and patients when they are deciding on a treatment plan to limit costs and patient exposure.

The PRESERVE trial was an induction/maintenance study of the biologic etanercept in which investigators assessed the consequences of etanercept dose reduction or withdrawal in adults with moderately active RA who achieved low disease activity (LDA) after 36 weeks of treatment with full-dose etanercept combined with methotrexate. The conventional full-dose or reduced-dose etanercept-methotrexate combination regimens were shown to be more effective in maintaining LDA than methotrexate alone after etanercept withdrawal [6]. Post hoc analyses of findings from the PRESERVE trial were conducted here to identify potential predictive markers for remission induction and loss after modification of etanercept dosing.

Methods

The methodology of the PRESERVE trial has been described in detail in a previous publication [6] and is briefly summarized in the following sections. In the last decade, a Disease Activity Score in 28 joints (DAS28, on the basis of erythrocyte sedimentation rate (ESR)) <2.6 was commonly considered to indicate remission in practice and clinical trials, including the PRESERVE trial [6, 7]. When the PRESERVE trial was designed and the statistical analyses planned, the American College of Rheumatology/European League Against Rheumatism (ACR/EULAR) Boolean definition of remission had not yet been published [8]. Although DAS28 < 2.6 no longer defines remission according to ACR/EULAR criteria, as it better represents minimal disease activity than remission [8], and other cut points for remission have been proposed [9–11], in these analyses, remission continues to be defined as DAS28 < 2.6 in agreement with the primary manuscript. However, ACR/EULAR index-based remission criteria were also evaluated.

Study design

All patients enrolled in the initial open-label period were treated with etanercept 50 mg once weekly (QW) plus methotrexate for 36 weeks. The dose of methotrexate at screening was continued in the open-label period, but dose adjustments were permitted at the investigator's discretion. Patients who achieved sustained LDA, defined as an average DAS28 ≤ 3.2 from weeks 12 to 36 and DAS28 ≤ 3.2 at week 36, after 36 weeks of combination etanercept-methotrexate treatment were randomized to continue weekly subcutaneous injections of etanercept 50 mg, reduce the etanercept dose to 25 mg, or withdraw etanercept and receive placebo injections, all in addition to background methotrexate, for the subsequent 52-week double-blind period. In the double-blind period, the same dose of methotrexate was administered as in the last 8 weeks of the open-label period.

Patients

Adults who were enrolled in this study had active RA with moderate disease activity (DAS28 > 3.2 and ≤5.1) at screening and baseline and had received stable methotrexate doses. Randomized patients who received double-blind treatment had completed the first 36 study weeks and achieved sustained LDA.

Post hoc analyses

The statistical analysis plans for the exploratory/post hoc predictor analyses are available in Additional file 1: Appendices 1 and 2.

Predictors of remission induction

Randomized patients were included in analyses of baseline variables; patients who were dosed and had week-36 visit data were included in post-baseline analyses. Patients who had week-36 DAS28/Simplified Disease Activity Index (SDAI)/Clinical Disease Activity Index (CDAI) values were included in the respective post hoc analysis of predictors of DAS28/SDAI/CDAI remission in the open-label period. Remission in this analysis was defined as DAS28 < 2.6, SDAI ≤3.3, or CDAI ≤2.8 after 36 weeks of full-dose combination therapy. Demographic characteristics and baseline disease characteristics—including clinical, patient-reported, and radiographic measures—were examined in the post hoc analyses as possible predictors of remission. Univariate logistic regression of each remission endpoint was conducted on each baseline predictor, treated as continuous (i.e., age, body mass index (BMI), and disease duration; anti-citrullinated peptide antibody (ACPA) and rheumatoid factor (RF) levels; C-

Table 1 Demographic and disease characteristics at baseline for the overall patient population (mITT) in the open-label period and for the treatment group subpopulations (mITT) in the randomized, double-blind period [6]

	Open-label population	Randomized population					
Demographic/disease characteristics at baseline	ETN 50 mg + MTX *N* = 834	ETN 50 mg + MTX *n* = 202		ETN 25 mg + MTX *n* = 202		MTX *n* = 200	
Age, years	48.4 (11.9)	48.1 (12.0)		46.4 (12.2)		48.3 (12.2)	
Female, *n* (%)	694 (83.2)	164 (81.2)		157 (77.7)		167 (83.5)	
Prior tobacco use, *n* (%)	158 (18.9)	42 (20.8)		31 (15.4)		39 (19.5)	
Disease duration, years	6.9 (7.0)	6.8 (7.2)		6.4 (7.1)		7.3 (6.7)	
ACPA positive, *n* (%)	642 (77.6)	161 (80.1)		156 (77.6)		156 (78.8)	
RF positive, *n* (%)	603 (72.7)	147 (73.1)		142 (70.7)		147 (74.2)	
Clinical and patient-reported characteristics at baseline and randomization	ETN 50 mg + MTX *N* = 834	ETN 50 mg + MTX *n* = 201		ETN 25 mg + MTX *n* = 201		MTX *n* = 197	
	Week 0	Week 0	Week 36	Week 0	Week 36	Week 0	Week 36
DAS28	4.4 (0.4)	4.3 (0.5)	2.0 (0.6)	4.4 (0.4)	2.1 (0.6)	4.3 (0.4)	2.1 (0.6)
SDAI	19.1 (5.1)	18.7 (4.8)	4.7 (3.6)	19.2 (5.1)	4.8 (3.2)	18.8 (5.4)	4.8 (3.2)
CDAI	17.8 (5.0)	17.5 (4.6)	4.1 (3.5)	17.9 (5.0)	4.2 (3.2)	17.8 (5.3)	4.3 (3.2)
TJC, 0–28	5.1 (2.9)	4.7 (2.7)	0.6 (1.2)	5.2 (2.9)	0.7 (1.3)	5.1 (2.9)	0.7 (1.2)
SJC, 0–28	3.8 (2.6)	3.9 (2.7)	0.6 (1.5)	3.8 (2.6)	0.6 (1.2)	4.0 (2.7)	0.6 (1.1)
CRP, mg/L	12.3 (16.4)	11.9 (13.9)	5.9 (5.9)	12.8 (18.0)	6.0 (6.5)	10.4 (13.1)	5.2 (3.3)
ESR, 0–100 mm/hour	22.2 (13.1)	22.2 (12.9)	9.9 (7.2)	21.7 (13.4)	10.7 (8.6)	20.4 (12.1)	9.6 (6.0)
PGA, 0–10	4.1 (1.3)	4.0 (1.3)	1.1 (0.9)	4.0 (1.3)	1.2 (1.1)	4.2 (1.3)	1.1 (0.8)
PtGA, 0–10	4.9 (1.7)	4.9 (1.8)	1.8 (1.7)	4.8 (1.7)	1.8 (1.5)	4.6 (1.7)	1.9 (1.6)
General health VAS, 0–100 mm	43.4 (17.0)	43.2 (17.3)	14.1 (15.8)	41.5 (15.5)	14.8 (15.0)	40.9 (15.6)	15.1 (15.5)
Pain VAS, 0–100 mm	45.5 (17.4)	46.1 (17.8)	12.8 (15.5)	43.1 (16.1)	13.8 (14.8)	44.1 (16.3)	14.2 (15.6)
Total HAQ, 0–3	1.1 (0.6)	1.1 (0.6)	0.5 (0.5)	1.1 (0.6)	0.5 (0.5)	1.1 (0.6)	0.5 (0.4)
Radiographic characteristics at baseline and randomization	ETN 50 mg + MTX *N* = 709	ETN 50 mg + MTX *n* = 184		ETN 25 mg + MTX *n* = 184		MTX *n* = 167	
	Week 0	Week 0	Week 36	Week 0	Week 36	Week 0	Week 36
mTSS (0–448)	39.3 (55.3)	42.6 (58.8)	42.7 (58.8)	39.1 (60.3)	38.9 (59.8)	42.3 (47.5)	42.4 (47.6)
Erosion score (0–280)	24.8 (33.2)	25.8 (34.6)	25.8 (34.6)	24.7 (36.8)	24.7 (36.5)	26.2 (28.1)	26.1 (28.1)
JSN score (0–168)	14.5 (23.6)	16.8 (25.3)	16.9 (25.4)	14.4 (24.8)	14.2 (24.6)	16.1 (21.1)	16.1 (21.2)

ACPA anti-citrullinated peptide antibody, *CDAI* Clinical Disease Activity Index, *CRP* C-reactive protein, *DAS28* Disease Activity Score based on a 28-joint count, *ESR* erythrocyte sedimentation rate, *ETN* etanercept, *HAQ* health assessment questionnaire, *JSN* joint space narrowing, *mITT* modified intention-to-treat, *mTSS* modified total Sharp score, *MTX* methotrexate, *PGA* physician global assessment, *PtGA* patient global assessment, *RF* rheumatoid factor, *SDAI* Simplified Disease Activity Index, *SJC* swollen joint count, *TJC* tender joint count, *VAS* visual analog scale

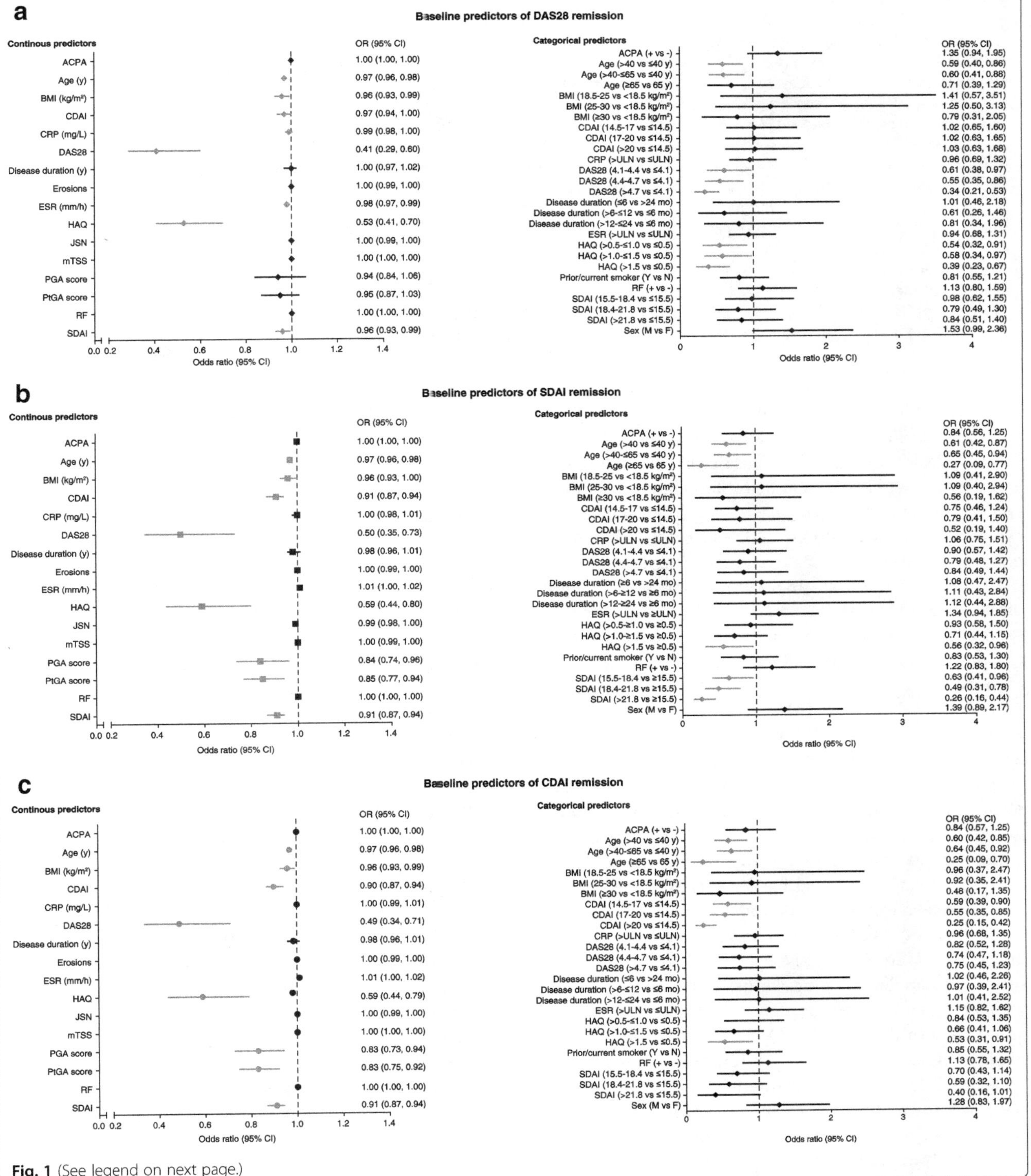

Fig. 1 (See legend on next page.)

(See figure on previous page.)
Fig. 1 Continuous and categorical baseline predictors of disease activity score based on 28 joints (DAS28) (**a**), Simplified Disease Activity Index (SDAI) (**b**), and Clinical Disease Activity Index (CDAI) (**c**) remission using univariate logistic regression (unadjusted). If the 95% CI does not contain the value 1.0, the predictor is statistically significant at α = 0.5. Non-significant predictors, black; significant predictors, gray. For continuous predictors with odds ratios >1, higher values are associated with a greater likelihood of remission. For numeric categorical predictors with odds ratios >1, higher numeric subgroups are associated a greater likelihood of remission (e.g., patients with body mass index (BMI) 18.5–25 kg/m^2 are more likely to achieve DAS28 remission than patients with BMI <18.5 kg/m^2); for nominal categorical predictors, the first named subgroup is associated with a greater likelihood of remission (e.g., anti-citrullinated peptide antibody (ACPA) + patients are more likely to achieve DAS28 remission than ACPA- patients). Conversely, for continuous predictors with odds ratios <1, lower values are associated with a greater likelihood of remission. For numeric categorical predictors with odds ratios <1, lower numeric subgroups are associated with a greater likelihood of remission (e.g., patients who are ≤40 years of age are more likely to achieve DAS28 remission than patients who are >40 years of age); for nominal categorical predictors with odds ratios <1, the second named subgroup is associated with a greater likelihood of remission (e.g., patients with erythrocyte sedimentation rate (ESR) levels ≤ upper limit of normal (ULN) are more likely to achieve DAS28 remission than patients with ESR > ULN). BL, baseline; CI, confidence interval; CRP, C-reactive protein; HAQ, Health Assessment Questionnaire; JSN, joint space narrowing: mTSS, modified total Sharp score: PGA, physician global assessment; PtGA patient global assessment; RF, rheumatoid factor. Analyses were adjusted for baseline DAS28, SDAI, and CDAI (respectively). Patients included in the DAS28, SDAI, and CDAI remission models: n = 763, n = 755, and n = 762, respectively. Radiographic variables were excluded from the stepwise analyses because 55 patients did not have radiographic data

reactive protein (CRP) and ESR levels; DAS28, SDAI, and CDAI; physician and patient global assessments (PGA and PtGA); Health Assessment Questionnaire (HAQ) score; and the van der Heijde modified total Sharp score (mTSS) and erosion and joint space narrowing (JSN) scores), or as categorical (i.e., age >40 vs. ≤40, >40 to ≤65 vs. ≤40, and ≥65 vs. <65 years; sex, male vs. female; BMI, 18.5–25 vs. <18.5 kg/m^2, 25–30 vs. <18.5 kg/m^2, ≥30 vs. <18.5 kg/m^2; disease duration, ≤6 vs. >24 months, >6 to ≤12 vs. ≤6 months, >12 to ≤24 vs. ≤6 months; ACPA and RF status, positive vs. negative; CRP and ESR, > vs. ≤ upper limit of normal (ULN); DAS28, 4.1–4.4 vs. ≤4.1, 4.4–4.7 vs. ≤4.1, and >4.7 vs. ≤4.1; SDAI, 15.5–18.4 vs. ≤15.5, 18.4–21.8 vs. ≤15.5, and >21.8 vs. ≤15.5; CDAI, 14.5–17 vs. ≤14.5, 17–20 vs. ≤14.5, and >20 vs. ≤14.5; and HAQ score, >0.5 to ≤1.0 vs. ≤0.5, >1.0 to ≤1.5 vs. ≤0.5, and >1.5 vs. ≤0.5; and prior/current smoker vs. non-smoker), and adjusted for the respective baseline DAS28, SDAI, or CDAI.

Stepwise logistic regression was performed on the following predictors selected by the authors based on their clinical relevance: age, ≤40, >40 to ≤65, and >65 years; BMI, <18.5 vs. ≥18.5 to <25 vs. ≥25 to <30 vs. ≥30; baseline CRP, ≤ULN vs. >ULN to 3*ULN vs. >3*ULN; sex, male and female; smoking status, prior/current vs. non-smoker; disease duration, ≤6, >6 to ≤12, >12 to ≤24, and >24 months; and HAQ score, ≤0.5, >0.5 to ≤1.0, >1.0 to ≤1.5, and >1.5. In addition, although radiographic variables were included in univariate analyses, they were excluded from the stepwise analyses because week-36 x-ray data were not available for approximately 65 patients.

Predictors of loss of remission

Patients in the modified intent-to-treat (mITT) population of the randomized treatment period (i.e., patients who received at least one dose of study drug and had at least one DAS28 evaluation in the randomized treatment period) who had achieved DAS28 remission (DAS28 < 2.6) at week 36 were examined to identify predictors of loss of DAS28 remission in this period. (As previously mentioned, more stringent definitions of remission have been proposed [8, 12]; however, the DAS28 < 2.6 cut point was used to define remission in the original PRESERVE trial and was therefore also applied in this publication for consistency.) Demographic and disease characteristics reported at baseline of the open-label period (week 0) and included in this predictor analysis were age, sex, BMI, disease duration, and ACPA and RF status. Clinical, functional, and radiographic outcomes observed at baseline of the randomized treatment period (week 36) and analyzed as week-36 predictors were DAS28 and change in DAS28 from baseline to week 36; tender joint count (TJC) and swollen joint count (SJC); CRP and ESR levels; PGA and PtGA; general health and pain scores (visual analog scale); HAQ score; and the mTSS, erosion, and JSN scores. With the exception of radiographic variables (mTSS, erosion, and JSN), which were not collected at week 40, all of these predictors were also analyzed at week 40, as well as change in the predictors from week 36 to week 40. The following categories of achievement of sustained remission in the open-label period were also analyzed as predictors: non-sustained vs. sustained remission (i.e., DAS28 < 2.6 at weeks 12, 20, 28, and 36) and sustained remission by duration (i.e., sustained remission at weeks 12, 20, 28, and 36 vs. weeks 20, 28, and 36 vs. weeks 28 and 36 vs. only at week 36).

Cox proportional hazards modeling, adjusted for baseline of the respective remission endpoints, was used to determine the relationship between the first loss of DAS28, SDAI, and CDAI clinical remission and the demographic and clinical predictors. A more stringent remission endpoint, loss of DAS28 remission plus a change in DAS28 ≥ 0.6 in the double-blind

Table 2 Summary of (a) significant baseline factors predictive of DAS28, SDAI, and CDAI remission induction after 36 weeks of full-dose etanercept-methotrexate therapy in the open-label period and (b) significant post-baseline factors predictive of DAS28, SDAI, and CDAI remission loss at a single time point in all treatment groups in the double-blind period of the PRESERVE trial

(a)		
Baseline predictors of remission induction		
DAS28	**SDAI**	**CDAI**
Continuous variables		
· **Younger age**	· **Younger age**	· **Younger age**
· **Lower BMI**	· **Lower BMI**	· **Lower BMI**
· **Lower DAS28, SDAI, and CDAI**	· **Lower DAS28, SDAI, and CDAI**	· **Lower DAS28, SDAI, and CDAI**
· **Lower HAQ**	· **Lower HAQ**	· **Lower HAQ**
	· Lower PGA and PtGA	· Lower PGA and PtGA
Categorical variables		
Younger age (>40 vs. ≤40 years; >40 to ≤65 vs. ≤40 years)	**Younger age (>40 vs. ≤40 years; >40 to ≤65 vs. ≤40 years**; ≥65 vs. <65 years)	**Younger age (>40 vs. ≤40 years; >40 to ≤65 vs. ≤40 years**; ≥65 vs. <65 years)
· Lower DAS28 (≤4.1)	· Lower SDAI (≤15.5)	· Lower CDAI (≤14.5)
· **Lower HAQ** (>0.5 to ≤1.0 vs. ≤0.5; >1.0 to ≤1.5 vs. ≤0.5; **>1.5 vs. ≤0.5**)	· **Lower HAQ (>1.5 vs. ≤0.5)**	· **Lower HAQ (>1.5 vs. ≤0.5)**
(b)		
Post-baseline predictors of remission loss		
DAS28	**SDAI**	**CDAI**
· Lack of sustained DAS28 remission		
· DAS28 at wk 36		
· **DAS28, SDAI, and CDAI at wk 40**	· **DAS28, SDAI, and CDAI at wk 40**	· **DAS28 and CDAI at wk 40**
· **Δ in DAS28,** SDAI, **and CDAI from wk 36-40**	· **Δ in DAS28,** SDAI, **and CDAI from wk 36 to 40**	· **Δ in DAS28 and CDAI from wk 36 to 40**
· TJC and SJC at wk 40		· TJC at wk 40
· Δ in TJC and SJC from wk 36 to 40		· Δ in TJC from wk 36 to 40
· ESR at wk 40		
· Δ in ESR from wk 36 to 40		
· Δ in HAQ from wk 36 to 40		· Δ in HAQ from wk 36-40
· **PGA, PtGA, general health VAS, and pain VAS at wk 40**	· **PGA, PtGA, general health VAS, and pain VAS at wk 40**	· **PGA, PtGA, general health VAS, and pain VAS at wk 40**
· **Δ in PGA, PtGA, general health VAS, and pain VAS from wk 36 to 40**	· **Δ in PGA, PtGA, general health VAS, and pain VAS from wk 36 to 40**	· **Δ in PGA, PtGA, general health VAS, and pain VAS from wk 36 to 40**

Bold face denotes predictors of remission induction and remission loss across all three sets of criteria, i.e., Disease Activity Score in 28 joints (DAS28), Simplified Disease Activity Index (SDAI), and Clinical Disease Activity Index (CDAI)

BMI body mass index, *HAQ* Health Assessment Questionnaire, *PGA* physician global assessment, *PtGA* patient global assessment, *TJC* tender joint count, *SJC* swollen joint count, *VAS* visual analog scale

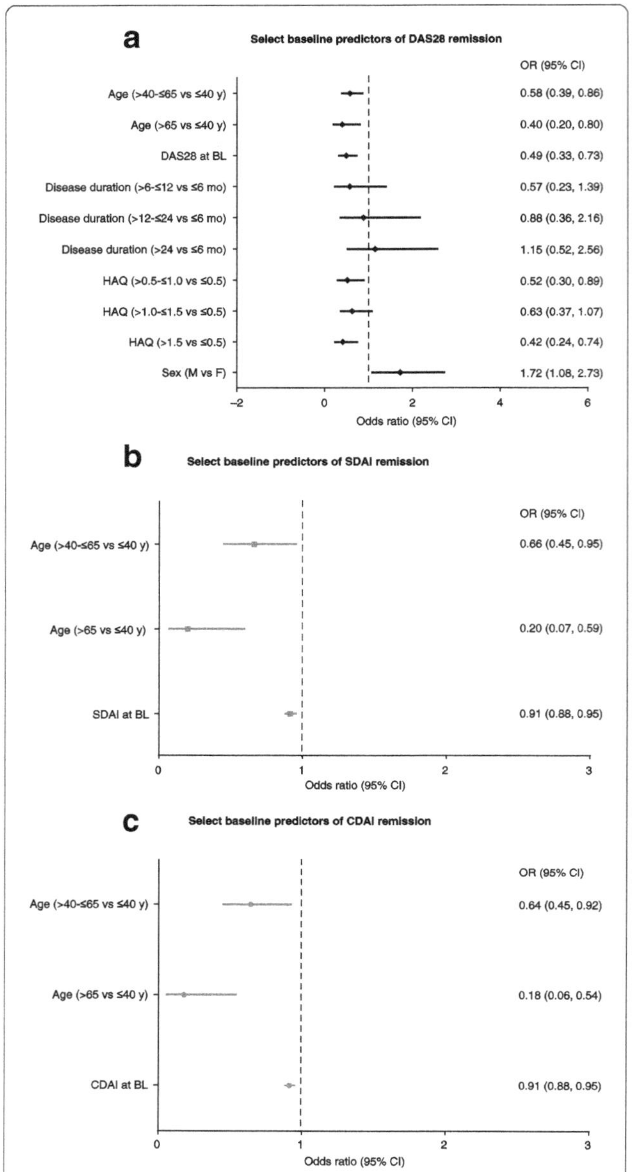

Fig. 2 Select continuous and categorical baseline predictors of Disease Activity Score based on a 28-joint count (DAS28) (**a**), Simplified Disease Activity Index (SDAI) (**b**), and Clinical Disease Activity Index (CDAI) (**c**) remission using stepwise models (adjusted for other variables). If the 95% confidence interval (CI) does not contain the value 1.0, the predictor is statistically significant at α = 0.5. Non-significant predictors, black; significant predictors, gray. HAQ, health assessment questionnaire

period, was also analyzed. Higher hazard ratios (HRs) denoted greater potential for the loss of remission. However, each predictor has a different range of values; because HRs are based on these ranges, HRs cannot be compared. Each predictor was analyzed for each treatment arm separately and therefore HRs cannot be compared between the treatment arms.

Stepwise models for each endpoint and each treatment were created to determine which subsets of predictors were the strongest. To explore the effects of clinical response to full-dose combination induction therapy on subsequent response after tapering or withdrawal of etanercept in the double-blind period, the relationships between week-36 DAS28, SDAI, and CDAI and the probability of loss of DAS28, SDAI, and CDAI remission or LDA in the double-blind period was analyzed in patients receiving reduced-dose combination therapy or methotrexate monotherapy after randomization, using univariate logistic regression models.

Descriptive summary statistics were also provided for mean DAS28 (95% confidence interval (CI)) during the double-blind period in patients who never lost remission at any time point during the period and those who did lose remission during the period, among patients who had achieved DAS28 remission at week 36.

Results

Patients

A detailed description of overall patient disposition in the PRESERVE study was previously published [6]; a summary of patients included in the current predictor analyses is provided in Additional file 2: Figure S1. Demographics and baseline disease characteristics of patients in the overall population in the open-label period and the randomized population of the double-blind period are shown in Table 1. At the start of the open-label period, 83% of patients were women, mean age was 48 years, and disease duration, 6.9 years; the mean DAS28, SDAI, and CDAI scores were 4.4 (standard deviation (SD), 0.4), 19.1 (SD, 5.1), and 17.8 (SD, 5.0), respectively. Disease, patient-reported, and radiographic characteristics were similar among the three treatment groups at baseline of both study periods.

Predictors of induction of remission

Based on univariate logistic regression, several continuous baseline factors were found to be predictive of DAS28, SDAI, and CDAI remission after 36 weeks of full-dose combination therapy when adjusting for their respective baseline DAS28, SDAI, and CDAI measurements (Fig. 1a–c; Table 2). Lower baseline DAS28 (unadjusted), SDAI (unadjusted), and CDAI (unadjusted), younger age (adjusted), BMI <30 kg/m^2 (adjusted), and lower HAQ score (adjusted) were significant predictors of achievement of all three remission endpoints.

When analyzed as continuous variables, lower DAS28, SDAI, and CDAI at baseline were significant predictors of week-36 DAS28, SDAI, and CDAI remission, respectively. Lower baseline SDAI and CDAI as continuous variables were also predictive of DAS28 remission, after adjusting for baseline DAS28. Lower baseline DAS28 and CDAI as continuous variables were predictors of SDAI remission after adjusting for baseline SDAI, and lower baseline DAS28 and SDAI as continuous variables were predictors of CDAI remission after adjusting for baseline CDAI. Lower baseline PGA and PtGA as continuous variables were significant predictors of SDAI and CDAI remission, but not DAS28 remission.

Logistic regression analyses of categorical predictors of DAS28, SDAI, and CDAI remission, shown in Fig. 1a–c, indicated that both younger age (≤40 years) and lower HAQ (≤0.5) were significant predictors for DAS28, SDAI, and CDAI remission, even after adjustment for baseline of the respective outcomes. Neither RF nor ACPA status, when analyzed as continuous predictors (i.e., RF and ACPA levels) or categories (i.e., negative or positive), was predictive of DAS28, SDAI, or CDAI remission at week 36.

In stepwise analyses of remission, including continuous and categorical analyses of baseline variables, age 40 years or younger at baseline and baseline DAS28, SDAI, and CDAI predicted achievement of the remission endpoints (Fig. 2a–c). Patients with a HAQ score ≤0.5 vs. >0.5 and who were male were significantly more likely to achieve DAS28 remission.

Loss of remission

At week 40 and thereafter in the double-blind period, approximately 25–34% of patients were not in DAS28 remission in the full-dose and reduced-dose combination therapy groups (Fig. 3). Although only patients who had achieved DAS28 remission were selected for the predictor analyses in the double-blind period, this rate of non-remission in the latter period was consistent with that observed at week 28 in the open-label period. At the first post-randomization visit (week 40), decreased DAS28 response was observed in all groups. In contrast, during this time frame, the proportion of patients in the etanercept withdrawal group who were not in DAS28 remission ranged from 52 to 65%. At week 88 at the end of the double-blind period, in the full-dose combination therapy group, the mean DAS28 (95% CI) in patients who never lost remission in the prior period was 1.7 (1.5, 1.8) compared with 2.7 (2.5, 2.9) in patients who lost remission at one or more time points in the period.

Predictors of loss of remission

As shown in Table 3 (and summarized in Table 2), several factors—including failure to achieve sustained remission in the open-label period and DAS28 level at weeks 36 and 40—were significant predictors of the loss of DAS28 remission at a single time point in the double-blind period in each treatment group. In addition, the components of DAS28 (e.g., CRP, ESR, TJC, and SJC), patient-reported outcomes (PROs) (e.g., HAQ, PGA, PtGA, and general health and pain scores), and SDAI and CDAI levels were significant predictors across most or all treatment groups but only at week 40. For predictive factors with odds ratios >1, higher values (i.e., greater worsening) were associated with greater likelihood of remission loss. Change from baseline from week 36 to week 40 for these predictors was also significant, with change in PROs being slightly weaker predictors than the best predictors (lack of sustained DAS28 remission,

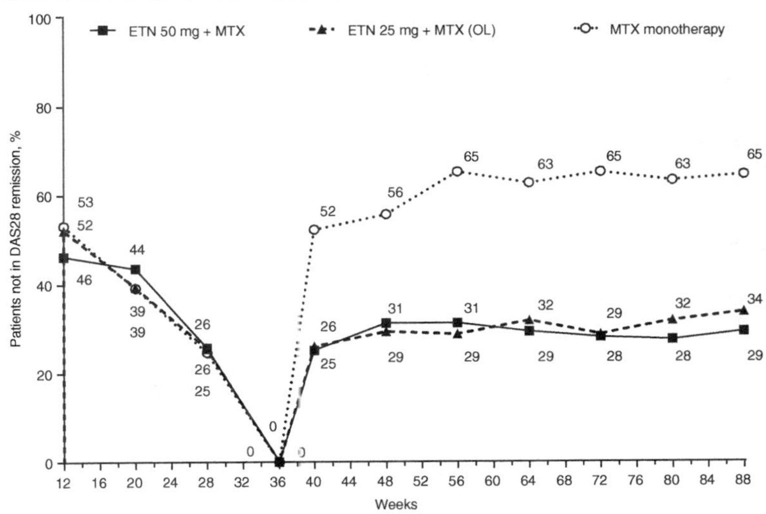

Fig. 3 Proportions of patients who were not in Disease Activity Score based on a 28-joint count (DAS28) remission in the double-blind period. ETN, etanercept; MTX, methotrexate

Table 3 Predictors of loss of remission in all treatment groups in the double-blind period

Predictor[a]	Adjusted hazard ratio[b] (95% CI)		
	ETN 50 mg + MTX *n* = 74	ETN 25 mg + MTX *n* = 56	MTX *n* = 66
Loss of DAS28 remission at single time point in double-blind period			
Lack of sustained DAS28 remission	2.32 (1.44, 3.73)	2.59 (1.48, 4.55)	1.85 (1.24, 2.77)
Sustained weighted DAS28 remission	0.67 (0.56, 0.80)	0.71 (0.59, 0.86)	0.79 (0.68, 0.92)
DAS28 at week 36	2.44 (1.59, 3.73)	2.81 (1.70, 4.63)	1.74 (1.20, 2.51)
DAS28 at week 40	3.24 (2.48, 4.23)	5.88 (4.05, 8.53)	2.26 (1.88, 2.71)
Change in DAS28 from week 36 to 40	3.24 (2.48, 4.23)	5.88 (4.05, 8.53)	2.26 (1.88, 2.71)
ESR at week 40	1.05 (1.02, 1.08)	1.05 (1.02, 1.07)	1.02 (1.01, 1.03)
Change in ESR from week 36 to 40	1.09 (1.06, 1.12)	1.07 (1.04, 1.10)	1.02 (1.01, 1.03)
Sustained weighted SDAI remission	*0.81 (0.58, 1.11)*	0.49 (0.30, 0.78)	*0.80 (0.60, 1.08)*
SDAI at week 40	1.12 (1.08, 1.16)	1.24 (1.17, 1.32)	1.08 (1.06, 1.11)
Change in SDAI from week 36 to 40	1.13 (1.09, 1.18)	1.23 (1.16, 1.30)	1.09 (1.06, 1.12)
Sustained weighted CDAI remission	*0.87 (0.65, 1.17)*	0.49 (0.32, 0.75)	*0.85 (0.64, 1.13)*
CDAI at week 40	1.12 (1.08, 1.16)	1.24 (1.17, 1.31)	1.09 (1.06, 1.12)
Change in CDAI from week 36 to 40	1.13 (1.09, 1.18)	1.23 (1.16, 1.30)	1.09 (1.07, 1.12)
PGA at week 40	1.50 (1.23, 1.81)	1.73 (1.40, 2.12)	1.26 (1.15, 1.39)
Change in PGA from week 36 to 40	1.52 (1.23, 1.88)	1.42 (1.10, 1.83)	1.25 (1.13, 1.38)
PtGA at week 40	1.27 (1.14, 1.42)	1.26 (1.11, 1.43)	1.25 (1.15, 1.36)
Change in PtGA from week 36 to 40	1.28 (1.14, 1.45)	1.49 (1.26, 1.78)	1.28 (1.17, 1.39)
General health VAS at week 40	1.03 (1.02, 1.04)	1.02 (1.01, 1.03)	1.02 (1.02, 1.03)
Change in general health VAS from week 36 to 40	1.04 (1.02, 1.05)	1.03 (1.02, 1.05)	1.03 (1.02, 1.04)
HAQ score at week 40	2.00 (1.31, 3.06)	*1.50 (0.94, 2.38)*	2.04 (1.47, 2.83)
Change in HAQ score from week 36 to 40	2.16 (1.11, 4.20)	3.40 (1.75, 6.59)	3.41 (2.12, 5.46)
TJC at week 40	1.15 (1.09, 1.22)	1.46 (1.31, 1.63)	1.22 (1.14, 1.30)
Change in TJC from week 36 to 40	1.15 (1.08, 1.22)	1.55 (1.37, 1.76)	1.24 (1.16, 1.32)
SJC at week 40	1.11 (0.98, 1.26)	1.44 (1.26, 1.65)	1.18 (1.09, 1.27)
Change in SJC from week 36 to 40	1.31 (1.14, 1.50)	1.40 (1.19, 1.64)	1.23 (1.13, 1.35)
Pain VAS at week 40	1.02 (1.01, 1.03)	1.03 (1.01, 1.04)	1.02 (1.01, 1.03)
Change in pain VAS from week 36 to 40	1.03 (1.01, 1.04)	1.05 (1.04, 1.07)	1.03 (1.02, 1.03)
Loss of DAS28 remission and change in DAS28 ≥ 0.6 in double-blind period			
Lack of sustained DAS28 remission	2.82 (1.64, 4.85)	2.59 (1.44, 4.66)	1.98 (1.33, 2.96)
Sustained weighted DAS28 remission	0.68 (0.57, 0.82)	0.68 (0.55, 0.83)	0.78 (0.67, 0.91)
DAS28 at week 36	*1.21 (0.80, 1.83)*	2.04 (1.25, 3.34)	*1.35 (0.95, 1.90)*
DAS28 at week 40	3.55 (2.67, 4.71)	7.18 (4.79, 10.75)	2.65 (2.17, 3.23)
Change in DAS28 from week 36 to 40	3.55 (2.67, 4.71)	7.18 (4.79, 10.75)	2.65 (2.17, 3.23)
ESR at week 40	1.05 (1.02, 1.08)	1.05 (1.02, 1.07)	1.02 (1.01, 1.03)
Change in ESR from week 36 to 40	1.09 (1.05, 1.12)	1.07 (1.04, 1.10)	1.02 (1.01, 1.03)
Sustained weighted SDAI remission	*0.71 (0.49, 1.01)*	0.47 (0.30, 0.76)	*0.81 (0.60, 1.09)*
SDAI at week 40	1.13 (1.09, 1.18)	1.29 (1.21, 1.38)	1.10 (1.07, 1.12)
Change in SDAI from week 36 to 40	1.15 (1.10, 1.20)	1.26 (1.19, 1.34)	1.11 (1.08, 1.14)
Sustained weighted CDAI remission	*0.80 (0.58, 1.10)*	0.48 (0.31, 0.74)	*0.85 (0.64, 1.14)*
CDAI at week 40	1.13 (1.09, 1.18)	1.28 (1.21, 1.36)	1.10 (1.07, 1.13)
Change in CDAI from week 36 to 40	1.14 (1.10, 1.19)	1.26 (1.19, 1.34)	1.11 (1.08, 1.14)

Table 3 Predictors of loss of remission in all treatment groups in the double-blind period *(Continued)*

Predictor[a]	Adjusted hazard ratio[b] (95% CI)		
	ETN 50 mg + MTX *n* = 74	ETN 25 mg + MTX *n* = 56	MTX *n* = 66
HAQ at week 40	1.74 (1.08, 2.80)	1.85 (1.15, 2.98)	2.17 (1.55, 3.04)
Change in HAQ from week 36 to 40	*1.74 (0.85, 3.56)*	4.21 (2.11, 8.39)	4.24 (2.61, 6.89)
PGA at week 40	1.55 (1.26, 1.91)	1.92 (1.54, 2.38)	1.30 (1.18, 1.43)
Change in PGA from week 36 to 40	1.70 (1.36, 2.11)	1.60 (1.23, 2.08)	1.30 (1.17, 1.43)
PtGA at week 40	1.25 (1.12, 1.40)	1.34 (1.17, 1.53)	1.30 (1.20, 1.41)
Change in PtGA from week 36 to 40	1.27 (1.12, 1.43)	1.52 (1.27 1.82)	1.35 (1.23, 1.47)
General health at week 40	1.03 (1.01, 1.04)	1.03 (1.01, 1.04)	1.03 (1.01, 1.04)
Change in general health from week 36 to 40	1.04 (1.02, 1.06)	1.03 (1.02, 1.05)	1.03 (1.02, 1.04)
TJC at week 40	1.16 (1.10, 1.23)	1.50 (1.34, 1.69)	1.25 (1.17, 1.34)
Change in TJC from week 36 to 40	1.16 (1.10, 1.23)	1.59 (1.39, 1.80)	1.28 (1.20, 1.37)
SJC at week 40	1.18 (1.03, 1.34)	1.51 (1.32, 1.73)	1.17 (1.08, 1.26)
Change in SJC from week 36 to 40	1.35 (1.16, 1.56)	1.49 (1.27, 1.75)	1.28 (1.17, 1.40)
Pain VAS at week 40	1.02 (1.01, 1.03)	1.03 (1.02, 1.05)	1.02 (1.01, 1.03)
Change in pain VAS from week 36 to 40	1.03 (1.01, 1.04)	1.05 (1.03, 1.07)	1.03, (1.02, 1.04)
	ETN 50 mg + MTX *n* = 72	ETN 25 mg + MTX *n* = 60	MTX *n* = 53
Loss of SDAI remission at single time point in double-blind period			
Lack of sustained SDAI remission	*2.57 (0.90, 7.32)*	*1.86 (0.55, 6.24)*	2.92 (1.08, 7.94)
Sustained weighted SDAI remission	0.67 (0.49, 0.90)	0.62 (0.45, 0.86)	0.68 (0.51, 0.90)
SDAI at week 36	1.56 (1.06, 2.29)	2.00 (1.34, 3.00)	*1.14 (0.80, 1.62)*
SDAI at week 40	1.13 (1.07, 1.19)	1.18 (1.09, 1.29)	1.05 (1.02, 1.08)
Change in SDAI from week 36 to 40	1.13 (1.07, 1.19)	1.18 (1.09, 1.29)	1.05 (1.02, 1.08)
Sustained weighted CDAI remission	0.71 (0.53, 0.95)	0.61 (0.44, 0.83)	0.71 (0.54, 0.92)
CDAI at week 40	1.12 (1.07, 1.18)	1.18 (1.09, 1.29)	1.05 (1.02, 1.08)
Change in CDAI from week 36 to 40	1.12 (1.07, 1.18)	1.19 (1.09, 1.29)	1.05 (1.02, 1.08)
Sustained weighted DAS28 remission	*0.81 (0.63, 1.03)*	*0.93 (0.71, 1.22)*	*0.86 (0.67, 1.10)*
DAS28 at week 40	1.76 (1.20, 2.59)	1.70 (1.05, 2.77)	1.46 (1.19, 1.79)
Change in DAS28 from week 36 to 40	2.09 (1.47, 2.96)	2.55 (1.52, 4.28)	1.62 (1.24, 2.11)
HAQ score at week 40	*1.76 (0.90, 3.44)*	*1.92 (0.86, 4.26)*	2.22 (1.17, 4.21)
Change in HAQ score from week 36 to 40	*2.66 (0.89, 7.96)*	6.13 (1.69, 22.26)	4.25 (1.83, 9.91)
PGA at week 40	1.77 (1.37, 2.29)	1.79 (1.32, 2.42)	1.27 (1.10, 1.47)
Change in PGA from week 36 to 40	1.69 (1.33, 2.14)	1.88 (1.30, 2.70)	1.26 (1.09, 1.46)
PtGA at week 40	1.37 (1.17, 1.61)	1.72 (1.32, 2.24)	1.30 (1.13, 1.50)
Change in PtGA from week 36 to 40	1.40 (1.20, 1.64)	1.73 (1.32, 2.27)	1.30 (1.14, 1.50)
General health VAS at week 40	1.04 (1.01, 1.07)	1.04 (1.01, 1.06)	1.02 (1.01, 1.04)
Change in general health VAS from week 36 to 40	1.05 (1.02, 1.07)	1.04, (1.01, 1.06)	1.03 (1.01, 1.04)
TJC at week 40	1.31 (1.10, 1.56)	1.36 (1.11, 1.68)	*1.05 (1.00, 1.11)*
Change in TJC from week 36 to 40	1.38 (1.14, 1.67)	1.38 (1.13, 1.69)	*1.06 (1.00, 1.12)*
SJC at week 40	1.31 (1.05, 1.63)	*1.15 (0.91, 1.44)*	1.17 (1.01, 1.36)
Change in SJC from week 36 to 40	1.30 (1.04, 1.63)	*1.15 (0.93, 1.44)*	1.17 (1.01, 1.35)
Pain VAS at week 40	1.03 (1.01, 1.05)	1.05 (1.02, 1.08)	1.03 (1.01, 1.04)
Change in pain VAS from week 36 to 40	1.04 (1.02, 1.06)	1.05 (1.03, 1.09)	1.03 (1.01, 1.05)

Table 3 Predictors of loss of remission in all treatment groups in the double-blind period *(Continued)*

Predictor[a]	Adjusted hazard ratio[b] (95% CI)		
	ETN 50 mg + MTX *n* = 74	ETN 25 mg + MTX *n* = 56	MTX *n* = 66
Loss of CDAI remission at single time point in double-blind period			
Lack of sustained CDAI remission	*2.10 (0.82, 5.40)*	*2.82 (0.83, 9.55)*	2.60 (1.04, 6.48)
Sustained weighted CDAI remission	0.69 (0.51, 0.92)	0.57 (0.42, 0.78)	0.71 (0.55, 0.93)
CDAI at week 36	1.49 (1.04, 2.15)	1.65 (1.14, 2.39)	*1.07 (0.76, 1.51)*
CDAI at week 40	1.15 (1.09, 1.21)	1.21 (1.11, 1.31)	1.05 (1.02, 1.09)
Change in CDAI from week 36 to 40	1.15 (1.09, 1.21)	1.21 (1.11, 1.31)	1.05 (1.02, 1.09)
Sustained weighted SDAI remission	0.63 (0.46, 0.87)	0.59 (0.42, 0.81)	(0.68 (0.51, 0.90)
Sustained weighted DAS28 remission	*0.78 (0.61, 1.00)*	*0.96 (0.76, 1.22)*	*0.81 (0.63, 1.04)*
DAS28 at week 40	1.95 (1.30, 2.91)	2.12 (1.32, 3.38)	1.51 (1.23, 1.86)
Change in DAS28 from week 36 to 40	2.11 (1.47, 3.01)	2.87 (1.77, 4.66)	1.71 (1.31, 2.22)
HAQ score at week 40	2.10 (1.10, 4.00)	*1.87 (0.85, 4.12)*	2.10 (1.10, 4.02)
Change in HAQ score from week 36 to 40	4.00 (1.38, 11.62)	10.88 (3.35, 35.34)	4.34 (1.86, 10.12)
PGA at week 40	1.93 (1.49, 2.49)	1.90 (1.40, 2.56)	1.30 (1.13, 1.50)
Change in PGA from week 36 to 40	1.83 (1.42, 2.35)	2.07 (1.48, 2.91)	1.30 (1.12, 1.51)
PtGA at week 40	1.45 (1.23, 1.70)	1.82 (1.40, 2.37)	1.32 (1.16, 1.51)
Change in PtGA from week 36 to 40	1.46 (1.24, 1.72)	1.75 (1.35, 2.28)	1.34 (1.17, 1.53)
General health VAS at week 40	1.05 (1.02, 1.08)	1.04 (1.02, 1.06)	1.03 (1.01, 1.04)
Change in general health VAS from week 36 to 40	1.05 (1.03, 1.08)	1.04 (1.02, 1.07)	1.03 (1.01, 1.04)
TJC at week 40	1.41 (1.18, 1.68)	1.41 (1.15, 1.74)	1.06 (1.01, 1.12)
Change in TJC from week 36 to 40	1.50 (1.24, 1.82)	1.45 (1.19, 1.76)	1.07 (1.01, 1.13)
SJC at week 40	1.40 (1.12, 1.74)	*1.19 (0.96, 1.49)*	1.20 (1.04, 1.39)
Change in SJC from week 36 to 40	1.39 (1.10, 1.74)	*1.20 (0.97, 1.49)*	1.20 (1.04, 1.39)
Pain VAS at week 40	1.04 (1.02, 1.06)	1.05 (1.03, 1.08)	1.03 (1.01, 1.04)
Change in pain VAS from week 36 to 40	1.04 (1.02, 1.06)	1.06 (1.03, 1.09)	1.03 (1.02, 1.05)

CDAI Clinical Disease Activity Index, *CI* confidence interval, *DAS28* Disease Activity Score based on a 28-joint count, *ESR* erythrocyte sedimentation rate, *ETN* etanercept, *HAQ* health assessment questionnaire, *MTX* methotrexate, *PGA* physician global assessment, *PtGA* patient global assessment, *SDAI* Simplified Disease Activity Index, *SJC* swollen joint count, *TJC* tender joint count, *VAS* visual analog scale

[a]Included factors were significant predictors of remission loss in at least one of the three treatment arms, except lack of sustained SDAI/CDAI remission, SJC at week 40, and change in SJC from week 30 to 40 for SDAI and CDAI loss of remission. Sustained remission predictors are weighted. Hazard ratios that are not statistically significant are reported in italics

[b]From Cox proportional hazards model for loss of response, adjusted for baseline of respective outcome (e.g., baseline DAS28, SDAI, or CDAI). Higher hazard ratios denote a higher likelihood of loss of remission. Results cannot be compared across treatment groups because separate models were used for each

continuous week-36 and week-40 DAS28, and change in DA28 from week 36 to week 40). These predictors were significant even after adjustment for week-36 DAS28, indicating that they explain additional variance beyond what is explained by week-36 DAS28. Similar results were generally found in analyses of predictors of the loss of DAS28 remission plus a change in DAS28 ≥ 0.6 in the double-blind period, as well as loss of SDAI and CDAI remission. However, failure to achieve sustained SDAI or CDAI remission was significantly predictive of the respective SDAI or CDAI loss of remission only in the placebo group, but not in either of the combination therapy groups; change in HAQ from week 36 to week 40 appeared to be one of the strongest predictors of both endpoints.

Based on a stepwise model, the strongest set of predictors of the loss of DAS28 remission in the double-blind period in patients maintained on full-dose combination therapy included higher DAS28 and PtGA at week 40; longer disease duration at baseline; less change from baseline in CDAI from week 36 to 40; and lack of sustained DAS28 remission in the open-label period (Fig. 4). In patients who received reduced-dose combination therapy, the strongest set of predictors of loss of DAS28 remission also included higher DAS28 at week 40 and prior lack of sustained DAS28 remission, in addition to ESR levels higher than the ULN at week 36, high SJC at week 36, and greater change in PtGA from weeks 36 to 40. The strongest set of predictors in patients who

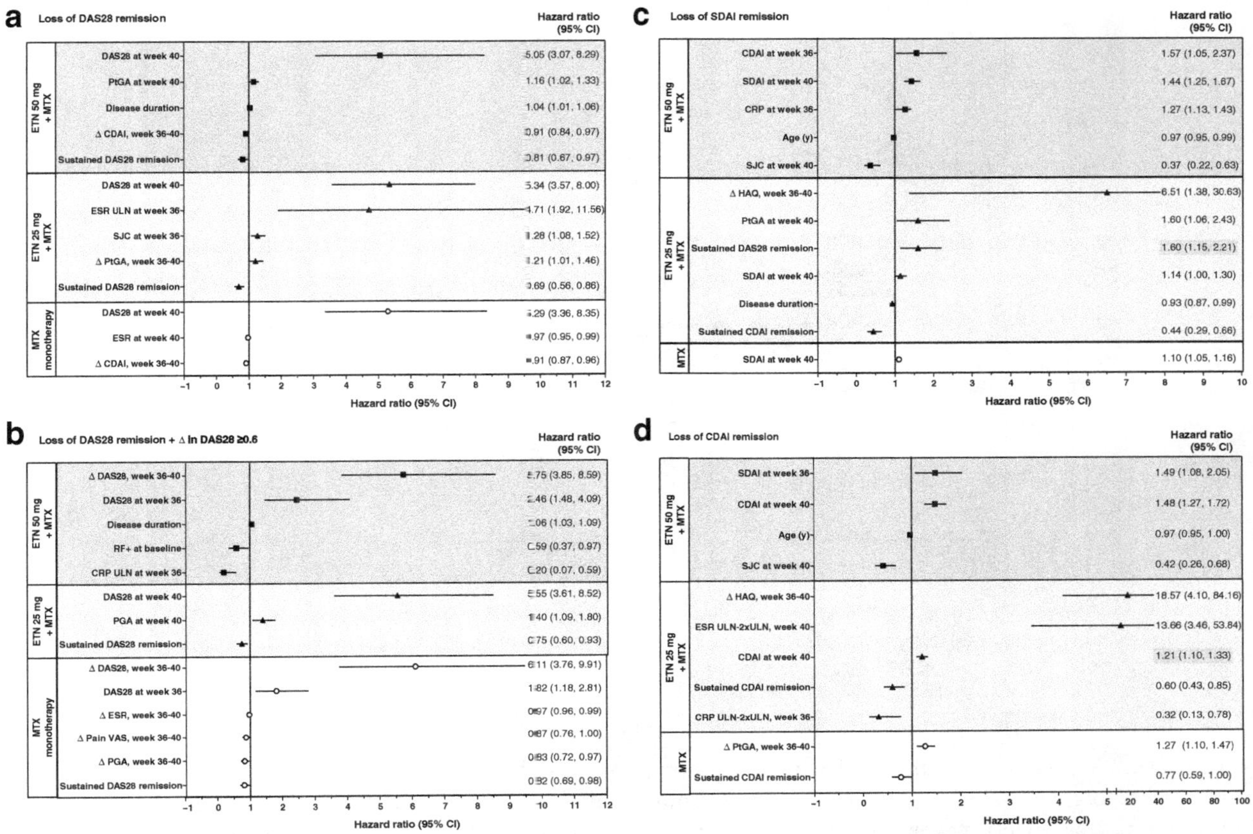

Fig. 4 Strongest sets of predictors of loss of Disease Activity Score based on a 28-joint count (DAS28) remission (**a**), DAS28 remission plus change in DAS28 ≥ 0.6 (**b**), Simplified Disease Activity Index (SDAI) remission (**c**), and Clinical Disease Activity Index (CDAI) remission (**d**) in the double-blind period by treatment group using stepwise models. CI, confidence interval; CRP, C-reactive protein; ESR, erythrocyte sedimentation rate; HAQ, health assessment questionnaire; PGA, physician global assessment; PtGA, patient global assessment; RF, rheumatoid factor; SJC, swollen joint count; ULN, upper limit of normal; VAS, visual analog scale

received methotrexate monotherapy in the double-blind period also included DAS28 at week 40, low ESR levels at week 40, and less change in CDAI from weeks 36 to 40. For loss of SDAI and CDAI remission, the strongest sets of predictors in patients maintained on full-dose combination therapy were similar, including high SDAI/CDAI at week 36 or 40, younger age at baseline, and lower SJC at week 40; however, less similarity was observed in the sets of predictors in the reduced-dose combination and methotrexate monotherapy groups (Fig. 4).

In analyses using logistic regression models conducted to determine which patients were most likely to experience sustained remission after tapering the etanercept dose or withdrawing the biologic agent, DAS28 after full-dose induction therapy was shown to predict the probability of subsequent loss of response. Patients receiving reduced-dose combination therapy or methotrexate monotherapy who had lower DAS28 at week 36 were less likely to lose remission or LDA in the double-blind period (Fig. 5). Although the relationship between week-36 DAS28 and loss of response in these treatment groups was strong, 95% CIs indicate that the prediction is not precise and no clear cut-point values predictive of loss of remission can be derived. The relationships between week-36 SDAI and CDAI and loss of remission/LDA were less consistent than those for DAS28 (Additional file 3: Figure S2).

Additional analyses showed that in all treatment groups, patients who achieved DAS28 remission only at week 36 or only at weeks 28 and 36 vs. weeks 12, 20, 28, and 36 were much more likely to lose remission at at least one time point after week 36 through week 88, regardless of the index used to measure disease activity (Fig. 6a–d). The trend was less prominent in the treatment group receiving methotrexate monotherapy during the latter period.

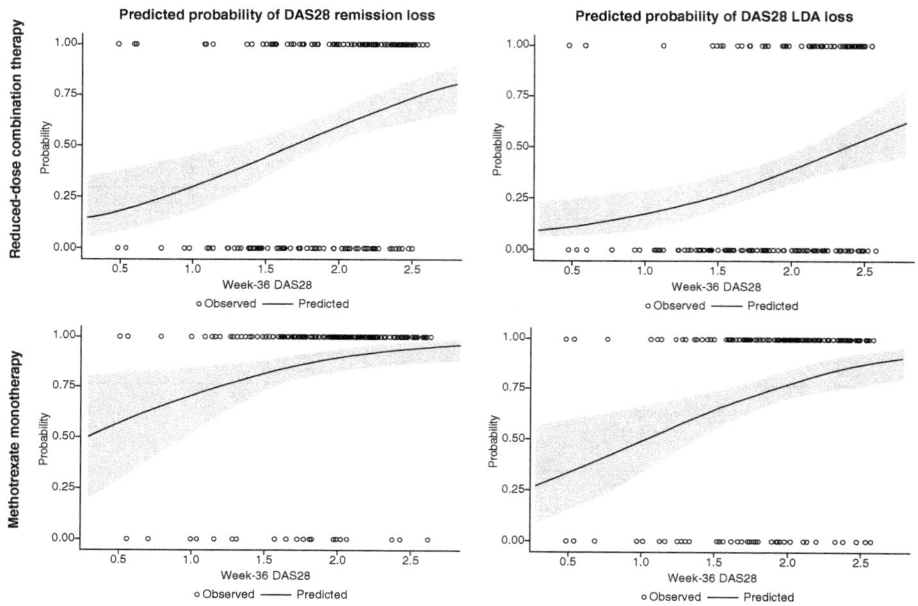

Fig. 5 Predicted probability (95% CI) of the loss of Disease Activity Score based on a 28-joint count (DAS28) remission and low disease activity (LDA) in patients receiving reduced-dose combination therapy or methotrexate monotherapy in the double-blind period based on mean DAS28 at week 36 of the open-label period, using logistic regression models. Circles at the top, patients who lost response; circles at the bottom, patients who did not lose response; smooth line, model-predicted probability of loss of response as a function of week-36 DAS28; shadowed area, 95% CI

Mean DAS28 levels were markedly higher among patients who lost remission at at least one time point than among those who never lost remission in all three treatment groups (Additional file 4: Figure S3). The difference in mean DAS28 between patients who did and did not lose remission was evident at week 36; at this time point, patients who lost remission had a mean DAS28 of approximately 2.2 and patients who never lost remission had a mean DAS28 of 1.6–1.7, which remained at this level even after reduction or withdrawal of etanercept. The difference in DAS28 levels between those who lost and never lost remission was greatest in the methotrexate monotherapy group.

Discussion

The PRESERVE trial was designed before the development of ACR/EULAR remission criteria and, therefore, DAS28 < 2.6 had been pre-specified as remission in accordance with the trends at that time. However, evidence suggests that patients in DAS28 remission may have substantial residual disease activity [13–15], which is further supported by the present analyses of findings from the PRESERVE trial, as the likelihood of maintaining a good outcome increased with decreasing DAS28 in the "remission" state. The findings of the PRESERVE trial presented in the current report reveal that a large proportion of patients with moderate RA were able to achieve DAS28 remission with full-dose combination etanercept-plus-methotrexate therapy by the end of the open-label period; however, withdrawal of etanercept after achievement of response resulted in a loss of remission in many patients in the double-blind period [6]. As derived from both the univariate and stepwise logistic regression models, patients with moderately active RA who had received full-dose etanercept and methotrexate as induction therapy were significantly more likely to achieve DAS28, SDAI, and CDAI remission if they had lower DAS28/CDAI/SDAI, younger age, BMI <30 kg/m^2, and lower HAQ score at baseline.

In a subpopulation of patients who were in remission at week 36, DAS28 response was found to be decreased in all treatment groups at the first post-randomization visit (week 40), possibly due to an artificially increased response at week 36 because achievement of DAS28 LDA was required for enrollment in the double-blind period and/or to the changeover from an open-label to a blinded, randomized study. Approximately 25–34% of patients in the full-dose or reduced-dose etanercept-plus-methotrexate groups were not in DAS28 remission at any visit in the double-blind period, having regressed toward their non-remission rate of approximately 25% at week 28 in the open-label period. Interestingly, the mean DAS28 (2.7 (2.5, 2.9)) in patients in the full-dose combination therapy group who lost remission at least once in the double-blind period suggests that patients who lost DAS28 remission at any time point in this period were, on average, near remission at week 88. In contrast, in the methotrexate monotherapy group, the mean

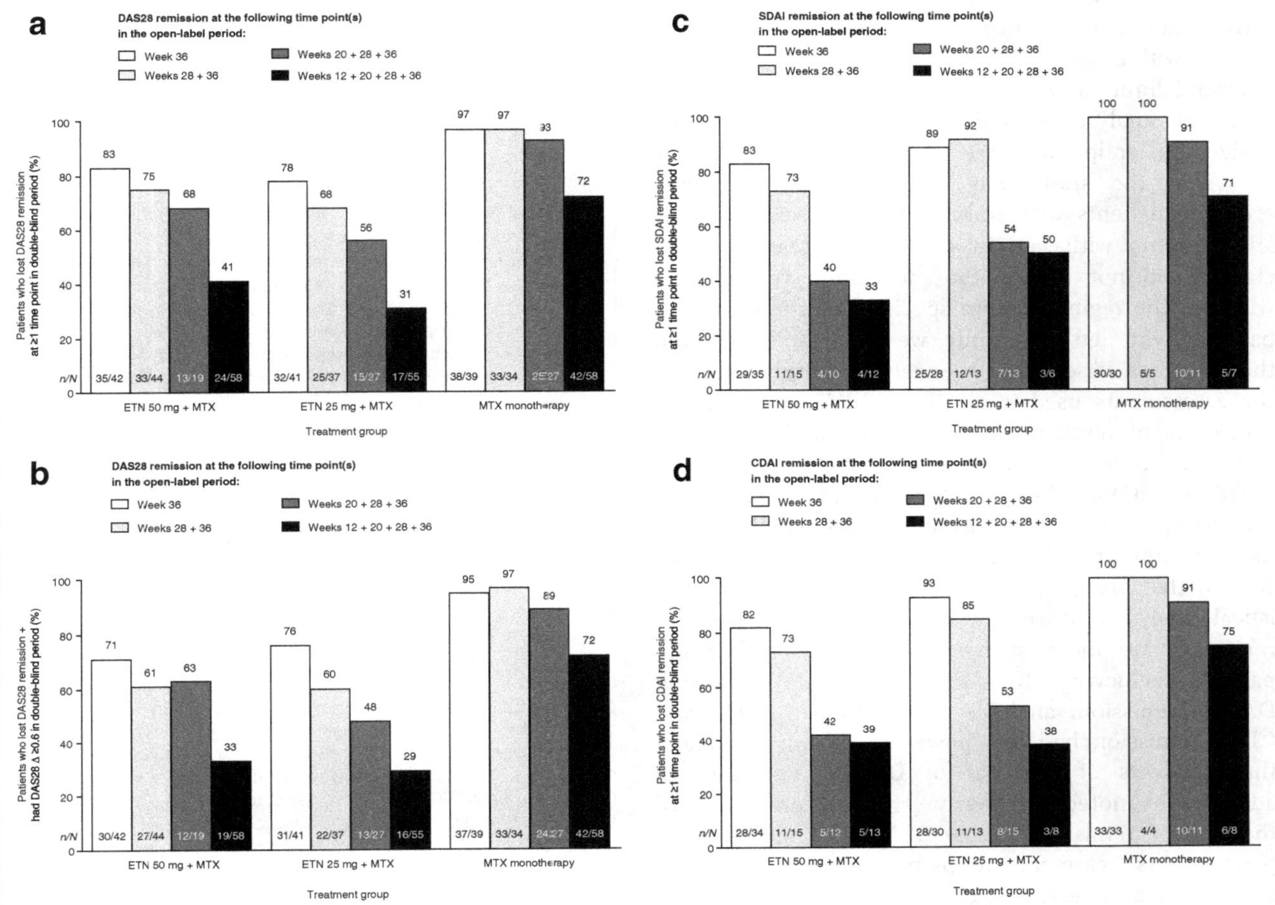

Fig. 6 Proportions of patients who lost Disease Activity Score based on a 28-joint count (DAS28) remission (**a**), DAS28 remission and had a change in DAS28 ≥ 0.6 (**b**), Simplified Disease Activity Index (SDAI) remission (**c**), and Clinical Disease Activity Index (CDAI) remission (**d**) at least once at any time point in the double-blind period by duration of remission in the open-label period. *n/N*, numbers of patients who lost remission in the double-blind period/numbers of patients who had remission at specified time points in the open-label period. Patients included in the loss of remission models (i.e., patients with remission at week 36). ETN, etanercept; MTX, methotrexate

DAS28 (3.7 (3.5, 3.9)) in patients who lost remission at least once in the double-blind period indicates a higher level of disease activity that did not similarly approach remission. Most patients who lost DAS28 remission in the double-blind period did so in the month between week 36 (randomization) and week 40; the greatest change in DAS28 scores among patients who lost remission in that period was also observed in this interval. These observations help explain the numerous significant predictors of remission loss identified at week 40 across remission endpoints.

Our findings suggest that patients who did not achieve sustained remission in the open-label period and had higher DAS28 at week 36 were more likely to lose remission with maintenance therapy in the double-blind period. Not surprisingly, patients who achieved remission at only week 36, those who sustained remission at only weeks 28 and 36, and those who sustained remission at only weeks 20, 28, and 36, were at higher risk for loss of remission than patients who sustained remission from week 12 to week 36, indicating that depth of disease control is an important predictor of remission loss. In line with the residual disease activity in patients with a DAS28 < 2.6 mentioned above, the lower the DAS28, and thus the lower the residual disease activity level, the greater the likelihood of sustained response. This result underscores and reinforces the current treat-to-target approach and the importance of adjusting treatment in patients who are not achieving the lowest levels of disease activity currently recommended in ACR/EULAR treatment guidelines [16, 17], as it suggests that the depth and duration of response are relevant. Predictors identified for the maintenance of SDAI and CDAI remission (with the exception of failure to achieve sustained SDAI or CDAI) further support the conclusion of a better outcome with lower disease activity and maintenance of a good response at the time of withdrawal.

Several limitations of the PRESERVE trial and these post hoc analyses should be considered. The study design and endpoints were contemporary at the time at which the study was initiated, and the study excluded patients with mild or severe disease activity and patients with certain comorbid diseases. Physicians could not modify the medication regimens at will (i.e., the regimens were specified by the protocol); patients who left the study were not followed and therefore not assessed. The analyses were limited to the assessments used in the PRESERVE trial and the predictors of remission analyses were limited to data collected in the first 36-week period of the study; in addition, patient follow up occurred at a fixed interval. Sample sizes were small in the methotrexate monotherapy group because most patients lost remission in that group, which resulted in less robust statistical analyses. Moreover, because SDAI and CDAI remission are more stringent endpoints, with fewer patients achieving them than patients achieving DAS28 remission, analyses of the loss of SDAI and CDAI remission had less power to detect differences than analyses of the loss of DAS28 remission. In addition, as noted previously, HRs for predictors of the loss of remission (Table 3) should not be compared across treatment groups because each treatment group has a different rate of loss of remission. Although similar proportions of patients treated with etanercept 50 mg and etanercept 25 mg maintained remission in the double-blind period, differences in HRs for some predictors of the loss of remission were seen between these groups (e.g., change in DAS28 at week 40, change in DAS28 from week 36 to 40).

Conclusion

The findings of the analyses in the current report suggest that targeting sustained and stringently defined clinical remission in patients receiving full-dose combination etanercept-plus-methotrexate therapy before considering dose or regimen changes may help improve the likelihood that patients will remain in clinical remission 1 year after the changes are made. Patients who are younger and have BMI <30 kg/m^2, lower HAQ scores, and lower disease activity, as measured by DAS28, SDAI, and CDAI, at baseline may be most likely to achieve a remission state with full-dose combination etanercept-methotrexate induction therapy, whereas those who achieve an early, strong, and durable response to induction therapy are most likely to experience a sustained response after biologic tapering or withdrawal.

Additional files

Additional file 1: Appendix 1 and Appendix 2. (DOCX 22 kb)

Additional file 2: Figure S1. Summary of patient disposition in the open-label and double-blind periods. *CDAI* Clinical Disease Activity Index, *DAS28* Disease Activity Score based on a 28-joint count, *ETN* etanercept, *LDA* low disease activity, *MTX* methotrexate, *QW* once weekly, *SDAI* Simplified Disease Activity Index. (EPS 1688 kb)

Additional file 3: Figure S2. Predicted probability (95% CI) of the loss of SDAI remission and LDA (**a**) and the loss of CDAI remission and LDA (b) in patients receiving reduced-dose combination therapy or methotrexate monotherapy in the double-blind period based on mean SDAI/CDAI at week 36 of the open-label period, using logistic regression models. Circles at the top indicate patients who lost response; circles at bottom indicate patients who did not lose response; smooth line, model-predicted probability of loss of response as a function of week-36 DAS28; shadowed area, 95% CI. (EPS 2683 kb)

Additional file 4: Figure S3. Mean DAS28 levels in patients who lost remission at ≥1 time point and who never lost remission in the double-blind period. mITT population in double-blind period who had remission at week 36. *CI* confidence interval, *DAS28* Disease Activity Score based on a 28-joint count, *ETN* etanercept, *mITT* modified intent-to-treat, *MTX* methotrexate. (EPS 1406 kb)

Abbreviations

ACPA: Anti-citrullinated peptide antibody; ACR/EULAR: American College of Rheumatology/European League Against Rheumatism; BMI: Body mass index; CDAI: Clinical Disease Activity Index; CI: Confidence interval; CRP: C-reactive protein; DAS28: Disease Activity Score in 28 joints; ESR: Erythrocyte sedimentation rate; ETN: Etanercept; HAQ: Health Assessment Questionnaire; JSN: Joint space narrowing; LDA: Low disease activity; mITT: Modified intent-to-treat; mTSS: Modified total Sharp score; MTX: Methotrexate; PGA: Physician global assessment; PRO: Patient-reported outcome; PtGA: Patient global assessment; QW: Once weekly; RA: Rheumatoid arthritis; RF: Rheumatoid factor; SD: Standard deviation; SDAI: Simplified Disease Activity Index; SJC: Swollen joint count; TJC: Tender joint count; TNF: Tumor necrosis factor; ULN: Upper limit of normal

Acknowledgements

PRESERVE trial investigators: we thank the PRESERVE investigators, their staff, and their patients for their participation in this clinical trial. In addition to the authors, the PRESERVE trial investigators included: Australia—P. Bird, R.R. Buchanan, M. Marabani, M. Smith, R. Will; Austria—J. Muellner, F. Rainer; Belgium—M. Malaise, F.E. van den Bosch; Chile—O.J. Neira; Colombia—M. Chalem, A.M. Dominguez, Antonio Guzmán Moreno, J.J. Jaller Raad; Czech Republic—D. Galatikova, L. Prochazkova, P. Vavrincova, P. Vitek; France—A. Cantagrel, B. Combe, L. Euller-Ziegler, P. Hilliquin, X. Mariette, O. Meyer, X. Puechal, J. Sibilia; Germany—G.-R. Burmester, U. Müller-Ladner, A. Rubbert-Roth, H.-P. Tony, H. Tremel, U. Wagner, J. Wollenhaupt; Hungary—P. Géher, L. Náfrádi, B. Rojkovich, Z. Szekanecz; Italy—A. Afeltra, B. Canesi, R. Carignola, R. Foti; Mexico—R. Burgos-Vargas, M. Garza Elizondo, J.J. Orozco Alcalá, F.A. Rosas-Lopez, J.A. Simon; Poland—M. Brzosko, A. Filipowicz-Sosnowska, S. Jeka, J. Lewandowicz, M. Majdanl, M. Rell-Bakalarska; Republic of Korea—H.-J. Baek, H.-A. Kim, I.J. Kim, S.-H. Lee, S.-C. Shim, D.-H. Yoo; Russia—L. Alexeeva, V.I. Mazurov, E.L. Nasonov, N. Sanina, E. Shmidt; Serbia—N. Damjanov, A. Dimic, D. Stefanovic; Spain— F.J. Blanco Garcia, A. Fernandez-Nebro, J.J. Gómez-Reino Carnota, J. Gratacós Masmitjá, F.J. López Longo, F.N. Sarabia, R. Sanmartí Sala; Sweden—J. Lysholm, A. Teleman; Taiwan—D.-M. Chang, J.-H. Yen; The Netherlands—E.J.A. Kroot, H.R.M. Peeters, D. Siewertsz van Reesema, H.R. van den Brink,E. van der Bijl; United Kingdom—C. Chattopadhyay, G.D. Kitas. Sponsored by Pfizer.

Funding

The PRESERVE trial was sponsored by Wyeth, which was acquired by Pfizer in October 2009 and which was responsible for collecting and analyzing the data. The sub-analyses of the PRESERVE trial conducted for this publication were sponsored by Pfizer. Editorial/medical writing support was provided by Kim Brown and Donna McGuire of Engage Scientific Solutions and was funded by Pfizer.

Availability of data and materials
Pfizer's policies on the provision of clinical trial data are available at: http://www.pfizer.com/research/clinical_trials/trial_data_and_results As described on this website, in addition to providing clinical trial results on the ClinicalTrials.gov registry, Pfizer provides secure access to anonymized patient-level data to qualified researchers in response to scientifically valid research proposals. Pfizer makes patient-level data available for globally conducted interventional trials in patients that complete after 27 September 2007, or initiated on or before that date and still ongoing as of 26 December 2007, as well as all such trials initiated after January 2014. Data are made available for trials of authorized medicines/indications, or terminated medicines, 2 years after clinical trial completion (defined as last subject last visit). Pfizer's practices adhere to the principles for responsible data sharing established by the European Federation of Pharmaceutical Industries and Associations (EFPIA) and the Pharmaceutical Research and Manufacturers of America (PhRMA): http://phrma.org/sites/default/files/pdf/PhRMAPrinciplesForResponsibleClinicalTrialDataSharing.pdf.

Authors' contributions
JSS, ASK, and TVJ made substantial contributions to the conception or design of the study. JSS, AS, ASK, TV, and LM contributed to the acquisition and interpretation of study data. AS conducted the statistical analyses. All authors (JSS, AS, ASK, TVJ, and LM) were involved in drafting the article or revising it for critically important intellectual content; all reviewed and approved the final manuscript to be published. All authors had full access to the study data and take responsibility for the integrity of the data and the accuracy of the data analysis.

Ethics approval and consent to participate
The PRESERVE trial was conducted in accordance with the ethical principles of the Declaration of Helsinki and the guidelines for Good Clinical Practice of the International Conference on Harmonisation. All patients were required to sign an informed consent form. The institutional review board or independent ethics committee at the following participating centers reviewed and approved all consent forms and the PRESERVE study protocol: Australia – Bellberry Limited, Dulwich, SA; Flinders Clinical Research Ethics Committee, Repatriation General Hospital, Daw Park, SA; The Austin Health Human Research Ethics Committee, Heidelberg, VIC. Austria – Ethikkommission der Stadt Wien, Wien. Belgium – Comite d'ethique Hospitalo-Facultaire Universitaire de Liege, Centre Hospitalier Universitaire du Sart Tilman, Liege; CHU Liege, Comité d'Ethique de la Faculté de Médicine, Centre Hospitalier Universitaire du Sart Tilman, Liege. Chile – Comite Etico Cientifico, Servicio de Salud Metropolitano Oriente, Santiago, RM. Colombia – Comite de etica de la fundacion instituto de reumatologia Fernando Chalem, Bogota, Cundinamarca; Comité de etica independiente centro de reumatologia y ortopedia, Barranquilla, Atlantico; Comite de Etica de la Investigacion Riesgo de Fractura S.A., Bogota, Cundinamarca. Czech Republic – Eticka komise Fakultni nemocnice Olomouc a Lekarske fakulty, Univerzity Palackeho, Olomouc Ethics Committee of Institute of Rheumatology, Praha; Eticka komise pro multicentricka klinicka hodnoceni Fakultni nemocnice v Motole, Praha; Multicentricka eticka komise Fakultni nemocnice u sv. Anny v Brne - decasovane pracoviste, Brno. France – Comité de Protection des Personnes, Sud-Ouest et Outre-Mer II Hôpital Purpan, Toulouse Cedex 9. Germany – Ethik-Kommission bei der Medizinischen Fakultaet der Universitaet Wuerzburg, Institut fuer Pharmakologie und Toxikologie, Wuerzburg. Hungary – Egeszsegugyi Tudomanyos Tanacs Klinikai Farmakologiai Etikai Bizottsaga, Budapest. Italy – Comitato Etico Scientifico dell'Azienda Ospedaliera Ospedale Niguarda Ca' Granda di Milano, Milano; Comitato Etico Azienda Ospedaliera Universitaria San Luigi Gonzaga di Orbassano, Orbassano; Comitato Etico dell'Universita' Campus Bio-Medico di Roma, Roma; Comitato Etico dell'Azienda Ospedali Vittorio Emanuele, Ferrarotto, S.Bambino, Catania. Republic of Korea – Institutional Review Board, Gangnam Severance Hospital, Seoul; Institutional Review Board/Ethics Commitee of Kangdong Sacred Heart Hospital, Seoul; Hallym University Sacred Heart Hospital Institutional Review Board, Anyang-Si, Gyeonggi-do; Institutional Review Board for Human Research, Konkuk University Hospital, Seoul; Institutional Review Board, Gachon Gil Medical Center, Incheon; Hanyang University Hospital IRB, Seoul; IRB of Eulji University Hospital, Daejeon. Mexico – Comite de Etica de la Facultad de Medidna de la UANL Hospital Universitario Dr Jose Eleuterio Gonzalez, Monterrey NL; Comite Bioetico para la Investigacion Clinica S. C., Puebla 422, Mexico, DF; Comite de Etica del Hospital San Javier, Guadalajara, Jalisco; Comité de Investigación del Hospital CEM, Merida, Yucatán. The Netherlands – Independent Review Board Nijmegen (IRBN) Nijmegen, Wijchen. Poland – Komisja Etyczna Przy Instytucie Reumatologicznym ul Spartanska 1, Warszawa. Russian Federation - Biomedical Ethics Committee at FGU "Severo-Zapadny District Medical Center of Rozdrav," St. Petersburg; Ethical council under responsibility of department of state regulation of circulation of medicines, Ministry of Public Health and Social Development of Russian Federation, Moscow; Local Ethics Committee at GU Institute of Rheumatology of RAMS, Moscow; Local Ethics Committee at GUZ "City Clinical Hospital #1 n.a., N.I.Pirogov," Rheumatology Department, Moscow; Local Ethics Committee at GUZ at Leningrad Regional Clinical Hospital, St. Petersburg; Local Ethics Committee at Moscow Regional Research Clinical Institute, n.a. M.F. Vladimirskogo, Moscow. Serbia and Montenegro – Ethics Committee of Institute of Rheumatology-Belgrade, Belgrade; Ethics Committee of Institute for Treatment and Rehabilitation "Niska Banja," Niska Banja; Ethics Committee Military Medical Academy, Belgrade. Spain – Hospital General Universitario Gregorio Marañon, Comite etico de Investigacion Clinica c/Doctor, Madrid. Sweden – Regionala etikprovningsnamnden i Uppsala, Uppsala. Taiwan – Institutional Review Board of Tri-Service General Hospital National Defense Medical Center, Neihu, Taipei; Kaohsiung Medical University Chung-Ho Memorial Hospital, Institutional Review Board, Kaohsiung. United Kingdom – Liverpool Adult Research Ethics Committee, Research Ethics Office, Liverpool; Wrightington, Wigan and Leigh LREC, Greater Manchester Strategic Health Authority, Manchester; West Midlands Research Ethics Committee, Redditch, Worcestershire.

Competing interests
JSS has received research grants and consulting fees from AbbVie, BMS, MSD, Pfizer, and Roche, and consulting fees from Astra-Zeneca, Boehringer Ingelheim, Celgene, Celtrion, GSK, ILTOO, Janssen, Lilly, Novartis-Sandoz, Samsung, and UCB. AS is an employee of inVentiv Health and was contracted by Pfizer to provide statistical support for the development of this paper. ASK, TVJ, and LM are employees of Pfizer and hold Pfizer stock. The authors do not report any non-financial conflicts of interest.

Author details
[1]Division of Rheumatology, Department of Medicine 3, Medical University of Vienna, Waehringer Guertel 18-20, 1090 Vienna, Austria. [2]Hietzing Hospital, Vienna, Austria. [3]inVentiv Health, Princeton, NJ, USA. [4]Pfizer, Collegeville, PA, USA.

References

1. Smolen JS, Aletaha D, Bijlsma JW, Breedveld FC, Boumpas D, Burmester G, Combe B, Cutolo M, de Wit M, Dougados M, et al. Treating rheumatoid arthritis to target: recommendations of an international task force. Ann Rheum Dis. 2010;69(4):631–7.
2. Pincus T, Sokka T, Kautiainen H. Patients seen for standard rheumatoid arthritis care have significantly better articular, radiographic, laboratory, and functional status in 2000 than in 1985. Arthritis Rheum. 2005;52(4): 1009–19.
3. Mierau M, Schoels M, Gonda G, Fuchs J, Aletaha D, Smolen JS. Assessing remission in clinical practice. Rheumatology (Oxford). 2007;46(6):975–9.
4. Smolen JS, Han C, van der Heijde DM, Emery P, Bathon JM, Keystone E, Maini RN, Kalden JR, Aletaha D, Baker D, et al. Radiographic changes in rheumatoid arthritis patients attaining different disease activity states with methotrexate monotherapy and infliximab plus methotrexate: the impacts of remission and tumour necrosis factor blockade. Ann Rheum Dis. 2009; 68(6):823–7.
5. van der Heijde D, Landewé R, van Vollenhoven R, Fatenejad S, Klareskog L. Level of radiographic damage and radiographic progression are determinants of physical function: a longitudinal analysis of the TEMPO trial. Ann Rheum Dis. 2008;67(9):1267–70.
6. Smolen JS, Nash P, Durez P, Hall S, Ilivanova E, Irazoque-Palazuelos F, Miranda P, Park MC, Pavelka K, Pedersen R, et al. Maintenance, reduction, or withdrawal of etanercept after treatment with etanercept and methotrexate in patients with moderate rheumatoid arthritis (PRESERVE): a randomised controlled trial. Lancet. 2013;381(9870):918–29.

7. Fransen J, Creemers MC, Van Riel PL. Remission in rheumatoid arthritis: agreement of the disease activity score (DAS28) with the ARA preliminary remission criteria. Rheumatology (Oxford). 2004;43(10):1252–5.
8. Felson DT, Smolen JS, Wells G, Zhang B, van Tuyl LH, Funovits J, Aletaha D, Allaart CF, Bathon J, Bombardieri S, et al. American College of Rheumatology/European League Against Rheumatism provisional definition of remission in rheumatoid arthritis for clinical trials. Arthritis Rheum. 2011;63(3):573–86.
9. Tanaka Y, Hirata S, Kubo S, Fukuyo S, Hanami K, Sawamukai N, Nakano K, Nakayamada S, Yamaoka K, Sawamura F, et al. Discontinuation of adalimumab after achieving remission in patients with established rheumatoid arthritis: 1-year outcome of the HONOR study. Ann Rheum Dis. 2015;74(2):389–95.
10. Tanaka Y, Takeuchi T, Mimori T, Saito K, Nawata M, Kameda H, Nojima T, Miyasaka N, Koike T. Discontinuation of infliximab after attaining low disease activity in patients with rheumatoid arthritis: RRR (remission induction by Remicade in RA) study. Ann Rheum Dis. 2010;69(7):1286–91.
11. Fleischmann R, van der Heijde D, Koenig A, Pedersen R, Szumski A, Marshall L, Bananis E. How much does Disease Activity Score in 28 joints ESR and CRP calculations underestimate disease activity compared with the Simplified Disease Activity Index? Ann Rheum Dis. 2015;74:1132–7.
12. Schoels M, Alasti F, Smolen JS, Aletaha D. Evaluation of newly proposed remission cut-points for disease activity score in 28 joints (DAS28) in rheumatoid arthritis patients upon IL-6 pathway inhibition. Arthritis Res Ther. 2017;19(1):155.
13. Mäkinen H, Kautiainen H, Hannonen P, Sokka T. Is DAS28 an appropriate tool to assess remission in rheumatoid arthritis? Ann Rheum Dis. 2005; 64(10):1410–3.
14. van der Heijde D, Klareskog L, Boers M, Landewé R, Codreanu C, Bolosiu HD, Pedersen R, Fatenejad S. Comparison of different definitions to classify remission and sustained remission: 1 year TEMPO results. Ann Rheum Dis. 2005;64(11):1582–7.
15. Smolen JS, Aletaha D. Interleukin-6 receptor inhibition with tocilizumab and attainment of disease remission in rheumatoid arthritis: the role of acute-phase reactants. Arthritis Rheum. 2011;63(1):43–52.
16. Singh JA, Saag KG, Bridges Jr SL, Akl EA, Bannuru RR, Sullivan MC, Vaysbrot E, McNaughton C, Osani M, Shmerling RH, et al. 2015 American College of Rheumatology Guideline for the Treatment of Rheumatoid Arthritis. Arthritis Rheumatol. 2016;68(1):1–26.
17. Smolen JS, Landewé R, Breedveld FC, Buch M, Burmester G, Dougados M, Emery P, Gaujoux-Viala C, Gossec L, Nam J, et al. EULAR recommendations for the management of rheumatoid arthritis with synthetic and biological disease-modifying antirheumatic drugs: 2013 update. Ann Rheum Dis. 2014;73(3):492–509.

8

Diagnostic value of a 3-day course of prednisolone in patients with possible rheumatoid arthritis – the TryCort study

Uta Kiltz[1†], Christine von Zabern[1†], Xenofon Baraliakos[1], Frank Heldmann[2], Bernd Mintrop[1], Michael Sarholz[1], Dietmar Krause[3], Friedrich Dybowski[4], Ludwig Kalthoff[5] and Jürgen Braun[1*]

Abstract

Background: In patients with tender and swollen finger joints, the differential diagnosis between rheumatoid arthritis (RA) and osteoarthritis (OA) of the hands can be initially difficult. This prospective study (the TryCort study) was performed to study the diagnostic value of prednisolone in differentiating between RA and hand OA. We present the results of this potentially diagnostic test in patients with possible RA in daily clinical practice by demonstrating the results of a pilot and a validation part of this 'prednisolone test' (pred-test).

Methods: We investigated the response to a 3-day course of 20 mg of prednisolone in patients with suspicion of RA. All patients received 1 g of paracetamol per day for 5 days for pain relief. On days 3–5, a morning dose of 20 mg of prednisolone was added. Hand pain was quantified on a 0–10 Numerical Rating Scale, and the subjective percentage of improvement (0–100%) was recorded. Thresholds for response to prednisolone were investigated in a pilot phase with differentiation in response between patients with RA and patients with OA of the hands, both with pain in the hands ≥4. In a validation phase, the best differentiating cut-off of the pilot phase was applied to discriminate responders from non-responders in consecutive patients with hand pain ≥4 referred because of suspected RA. Final diagnoses were made by the expert upon re-examination at week 12. Primary outcomes were the sensitivity and specificity of a positive test in relation to the diagnosis.

Results: A percentage of 40% subjective improvement of pain in the hands on day 3 discriminated best between RA and OA in the pilot phase. Among 95 patients with complete data in the validation phase, RA was diagnosed in about 50%. Patients with RA had more swollen joints, higher C-reactive protein levels and slightly higher Health Assessment Questionnaire scores. The pred-test was positive in 42.1% of all patients (40 of 95). The median percentage of improvement on day 5 was higher in RA than in non-RA: 50% (IQR 30–60%) vs. 20% (IQR 10–30%) ($p < 0.001$). The sensitivity and specificity of the pred-test were 0.6 (95% CI 0.5–0.8) and 0.8 (95% CI 0.7–0.9), respectively, and the positive and negative predictive values were 0.77 and 0.70, respectively.

Conclusions: To our knowledge, this is the first evaluation of the widely used pred-test that has ever been performed. The pred-test had a moderate sensitivity and a good specificity. We conclude that rheumatologists may use this test in unclear clinical situations to better differentiate between inflammatory and other conditions.

* Correspondence: juergen.braun@elisabethgruppe.de
[†]Equal contributors
[1]Rheumazentrum Ruhrgebiet, Claudiusstraße 45, 44649 Herne, Germany
Full list of author information is available at the end of the article

Background

Joint pain of the hands is among the most frequent symptoms and reasons for admission in rheumatology. The biggest problem is arthralgia of the hands caused by rheumatoid arthritis (RA) and/or hand osteoarthritis (OA) [1]. In patients with tender and swollen finger joints, the differential diagnosis between RA and OA can be difficult, especially in relatively early disease stages and also when the diseases overlap, and there is no evidence that RA protects against OA or vice versa. Current classification criteria are of limited help because of their poor diagnostic utility in early and more advanced disease stages [2, 3]. Similarly, the specificity of the RA classification criteria was 0.61, suggesting that 39% of the patients have a diagnosis other than RA [4]. In addition, many patients are initially diagnosed with undifferentiated arthritis, and some of these patients will fulfil RA classification criteria at later time points [5].

For the differential diagnosis between RA and OA, the main question is usually whether the cause of arthralgia is related to inflammation or to degenerative mechanisms. However, even this differentiation is not so straightforward anymore, because magnetic resonance imaging (MRI) findings of synovitis and osteitis have also been described in patients with OA [6]. Furthermore, involvement of the distal interphalangeal joints may indicate OA rather than RA. However, even this important clinical feature may be misleading because the patient may well have both diseases [7]. Clinically, there are different ways to potentially answer the question of RA vs. OA – a clinically relevant question because of the largely different therapeutic options [6, 8]. Of potential help for the differential diagnosis are patient history and the presence of morning stiffness for >30 minutes, the joint pattern in the physical examination and/or the patient history, and the obvious presence of swelling and tenderness of joints. When taking technical procedures into account, the measurement of biomarkers of inflammation, erythrocyte sedimentation rate (ESR) and C-reactive protein (CRP) may be useful to differentiate OA from RA. For RA, there are even specific tests available, such as anti-citrullinated peptide antibody (ACPA), which are also believed to be of pathophysiological importance in terms of their pathogenetic mechanism, which in part is also connected to smoking habits of patients [8]. Finally, imaging procedures may be helpful, especially those with the capacity to visualize inflammation. MRI and ultrasound techniques are now increasingly used to search for arthritis and synovitis in both RA and OA [9, 10]. However, clinical diagnosis is still considered the gold standard for a diagnosis of these two most frequent rheumatic diseases.

However, there are patients and clinical situations where even the totality of the evidence these tests and examinations provide cannot definitively answer the clinical question posed. At this point in time, many rheumatologists are accustomed to just performing a short therapeutic attempt with glucocorticoids (GCs). The effect of GCs in reducing the inflammatory burden of arthritic conditions has been well known for almost 70 years [11]. GCs still play an important role in international recommendations for the treatment of RA [12, 13], and they are still frequently used in daily practice [14]. The mechanisms of action are now far better understood [15, 16]. The basic idea is that RA is due to inflammation, whereas OA is either not based on the same pathophysiology, or at least not to the same degree. However, a short therapeutic attempt with GCs is a clinical test whose diagnostic value has never been evaluated. This prospective study (the TryCort study) was performed to evaluate the diagnostic value of prednisolone in differentiating between RA and hand OA.

Methods

Study design

The TryCort study was performed as a monocentric, prospective clinical study to add another tool to improve the diagnosis of RA. The study was planned in two phases: a pilot and a validation study. The pilot part was designed as a proof-of-concept study to investigate the effect of a 3-day treatment intervention with 20 mg of prednisolone (the 'pred-test') in patients with established RA and hand OA. In detail, we wanted to determine the 'cut-off' for response, and we also aimed to gain first insight into the percentage of responders. The validation study was designed to test the diagnostic utility of the pred-test and to confirm the threshold of the treatment effect.

The ethics committee of the University of Muenster approved the study protocol, and all patients gave informed consent before participation. This study is registered with EudraCT (2011-002633-19).

Study populations

Consecutive patients aged >18 years and <80 years presenting to our hospital or two private practice offices of cooperating rheumatologists were included in the study between January 2012 and November 2014. In the pilot phase, patients with pain in their fingers and/or hands and either an established diagnosis of RA or an established diagnosis of hand OA according to the treating rheumatologist were eligible for enrolment into this first phase. Patients with RA had to fulfil the American College of Rheumatology (ACR)/European League Against Rheumatism (EULAR) 2010 criteria for RA [2], and patients with OA had to fulfil the ACR classification criteria for OA [3].

In the validation phase, patients with suspicion of RA were eligible for enrolment into this phase. Suspicion of RA was defined as chronic pain in fingers and hands lasting >6 weeks without other causality. The presence of pain in finger joints was mandatory; pain in the hands (palm and wrist) was not. Patients with hand OA fulfilling ACR classification criteria for OA but who were positive for ACPA were not included in the trial. We excluded patients with triggering factors for inflamed joints, such as tophi, psoriasis or accidents.

For both groups, the degree of pain had to be ≥4 on a 0–10 Numerical Rating Scale (NRS). Patients receiving concomitant treatment with oral GCs were not eligible. In addition, patients who had been treated with oral GCs of any dose within the 2 weeks before their baseline visit were not included in the trial. In addition, patients with uncontrolled diabetes mellitus, hypertension and glaucoma, as well as those with pregnancy or desire to become pregnant, were not eligible.

Interventions

All patients received 1 g of paracetamol/day for 5 days (days 1–5) during the pilot and validation study to provide a background of pain reduction for ethical reasons and comparability (Fig. 1). Rationale for paracetamol was the low analgesic potency and the absence of an anti-inflammatory effect so that medication could serve as background medication without disturbing response to GC therapy. Patients with an insufficient reduction of pain could ask for an additional dose of paracetamol up to a maximum of 2 g of paracetamol/day. Other analgesics or non-steroidal anti-inflammatory drugs were not allowed and were discontinued before the start of the study.

On days 3–5, a morning dose of 20 mg of prednisolone was added. An intervention phase lasting about 3 days was considered sufficient because prednisolone mediates a quick anti-inflammatory response, but prednisolone requires a 3-day interval to influence inflammation in joints. Patients in the validation phase received the same trial medication (paracetamol on days 1–5, prednisolone on days 3–5) as patients in the pilot phase. Intervention on days 1–5 in the validation phase was followed by an observational phase up to week 12. In this observational phase, the patients did not receive study medication but might receive therapy with disease-modifying anti-rheumatic drugs (DMARDs) if RA had been diagnosed. The choice of DMARD therapy was not pre-defined in the study protocol, and the decision was up to the treating rheumatologist (Fig. 1). Patients underwent re-examination by a rheumatologist in week 12 to confirm the diagnosis made on day 5. Re-examination consists of history, physical examination, assessment of patient-reported outcomes and safety signals and CRP measurement.

Outcome assessments

Pain in the hands was assessed on the basis of an NRS score of 0–10 (0 = no pain, 10 = severe pain). The improvement of pain was determined on a percentage scale of 0–100% (0 = no improvement, 100% = optimal improvement). The 68-joint count for swelling and tenderness was performed by one rheumatologist blinded to laboratory and imaging data to exclude an influence of these results on the physical examination.

Disease activity was measured using the 28-joint Disease Activity Score (DAS28) [17] and the Rheumatoid Arthritis Disease Activity Index (RADAI) [18]. Functional disability was assessed by the Funktionsfragebogen Hannover (FFbH) score, which strongly correlates with the Health Assessment Questionnaire (HAQ) [19]. Values of FFbH were converted into HAQ values by the published formula: HAQ score = 3.16 – (0.028 × FFbH score). Grip strength was evaluated by using a standard dynamometer. All clinical measurements were recorded at each visit (days 1, 3 and 5 and week 12) in the afternoon. Time of day was important to assess treatment response of the morning prednisolone dose. Laboratory parameters measured

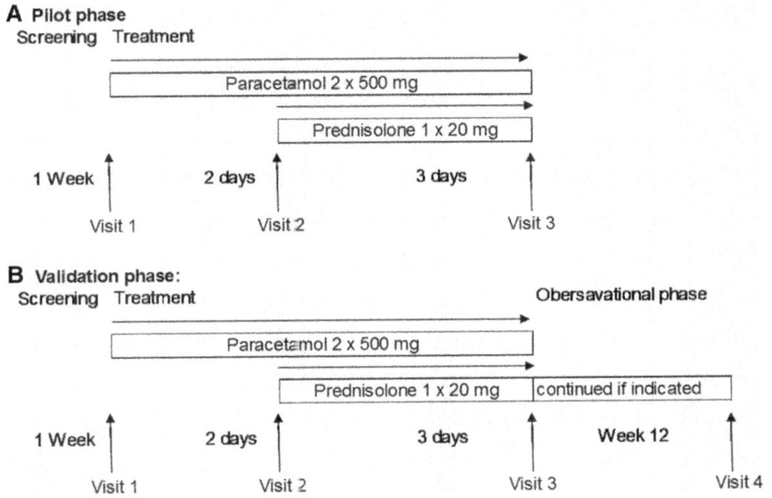

Fig. 1 Study design of the pilot (**a**) and validation (**b**) phases

included CRP measured at days 1 and 5 and week 12, and ACPA and rheumatoid factor measured at day 1.

Furthermore, all patients underwent the usual diagnostic procedures performed in our centre, independent of the study design. The evaluation of conventional radiographs and MRI was performed by an experienced radiologist in our centre. Safety assessments were based on reports of adverse events (AEs), routine physical examinations and vital signs, and laboratory test results were documented in each visit. The clinical diagnosis of an independent and experienced rheumatologist after 3 months was used as a gold standard.

Evaluation

The primary endpoint of the pilot phase was the proportions of patients with RA and patients with OA with positive pred-tests. The pre-defined cut-off of 40% improvement was applied to differentiate between responders and non-responders. Thus, the pred-test was defined as being positive if patients had an improvement of ≥40% on day 5. The primary endpoint of the validation phase was the sensitivity, specificity and predictive value of the pred-test.

Statistical analysis

Descriptive data are presented as absolute values and their proportions when referring to qualitative variables. Continuous variables are expressed as the mean ± SD or as the median with IQR (25–75% range) where appropriate. The Mann-Whitney *U* test was used to compare the data between subgroups at single time points. A *p* value <0.05 was considered statistically significant. The diagnostic utility of the pred-test was determined by calculating the sensitivity, specificity and positive and negative predicative values. AUC was analysed and graphically plotted by using ROC curve analysis to show performance of the cut-off values. For the statistical analysis, IBM SPSS Statistics version 22 software (IBM, Armonk, NY, USA) was used.

Results

A total of 132 patients were eligible for the study, 125 of whom were included in the study: 30 in the pilot and 95 in the validation study (Fig. 2).

Pilot phase

A total of 15 patients with a confirmed diagnosis of RA and 15 patients with a confirmed diagnosis of OA, respectively, were included. In the RA group, there were 13 women (86.7%), and in the OA group, there were 11 women (73.3%). Demographic and clinical characteristics of the patients are presented in Table 1.

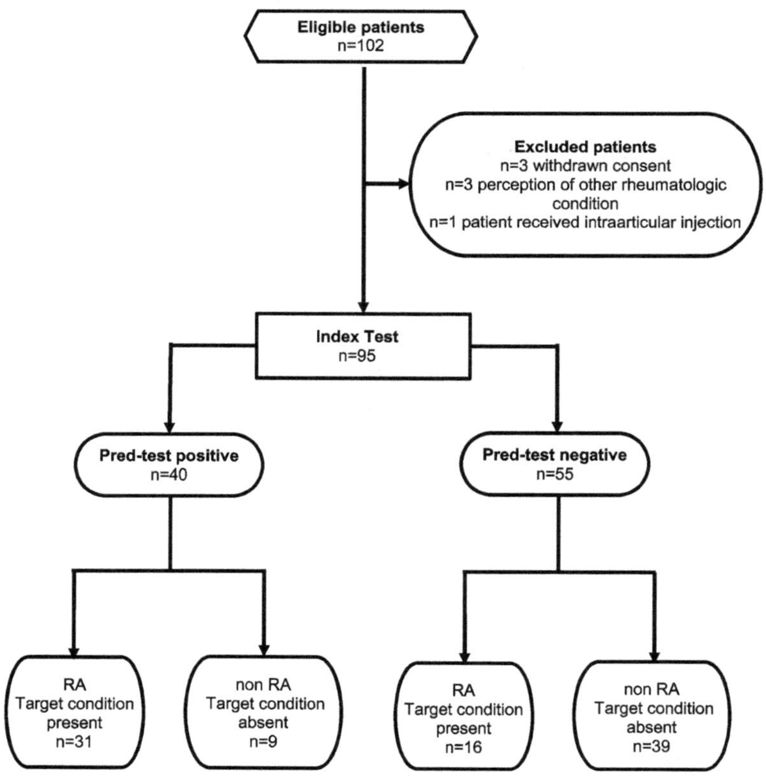

Fig. 2 Flow diagram of the validation phase. *RA* Rheumatoid arthritis

Table 1 Demographic characteristics of the patients with rheumatoid arthritis, osteoarthritis in the pilot study and of patients with rheumatoid arthritis and patients without rheumatoid arthritis in the validation study

	Pilot phase		Validation phase	
	RA ($n = 15$)	OA ($n = 15$)	RA ($n = 47$)	Non-RA ($n = 48$)
Mean age, years	59.3 ± 6.3	66.8 ± 10.3	57.6 ± 12.2	54.5 ± 9.2
Female sex	86.7%	73.3%	70.2%	83.3%
Symptom duration, years	4.0 ± 3.5	10.8 ± 13.9	5.3 ± 10.2	4.9 ± 5.7

OA Osteoarthritis, *RA* Rheumatoid arthritis
Values are given as mean ± SD

The mean age and symptom duration of the patients with OA were somewhat higher than those of patients with RA. The mean pain scores were similar in patients with RA (5.4 ± 1.6) and patients with OA (5.3 ± 1.4). However, patients with RA experienced a greater reduction in pain scores between days 1 and 5 to 2.9 ± 1.8 (RA) and 4.1 ± 1.5 (OA), respectively. The mean percentages of improvement at day 5 (after 3 days of 20-mg prednisolone therapy) were 52.3 ± 27.9% in the RA group and 22.0 ± 20.1% in the OA group (Fig. 3).

The sensitivity and specificity for the cut-offs of subjective improvement of 20%, 30%, 40% and 50% are given in Table 2. The threshold of 40% of subjective improvement was selected as the best-performing cut-off, so the pred-test was defined as being positive if the patient reported a subjective improvement in hand pain ≥40%. Applying this threshold, the pred-test was positive in 11 patients with RA (73.3%) and 4 patients with OA (26.7%) (Table 2) ($p = 0.012$). The sensitivity and specificity for a diagnosis of RA were both 73.3%.

Validation phase

A total of 95 patients with pain in their fingers and hands without a clear diagnosis were enrolled in the validation phase and completed the 5 days of the intervention. Of these 95 patients, 78 (82%) participated in the final visit at week 12. According to the judgement of the rheumatologist at week 12, 47 patients were diagnosed with RA and 48 with non-RA. The mean age and symptom duration of the patients were rather similar in patients with RA and subjects with non-RA (Table 1). Patients with RA had more swollen joints, higher CRP levels and comparable HAQ scores assessed on day 1 (Table 3).

Patients with RA experienced a more severe reduction of pain during the treatment course with prednisolone. Similarly, the median percentage of improvement at day 5 was higher in patients with RA than in those with non-RA: 50% (IQR 30–60%) vs. 20% (IQR 10–30%) ($p = 0.001$) (Fig. 3).

Overall, 40 (42.1%) of 95 patients had an improvement of ≥40% on day 5, fulfilling the criteria of a positive pred-test. More patients with RA than patients with non-RA had a positive pred-test (31 patients with RA [77.5%] vs. 9 patients with non-RA [22.5%]; $p < 0.001$). The sensitivity of the pred-test for a diagnosis of RA was 0.6 (95% CI 0.5–0.8), and the specificity was 0.8 (95% CI 0.7–0.9). The positive and negative predictive values were 0.77 and 0.70, respectively. The ROC analysis showed an AUC of 0.77 (95% CI 0.65–0.85) (Fig. 4).

The safety analysis showed that 23 patients (24.2%) had AEs, and 16 AEs were considered drug-related (5 headaches, 5 flushings, 2 tachycardia, 2 hypertension, and 2 dizziness). There were no serious AEs.

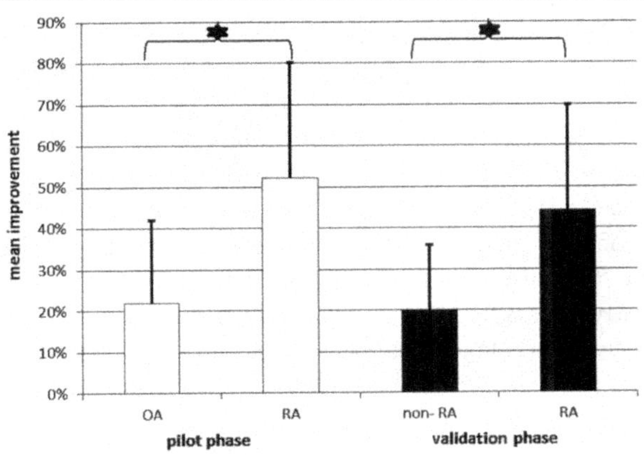

Fig. 3 Difference between RA and non-RA regarding the mean improvement of pain in the hands after prednisolone test in the pilot and validation phases. *RA* Rheumatoid arthritis, *OA* Osteoarthritis

Table 2 Diagnostic utility of the different cut-offs

Cut-off of subjective improvement	Pilot phase		Validation phase	
	Sensitivity[a]	Specificity	Sensitivity	Specificity
20%	93.3%	37.5%	79.2%	41.7%
30%	80.0%	66.7%	76.6%	58.3%
40%	73.3%	73.3%	66.0%	81.3%
50%	60.0%	80.0%	57.5%	91.7%

[a]Based on fourfold table
The safety analysis showed that ten patients (30%) had adverse events (AEs), five of them with gastrointestinal complaints which were considered drug-related AEs. No serious AEs were recognized

Table 3 Clinical characteristics of patients with rheumatoid arthritis and non-rheumatoid arthritis in the validation phase

	Day 1			Day 5		
Characteristic	RA ($n = 47$)	Non-RA ($n = 48$)	*p* Value	RA ($n = 47$)	Non-RA ($n = 48$)	*p* Value
Pain	6.1 ± 1.6	5.8 ± 1.6	0.3	3.4 ± 2.3	4.3 ± 1.8	<0.05
Swollen joint count	2.3 ± 2.4	1.4 ± 2.3	0.02	2.3 ± 4.3	1.1 ± 2.0	0.06
Tender joint count	13.0 ± 8.5	13.9 ± 10.5	0.7	12.0 ± 13.1	11.1 ± 8.9	0.8
CRP, mg/dl	0.5 ± 0.6	0.2 ± 0.3	0.03	0.4 ± 0.6	0.2 ± 0.1	0.1
DAS28	3.7 ± 0.8	3.3 ± 0.8	0.1	3.2 ± 1.0	3.1 ± 0.8	0.7
RADAI	5.0 ± 1.4	4.6 ± 1.2	0.2	3.7 ± 1.53	4.0 ± 1.33	0.4
HAQ	1.2 ± 0.6	1.1 ± 0.4	0.8	1.0 ± 0.5	1.1 ± 0.4	0.2
Grip strength, Pascal	40.2 ± 21.8	35.8 ± 17.6	0.4	38.4 ± 22.1	43.4 ± 26.2	0.5

Abbreviations: CRP C-reactive protein, *DAS28* 28-Joint Disease Activity Score, *HAQ* Health Assessment Questionnaire, *RA* Rheumatoid arthritis, *RADAI* Rheumatoid Arthritis Disease Activity Index

Values are given as mean ± SD

Assessment: CRP <0.5 mg/dl, DAS28 range 0–10, grip strength range 0–1.0, HAQ range 0–3, pain NRS range 0–10, RADAI range 0–10, swollen joint count range 0–66, Tender joint count range 0–68

Discussion

The TryCort study is the first evaluation of a widely used test, the pred-test, that has ever been performed to systematically investigate its diagnostic value in patients with possible RA. The data document a statistically significant association between positive responses to GCs and a diagnosis of RA. Our hypothesis that more patients with RA than patients with non-inflammatory rheumatic conditions will improve when treated with GCs was clearly confirmed and substantiated in both study phases.

The anti-inflammatory properties of GCs are certainly well established, and they are widely used to treat inflammatory rheumatic conditions such as RA [14, 20].

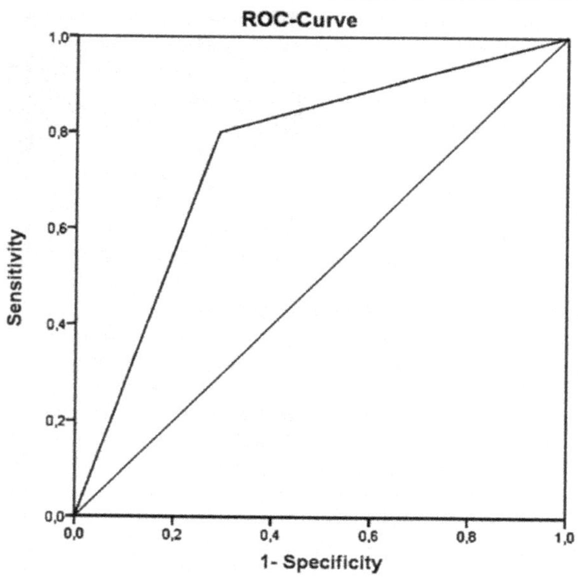

Fig. 4 ROC curve of the diagnostic utility of the prednisolone test in the validation phase

Accordingly, in a recent early arthritis cohort study, the response to a GC bridging therapy at 2 weeks was clearly predictive of having active disease at 3 months [21]. In contrast to our study, the duration of the intervention was much longer. Furthermore, the main question of our study was different, because we studied the diagnostic utility of GCs to diagnose inflammatory arthritis and to differentiate RA from non-RA.

For many years, rheumatologists have been using a short therapeutic attempt with prednisolone in unclear clinical situations to differentiate between inflammatory arthritis and non-inflammatory conditions. Our results confirm that this test may indeed be useful in this regard. The assumption that systemic GCs do not really work in OA has recently been backed by the results of a study in OA in which patients with OA reported no significant pain reduction after treatment with 5 mg of prednisolone for 4 weeks, although some synovitis had been initially detected by MRI [6]. This is in contrast to RA, where even low doses of prednisolone were shown to be efficacious by reducing disease activity and to even inhibit radiographic progression [14, 22, 23]. Therefore, GCs have even been considered as DMARDs in RA [23], and recent international recommendations have addressed all issues in connection with the use of prednisolone in RA [12, 24, 25]. Of interest, to provide help for the clinical diagnosis, the diagnostic utility of prednisolone has also been studied in patients with chronic obstructive pulmonary disease (COPD) [26], but no meaningful diagnostic value was found. This may be explained by the pathophysiologic differences between COPD and RA.

Could the patients with early arthritis and arthralgia involving hands and feet in our study have had rheumatologic diagnoses other than RA? Several other inflammatory rheumatic diseases, such as psoriatic arthritis, connective tissue diseases and even vasculitides, are known to possibly present with a similar picture [27]. Establishing a differential diagnosis was therefore one of the key elements before including patients in the study. However, because the gold standard of our test was a clinical diagnosis of an independent and experienced rheumatologist after 3 months, we cannot be perfectly sure that we included patients with other inflammatory arthritic conditions of the hand. As stated in the Methods section above, we tried to minimize this bias by performing a standard diagnostic work-up for every patient. Furthermore, many patients have to be classified as having undifferentiated arthritis because they do not fit into one of the well-defined categories. However, patients may well progress from an initial classification of undifferentiated arthritis to RA [5]. In any case, the response to therapy was similar in a large recent study [28].

Because the early classification of RA may be difficult, in this study we decided to rely on an expert's diagnosis after an observational period of 12 weeks. However, we are aware that even this period of time may not be long enough to finally ascertain a diagnosis of RA. Thus, we cannot exclude that some patients with a diagnosis of possible RA would have been diagnosed differently at later time points. Other diagnoses would include, for example, psoriatic arthritis and undifferentiated arthritis. Because there is some evidence that MRI does not differentiate patients with established RA from other forms of early arthritis, we could not use such results for this purpose [29]. We are aware that symptom duration of approximately 5 years in our patient population (validation cohort) might be a matter of debate. However, in patients with arthralgia but without clear synovitis, diagnosis is often delayed and is even seen in registry cohorts [30].

The ACR/EULAR classification criteria for RA require at least one swollen joint [2]. The data of our study showed that one-third of the patients diagnosed with RA initially had clinically no clear swollen joints (the main inclusion criterion for this study was finger and hand pain) but MRI changes suggestive of synovitis. Because it is now well established that early diagnosis and treatment are critical for patients with RA [8, 31], we think that our study gives a first hint that the response to GCs could become an important component of diagnosing and treating patients with RA at early time points and when the ACR/EULAR criteria are not reliably fulfilled. Of course, the prognostic significance of this test needs to be assessed in studies with a different design.

Our pilot study revealed that a 40% improvement was the best choice between sensitivity and specificity regarding a diagnosis of RA. The ACR 20% improvement criteria (ACR20) are widely used in RA trials [32, 33]. However, their performance related to discrimination is known not to be optimal [34]. Indeed, the ACR50 criteria seem to be superior [35]. Our evaluation for this diagnostic test showed a moderate sensitivity of 65.9% with a good specificity of 81.2%. Thus, our pred-test performed well, but it did not perform perfectly well. Possible reasons are our inhomogeneous patient cohort, lack of an objective gold standard for diagnosis and arbitrarily chosen time point for diagnostic testing. Some of these aspects (e.g., symptom duration) might have had an impact on test accuracy, but this cannot be quantified within our study design.

We are aware that the pred-test without confirmation of other surrogate markers is not helpful in clinical decision-making processes. We therefore recommend use of the test in light of other confirming factors, such as history, physical examination, imaging and laboratory results. Whether the test is useful in the hands of primary care doctors cannot be answered by our study. However, we think that the pred-test can triage patients from primary care to rheumatology specialists.

On one hand, a positive test result will help to identify patients with inflammatory arthritis, especially RA, who are then subject to proper treatment. In case of a negative test result, the likelihood of RA is low. However, a re-evaluation may still be necessary if suggestive symptoms appear. Nevertheless, may a negative test result prevent patients from receiving unnecessary treatment with GCs?

On the other hand, our study also shows that 4 of 15 patients in the pilot phase and 15 of 47 patients diagnosed with RA in the validation phase had a negative test result. One possible explanation for this is that some patients may need higher doses of GCs. Indeed, the Combination Therapy for Rheumatoid Arthritis (COBRA) study showed that a high GC dose of 60 mg/day worked well in many patients with RA [36]. Ever since then, also starting doses of 10 mg/day have been used to reach remission [37, 38], but for maintenance therapy, even dosages <5 mg/day have been successful in some patients [39]. In an ongoing study, the performance of two GC doses were compared in patients with early RA [40]. Different tapering strategies have been proposed [24]. Especially, the questions of which patients may need higher dosages of prednisolone and why deserve further study. GC receptors may have a role in this [16]. Another possibility is that, in addition to RA, there may be other reasons for pain, such as OA, and the patient is unable to differentiate between the two.

Conclusions

This study shows that the pred-test can support clinical decision-making as a diagnostic aid in differentiating between RA and non-RA. These data also confirm a cut-off point of ≥40% improvement with good sensitivity and specificity. The study also clearly shows that a positive response to prednisolone cannot be taken as evidence that a diagnosis of RA is a given. Further studies are needed to confirm the diagnostic utility of the pred-test with larger patient groups in rheumatology as well as in primary care. Future research can be focused on test accuracy in the light of possible influencing factors.

Abbreviations

ACPA: Anti-citrullinated peptide antibody; ACR: American College of Rheumatology; ACR20: American College of Rheumatology 20% improvement criteria; ACR50: American College of Rheumatology 50% improvement criteria; AE: Adverse event; COPD: Chronic obstructive pulmonary disease; CRP: C-reactive protein; DAS28: 28-joint Disease Activity Score; DMARD: Disease-modifying anti-rheumatic drug; ESR: Erythrocyte sedimentation rate; EULAR: European League Against Rheumatism; FFbH: Funktionsfragebogen Hannover; GC: Glucocorticoid; HAQ: Health Assessment Questionnaire; MRI: Magnetic resonance imaging; NRS: Numerical Rating Scale; OA: Osteoarthritis; pred-test: Prednisolone test; RA: Rheumatoid arthritis; RADAI: Rheumatoid Arthritis Disease Activity Index; RF: Rheumatoid factor

Acknowledgements

We thank all patients who participated in the TryCort study. We also thank all other rheumatologists and fellows who enrolled patients in this study.

Funding

This study was financially supported by Rheumazentrum Ruhrgebiet, Herne, Germany.

Authors' contributions

JB, UK, CvZ and FH designed the study. CvZ, UK, FH, FD, LK and DK contributed to patient recruitment. CvZ, UK, FH, BM and MS contributed to patient investigation. UK, CvZ, XB and JB contributed to data management and analysis. CvZ and UK designed the tables and figures. CvZ, UK and JB drafted the manuscript for this publication. All authors were involved in revising the manuscript critically for important intellectual content. JB had full access to all the data in the study and had final responsibility for the decision to submit the manuscript for publication. All authors read and approved the final manuscript.

Competing interests

The authors declare that they have no competing interests.

Author details

[1]Rheumazentrum Ruhrgebiet, Claudiusstraße 45, 44649 Herne, Germany. [2]Zeisigwaldklinik Bethanien Chemnitz, Zeisigwaldstraße 101, 09130 Chemnitz, Germany. [3]Rheumatology private office in Gladbeck, Friedrich-Ebert-Straße 2, 45964 Gladbeck, Germany. [4]Rheumatology private office in Herne, Claudiusstraße 45, 44649 Herne, Germany. [5]Rheumatology private office in Bochum, Gudrunstrasse 56, 44791 Bochum, Germany.

References

1. Jakobsson U, Hallberg IR. Pain and quality of life among older people with rheumatoid arthritis and/or osteoarthritis: a literature review. J Clin Nurs. 2002;11(4):430–43.
2. Aletaha D, Neogi T, Silman AJ, Funovits J, Felson DT, Bingham 3rd CO, et al. 2010 Rheumatoid arthritis classification criteria: an American College of Rheumatology/European League Against Rheumatism collaborative initiative. Arthritis Rheum. 2010;62(9):2569–81.
3. Altman R, Alarcón G, Appelrouth D, Bloch D, Borenstein D, Brandt K, et al. The American College of Rheumatology criteria for the classification and reporting of osteoarthritis of the hand. Arthritis Rheum. 1990;33(11):1601–10.
4. Radner H, Neogi T, Smolen JS, Aletaha D. Performance of the 2010 ACR/EULAR classification criteria for rheumatoid arthritis: a systematic literature review. Ann Rheum Dis. 2014;73(1):114–23.
5. van Aken J, van Dongen H, Le Cessie S, Allaart CF, Breedveld FC, Huizinga TW. Comparison of long term outcome of patients with rheumatoid arthritis presenting with undifferentiated arthritis or with rheumatoid arthritis: an observational cohort study. Ann Rheum Dis. 2006;65(1):20–5.
6. Wenham CYJ, Hensor EMA, Grainger AJ, Hodgson R, Balamoody S, Doré CJ, et al. A randomized, double-blind, placebo-controlled trial of low-dose oral prednisolone for treating painful hand osteoarthritis. Rheumatology (Oxford). 2012;51(12):2286–94.
7. Frisell T, Hellgren K, Alfredsson L, Raychaudhuri S, Klareskog L, Askling J. Familial aggregation of arthritis-related diseases in seropositive and seronegative rheumatoid arthritis: a register-based case-control study in Sweden. Ann Rheum Dis. 2016;75(1):183–9.
8. Scott DL, Wolfe F, Huizinga TW. Rheumatoid arthritis. Lancet. 2010;376(9746):1094–108.
9. Nieuwenhuis WP, Krabben A, Stomp W, Huizinga TW, van der Heijde D, Bloem JL, et al. Evaluation of magnetic resonance imaging-detected tenosynovitis in the hand and wrist in early arthritis. Arthritis Rheumatol. 2015;67(4):869–76.
10. Glimm AM, Werner SG, Burmester GR, Backhaus M, Ohrndorf S. Analysis of distribution and severity of inflammation in patients with osteoarthritis compared to rheumatoid arthritis by ICG-enhanced fluorescence optical imaging and musculoskeletal ultrasound: a pilot study. Ann Rheum Dis. 2016;75(3):566–70.
11. Ward LE, Polley HF, Power MH, Mason HL, Slocumb CH, Hench PS. Prednisone in rheumatoid arthritis: metabolic and clinical effects. Ann Rheum Dis. 1958;17(2):145–59.
12. Gorter SL, Bijlsma JW, Cutolo M, Gomez-Reino J, Kouloumas M, Smolen JS, et al. Current evidence for the management of rheumatoid arthritis with glucocorticoids: a systematic literature review informing the EULAR recommendations for the management of rheumatoid arthritis. Ann Rheum Dis. 2010;69(6):1010–4.
13. Dernis E, Ruyssen-Witrand A, Mouterde G, Maillefert JF, Tebib J, Cantagrel A, et al. Use of glucocorticoids in rheumatoid arthritis – practical modalities of glucocorticoid therapy: recommendations for clinical practice based on data from the literature and expert opinion. Joint Bone Spine. 2010;77(5):451–7.
14. Bijlsma JW. Disease control with glucocorticoid therapy in rheumatoid arthritis. Rheumatology (Oxford). 2012;51 Suppl 4:iv9–13.
15. Baschant U, Lane NE, Tuckermann J. The multiple facets of glucocorticoid action in rheumatoid arthritis. Nat Rev Rheumatol. 2012;8(11):645–55.
16. Strehl C, Gaber T, Löwenberg M, Hommes DW, Verhaar AP, Schellmann S, et al. Origin and functional activity of the membrane-bound glucocorticoid receptor. Arthritis Rheum. 2011;63(12):3779–88.
17. Prevoo ML, van 't Hof MA, Kuper HH, van Leeuwen MA, van de Putte LB, van Riel PL. Modified disease activity scores that include twenty-eight-joint counts: development and validation in a prospective longitudinal study of patients with rheumatoid arthritis. Arthritis Rheum. 1995;38(1):44–8.
18. Stucki G, Liang MH, Stucki S, Brühlmann P, Michel BA. A self-administered rheumatoid arthritis disease activity index (RADAI) for epidemiologic research: psychometric properties and correlation with parameters of disease activity. Arthritis Rheum. 1995;38(6):795–8.
19. Lautenschläger J, Mau W, Kohlmann T, Raspe HH, Struve F, Brückle W, et al. Comparative evaluation of a German version of the Health Assessment Questionnaire and the Hannover Functional Capacity Questionnaire [in German]. Z Rheumatol. 1997;56(3):144–55.
20. Buttgereit F, Straub RH, Wehling M, Burmester G. Glucocorticoids in the treatment of rheumatic diseases: an update on the mechanisms of action. Arthritis Rheum. 2004;50(11):3408–17.
21. de Jong PHP, Quax RA, Huisman M, Gerards AH, Feelders RA, de Sonnaville PB, et al. Response to glucocorticoids at 2 weeks predicts the effectiveness of DMARD induction therapy at 3 months: post hoc analyses from the tREACH study. Ann Rheum Dis. 2013;72(10):1659–63.
22. Wassenberg S, Rau R, Steinfeld P, Zeidler H. Very low-dose prednisolone in early rheumatoid arthritis retards radiographic progression over two years: a multicenter, double-blind, placebo-controlled trial. Arthritis Rheum. 2005;52(11):3371–80.

23. van Everdingen AA, Jacobs JWG, Siewertsz van Reesema DR, Bijlsma JWJ. Low-dose prednisone therapy for patients with early active rheumatoid arthritis: clinical efficacy, disease-modifying properties, and side effects: a randomized, double-blind, placebo-controlled clinical trial. Ann Intern Med. 2002;136(1):1–12.
24. Gaujoux-Viala C, Gossec L. When and for how long should glucocorticoids be used in rheumatoid arthritis? International guidelines and recommendations. Ann N Y Acad Sci. 2014;1318:32–40.
25. Gaujoux-Viala C, Nam J, Ramiro S, Landewé R, Buch MH, Smolen JS, et al. Efficacy of conventional synthetic disease-modifying antirheumatic drugs, glucocorticoids and tofacitinib: a systematic literature review informing the 2013 update of the EULAR recommendations for management of rheumatoid arthritis. Ann Rheum Dis. 2014;73(3):510–5.
26. Broekhuizen BDL, Sachs APE, Moons KGM, Cheragwandi SAA, Damsté HEJ, Wijnands GJA, et al. Diagnostic value of oral prednisolone test for chronic obstructive pulmonary disorders. Ann Fam Med. 2011;9(2):104–9.
27. Tehlirian CV, Bathon JM, Waldburger JM, Firestein GS, Oliver AM, St Clair EW. Rheumatoid arthritis. In: Klippel JH, Stone JH, Crofford LJ, White PH, editors. Primer on the rheumatic diseases. 13th ed. New York: Springer Science + Business Media; 2008. p. 114–41.
28. Wevers-de Boer K, Visser K, Heimans L, Ronday HK, Molenaar E, Groenendael JH, et al. Remission induction therapy with methotrexate and prednisone in patients with early rheumatoid and undifferentiated arthritis (the IMPROVED study). Ann Rheum Dis. 2012;71(9):1472–7.
29. Stomp W, Krabben A, van der Heijde D, Huizinga TW, Bloem JL, van der Helm-van Mil AH, et al. Are rheumatoid arthritis patients discernible from other early arthritis patients using 1.5T extremity magnetic resonance imaging? A large cross-sectional study. J Rheumatol. 2014;41(8):1630–7.
30. Pappas DA, Kent JD, Greenberg JD, Mason MA, Kremer JM, Holt RJ. Delays in initiation of disease-modifying therapy in rheumatoid arthritis patients: data from a US-based registry. Rheumatol Ther. 2015;2(2):153–64.
31. McInnes IB, O'Dell JR. State-of-the-art: rheumatoid arthritis. Ann Rheum Dis. 2010;69(11):1898–906.
32. Felson DT, Anderson JJ, Boers M, Bombardier C, Furst D, Goldsmith C, et al. American College of Rheumatology preliminary definition of improvement in rheumatoid arthritis. Arthritis Rheum. 1995;38(6):727–35.
33. American College of Rheumatology Committee to Reevaluate Improvement Criteria. A proposed revision to the ACR20: the hybrid measure of American College of Rheumatology response. Arthritis Rheum. 2007;57(2):193–202.
34. Pincus T, Sokka T. Quantitative measures for assessing rheumatoid arthritis in clinical trials and clinical care. Best Pract Res Clin Rheumatol. 2003;17(5):753–81.
35. Chung CP, Thompson JL, Koch GG, Amara I, Strand V, Pincus T. Are American College of Rheumatology 50% response criteria superior to 20% criteria in distinguishing active aggressive treatment in rheumatoid arthritis clinical trials reported since 1997? A meta-analysis of discriminant capacities. Ann Rheum Dis. 2006;65(12):1602–7.
36. Landewé RBM, Boers M, Verhoeven AC, Westhovens R, van de Laar MA, Markusse HM, et al. COBRA combination therapy in patients with early rheumatoid arthritis: long-term structural benefits of a brief intervention. Arthritis Rheum. 2002;46(2):347–56.
37. den Uyl D, ter Wee M, Boers M, Kerstens P, Voskuyl A, Nurmohamed M, et al. A non-inferiority trial of an attenuated combination strategy ('COBRA-light') compared to the original COBRA strategy: clinical results after 26 weeks. Ann Rheum Dis. 2014;73(6):1071–8.
38. Bakker MF, Jacobs JWG, Welsing PMJ, Verstappen SM, Tekstra J, Ton E, et al. Low-dose prednisone inclusion in a methotrexate-based, tight control strategy for early rheumatoid arthritis: a randomized trial. Ann Intern Med. 2012;156(5):329–39.
39. Pincus T, Castrejón I. Effective initial and long-term prednisone in doses of less than 5 mg/day to treat rheumatoid arthritis: documentation using a patient self-report Multidimensional Health Assessment Questionnaire (MDHAQ). Bull NYU Hosp Jt Dis. 2012;70 Suppl 1:14–20.
40. Trampisch US, Krause D, Trampisch HJ, Klaassen-Mielke R, Baraliakos X, Braun J. Comparison of the efficacy and safety of two starting dosages of prednisolone in early active rheumatoid arthritis (CORRA): study protocol for a randomized controlled trial. Trials. 2014;15:344.

9

Thinking BIG rheumatology: how to make functional genomics data work for you

Deborah R. Winter

Abstract

High-throughput sequencing assays have become an increasingly common part of biological research across multiple fields. Even as the resulting sequences pile up in public databases, it is not always obvious how to make use of these data sets. Functional genomics offers approaches to integrate these "big" data into our understanding of rheumatic diseases. This review aims to provide a primer on thinking about big data from functional genomics in the context of rheumatology, using examples from the field's literature as well as the author's own work to illustrate the execution of functional genomics research. Study design is crucial to ensure the right samples are used to address the question of interest. In addition, sequencing assays produce a variety of data types, from gene expression to 3D chromatin structure and single-cell technologies, that can be integrated into a model of the underlying gene regulatory networks. The best approach for this analysis uses the scientific process: bioinformatic methods should be used in an iterative, hypothesis-driven manner to uncover the disease mechanism. Finally, the future of functional genomics will see big data fully integrated into rheumatology, leading to computationally trained researchers and interactive databases. The goal of this review is not to provide a manual, but to enhance the familiarity of readers with functional genomic approaches and provide a better sense of the challenges and possibilities.

Keywords: Functional genomics, Big data, High-throughput sequencing assays, Gene expression, Epigenomics, Chromatin

Background

The medical sciences are abuzz with big data. Across virtually every field and discipline there are projects to collect data from "omics" assays. The resulting data sets are characterized as "big data" and may involve thousands to billions of measurements for a handful to thousands of individual samples. In the field of functional genomics, the traditional omics assay makes use of next-generation sequencing technology. Such assays tend to relate to genomics, transcriptomics, and epigenomics although these data sets may be linked to everything from metabolomics and proteomics to microbiomics and clinical "omics". These high-throughput assays generate libraries of DNA fragments that are "read" by the sequencer. These sequence reads must be computationally linked to generate a de novo genome (usually in the case where the source genome is unknown) or aligned to the reference genome. In the case of patient data, this means aligning millions or billions of reads—depending on the desired coverage—to the approximately 3 billion base-pair human genome. At later stages, these data may be simplified into summary files listing only the genes or regions of interest: however, the final list is still likely to contain thousands of entries. Although the simplest experiment may only have two conditions each with a few replicates, it is rapidly becoming common for studies to include several populations under changing conditions or across time. Moreover, studies involving human patients may wish to include large cohorts to address individual variation. Finally, with the expanding popularity and ease of single-cell technologies, each individual cell may represent its own sample and may number in the thousands and counting.

Several consortiums exist that collect these types of big data in a systematic way and make it publicly available. The ENCyclopedia of DNA Elements (ENCODE) is an example of a consortium that seeks to build a comprehensive list of functional elements in the human

Correspondence: Deborah.winter@northwestern.edu
Department of Medicine, Division of Rheumatology, Northwestern University Feinberg School of Medicine, Chicago, IL 60611, USA

genome [1]. The ENCODE pilot began with 1% of the genome across a small defined set of common human cell lines [2], but it rapidly expanded to include a variety of cell types and then spun off into the Epigenomics Roadmap to catalog human variation by collecting tissue samples from many individuals [3]. Together, ENCODE and Roadmap represent data from gene expression, protein binding, chromatin state, and other assays and are accompanied by a host of quality standards, computational tools, and annotations resulting from the processing and analysis [4]. Another consortium, Genotype-Tissue Expression project (GTex), focuses specifically on the interactions between genotype and gene expression in vivo by collecting multiple tissues from human donors [5]. In contrast, the NIH Library of Integrated Network-based Cellular Signatures (LINCS) is cataloging the generalized response profiles by measuring changes in gene expression in multiple cell types exposed to a variety of induced perturbations [6]. For immunology specifically, the Immunological Genome Project (ImmGen) [7] and the European Blueprint Epigenome [8] provide databases for gene expression and epigenomics, respectively. These examples are valuable resources of quality-controlled data that may obviate the requirement to repeat assays in individual laboratories. However, it is one thing to catalog these data and another to use them to test a hypothesis. This is the difference between descriptive genomics and functional genomics.

Functional genomics makes use of high-throughput sequencing data to describe how genes contribute to the identity, function, and activity of cells. It is often used interchangeably with the term "systems biology" because both tend to involve modeling of multiple interacting components and use a variety of techniques from different fields to study the resulting networks. In functional genomics, the collection of interactions can be described as the Gene Regulatory Network (GRN) of the cell. Gene expression as reflected by RNA transcription is the typical output of GRNs while the interactors are cis-regulatory elements within the noncoding genome and the transcription factors (TFs) that bind them. Because the transcription of RNA is not perfectly correlated with protein translation, it may not directly reflect the cell's phenotype. However, the cell's GRN is critical to understanding the underlying programming of the cell regardless of the exact impact on function. High-throughput sequencing assays provide the raw data with which to model these GRNs. The goal of functional genomics is to inform how cells evolved to fulfill their roles and the pathways to which they devote their energy.

The aim of this review to provide a primer on big data in functional genomics in the context of rheumatology. Although other articles cover similar topics, this review is meant to be accessible to researchers whose focus is rheumatic disease by highlighting field-specific issues and using examples from the literature. It is not intended to present a step-by-step manual, but rather to draw attention to key features of big data studies and provide information on the critical techniques. The first section discusses several options that should be considered when designing a functional genomics study to optimize the relevance to the question. Next follows a description of functional genomic data types and the assays commonly used to generate these data. In these studies, how the data are analyzed is as important as how they are collected. Thus, the third section gives an overview of the key approaches involved in bioinformatic analysis. Finally, the author shares her vision for the future of big data in rheumatology. For a precise description of the methods mentioned, please refer to the specific references throughout the text. For the most part, the goal is to present studies in rheumatology as examples, but other functional genomics research is used in order to cover a wider variety of approaches. Due to space constraints, the review does not cover some topics in functional genomics in detail—including noncoding RNA, splicing, and other post-transcriptional regulation. While not all relevant studies could be mentioned, the goal is to convey the big potential associated with these approaches and increase awareness of the possibilities and considerations involved.

Main text

Big study design

The key to successful research in functional genomics is designing the study to effectively address the question of interest. This is true even when the data are downloaded from a public database. However, in some cases it might be necessary to generate new data in order to have access to the most relevant data. In the world of functional genomics, study design boils down to what populations of cells are chosen as samples for the assay. Here, the major choices involved are discussed.

In vitro vs in vivo

This review refers to cell populations assayed directly after isolation from either the patient or the model organism as in vivo samples. Alternatively, cells may be first cultured or differentiated in vitro. The main advantage of in vitro populations is the ease in obtaining enough cells for the desired assay. For example, bone-marrow-derived macrophages (BMDMs) are commonly used to test hypotheses about immune response [9, 10]. However, recent work has shown systematically that BMDMs and the related dendritic cells (DCs) that are differentiated by culturing bone marrow cells with granulocyte–macrophage colony-stimulating factor (GMCSF) do not fully resemble any in vivo population [11]. Moreover, even the GRN of mature cells are influenced by their local environment:

thus, cells such as macrophages, when removed from the culture, tend to lose their distinct regulatory landscape [12, 13]. Similarly, Gardner et al. [14] showed that gene expression profiles obtained using explanted fibroblasts from patients and controls are a poor substitute for skin biopsies. There may be cases where assays on in vitro cells may be sufficient, or even preferable, for the question of interest. Using cultured cells may help distinguish between cell-autonomous and environmental effects. Also, in vitro cells are useful for proof-of-principle studies and to establish gene editing.

Mouse model vs patient sample

In rheumatology, mouse models are commonly used to approximate human diseases, such as systemic lupus erythematosus (SLE), systemic sclerosis (SSc), and rheumatoid arthritis (RA) [15–17]. Researchers have studied gene expression profiles of both genetic models, such as NZB/W mice that are SLE prone [18, 19], and chemical models, such as bleomycin-induced pulmonary fibrosis [20, 21]. Mouse models have the obvious advantage of being easier to manipulate and genetically identical mice minimize the individual variation. In addition, cells from any tissue or organ may be obtained for study at any stage of disease. On the other hand, it is often difficult to obtain human tissues, other than blood, at multiple time points. For example, skin biopsies have been used to study gene expression in SSc patients and controls [22], although the small sample size may limit the ability to study individual cell populations without first culturing the cells (e.g., fibroblasts [14]). Alternatively, researchers can take advantage of transplants to access donor and explanted tissue [23]; however, these samples typically represent end-stage disease. Several studies have shown high homology between both the definition of cell populations [24, 25] and their key regulatory factors [26] across mice, human, and other primates. Furthermore, kidney mononuclear cells from mouse models of lupus demonstrated significant overlap of GRNs and activated genes with human lupus nephritis samples [27]. The main shortcoming of mouse models arises for studies interested in the causative signals behind rheumatic disease; there is often a lack of evidence that the conditions by which symptoms were initiated in mice will reflect the real etiology of disease. For a given study, one must be clear on whether the intention is to study the cause or behavior of cells in disease.

Whole tissue vs cell-type specific

For the purposes of bulk assays in functional genomics, it is generally preferable to aim for homogeneous cell populations as opposed to whole tissue or mixed populations. Notably, single-cell technologies are the exception to this rule, as will be explained in the following. In bulk assays of hundreds to millions of cells, the resulting data represent an average across all cells and it is difficult to parse out the effect of specific cell types. Without sophisticated algorithms, it is impossible to distinguish between changes in expression within a single cell type and changes to the proportion of that cell type within the population. Using a network approach in a meta-analysis of other SSc expression studies, Mahoney et al. [28] implicated the interferon pathway, M2 macrophage polarization, adaptive immunity, and cell proliferation. However, while enriched pathways may be found in tissue samples, one cannot be sure that any group of genes is expressed in the same cell type. Moreover, it is conceivable that different cell types may regulate genes in opposite directions that then cancel each other out. Similarly, in our studies of RA, we have observed that changes in some less highly expressed genes within a single population, such as macrophages, may be drowned out by the remaining population in whole joint synovium (Mandelin et al, accepted). Thus, it is not feasible to model a coherent GRN of the interactions between genes and regulatory elements. Even with deconvolution, one must define a characteristic set of genes to attribute to each discoverable cell type [29, 30]. This approach may reveal the proportion of different cell types within the sample, but cannot then define the changes in the gene expression within these cell types without begging the question, since this data was used in the model's assumptions. Thus, in order to model the GRN of a cell type, each study should aim to assay the purest populations of cells possible.

Control, reference, and outgroup

A key aspect of study design in functional genomics is to choose one or more auxiliary samples that will underscore the feature of interest in the test sample. In the most common and straightforward cases for studying rheumatic disease, the test sample would be derived from patients while the control sample would come from healthy volunteers. This approach is seen in a study of lung tissue samples from patients with SSc and healthy controls [31]. Similarly, the mouse equivalent would compare the mouse model with mice given sham treatment of the same age and genetic background as the control. In the case of bleomycin treatment, the control mice would be intubated with PBS as in traditional experiments measuring changes in surface marker expression [21]. In contrast, the reference is defined as a sample that provides necessary context for an experiment. This may be the sample from "Day 0" in a time course of serum-transfer induced arthritis (STIA) vs control [25]; the population of monocytes that is thought to be the precursor of macrophages in SSc-associated skin fibrosis vs healthy skin [32]; or skin biopsies from controls in a study of response to mycophenolate in SSc patients [33]. These populations are assayed in addition to the typical control as they may be necessary to distinguish between regulatory factors that are involved in the main comparison vs other confounding variables. In another instance, skin samples from the unaffected back of SSc patients were used as a reference to define "intrinsic" genes that exhibited consistent expression with their affected forearm before comparison across patients [22]. Finally, in some experiments it may be helpful to include a population of cells as an outgroup. The purpose of an outgroup is to provide perspective about the relationship between the main population of a comparison. For example, in comparing tissue-resident macrophages, we included neutrophils as an outgroup to demonstrate the difference between macrophages compared to that between cell types that shared a common myeloid lineage [13]. As experiments become more complicated and involve multidimensional comparisons, the distinction between controls, references, and outgroups may be blurred. How these experimental tools are used should be evaluated on a case-by-case basis.

Replicates and batch effect

Once the identities of the comparison samples are chosen, one should consider including replicates whenever possible. The statistical power of high-throughput sequencing assays is relatively insensitive to the replicate number because they involve millions of measurements for thousands of genes and regulatory elements. Any single gene may fall below the cutoff value for the false discovery rate (FDR), but, globally, the set of differential genes represents a substantial effect size [34, 35]. Nonetheless, replicates are crucial to account for technical variation, experimental error, signal-to-noise ratio, and batch effect. Biological replicates generally refer to distinct samples either taken subsequently from the same patient or from genetically identical mice undergoing the same treatment. These can be used to account for variability in the experimental conditions and can help to control for artifacts in the data. On the other hand, a technical replicate occurs when a single sample is divided for the purposes of the assay. A technical replicate can be useful, especially when it is difficult or cost-prohibitive to obtain biological replicates of human samples, to estimate the amount of noise or to help optimize library protocols during development [36]. Another use of replicates is to provide robust results: the activity of a tissue-specific macrophage cis-regulatory element may be confirmed by enrichment in two replicates [13] and the identification of immune cell subsets in human blood can be validated across patients [37]. The other benefit of multiple replicates is to control for batch effect. The batch effect describes technical variation that arises between groups of samples that are prepared at different times. While this may sometimes be unavoidable based on the availability of samples for the throughput of the experiment, replicates can help to mediate the impact on the data. For both bulk and single-cell genomic assays, replicates should be spread out across groups so that batch effects are not confounded with the differences between the samples being compared [38, 39]. For example, in a single-cell study of microglia development, we replicated the single-cell population for each time point so that we could distinguish time-dependent differences from the batch effect [40]. Alternatively, long-term studies, such as longitudinal patient studies, may choose to use a reference sample (some are commercially available) that is included in each run.

Big data types

High-throughput sequencing assays come in multiple flavors depending on the feature being measured. Regardless of the assay, the output is a library of DNA fragments or reads that are enriched for the feature of interest, whether that is expressed genes or epigenetically modified regions. A functional genomics study may combine two or more different assays on the same samples in order to gain a better picture of the underlying GRN. The relationship between different data types and their biological significance is shown in Fig. 1.

Gene expression

The expression level of a gene is determined by the number of times the DNA sequence of the gene is transcribed by RNA Polymerase II (PolII) into RNA and can be thought of as the output of GRNs. In the past, microarrays were commonly used to measure gene expression, but, more recently, RNA-seq has taken over as a more exact digital measurement for clinical applications [41, 42]. Typical RNA-seq measures the steady-state number of transcripts for each gene and may be full length with reads covering the whole sequence of the gene or end biased with reads starting at only the 5′ or 3′ end of the gene. Both methods have their advantages and disadvantages, with full-length reads allowing for analysis of allele-specific expression and alternative splicing, while end-biased reads are typically cheaper and provide a more accurate quantification of expression level [42]. Recently, advances in RNA-seq have allowed for high-throughput processing of samples with low cell numbers, such as one used on hematopoietic progenitors [36]. In addition, Global Run-on sequencing (GRO-seq) and similar assays were developed to measure nascent transcripts as they are transcribed and enrich for noncoding RNAs that play regulatory roles in the GRNs [43].

DNA methylation

DNA methylation, which primarily occurs on the cytosine (C) base of CpG sites, is an epigenetic mechanism associated with gene regulation. Genome-wide DNA methylation is typically measured by bisulfite sequencing (BS-seq),

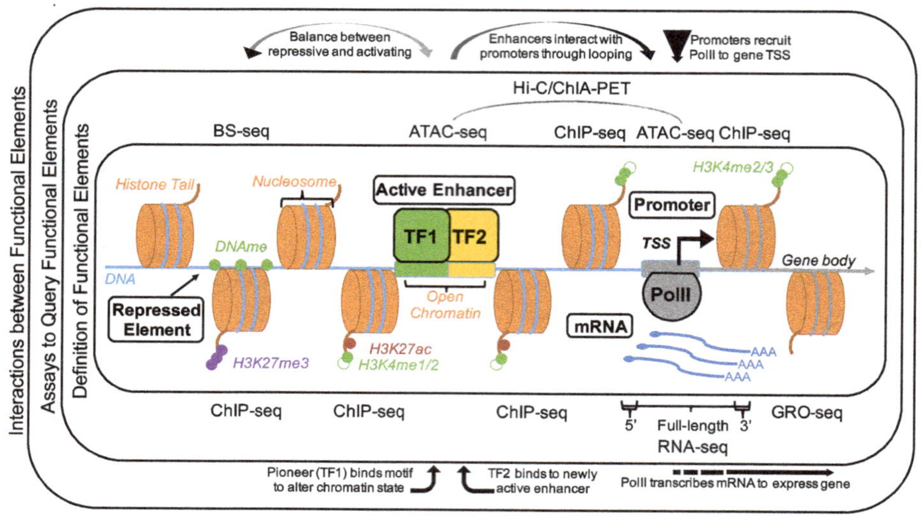

Fig. 1 Common functional elements. Inner box: definitions of various functional elements (left to right): repressed element with methylated DNA (DNAme) and repressive modification of the histone tail of a nearby nucleosome (H3K27me3); active enhancer in an open chromatin region bound by two transcription factors (TF1, TF2) and marked by H3K4me1 or H3K4me2 (enhancer) and H3K27ac (activity); promoter bound by RNA Polymerase II (PolII) in an open chromatin region around the transcription start site (TSS, black arrow) of a gene body and marked by H3K4me2 or H3K4me3; and mRNA molecules transcribed from the gene with 5′ caps and 3′ poly (A) tails. Middle box: list of high-throughput sequencing assays used to annotate these functional elements, including bisulfite sequencing (BS-seq) for DNA methylation, Assay for Transposase Accessible Chromatin (ATAC-seq) for open chromatin, high-throughput chromosome conformation capture (Hi-C) or Chromatin Interaction Analysis by Paired-End Tag Sequencing (ChIA-PET) for interactions between regions, chromatin immunoprecipitation (ChIP-seq) for histone modifications, RNA-sequencing (RNA-seq) for mature mRNA (either 5′ biased, full length, or 3′ biased), and Global Run-On (GRO-seq) for nascent mRNA. Outer box: interactions between functional elements

where bisulfite selectively converts unmethylated cytosine (C) into uracil that is then read by the sequencer as aberrant thymine (T) [44]. The biological significance arises from sites that are differentially methylated between cell types or conditions [45]. Extended regions of differential methylation (DMRs) between cell types are likely to occur in cis-regulatory elements and may reflect cell ontogeny [46]. In particular, regions enriched for CpGs, known as CpG islands, are often found around promoters and tend to be hypomethylated [45]. Methylation of CpG islands is associated with repressed genes; for example, a signature of methylation within these regions in fibroblast-like synoviocytes is thought to distinguish RA from osteoarthritis [47]. Moreover, differential methylation in blood is associated with genes in monozygotic twins who were discordant for SLE [48]. Outside of promoters, methylation has a more complex relationship with gene expression. For example, gene bodies may be heavily methylated in patterns that are associated with nucleosome positioning, binding of structural proteins (e.g., CTCF), intron–exon boundaries, and splicing [49, 50]. This dynamic is regulated by the opposing activity of DNA methyltransferases and demethylases whose expression may be altered in autoimmune disease, such as SLE [51]. Similarly, there is a close association between DNA methylation and histone modifications since hypermethylation tends to overlap repressive marks while hypomethylation is associated with activating marks at cis-regulatory elements [52].

Chromatin state

Along with DNA methylation, the genome-wide chromatin state of a cell is part of its epigenomic profile and may be used to annotate its cis-regulatory elements. When compared with gene expression, the chromatin state tends to give a broader picture of the cell's GRN by highlighting the relevant interactors. Much of the genome consists of nucleosomes, approximately 150 bp of DNA wrapped around a histone octamer, that form the fundamental unit of chromatin [53]. Open chromatin, accessible regions of the genome that are depleted of nucleosomes, is associated with functional regulatory elements [54, 55]. The Assay for Transposase Accessible Chromatin (ATAC-seq) has emerged as an easy and versatile protocol for identifying open chromatin regions at low cell numbers [56]. Furthermore, specific post-translational modifications to histone tails have been associated with different regulatory elements [57]. The first genome-wide study of multiple histone modifications in human CD4$^+$ T cells showed that, among other marks, variable levels of methylation of the fourth lysine on histone 3 were associated with different cis-regulatory elements: tri-methylation (H3K4me3) was highest at proximal elements, known as promoters, while monomethylation (H3K4me1) was more commonly found near distal enhancers. H3K4me2 acts as a hybrid and has been used with other marks and gene contexts to mark both promoters or enhancers [12, 13]. Histone acetylation is typically associated with gene activation: for example, the combination of H3K27ac and H3K4me1 marks active enhancers while H3K4me1 alone is a mark of poised enhancers [58]. In contrast, H3K27me3 is found at repressed elements or, in combination with H3K4me3, bivalent domains, that occur specifically at the promoters of genes poised in stem cells [59, 60]. Together, the profiles of multiple histone modifications can be used to infer the chromatin state of genomic regions: in fact, ChromHMM was designed to automate this process using a machine-learning algorithm [61]. Chromatin immunoprecipitation (ChIP-seq) is used to generate a genome-wide map of these histone modifications, as well as the binding of specific TFs, based on the affinity of antibodies. Gosselin et al. [12] combined ChIP-seq of histone modifications and the myeloid TF, PU.1, to identify tissue-specific factors in macrophages. These chromatin assays have not yet been widely used in rheumatology: this is likely because of the inability to collect sufficient cell numbers in the models of interest. A recently developed protocol of ChIP-seq, named indexing-first ChIP (iChIP), enables parallelization of multiple modifications and samples with low input [36].

Chromatin interactions

In addition to the chromatin state of an individual region, it can be informative to assay the interactions of that region with the rest of the genome. Interacting regions include enhancer-to-promoter loops and topologically associated domains (TADs), which are thought to bring together distant genomic regions that are coregulated [62]. This three-dimensional structure of the chromatin has been widely assayed with Hi-C [63], a high-throughput successor of earlier chromosome conformation capture (3C) methods, and Chromatin Interaction Analysis by Paired-End Tagging (ChIA-PET) [64], an extension of ChIP to capture chromatin interactions. These technologies are at the forefront of innovation with new development in both experimental and computational approaches being put forward regularly. A new method, known as genome architecture mapping, represents an innovative approach to mapping chromatin interactions based on the principle that interacting regions should be frequently found in the same nuclear slice [65].

Single-cell technology

As opposed to the bulk assays already described that represent whole cell populations, single-cell technologies are aimed at assaying individual cells. The goal of single-cell approaches is to discern the heterogeneity of a population of cells without relying on *a priori* sorting. Thus, unlike the bulk assays, single-cell samples should be designed to contain a variable population. Typically, this variation is used to identify subpopulations of cells, which are then compared to reference bulk data sets or isolated as input for future assays. In particular, single-cell RNA-seq, which may be called scRNA-seq generically, has become quite popular in many fields including immunology [66], although other single-cell functional genomic protocols exist [67–71]. There are high hopes for the applicability of scRNA-seq to clinical rheumatology and precision medicine in the near future [66]. Single-cell protocols are generally just scaled-down versions of bulk protocols that are adapted for very low input. A few different versions of scRNA-seq exist that vary by the exact RNA-seq protocol (i.e., end biased or full length), the isolation of single cells, and the use of unique molecular identifiers (UMIs). For example, MARS-seq [40] and SMART-seq2 [37] both use fluorescence-activated cell sorting (FACS) to isolate single cells and deposit them in the wells of a cell-capture plate. While SMART-seq2 provides the additional information of full-length reads, MARS-seq uses 3′-biased reads with UMIs, which reduce noise by enabling the discrimination of true biological copies from amplification duplicates. Other versions of scRNA-seq rely on microfluidics (CEL-seq2 [72]) or microdroplets (Drop-seq [73]) to ensure single-cell reactions. Because of technical and biological limitations, single-cell technologies tend to have low coverage and depth, leading to sparse data sets and high noise [74]: thus, they will likely fall short of modeling the GRNs of individual cells. However, single-cell approaches are effective at assigning cells to different GRNs based on clustering or other algorithms that organize cells by similar cellular states, especially when used in combination with bulk assays or databases. These cellular states may differ based on cell type [37], development [40], cell cycle [75], spatial niche [76], response to stimuli [77], and so forth. For example, single-cell analysis of old and young hematopoietic stem cells demonstrated fewer old cells in the G1 phase and an inverse relationship between differentiation and age [75]. At present, single-cell analysis is fairly complicated owing to the large, complex data sets, but the bioinformatics support is rapidly catching up.

Big bioinformatics

The utility of high-throughput sequencing assays is dependent on the ability to analyze and model the resulting data. Fortunately, development of bioinformatic methods has progressed steadily, giving rise to a variety of standard techniques and publicly available software for the common approaches. For conciseness, this review begins with an analysis of the processed data (see Table 1) assuming that alignment, normalization,

Table 1 Different assays for functional genomics, common protocols, format of the data after processing, and application to the GRN

Assay	Protocol	Processed data format	Direct application to GRN
Gene expression	RNA-seq, microarray	Table of samples (columns) by genes (rows)	Output
Chromatin state	ChIP-seq, ATAC-seq	List of peaks	Nodes
Chromatin interactions	Hi-C, ChIA-PET, GAM	Matrix of interactions	Edges
DNA methylation	BS-seq	List of methylated sites	Nodes
Single-cell technology	scRNA-seq	Table of cells (columns) by genes (rows)	Discriminate different GRNs

GRN gene regulatory network, *RNA-seq* RNA-sequencing, *ChIP-seq* chromatin immunoprecipitation followed by high-throughput sequencing, *ATAC-seq* Assay for Transposase Accessible Chromatin followed by high-throughput sequencing, *Hi-C* high-throughput chromosome conformation capture, *ChIA-PET* Chromatin Interaction Analysis by Paired-End Tag Sequencing, *GAM* genome architecture mapping, *BS-seq* bisulfite sequencing, *scRNA-seq* single-cell RNA-sequencing

and filtering has occurred as necessary. In fact, these early processing steps are well covered by the literature and the related algorithms have already undergone several iterations of development since the dawn of high-throughput genomic assays. Readers are encouraged to approach the analysis as an extension of the experiment in which the various steps must be optimized, reproducible, and confirmed by multiple pieces of evidence. As in "wet" laboratory protocols, there is often no universally correct choice: the parameters must be decided based on the question and the data. The results should be presented given the implicit assumptions of the methods. Figure 2 shows sample output from RNA-seq, ATAC-seq, and ChIP-seq to give the reader an idea of what the data look like.

Differential analysis

The simplest analysis involves a pairwise comparison between two samples or sets of samples. In the field of rheumatology, this will often, but not always, involve comparison of healthy to diseased cells. For gene expression, several algorithms exist to test, for each gene, the null hypothesis that the expression across the replicates of two samples is derived from the same distribution [78]. Because thousands of genes are compared in parallel, these algorithms often report a FDR to account for multiple hypotheses. In SSc, one might ask which genes are differentially expressed between fibrotic patients vs healthy control tissue [31] or treated vs untreated patients [33]. For DNA methylation, DMRs reflect changes in the methylation rate across windows covering many individual methylation sites [44]. For example, changes in the methylation status between T cells in lupus compared with health are thought to reflect changes to the regulation of adaptive immunity [51]. Pairwise comparison of peaks, regions of enrichment for the feature of interest, reflecting the chromatin state is less well defined. Complexity arises when determining which regions to compare since the peaks calls from one sample will not necessarily align with those in another. Simply assessing overlap of peaks is vulnerable to thresholding issues and differing levels of signal-to-noise ratios across samples: thus, peaks across samples are generally merged and the relevant scores are recalculated for the merged regions. Differential chromatin state reflects the opening, closing, or activation of cis-regulatory elements between samples, but these patterns may be more complicated than can be captured by a pairwise comparison.

Beyond pairwise comparisons

Often, differential analysis is not sufficient to cover the diversity or dimensionality of the samples in rheumatology. This may be the case when comparing multiple patient samples with disease subtypes [22] or when collecting multiple samples from different tissues or differentiation states [13, 36]. In these cases, supervised classification may be used when the labeling (e.g., clinical subtype) of samples is known. Otherwise, clustering provides an unsupervised option that does not rely on prior assumptions in order to address the question. Both samples and genes may be clustered based on their similarity by Pearson's correlation, although there are alternative distance metrics. Milano et al. [22] used hierarchical clustering to group SSc patients by intrinsic gene expression. In contrast, *k*-means clustering was used to group enhancers based on H3K4me1 intensity across hematopoiesis [36]. Clustering of genes can also be used to categorize the coregulation of genes or regulatory elements. ImmGen executed a substantial effort of this sort to identify modules of coregulated genes across numerous immune cell types and link them to candidate regulators [79]. In human disease, we used the correlation of expression across macrophage samples isolated from the joints of RA patients to identify gene modules that may be associated with disease subtype (Mandelin et al, accepted). Similarly, Olsson et al. [80] use an iterative filtering approach to identify the most coregulated genes for clustering of single-cell data. Alternatively, assignment to meta-genes (or regulatory profiles) can be used to capture the major patterns of regulation across conditions, such as that seen by non-negative matrix factorization of gene expression through microglia development [40]. As the data sets get larger, dimension reduction methods enable visualization of samples as points in a graph of two-dimensional space. For

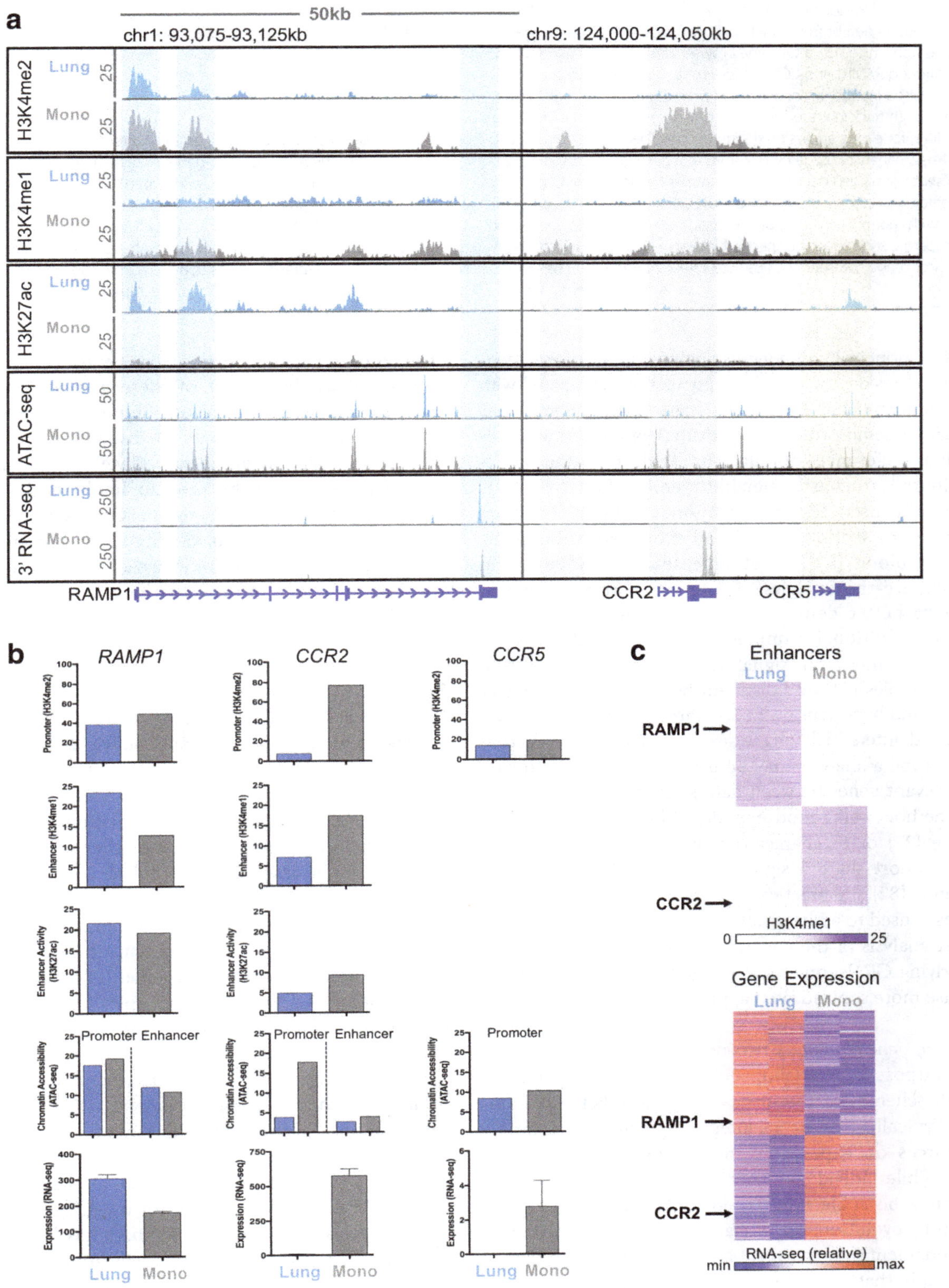

Fig. 2 (See legend on next page.)

(See figure on previous page.)
Fig. 2 Sample output from functional genomic assays. Data generated from lung alveolar macrophages (blue) and bone marrow monocytes (grey) isolated from mice [13]. **a** Genome browser view of raw data from ChIP-seq (H3K4me2, H3K4me1, H3K27ac), ATAC-seq, and 3′-biased RNA-seq in 50 kb locus around RAMP1 and CCR2/CCR5. Highlighted regions from left to right represent: promoter, active intragenic enhancer, and 3′ end of RAMP1 (blue); poised intergenic enhancer and promoter/3′ end of CCR2 (gray); and promoter/3′ end of CCR2 (yellow). Genomic coordinates given above and scale of each track indicated on the left. Genes represented by blue lines below: thin lines for introns, medium lines for untranslated regions (UTRs), thick lines for exons; arrows on the gene body specify gene direction. **b** Quantitative measures of functional elements in **a**. Promoter usage is given by H3K4me2, enhancer usage by H3K4me1, enhancer activity by H3K27ac, chromatin accessibility by ATAC-seq, and gene expression by RNA-seq. Values represent normalized density (read count per kb region length per million reads) for ATAC-seq and ChIP-seq, and normalized CPM (counts per million reads) for RNA-seq (note varying scale). RAMP1, example of lung-specific gene with constitutive promoter. CCR2, example of highly monocyte-specific gene with monocyte-specific promoter and enhancer. CCR5, example of nonexpressed gene with low promoter activity. **c** Heatmaps clustered into lung-specific and monocyte-specific functional elements indicating how data from individual genes are integrated into global analyses. Differential enhancer usage measured by absolute value of H3K4me1 in 6575 regions and differential gene expression measured by relative value of RNA-seq in 3348 genes. ATAC-seq Assay for Transposase Accessible Chromatin followed by high-throughput sequencing, RNA-seq RNA-sequencing

instance, principal components analysis (PCA) of endogenous tissue-resident macrophage populations compared with those differentiated from bone marrow transplants after irradiation demonstrated the proximity of the chimera cells to their reference populations [13]. In addition, t-distributed stochastic neighbor embedding (tSNE) is commonly used for visualization of single-cell data, as in the dissection of DC and monocyte subpopulations in blood [37]. In other cases, it may be useful to compare the samples of interest to related data in order to better demarcate the genes involved. By including additional samples, researchers identified a consistent interferon signature between SSc and SLE blood samples [81] and distinguished between pulmonary fibrosis and hypertension in SSc through comparison with unrelated interstitial lung disease samples [23]. Alternatively, a meta-analysis may be used to indirectly compare the relevant genes between data sets; for example, to determine how well a mouse model of lupus reflects human disease [27] or to characterize which patients in a published cohort share a signature associated with imatinib response [82]. In practice, a combination of these techniques is used to address different questions and provide a robust analysis of the data. However, to fully capture the underlying GRNs, one must integrate different data types and use more sophisticated approaches.

Modeling gene regulatory networks

The purpose of modeling GRNs is to understand the overall scheme for the observed changes between samples. Typically, this means integrating data from a variety of sources on expression, methylation, and chromatin state. While individual changes in any one of these profiles may be subject to random change and not conserved by evolution, the global shape of the GRN should be fundamental to the identity of the cell. The nodes of the graph that constitute the GRN represent the cis-acting and trans-acting regulatory factors, while the edges represent interactions between them, such as the binding of TFs to regulatory elements or the looping of promoters and enhancers. Gene expression can be thought of as the output of these graphs; changes in expression indicate changes in the GRN, but may be of limited utility on their own in distinguishing between the many possible explanations. Given enough samples, gene expression may be used to implicate TF activity within a network as done by the Ontogenet algorithm developed by ImmGen to identify lineage-specific regulation [7] and by a network approach to a meta-analysis SSc cohort [28]. Alternatively, the chromatin state can provide additional depth and the ability to quantify the changes between conditions. By first choosing an assay to anchor the analysis—for example, peaks identified from the ATAC-seq data—one can then annotate these regions based on the remaining assays to identify promoters, poised enhancers, and active enhancers. The next step is to categorize the regions that change state between conditions. This method can be used to assess the degree of change across differentiation [83], environment [12, 13], or time [40]. One challenge in constructing the GRN is assigning cis-regulatory elements to the genes they regulate [84]. This is typically done by physical proximity, although this may not be reliable [55]. Another option is to use Hi-C or ChIA-PET data as proof of interactions between enhancers and gene promoters [63, 64]. Nodes at the apex of the GRN are enhancers or TFs that are involved in the regulation of other regulatory factors, such as lineage-determining TFs that specify the cell's identity and pioneer TFs that bring about changes in the chromatin state [46]. Identification of these factors may be tantamount to defining the whole GRN. For example, identification of overrepresented TF binding motifs in the DNA sequence of enhancers based on their pattern of usage and expression of the associated TF family members has been used to implicate TFs associated with specification of cell types in hematopoiesis and environmental signals in tissue specificity [13, 36]. Similarly, by comparing gene expression and the dynamics of enhancers through T-cell development, Kitagawa et al. [83] implicated Satb1 in regulatory T-cell specification. The key factors of GRNs are likely to provide effective therapeutic targets depending on their relationship to disease.

Understanding the disease mechanism

Given a well-designed study, the differences in GRNs between samples should reflect the underlying disease mechanism. In effector cells, the GRN will explain how the cells are malfunctioning to enact disease and may even account for the cause, offering an attractive target for therapies. Sets of genes, whether arrived at through differential analysis, clustering, or other approach, may be compared to gene annotations to find enriched pathways or processes, as done to label gene modules in an SSc meta-analysis [28]. The gene ontology (GO) annotation is popularly used for this purpose, although it is limited by the underlying database (some genes may be unannotated) and biased by the more common cell types used to build this database. There has been some success in linking key sets of genes to disease severity [85] or response to treatment [33] using training (to identify the predictive genes) and testing (to validate their efficacy) cohorts. These approaches are likely to be improved with more data on cell-type-specific and tissue-specific populations. Moreover, changes in the GRN of a cell may be compared to publicly available databases to find similarities associated with shared triggers. For example, the LINCS website offers a similar function to recognize common signatures caused by specific cellular perturbations [6]. In rheumatic diseases with a genetic component, the causative single nucleotide polymorphisms (SNPs) are often found in noncoding regions where they have an impact on epigenomic regulation by directly or indirectly affecting TF binding [46]. When these SNPs are associated with changes in gene expression, termed eQTLs, they can be used to implicate cell types that are likely to play a role in disease, such as T-cell genes in RA and B cells in lupus [86, 87], although the underlying mechanism is not always clear. To uncover the molecular link between SNPs and disease, two studies which used data from genome-wide association studies (GWAS) and chromatin assays of multiple cell types found were able to implicate high-confidence causal SNPs that have the potential to disrupt regulatory elements [88–90]. But these studies, limited as they are by the sensitivity of GWAS and generic chromatin profiles from unrelated donors, are just the beginning.

Big future

In the future, functional genomics approaches will become more prevalent in rheumatology. Certainly, the next review on a similar topic will have many more examples within the field on which to draw. Advances in other fields will influence how we view rheumatic disease and vice versa. As these assays become more popular, there are likely to be changes in their uses and scope.

Even bigger data

As the technology matures, the experiments will become cheaper and of even higher throughput. Rather than pairwise comparisons of test vs control, this will lead to larger data sets as more samples or single cells are assayed in a given experiment. In mouse models, this will enable more thorough modeling of GRNs by comparing the evolution of closely related populations at multiple conditions or time points. Human studies should include larger cohorts of patients and focus on identifying clinical subtypes in the pathogenesis of disease. Moreover, multiple forms of genomic data will be collected for each individual sample so that genetic variation can be directly associated with changes in the transcriptional and epigenomic profile. This is in contrast with the current situation where most epigenomic data from humans treat different individuals as replicates without the power to characterize individual variation. Similarly, whole tissue samples and in vitro cultures will be abandoned in favor of assays that focus on the cell type(s) of interest at multiple time points, states of differentiation/activation, or disease progression. With the advance in efficiency of assays, there will be a corresponding expansion in data available online.

Interactive public databases and user-friendly analysis programs

As already described, several concerted efforts already exist to collect data sets for public consumption. Currently, they are limited in the scope of the samples and the usefulness to the average researcher. Although most journals require authors to submit their data to a publicly available database, most biologists do not have the skills, time, or interest to find and use this raw data. In the future, when these databases reach a critical mass in the field of rheumatology, it will increasingly become more valuable for researchers to interact with them. Likewise, the databases will evolve to offer more user-friendly interfaces so that even the less tech-savvy users can find the information for which they are searching. Moreover, as the technology matures, increasingly more programs have become available that allow amateurs to peruse data and perform conventional analyses. Online programs to identify enriched GO terms and pathways are particularly prevalent, even for intergenic genomic regions [84]. There is even software with graphical user interfaces for sequencing pipelines (https://usegalaxy.org/) and clustering (https://software.broadinstitute.org/morpheus/). The challenge here is that they can be so easy to run that the user is unaware of the assumptions being made: this is why they do not replace training in functional genomics analysis. As the amount of data available increases and the bioinformatics methods become popularized, the skill set of researchers will evolve in kind.

Integration of computational approaches

At some point in the future, the distinction between computational biologists and other biologists will disappear. Already, young scientists are being taught quantitative methods and how to use bioinformatics tools as part of their general training in biology. In the future, a degree in biology will de facto include an education on computer science and statistics. As the average level of computational aptitude is raised, researchers will handle their own data throughout the processing and analysis stages. The bioinformatics capabilities of biologists and the accessibility of computational tools will dovetail to empower a progressively larger proportion of the community. Any competent researcher in functional genomics will be proficient at both the "wet" and "dry" components, meaning that advances in analysis will be synonymous with advances in experimental technique. As a result, the field of computational biology will become obsolete along with the value of so-called bioinformatics cores. Research in the intersection of rheumatology and genomics will be performed by interdisciplinary researchers or equal collaborations between rheumatologists and genomic investigators specializing in the cell type or tissue of interest.

Conclusions

The goal of this review is to provide an overview of functional genomics and the challenges and possibilities inherent in big data. This overview comes at a time when genomics assays are widespread throughout biological fields but have yet to be fully taken advantage of in the field of rheumatology. This may be because it is not obvious to researchers how to make use of these data in a manner that extends beyond an exploratory study with descriptive results, or it may be because researchers are overwhelmed by the plethora of options and do not know where to begin. Therefore, the review has broken down functional genomics research into several stages. First, designing the study to best reflect the question of interest. Next, understanding the diverse data types that can be integrated into the following analysis. The bioinformatics section covers multiple approaches to be used in tandem to better model the underlying GRNs of disease. Finally, the review offers a future vision of the inevitable expansion of functional genomics into rheumatology.

Abbreviations

ATAC-seq: Assay for Transposase Accessible Chromatin followed by high-throughput sequencing; BMDM: Bone-marrow-derived macrophage; BS-seq: BiSulfite sequencing; ChIA-PET: Chromatin Interaction Analysis by Paired-End Tag Sequencing; ChIP-seq: Chromatin Immuno Precipitation followed by high-throughput sequencing; DC: Dendritic cell; DMR: Differentially methylated regions; ENCODE: ENCyclopedia of DNA Elements; FDR: False discovery rate; GAM: Genome architecture mapping; GMCSF: Granulocyte–macrophage colony-stimulating factors; GRN: Gene regulatory network; GRO-seq: Global Run-On sequencing; GTex: Genotype-Tissue Expression project; GWAS: Genome-wide association study; Hi-C: High-throughput chromosome conformation capture; iChIP: Indexing first ChIP-seq; ImmGen: Immunological Genome Project; LINCS: Library of Integrated Network-based Cellular Signatures; PCA: Principal components analysis; PolII: RNA Polymerase II; RA: Rheumatoid arthritis; SNP: Single nucleotide polymorphism; SSc: Systemic sclerosis; STIA: Serum-transfer induced arthritis; TAD: Topologically associated domains; TF: Transcription factor

Acknowledgements

The author thanks Dr Daniel Fleisher for critical reading of the manuscript and Dr Harris Perlman for inspiring her personal application of functional genomics to the study of rheumatology.

Funding

Research in the Winter Lab is funded by the Northwestern Memorial Foundation Dixon Award, Arthritis National Research Foundation, and the American Lung Association.

Author's information

DRW obtained a PhD in Computational Biology from Duke University studying basic gene regulation. Her research turned to immunology with her postdoctorate in the laboratory of Ido Amit. Currently, she is an Assistant Professor in the Division of Rheumatology, manages the Winter Lab of Functional Genomics to apply genomic approaches to study the role of immune cells in health and rheumatic disease, and is a member of the American College of Rheumatology.

Competing interests

The authors declare that they have no competing interests.

References

1. Consortium EP, Bernstein B, Birney E, Dunham I, Green E, Gunter C, Snyder M. An integrated encyclopedia of DNA elements in the human genome. Nature. 2012;489(7414):57–74.
2. Consortium EP, Birney E, Stamatoyannopoulos J, Dutta A, Guigó R, Gingeras T, Margulies E, Weng Z, Snyder M, Dermitzakis E, et al. Identification and analysis of functional elements in 1% of the human genome by the ENCODE pilot project. Nature. 2007;447(7146):799–816.
3. Kundaje A, Meuleman W, Ernst J, Bilenky M, Yen A, Heravi-Moussavi A, Kheradpour P, Zhang Z, Wang J, Ziller MJ, et al. Integrative analysis of 111 reference human epigenomes. Nature. 2015;518(7539):317–30.
4. Consortium EP. A user's guide to the encyclopedia of DNA elements (ENCODE). PLoS Biol. 2011;9(4):e1001046.
5. Mele M, Ferreira PG, Reverter F, DeLuca DS, Monlong J, Sammeth M, Young TR, Goldmann JM, Pervouchine DD, Sullivan TJ, et al. Human genomics. The human transcriptome across tissues and individuals. Science. 2015; 348(6235):660–5.
6. Duan Q, Flynn C, Niepel M, Hafner M, Muhlich JL, Fernandez NF, Rouillard AD, Tan CM, Chen EY, Golub TR, et al. LINCS Canvas Browser: interactive web app to query, browse and interrogate LINCS L1000 gene expression signatures. Nucleic Acids Res. 2014;42:W449–60.
7. Heng TS, Painter MW, Immunological Genome Project Consortium. The Immunological Genome Project: networks of gene expression in immune cells. Nat Immunol. 2008;9(10):1091–4.
8. Martens JHA, Stunnenberg HG. BLUEPRINT: mapping human blood cell epigenomes. Haematologica. 2013;98(10):1487–9.
9. Ostuni R, Piccolo V, Barozzi I, Polletti S, Termanini A, Bonifacio S, Curina A, Prosperini E, Ghisletti S, Natoli G. Latent enhancers activated by stimulation in differentiated cells. Cell. 2013;152(1–2):157–71.

10. Heinz S, Benner C, Spann N, Bertolino E, Lin Y, Laslo P, Cheng J, Murre C, Singh H, Glass C. Simple combinations of lineage-determining transcription factors prime cis-regulatory elements required for macrophage and B cell identities. Mol Cell. 2010;38(4):576–89.
11. Helft J, Bottcher J, Chakravarty P, Zelenay S, Huotari J, Schraml BU Goubau D. Reis e Sousa C. GM-CSF mouse bone marrow cultures comprise a heterogeneous population of CD11c(+)MHCII(+) macrophages and dendritic cells. Immunity. 2015;42(6):1197–211.
12. Gosselin D, Link VM, Romanoski CE, Fonseca GJ, Eichenfield DZ, Spann NJ, Stender JD, Chun HB, Garner H, Geissmann F, et al. Environment drives selection and function of enhancers controlling tissue-specific macrophage identities. Cell. 2014;159(6):1327–40.
13. Lavin Y, Winter D, Blecher-Gonen R, David E, Keren-Shaul H, Merad M, Jung S, Amit I. Tissue-resident macrophage enhancer landscapes are shaped by the local microenvironment. Cell. 2014;159(6):1312–26.
14. Gardner H, Shearstone JR, Bandaru R, Crowell T, Lynes M, Trojanowska M, Pannu J, Smith E, Jablonska S, Blaszczyk M, et al. Gene profiling of scleroderma skin reveals robust signatures of disease that are imperfectly reflected in the transcript profiles of explanted fibroblasts. Arthritis Rheum. 2006;54(6):1961–73.
15. Bessis N, Decker P, Assier E, Semerano L, Boissier MC. Arthritis models: usefulness and interpretation. Semin Immunopathol. 2017;39(4):469–86.
16. Marangoni RG, Varga J, Tourtellotte WG. Animal models of scleroderma: recent progress. Curr Opin Rheumatol. 2016;28(6):561–70.
17. Bender AT, Wu Y, Cao Q, Ding Y, Oestreicher J, Genest M, Akare S, Ishizaka ST, Mackey MF. Assessment of the translational value of mouse lupus models using clinically relevant biomarkers. Transl Res. 2014;163(6):515–32.
18. Rose S, Eren M, Murphy S, Zhang H, Thaxton CS, Chowaniec J, Waters EA, Meade TJ, Vaughan DE, Perlman H. A novel mouse model that develops spontaneous arthritis and is predisposed towards atherosclerosis. Ann Rheum Dis. 2013;72(1):89–95.
19. Bethunaickan R, Berthier CC, Ramanujam M, Sahu R, Zhang W, Sun Y, Bottinger EP, Ivashkiv L, Kretzler M, Davidson A. A unique hybrid renal mononuclear phagocyte activation phenotype in murine systemic lupus erythematosus nephritis. J Immunol. 2011;186(8):4994–5003.
20. Mouratis MA, Aidinis V. Modeling pulmonary fibrosis with bleomycin. Curr Opin Pulm Med. 2011;17(5):355–61.
21. Misharin AV, Morales-Nebreda L, Reyfman PA, Cuda CM, Walter JM, McQuattie-Pimentel AC, Chen CI, Anekalla KR, Joshi N, Williams KJN et al. Monocyte-derived alveolar macrophages drive lung fibrosis and persist in the lung over the life span. J Exp Med. 2017;214(8):2387–404.
22. Milano A, Pendergrass SA, Sargent JL, George LK, McCalmont TH, Connolly MK, Whitfield ML. Molecular subsets in the gene expression signatures of scleroderma skin. PLoS One. 2008;3(7):e2696.
23. Hsu E, Shi H, Jordan RM, Lyons-Weiler J, Pilewski JM, Feghali-Bostwick CA. Lung tissues in patients with systemic sclerosis have gene expression patterns unique to pulmonary fibrosis and pulmonary hypertension. Arthritis Rheum. 2011;63(3):783–94.
24. Bharat A, Bhorade SM, Morales-Nebreda L, McQuattie-Pimentel AC, Soberanes S, Ridge K, DeCamp MM, Mestan KK, Perlman H, Budinger GR, et al. Flow cytometry reveals similarities between lung macrophages in humans and mice. Am J Respir Cell Mol Biol. 2016;54(1):147–9.
25. Misharin AV, Cuda CM, Saber R, Turner JD, Gierut AK, Haines 3rd GK Berdnikovs S, Filer A, Clark AR, Buckley CD, et al. Nonclassical Ly6C(-) monocytes drive the development of inflammatory arthritis in mice Cell Rep. 2014;9(2):591–604.
26. Bernstein BE, Kamal M, Lindblad-Toh K, Bekiranov S, Bailey DK, Huebert DJ, McMahon S, Karlsson EK, Kulbokas 3rd EJ, Gingeras TR, et al. Genomic maps and comparative analysis of histone modifications in human and mouse. Cell. 2005;120(2):169–81.
27. Berthier CC, Bethunaickan R, Gonzalez-Rivera T, Nair V, Ramanujam M, Zhang W, Bottinger EP, Segerer S, Lindenmeyer M, Cohen CD, et al. Cross-species transcriptional network analysis defines shared inflammatory responses in murine and human lupus nephritis. J Immunol. 2012;189(2):988–1001.
28. Mahoney JM, Taroni J, Martyanov V, Wood TA, Greene CS, Pioli PA, Hinchcliff ME, Whitfield ML. Systems level analysis of systemic sclerosis shows a network of immune and profibrotic pathways connected with genetic polymorphisms. PLoS Comput Biol. 2015;11(1):e1004005.
29. Altboum Z, Steuerman Y, David E, Barnett-Itzhaki Z, Valadarsky L, Keren-Shaul H, Meningher T, Mendelson E, Mandelboim M, Gat-Viks I, et al. Digital cell quantification identifies global immune cell dynamics during influenza infection. Mol Syst Biol. 2014;10(2):720.
30. Becht E, Giraldo NA, Lacroix L, Buttard B, Elarouci N, Petitprez F, Selves J, Laurent-Puig P, Sautes-Fridman C, Fridman WH, et al. Estimating the population abundance of tissue-infiltrating immune and stromal cell populations using gene expression. Genome Biol. 2016;17(1):218.
31. Christmann RB, Sampaio-Barros P, Stifano G, Borges CL, de Carvalho CR, Kairalla R, Parra ER, Spira A, Simms R, Capellozzi VL, et al. Association of Interferon- and transforming growth factor beta-regulated genes and macrophage activation with systemic sclerosis-related progressive lung fibrosis. Arthritis Rheumatol. 2014;66(3):714–25.
32. Higashi-Kuwata N, Jinnin M, Makino T, Fukushima S, Inoue Y, Muchemwa FC, Yonemura Y, Komohara Y, Takeya M, Mitsuya H, et al. Characterization of monocyte/macrophage subsets in the skin and peripheral blood derived from patients with systemic sclerosis. Arthritis Res Ther. 2010;12(4):R128.
33. Hinchcliff M, Huang CC, Wood TA, Matthew Mahoney J, Martyanov V, Bhattacharyya S, Tamaki Z, Lee J, Carns M, Podlusky S, et al. Molecular signatures in skin associated with clinical improvement during mycophenolate treatment in systemic sclerosis. J Invest Dermatol. 2013;133(8):1979–89.
34. Ching T, Huang S, Garmire LX. Power analysis and sample size estimation for RNA-Seq differential expression. RNA. 2014;20(11):1684–96.
35. Lee ML, Whitmore GA. Power and sample size for DNA microarray studies. Stat Med. 2002;21(23):3543–70.
36. Lara-Astiaso D, Weiner A, Lorenzo-Vivas E, Zaretsky I, Jaitin D, David E, Keren-Shaul H, Mildner A, Winter D, Jung S, et al. Chromatin state dynamics during blood formation. Science. 2014;345(6199):943–9.
37. Villani AC, Satija R, Reynolds G, Sarkizova S, Shekhar K, Fletcher J, Griesbeck M, Butler A, Zheng S, Lazo S et al. Single-cell RNA-seq reveals new types of human blood dendritic cells, monocytes, and progenitors. Science. 2017;356(6335): eaah4573.
38. Leek J, Scharpf R, Bravo H, Simcha D, Langmead B, Johnson W, Geman D, Baggerly K, Irizarry R. Tackling the widespread and critical impact of batch effects in high-throughput data. Nat Rev Genet. 2010;11(10):733–9.
39. Oytam Y, Sobhanmanesh F, Duesing K, Bowden JC, Osmond-McLeod M, Ross J. Risk-conscious correction of batch effects: maximising information extraction from high-throughput genomic datasets. BMC Bioinf. 2016;17(1):332.
40. Matcovitch-Natan O, Winter DR, Giladi A, Vargas Aguilar S, Spinrad A, Sarrazin S, Ben-Yehuda H, David E, Zelada González F, Perrin P, et al. Microglia development follows a stepwise program to regulate brain homeostasis. Science. 2016;353(6301):aad8670.
41. Zhang W, Yu Y, Hertwig F, Thierry-Mieg J, Zhang W, Thierry-Mieg D, Wang J, Furlanello C, Devanarayan V, Cheng J, et al. Comparison of RNA-seq and microarray-based models for clinical endpoint prediction. Genome Biol. 2015;16:133.
42. Conesa A, Madrigal P, Tarazona S, Gomez-Cabrero D, Cervera A, McPherson A, Szczesniak MW, Gaffney DJ, Elo LL, Zhang X, et al. A survey of best practices for RNA-seq data analysis. Genome Biol. 2016;17:13.
43. Lopes R, Agami R, Korkmaz G. GRO-seq, a tool for identification of transcripts regulating gene expression. Methods Mol Biol. 2017;1543:45–55.
44. Beck S, Rakyan V. The methylome: approaches for global DNA methylation profiling. Trends Genet. 2008;24(5):231–7.
45. Viatte S, Plant D, Raychaudhuri S. Genetics and epigenetics of rheumatoid arthritis. Nat Rev Rheumatol. 2013;9(3):141–53.
46. Winter DR, Jung S, Amit I. Making the case for chromatin profiling: a new tool to investigate the immune-regulatory landscape. Nat Rev Immunol. 2015;15(9):585–94.
47. Nakano K, Whitaker JW, Boyle DL, Wang W, Firestein GS. DNA methylome signature in rheumatoid arthritis. Ann Rheum Dis. 2013;72(1):110–7.
48. Javierre BM, Fernandez AF, Richter J, Al-Shahrour F, Martin-Subero JI, Rodriguez-Ubreva J, Berdasco M, Fraga MF, O'Hanlon TP, Rider LG, et al. Changes in the pattern of DNA methylation associate with twin discordance in systemic lupus erythematosus. Genome Res. 2010;20(2):170–9.
49. Chodavarapu R, Feng S, Bernatavichute Y, Chen P-Y, Stroud H, Yu Y, Hetzel J, Kuo F, Kim J, Cokus S, et al. Relationship between nucleosome positioning and DNA methylation. Nature. 2010;466(7304):388–92.
50. Shukla S, Kavak E, Gregory M, Imashimizu M, Shutinoski B, Kashlev M, Oberdoerffer P, Sandberg R, Oberdoerffer S. CTCF-promoted RNA polymerase II pausing links DNA methylation to splicing. Nature. 2011; 479(7371):74–9.
51. Hedrich CM, Mabert K, Rauen T, Tsokos GC. DNA methylation in systemic lupus erythematosus. Epigenomics. 2017;9(4):505–25.
52. Cedar H, Bergman Y. Linking DNA methylation and histone modification: patterns and paradigms. Nat Rev Genet. 2009;10(5):295–304.

53. Richmond T, Davey C. The structure of DNA in the nucleosome core. Nature. 2003;423(6936):145–50.
54. Gross D, Garrard W. Nuclease hypersensitive sites in chromatin. Annu Rev Biochem. 1988;57:159–97.
55. Thurman R, Rynes E, Humbert R, Vierstra J, Maurano M, Haugen E, Sheffield N, Stergachis A, Wang H, Vernot B, et al. The accessible chromatin landscape of the human genome. Nature. 2012;489(7414):75–82.
56. Buenrostro J, Giresi P, Zaba L, Chang H, Greenleaf W. Transposition of native chromatin for fast and sensitive epigenomic profiling of open chromatin, DNA-binding proteins and nucleosome position. Nat Methods. 2013;10(12): 1213–8.
57. Kouzarides T. Chromatin modifications and their function. Cell. 2007;128(4): 693–705.
58. Creyghton M, Cheng A, Welstead G, Kooistra T, Carey B, Steine E, Hanna J, Lodato M, Frampton G, Sharp P, et al. Histone H3K27ac separates active from poised enhancers and predicts developmental state. Proc Natl Acad Sci U S A. 2010;107(50):21931–6.
59. Barski A, Cuddapah S, Cui K, Roh T-Y, Schones D, Wang Z, Wei G, Chepelev I, Zhao K. High-resolution profiling of histone methylations in the human genome. Cell. 2007;129(4):823–37.
60. Cui K, Zang C, Roh T-Y, Schones DE, Childs RW, Peng W, Zhao K. Chromatin signatures in multipotent human hematopoietic stem cells indicate the fate of bivalent genes during differentiation. Cell Stem Cell. 2009;4(1):80–93.
61. Ernst J, Kellis M. ChromHMM: automating chromatin-state discovery and characterization. Nat Methods. 2012;9(3):215–6.
62. Dixon J, Selvaraj S, Yue F, Kim A, Li Y, Shen Y, Hu M, Liu J, Ren B. Topological domains in mammalian genomes identified by analysis of chromatin interactions. Nature. 2012;485(7398):376–80.
63. Lieberman-Aiden E, van Berkum N, Williams L, Imakaev M, Ragoczy T, Telling A, Amit I, Lajoie B, Sabo P, Dorschner M, et al. Comprehensive mapping of long-range interactions reveals folding principles of the human genome. Science. 2009;326(5950):289–93.
64. Kieffer-Kwon K-R, Tang Z, Mathe E, Qian J, Sung M-H, Li G, Resch W, Baek S, Pruett N, Grøntved L, et al. Interactome maps of mouse gene regulatory domains reveal basic principles of transcriptional regulation. Cell. 2013; 155(7):1507–20.
65. Beagrie RA, Scialdone A, Schueler M, Kraemer DC, Chotalia M, Xie SQ, Barbieri M, de Santiago I, Lavitas LM, Branco MR, et al. Complex multi-enhancer contacts captured by genome architecture mapping. Nature. 2017;543(7646):519–24.
66. Jaitin DA, Keren-Shaul H, Elefant N, Amit I. Each cell counts: hematopoiesis and immunity research in the era of single cell genomics. Semin Immunol. 2015;27(1):67–71.
67. Buenrostro JD, Wu B, Litzenburger UM, Ruff D, Gonzales ML, Snyder MP, Chang HY, Greenleaf WJ. Single-cell chromatin accessibility reveals principles of regulatory variation. Nature. 2015;523(7561):486–90.
68. Rotem A, Ram O, Shoresh N, Sperling RA, Goren A, Weitz DA, Bernstein BE. Single-cell ChIP-seq reveals cell subpopulations defined by chromatin state. Nat Biotechnol. 2015;33(11):1165–72.
69. Farlik M, Sheffield NC, Nuzzo A, Datlinger P, Schonegger A, Klughammer J, Bock C. Single-cell DNA methylome sequencing and bioinformatic inference of epigenomic cell-state dynamics. Cell Rep. 2015;10(8):1386–97.
70. Smallwood SA, Lee HJ, Angermueller C, Krueger F, Saadeh H, Peat J, Andrews SR, Stegle O, Reik W, Kelsey G. Single-cell genome-wide bisulfite sequencing for assessing epigenetic heterogeneity. Nat Methods. 2014; 11(8):817–20.
71. Cusanovich DA, Daza R, Adey A, Pliner HA, Christiansen L, Gunderson KL, Steemers FJ, Trapnell C, Shendure J. Multiplex single cell profiling of chromatin accessibility by combinatorial cellular indexing. Science. 2015; 348(6237):910–4.
72. Hashimshony T, Senderovich N, Avital G, Klochendler A, de Leeuw Y, Anavy L, Gennert D, Li S, Livak KJ, Rozenblatt-Rosen O, et al. CEL-Seq2: sensitive highly-multiplexed single-cell RNA-Seq. Genome Biol. 2016;17:77.
73. Macosko EZ, Basu A, Satija R, Nemesh J, Shekhar K, Goldman M, Tirosh I, Bialas AR, Kamitaki N, Martersteck EM, et al. Highly parallel genome-wide expression profiling of individual cells using nanoliter droplets. Cell. 2015; 161(5):1202–14.
74. Kim JK, Kolodziejczyk AA, Ilicic T, Teichmann SA, Marioni JC. Characterizing noise structure in single-cell RNA-seq distinguishes genuine from technical stochastic allelic expression. Nat Commun. 2015;6:8687.
75. Kowalczyk MS, Tirosh I, Heckl D, Rao TN, Dixit A, Haas BJ, Schneider RK, Wagers AJ, Ebert BL, Regev A. Single-cell RNA-seq reveals changes in cell cycle and differentiation programs upon aging of hematopoietic stem cells. Genome Res. 2015;25(12):1860–72.
76. Halpern KB, Shenhav R, Matcovitch-Natan O, Toth B, Lemze D, Golan M, Massasa EE, Baydatch S, Landen S, Moor AE, et al. Single-cell spatial reconstruction reveals global division of labour in the mammalian liver. Nature. 2017;542(7641):352–6.
77. Gury-BenAri M, Thaiss CA, Serafini N, Winter DR, Giladi A, Lara-Astiaso D, Levy M, Salame TM, Weiner A, David E, et al. The spectrum and regulatory landscape of intestinal innate lymphoid cells are shaped by the microbiome. Cell. 2016;166(5):1231–46. e1213.
78. Zhang ZH, Jhaveri DJ, Marshall VM, Bauer DC, Edson J, Narayanan RK, Robinson GJ, Lundberg AE, Bartlett PF, Wray NR, et al. A comparative study of techniques for differential expression analysis on RNA-Seq data. PLoS One. 2014;9(8):e103207.
79. Jojic V, Shay T, Sylvia K, Zuk O, Sun X, Kang J, Regev A, Koller D, Immunological Genome Project C, Best AJ, et al. Identification of transcriptional regulators in the mouse immune system. Nat Immunol. 2013; 14(6):633–43.
80. Olsson A, Venkatasubramanian M, Chaudhri VK, Aronow BJ, Salomonis N, Singh H, Grimes HL. Single-cell analysis of mixed-lineage states leading to a binary cell fate choice. Nature. 2016;537(7622):698–702.
81. Assassi S, Mayes MD, Arnett FC, Gourh P, Agarwal SK, McNearney TA, Chaussabel D, Oommen N, Fischbach M, Shah KR, et al. Systemic sclerosis and lupus: points in an interferon-mediated continuum. Arthritis Rheum. 2010;62(2):589–98.
82. Chung L, Fiorentino DF, Benbarak MJ, Adler AS, Mariano MM, Paniagua RT, Milano A, Connolly MK, Ratiner BD, Wiskocil RL, et al. Molecular framework for response to imatinib mesylate in systemic sclerosis. Arthritis Rheum. 2009;60(2):584–91.
83. Kitagawa Y, Ohkura N, Kidani Y, Vandenbon A, Hirota K, Kawakami R, Yasuda K, Motooka D, Nakamura S, Kondo M, et al. Guidance of regulatory T cell development by Satb1-dependent super-enhancer establishment. Nat Immunol. 2017;18(2):173–83.
84. McLean C, Bristor D, Hiller M, Clarke S, Schaar B, Lowe C, Wenger A, Bejerano G. GREAT improves functional interpretation of cis-regulatory regions. Nat Biotechnol. 2010;28(5):495–501.
85. Lofgren S, Hinchcliff M, Carns M, Wood T, Aren K, Arroyo E, Cheung P, Kuo A, Valenzuela A, Haemel A, et al. Integrated, multicohort analysis of systemic sclerosis identifies robust transcriptional signature of disease severity. JCI Insight. 2016;1(21):e89073.
86. Hu X, Kim H, Raj T, Brennan PJ, Trynka G, Teslovich N, Slowikowski K, Chen WM, Onengut S, Baecher-Allan C, et al. Regulation of gene expression in autoimmune disease loci and the genetic basis of proliferation in CD4+ effector memory T cells. PLoS Genet. 2014;10(6):e1004404.
87. Hu X, Kim H, Stahl E, Plenge R, Daly M, Raychaudhuri S. Integrating autoimmune risk loci with gene-expression data identifies specific pathogenic immune cell subsets. Am J Hum Genet. 2011;89(5):682.
88. Farh KK-H, Marson A, Zhu J, Kleinewietfeld M, Housley WJ, Beik S, Shoresh N, Whitton H, Ryan RJH, Shishkin AA et al. Genetic and epigenetic fine mapping of causal autoimmune disease variants. Nature 2014, advance online publication.
89. Trynka G, Sandor C, Han B, Xu H, Stranger B, Liu X, Raychaudhuri S. Chromatin marks identify critical cell types for fine mapping complex trait variants. Nat Genet. 2013;45(2):124–30.
90. Hui-Yuen JS, Zhu L, Wong LP, Jiang K, Chen Y, Liu T, Jarvis JN. Chromatin landscapes and genetic risk in systemic lupus. Arthritis Res Ther. 2016;18(1):281.

10

Doctors' preferences in de-escalating DMARDs in rheumatoid arthritis: a discrete choice experiment

T. Martijn Kuijper[1*†], Riëtte Folmer[1†], Elly A. Stolk[2], Johanna M. W. Hazes[1] and Jolanda J. Luime[1]

Abstract

Background: Current guidelines suggest reduction of DMARDs can be considered in RA patients in remission. Objectives were (1) to estimate the relative importance of patient characteristics rheumatologists consider in their decision to de-escalate (2) to assess whether heterogeneity exists among rheumatologists with respect to de-escalation and (3) to identify the preferred de-escalation strategy.

Methods: A discrete choice experiment (DCE) was conducted. All rheumatologists and trainees in The Netherlands were invited to participate. A conditional logit model was estimated to assess overall preference for de-escalation and its determinants. Heterogeneity was estimated by latent class analysis.

Results: The DCE questionnaire was completed by 156 doctors. This questionnaire was constructed using the results of semi-structured interviews with 12 rheumatologists that identified five patient characteristics relevant for de-escalation: number of swollen joints (SJC), presence of DAS remission/low disease activity (LDA), patient history, duration of remission/LDA and patient willingness to de-escalate DMARDs. Overall SJC and patient history were most important. Latent class analysis revealed five subgroups of doctors, showing differences regarding willingness to de-escalate and relative importance of patient characteristics. De-escalation of the TNF inhibitor rather than methotrexate first was the most preferred strategy.

Conclusions: Rheumatologists are not uniform in their decision on whom to de-escalate. Differences emerged in which characteristics they traded off resulting in five subgroups: those that taper (1) always, (2) in absence of swollen joints, (3) in absence of swollen joints and presence of favorable patient history, (4) in DAS remission and favorable patient history, and (5) taking into account all factors.

Keywords: Discrete choice experiment, Rheumatoid arthritis, Treatment de-escalation, Preferences

Background

Treatment of rheumatoid arthritis (RA) has advanced greatly during the past decades. The introduction of combination therapy with disease-modifying anti-rheumatic drugs (DMARDs), the recognition of early, tightly controlled treatment, and the introduction of biologic agents have contributed to improved outcomes for patients suffering from RA [1]. With intensive use of (a combination of) DMARDs, a state of low disease activity (LDA) or remission can be achieved by many patients while preventing erosions and functional impairment [2, 3]. Although DMARD therapy is essential to obtain disease control, continuous use comes with several disadvantages. Apart from obvious drawbacks such as drug toxicity and side effects, medication use by itself may be perceived as burdensome and unhealthy by patients. Hence many patients view medication use as a necessary burden and wish to minimize its use. Also medication costs, especially for expensive biological treatments, are of increasing concern for governments. From this viewpoint tapering or discontinuation of DMARDs is preferable once disease control has been obtained.

Current guidelines suggest that reduction of biological (b)DMARDs can be considered, especially if this treatment

* Correspondence: t.kuijper@erasmusmc.nl
†Equal contributors
[1]Department of Rheumatology, Erasmus Medical Center, Room Na-609, PO Box 20403000 CA Rotterdam, The Netherlands
Full list of author information is available at the end of the article

is combined with a conventional synthetic (cs)DMARD, once sustained remission has been achieved and glucocorticoids have been tapered first [4, 5]. In addition, guidelines state that a cautious reduction of csDMARDs could be considered, as a shared decision between patient and physician, after glucocorticoids and bDMARDs have been successfully withdrawn [5]. Furthermore, a general recommendation is included that, apart from disease activity, other factors should be taken into account such as progression of structural damage, comorbidities, and safety issues [5].

Indeed, evidence from a range of clinical studies suggests that de-escalation of DMARDs is feasible in a large number of patients in LDA or disease remission [6–8]. However, to date there is no standardized way to determine the patient for whom de-escalation of DMARD therapy is appropriate [8]. Also, adherence of rheumatologists to the guidelines that are currently available for de-escalation may not be optimal [9]. Therefore large differences are expected to exist between rheumatologists with respect to whether, when, and in which patients they will de-escalate therapy. Obtaining insight in these differences may assist in future guideline development and guide further research into this topic. In the assessment whether a patient is a suitable candidate for treatment de-escalation, rheumatologists weigh several patient characteristics together at the same time. Hence a simple questionnaire in which the importance of patient characteristics is rated separately does not reflect a real-life decision. A discrete choice experiment (DCE) is a method that allows for the analysis of such complex decisions. It does so by presenting a series of "choice tasks" to the participant. Each choice task consists of two hypothetical patients with varying characteristics. The participant must then choose the patient with the most favorable combination of characteristics. By analyzing the choices participants made based on the characteristics, the relative importance of patient characteristics on the decision to de-escalate treatment can be assessed. A technique very similar to that of a discrete choice experiment was used in the process of the development of the American College of Rheumatology/European League Against Rheumatism (ACR/EULAR) 2010 criteria for RA [10].

Objectives of this study were (1) to estimate the relative importance of patient characteristics rheumatologists consider in their decision to de-escalate medication, (2) to quantify how these characteristics influence doctor's preferences for de-escalating DMARDs, (3) to assess whether heterogeneity exists among rheumatologists with respect to their preference for de-escalation and the patient characteristics influencing this decision, and (4) to identify the most preferred de-escalation strategy.

Methods

DCE

In a DCE it is assumed that the analyzing process leading to a decision to medically intervene, such as de-escalation of medication, can be described by features relevant for making that decision (patient and disease characteristics) [11, 12]. In the case of a rheumatologist deciding whether to de-escalate DMARDs for a certain patient, these characteristics are likely disease related (e.g., presence of swollen joints indicating active disease). Each characteristic can then be further described by specific variants or levels (e.g., presence of no, one or two swollen joints) [11, 12]. Another assumption is that an individual's preference for the intervention is determined by the levels of these characteristics [11, 12]. By offering a series of choices between two options with different characteristics (patients with different characteristics), the relative importance of the characteristics on the decision can be determined [11].

Questionnaire design

To identify patient characteristics that determine the decision-making for DMARD de-escalation, 12 rheumatologists were randomly selected for interviews stratified by region and type of hospital (university or general). A semi-structured interview schedule (Additional file 1) was designed based on characteristics identified by pilot interviews of rheumatologists and literature [7]. During the semi-structured interviews, rheumatologists were questioned by telephone about their personal opinion and attitude with respect to DMARD de-escalation. The number of interviews was deemed sufficient as no new themes were mentioned during the final interviews, and therefore no other rheumatologists were approached. Based on the interviews, five patient characteristics with corresponding levels were developed (Table 1).

Study design and questionnaire

A questionnaire containing 16 choice tasks, each consisting of two hypothetical patients, was deemed feasible to complete by rheumatologists attending the annual convention of the Dutch Society of Rheumatology (Nederlandse Vereniging voor Reumatologie, NVR). All hypothetical patients were assumed to use the combination of methotrexate 20–25 mg/week and a tumor necrosis factor (TNF) blocker, without additional glucocorticoids. In order to gain as much information as possible (enhancing precision) from a limited number of choice sets and sample size, computer software using experimental design theory (Ngene 1.1.2, 2014 ChoiceMetrics software, Sydney, NSW, Australia) was used to generate the most efficient sets of choices given the characteristics as defined previously (optimized for a main effect model with full dummy specification). To further optimize this process, priors were

Table 1 Choice task example

	Patient A	Patient B
Duration of remission[1]	6 months	1 year
Patient preference for de-escalation at the start of the consult[2]	Patient is not willing to de-escalate	Patient is willing to de-escalate
Number of swollen joints[3]	1	2
DAS28[4]	≤3.2	<2.6
Medical history[5]	Difficult to accomplish remission	Easy to accomplish remission
	Non-erosive	Erosive

Participants were required to choose the patient they deemed most suitable for de-escalation or neither (opt-out). For each choice task patient characteristics were varied by assigning different levels. Possible levels are indicated in the subscript. All patients were assumed to use the combination of methotrexate 20–25 mg/week and a TNF blocker

DAS Disease Activity Score

[1]Levels were "6 months" and "12 months"

[2]Levels were "patient is not willing to de-escalate" and "patient is willing to de-escalate"

[3]Levels were "0", "1" and "2"

[4]Levels were "≤3.2" and "<2.6"

[5]Levels were "difficult to accomplish remission, erosive", "difficult to accomplish remission, non-erosive", "easy to accomplish remission, erosive" and "easy to accomplish remission, non-erosive"

chosen reflecting the expected direction of characteristic levels on preference (Additional file 2), but not imposing any strong assumptions about the weight of each characteristic in the decision that might (dis)favor identification of some effects over others.

Choice sets consisted of two hypothetical patients and an opt-out option (Additional file 3). From each choice set, rheumatologists were asked to choose the patient they deemed most suitable to de-escalate DMARDs. The opt-out option was included in case respondents deemed neither patient suitable for de-escalation, resembling real-life decision-making. Of note, only after rheumatologists chose to de-escalate treatment in either patient they were offered a second question to select the strategy they most preferred. If de-escalation was deemed appropriate, a second choice was given on how they would de-escalate DMARDs. To make respondents familiar with the concept of DCE, two introductory questions were included. To avoid bias by presentation, the order of choice sets and order of attributes were randomized for each participant [13]. An English translation of a complete questionnaire was included (Additional file 4).

Study sample

All rheumatologists and rheumatology trainees active in the Netherlands were eligible for participation.

Invitation of subjects

A list of active rheumatologists was kindly provided by the Dutch Society of Rheumatology (NVR). Doctors were recruited during the annual meeting of the NVR on 25 and 26 September 2014. Questionnaires were provided electronically on iPads. Non-attending rheumatologists received an invitation by e-mail to complete the questionnaire at their own computer.

Statistical analyses

We estimated a conditional logit model to assess overall preference for de-escalation of DMARDs and its determinants (Additional file 5).

To assess whether preferences for de-escalation and relative importance of patient characteristics determining this decision differed among rheumatologists, a subgroup analysis (latent class model) was performed as well (Additional file 3). With this model, subgroups of rheumatologists (clusters or classes) can be identified. To determine the optimal number of classes, we selected the model with the best fit on the consistent Akaike information criterion (cAIC). This measure deals with the trade-off between increase in goodness of fit of the model and the increase in complexity by the addition of clusters. Analyses were performed using the clogit and lclogit function in STATA (version 13.1, StataCorp, College Station, TX, USA).

Results

In total 156 doctors completed the questionnaire (128 rheumatologists and 28 trainees), 128 of which completed the questionnaire at the annual conference Of 174 rheumatologists that had not participated at the annual conference and received an invitation by e-mail, 28 (16%) completed the questionnaire online. Eleven rheumatologists did not provide demographic data because of technical problems or by their own wishes. Characteristics of the study sample are shown in Table 2.

De-escalation of therapy was preferred in 74% of the patient choice sets evaluated by the rheumatologists. To quantify how patient characteristics influence doctor's preferences for de-escalating DMARDs, a conditional logit model was estimated (Table 3). The interpretation of such a model is somewhat different than of a linear or logit regression model. Each of the patient characteristics played

Table 2 Characteristics of study sample

	Rheumatologists ($n = 117$)[a]	Trainee ($n = 28$)
Age (years), median (IQR)	47 (40–57)	34 (31–36)
Female, n (%)	60 (51%)	20 (71%)
Work experience (years), median (IQR)	10 (5–23)	-
Self-reported number of RA patients in practice, median (IQR)	350 (200–1000)	70 (25–100)
Self-reported prevalence of biological treatment among RA patients in practice, median (IQR)	25 (20–30)	30 (20–35)
Working in academic hospital, n (%)	19 (16%)	10 (36%)

[a]Eleven out of 128 rheumatologists did not provide information due to technical problems or by their own wish

a role in the decision to de-escalate DMARDs, as all coefficients of the model showed significance. The opt-out option was chosen if a rheumatologist deemed neither patient of a pair suitable for treatment de-escalation. De-escalation was chosen in 74% of cases, while the opt-out was chosen in 26% of cases. Therefore, in general, the opt-out was less preferred than de-escalation (the reference category), which is reflected by a negative sign for the opt-out (Table 1). Coefficients for the other factors have a similar interpretation, as will be further explained.

For each characteristic, we chose the level we expected to be most preferable for de-escalation to be the reference level, e.g., no swollen joints, Disease Activity Score (DAS) < 2.6 (see footnotes Table 3). Therefore, the ideal patient that doctors would like to consider for de-escalation of DMARDs is a patient having all the reference characteristics, i.e., came in remission easily, has no erosions, a remission duration of 1 year, no swollen joints, and has DAS remission rather than DAS LDA. Hence, the coefficients represent the relative decrease in de-escalation preference when a patient presents with that feature (e.g., two swollen joints) relative to the reference of that feature (no swollen joints). Presence of two swollen joints (-1.68, $p < 0.001$) and a patient history of erosive disease in combination with difficulties achieving remission (-1.64, $p < 0.001$) had the strongest influence on the decision not to de-escalate (Table 3). It should be emphasized that above results did not depend on the fashion in which DMARDs were de-escalated, as this was not specified in the questionnaire. Only after rheumatologists chose to de-escalate treatment in either patient they were offered a second question to select the strategy they most preferred (see below).

Table 3 Overall preference of doctors for de-escalation based on a conditional logit model

	Overall $n = 156$	
	β	SE
Opt out[1] chosen	26%	
Opt out[1]	-2.96***	0.11
DAS ≤ 3.2[2]	-0.98***	0.07
Swollen joint count		
1[3]	-1.15***	0.08
2[3]	-1.68***	0.09
Patient history		
Erosive disease[4]	-0.69***	0.11
Remission difficult[4]	-0.80***	0.09
Erosive + remission difficult[4]	-1.64***	0.10
Remission duration 6 months[5]	-0.52***	0.06
Patient not willing to de-escalate at start of visit[6]	-1.09***	0.07

β beta coefficient, *SE* standard error, *DAS* Disease Activity Score

***$p < 0.001$

[1]This option was included in case a rheumatologist did not want to de-escalate DMARDs in either of the patients presented in a pair

[2]Reference DAS < 2.6

[3]Reference no swollen joints

[4]Reference easy remission and no erosions

[5]Reference remission duration 1 year

[6]Reference patient willing to de-escalate DMARDs at start of visit

Although this model describes the preferences of rheumatologists for de-escalation of DMARDs on average, in reality subgroups of doctors may exist that weigh patient characteristics differently. Therefore we looked whether we could distinguish subgroups based on answering patterns. Using a latent class model, we identified five subgroups of rheumatologists as shown in Table 4. Each of the groups made different trade-offs in whom to de-escalate DMARDs given the relative weight in the patient characteristics and opt-out. Opt-out preference ranged from 1% in class 4 to 53% in class 5. For each subgroup the relative weights of the patient characteristics that drove de-escalation were analyzed (absolute weights of coefficients cannot be directly compared between subgroups because coefficients are on different scales). Table 4 shows that presence of swollen joints was the most important characteristic for rheumatologists to consider in subgroups 2 and 5, whereas in subgroups 1 and 3 patient history was most important. Of note, in subgroup 4 none of the patient characteristics dominated the decision to de-escalate, while their preference for de-escalation was strong. To further illustrate differences between the subgroups, 96 unique patient profiles were created, using the characteristics and levels as defined in Table 1. As shown in Fig. 1, overall, patients 1–10 had a high probability to be considered for de-escalation (>80%) and patients 83–96 had a low

Table 4 Preference of doctors for de-escalation of DMARDs by subgroups based on answering patterns

	Group 1 *n* = 48		Group 2 *n* = 22		Group 3 *n* = 26		Group 4 *n* = 30		Group 5 *n* = 30	
	β	SE	β	SE	β	SE	β	SE	β	SE
Opt-out[1] chosen	38%		21%		9%		1%		53%	
Opt-out[1]	-2.78^{***}	0.23	-5.33^{***}	0.97	-4.98^{***}	0.83	-5.70^{***}	0.64	-4.72^{***}	0.41
DAS ≤ 3.2[2]	-0.59^{***}	0.15	-1.60^{**}	0.49	-2.55^{***}	0.57	-0.59^{***}	0.15	-1.87^{***}	0.27
Swollen joint count										
1[3]	-1.01^{***}	0.19	-3.24^{***}	0.59	-1.02	0.53	-0.79^{***}	0.19	-3.53^{***}	0.48
2[3]	-1.90^{***}	0.22	-6.06^{***}	0.99	-0.63^{*}	0.28	-1.25^{***}	0.21	-3.92^{***}	0.51
Patient history										
Erosive disease[4]	-1.27^{***}	0.20	-0.73	0.40	-1.23^{**}	0.38	-0.58^{*}	0.24	-1.29^{***}	0.43
Remission difficult[4]	-1.08^{***}	0.20	-0.95^{*}	0.46	-1.42^{**}	0.42	-0.44	0.27	-1.79^{***}	0.37
Erosive + remission difficult[4]	-2.80^{***}	0.25	-1.14	0.62	-2.99^{***}	0.60	-1.29^{***}	0.30	-2.79^{***}	0.40
Remission duration 6 months[5]	-0.41^{*}	0.16	-1.17^{***}	0.40	-0.52	0.31	-0.17	0.14	-3.74	-
Patient not willing to de-escalate at start of visit[6]	-1.61^{***}	0.20	-1.05^{***}	0.30	-0.98^{**}	0.30	-1.14^{***}	0.13	-1.49^{***}	0.27
Class probabilities, median (range)	0.99 (0.55 – 0.99)		0.99 (0.55 – 0.99)		0.94 (0.58 – 0.99)		0.99 (0.77 – 0.99)		0.98 (0.57 – 0.99)	

β beta coefficient, *SE* standard error, *DAS* Disease Activity Score
$^{*}p < 0.05$; $^{**}p < 0.01$; $^{***}p < 0.001$
[1]This option was included in case a rheumatologist did not want to de-escalate DMARDs in either of the patients presented in a pair
[2]Reference DAS < 2.6
[3]Reference no swollen joints
[4]Reference easy remission and no erosions
[5]Reference remission duration 1 year
[6]Reference patient willing to de-escalate DMARDs at start of visit

probability (<20%). For the other patients (11–82), probabilities to be considered for de-escalation were variable among subgroups. Comparing subgroups with respect to their willingness to de-escalation, group 4 had the greatest willingness to de-escalate and group 5 was least willing to de-escalate medication. Given the diagonal in Fig. 1, group 3 had above average willingness to de-escalate, whereas group 1 was somewhat below average. Willingness to de-escalate for group 2 was in general above average for patients at the left side of the figure (patients 1–48) and less than average for patients at the right side (patients 49–96). A simple analysis to see whether differences related to age, sex or practice-related factors (Table 5) did not reveal particular

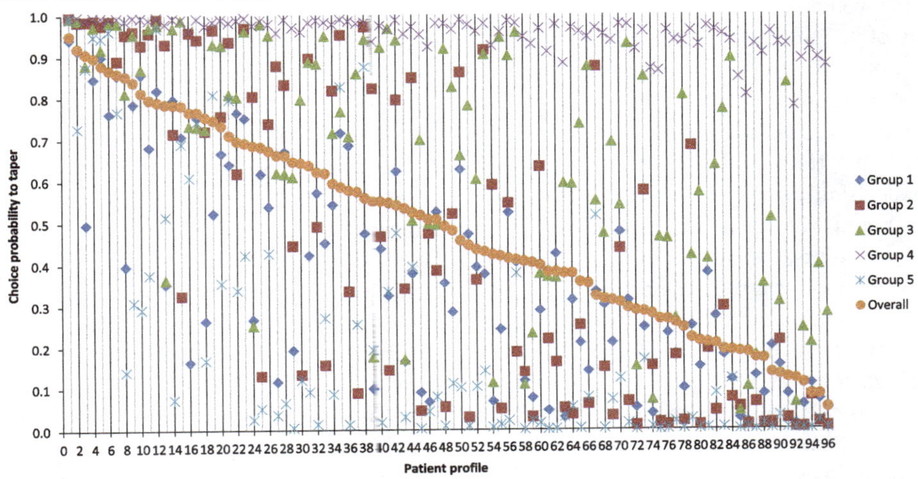

Fig. 1 The probability rheumatologists choose to taper specific patients, shown for 96 unique patient profiles. Overall probability (average for all rheumatologists, *orange rounds*) and probabilities by subgroups (*other shapes*) are shown

Table 5 Characteristics of subgroups

	Group 1 $n=48$	Group 2 $n=22$	Group 3 $n=26$	Group 4 $n=30$	Group 5 $n=30$	p^*
Age (years), median (IQR)	43 (35–51)	49 (40–56)	39 (35–45)	50 (40–60)	41 (37–52)	0.038
Female, n (%)	22 (51%)	12 (55%)	15 (60%)	15 (50%)	20 (67%)	0.663
Trainee, n (%)	11 (26%)	2 (9%)	7 (29%)	1 (3%)	7 (26%)	0.051
Work experience (years), median (IQR)	7 (0–15)	13 (5–25)	5 (0–8)	12 (5–25)	4 (0–18)	0.027
Self-reported number of RA patients in practice, median (IQR)	375 (100–800)	425 (200–1100)	450 (100–2000)	300 (200–1000)	300 (100–500)	0.492
Self-reported prevalence of biological treatment among RA patients in practice, median (IQR)	23 (20–30)	20 (20–33)	30 (20–30)	29 (20–33)	20 (15–30)	0.641
Working in academic hospital, n (%)	9 (21%)	4 (18%)	6 (24%)	5 (17%)	7 (23%)	0.955
No data, n (%)	5 (10%)	0 (0%)	2 (8%)	1 (3%)	3 (10%)	<0.001

RA rheumatoid arthritis
*Kruskall-Wallis test

characteristics of doctors. Being a trainee was associated with lower preference to de-escalate.

After the decision whether to de-escalate or not, the rheumatologists were presented with the choice which DMARDs to de-escalate. Three options were presented: de-escalating the TNF blocker, de-escalating methotrexate (MTX) or de-escalating MTX to half the dose followed by de-escalating the TNF blocker. Of de-escalation strategies, rheumatologists chose de-escalating the TNF blocker in the majority of cases (61%), followed by de-escalating the TNF blocker after de-escalating MTX to half dosage (33%).

Discussion

By semi-structured interviews, we identified five patient characteristics rheumatologists take into account in their decision to de-escalate DMARDs: number of swollen joints, presence of DAS remission/LDA, patient history, duration of remission/LDA and patient willingness to de-escalate. Using a discrete choice experiment among Dutch rheumatologists, number of swollen joints and patient history were identified as factors of greatest importance. However, rheumatologists were not uniform in their decision to de-escalate DMARDs. Based on a further (latent class) analysis of the answering patterns, five subgroups of rheumatologists were identified that traded off patient characteristics differently in their decision to de-escalate: (1) rheumatologists that always tapered, (2) rheumatologists tapering in the absence of swollen joints, (3) rheumatologists tapering in the absence of swollen joints and in the presence of a favorable patient history, (4) rheumatologists tapering in case of DAS remission and favorable patient history, and (5) rheumatologists taking into account all factors. That heterogeneity among rheumatologists exists with respect to decision-making was further demonstrated by calculating the probability rheumatologists would decide to de-escalate medication for 96 unique patient profiles (Fig. 1). This showed that subgroup probabilities were highly variable for most of the profiles, especially those for which one or more characteristics were less favorable (e.g., presence of one rather than no swollen joints or DAS LDA rather than DAS remission). This means that no general consensus exists on which patients are suitable for de-escalation. Eliciting details on rheumatologist subgroups resulted in mixed demographic characteristics, so other person-related factors are likely to play a role. We only observed that trainees were less willing to taper, possibly due to lack of experience and confidence. Of de-escalation strategies rheumatologists could choose from, de-escalating the TNF blocker first and de-escalating the TNF blocker after reducing MTX to half dosage were chosen in 94% of cases.

To date there is no standardized way to determine the patient for whom de-escalation of DMARD therapy is appropriate [8]. Of clinical factors, conflicting results have been reported for deeper remission [14, 15] and shorter disease duration [14–16] to be associated with successful tapering, while observations from the CORRONA registry suggested that a rapid response to DMARDs is associated with better maintenance of remission when the agents are tapered later on [8, 17]. In this DCE, rheumatologists regarded presence of swollen joints, a patient history of erosive disease and difficulties achieving remission and patient fulfilling DAS LDA rather than remission as most important factors to not de-escalate. Although swollen joints may be regarded as a direct indication of inflammation and contraindication for de-escalation, this is not necessarily true for the DAS28 score itself, which could be high because of psychosocial distress or comorbidities. Rheumatologists in clinical practice may therefore sometimes decide to de-escalate in case of DAS LDA in the absence of other signs of inflammation. Future research may aid to clarify which clinical factors are really important for predicting successful de-escalation. Ultrasound [18–20] or biomarkers [14, 21] may have an additional role in detecting in which patients subclinical synovitis is still present increasing the risk of flare after treatment withdrawal. It would also be of interest to study whether (a combination of) clinical, ultrasonographic and/or serum factors can adequately predict which patients can successfully de-escalate treatment.

This study was conducted using a DCE, which in comparison to other quantified preference techniques, bears most resemblance to real-world decision-making [22]. A strength of this design is that several patient characteristics can be evaluated at once in which the weight of each characteristic contributes to the decision to de-escalate medication. Another strength of this study is that we identified relevant characteristics using semi-structured interviews with a random sample of rheumatologists to identify relevant factors (characteristics and levels) for the DCE questionnaire. As no new factors were mentioned during the final interviews, we assumed that saturation was reached and hence no important factors had been missed. One inherent limitation of a DCE is that rheumatologists were asked to evaluate virtual RA patients on screen. Consequently, as the decision to de-escalate does not have real clinical implications, rheumatologists may have been more risk-taking than they would be when dealing with real patients. This could then have resulted in an overestimation of rheumatologists' willingness to de-escalate. Another limitation of this study is that, although the majority of rheumatologists attending the annual conference participated in the study, response rates were low for rheumatologists not attending the conference that were invited to participate from home. Although this could for a large part be explained by the method of recruitment, we could not fully exclude the possibility of a relationship between non-responders and tendency to de-escalate DMARDs.

In designing the questions for the DCE we made several choices that need clarification. We refrained from including side effects in the decision to de-escalate. Several rheumatologists remarked that presence of side effects is relevant in the decision of de-escalation therapy. Although we agree, this is likely to influence the decision to de-escalate a particular medicine first due to side effects, it not necessarily relates to the decision of de-escalation in patients achieving LDA or remission. The presence of severe side effects would likely result in de-escalation or switching medication before sustained remission or LDA is achieved.

Second, a simple choice was given on what to de-escalate. Rheumatologists could choose between de-escalating the TNF inhibitor or MTX completely, or to de-escalate the TNF inhibitor completely after reducing MTX to half dosage. As more strategies are imaginable, different strategies can and will be adopted in reality. Therefore, more work on preference of what to de-escalate first given both the medication characteristics and patient characteristics would help to further understand de-escalation of therapy decisions.

Third, due to the definition of levels assigned to the disease characteristics, the relative importance of characteristics could change if levels had been defined differently (e.g., remission duration of 2 years rather than 1 year). Therefore, the relative importance of characteristics can only be interpreted taking the definition of the levels into consideration.

Conclusions

Swollen joint count (SJC) and patient history were the most important characteristics rheumatologists take into consideration in the decision to de-escalate. However rheumatologists are not uniform in their decision on whom to de-escalate. Five subgroups of rheumatologists could be identified: those that taper (1) always, (2) in absence of swollen joints, (3) in absence of swollen joints and favorable patient history, (4) if DAS remission and favorable patient history, and (5) taking into account all factors.

To improve uniform decision-making in the future, more research is needed assessing the predictive value of patient characteristics for successful de-escalation of DMARDs.

Additional files

Additional file 1: Topics for semi-structured interview. List of topics that were discussed in the semi-structured interviews. (DOCX 18 kb)

Additional file 2: Priors for the levels of patient characteristics. Priors used in the design of the questionnaire. (DOCX 24 kb)

Additional file 3: Choice set example. Example of a choice set as presented in the questionnaire. (DOCX 23 kb)

Additional file 4: English translation of DCE questionnaire (questionnaire was taken in Dutch). English translation of a complete DCE questionnaire. The original questionnaire was taken in Dutch. (DOCX 89 kb)

Additional file 5: Utility functions for the conditional logit and latent class models. (DOCX 23 kb)

Abbreviations

ACR: American College of Rheumatology; cAIC: Consistent Akaike Information Criterion; DAS: Disease Activity Score; DCE: Discrete Choice Experiment; DMARDs: Disease-modifying anti-rheumatic drugs; EULAR: European League Against Rheumatism; LDA: Low disease activity; MTX: Methotrexate; NVR: Nederlandse Vereniging voor Reumatologie (Dutch Society of Rheumatology); RA: Rheumatoid arthritis; SJC: Swollen joint count; TNF: Tumor necrosis factor

Acknowledgements

The authors express their gratitude towards the Rheumatology Association of the Netherlands for allowing us to collect our data during the conference. A special thanks goes to Marcel Jonker for his support with the analyses.

Funding

No external funding was received for the realization of this project

Authors' contributions

TMK contributed to study design, data acquisition, data analysis, drafting and revising the manuscript, and final approval of the manuscript. RF contributed to study design, data acquisition, data analysis, drafting and revising the manuscript, and final approval of the manuscript. EAS contributed to study design, data analysis, drafting and revising the manuscript, and final approval of the manuscript. JJL contributed to study design, data acquisition, data analysis, drafting and revising the manuscript, and final approval of the manuscript. JMWH contributed to study design, data acquisition, data analysis, drafting and revising the manuscript, and final approval of the manuscript.

Competing interests

The authors declare that they have no competing interests.

Author details

[1]Department of Rheumatology, Erasmus Medical Center, Room Na-609, PO Box 20403000 CA Rotterdam, The Netherlands. [2]Institute for Medical Technology Assessment, Erasmus University, Rotterdam, The Netherlands.

References

1. McInnes IB, O'Dell JR. State-of-the-art: rheumatoid arthritis. Ann Rheum Dis. 2010;69:1898–906.
2. de Jong PH, Hazes JM, Han HK, Huisman M, van Zeben D, van der Lubbe PA, et al. Randomised comparison of initial triple DMARD therapy with methotrexate monotherapy in combination with low-dose glucocorticoid bridging therapy; 1-year data of the tREACH trial. Ann Rheum Dis. 2014;73:1331–9.
3. Goekoop-Ruiterman YP, de Vries-Bouwstra JK, Allaart CF, van Zeben D, Kerstens PJ, Hazes JM, et al. Clinical and radiographic outcomes of four different treatment strategies in patients with early rheumatoid arthritis (the BeSt study): a randomized, controlled trial. Arthritis Rheum. 2008;58:S126–35.
4. Singh JA, Saag KG, Bridges Jr SL, Akl EA, Bannuru RR, Sullivan MC, et al. 2015 American College of Rheumatology guideline for the treatment of rheumatoid arthritis. Arthritis Rheumatol. 2016;68:1–26.
5. Smolen JS, Landewe R, Breedveld FC, Buch M, Burmester G, Dougados M, et al. EULAR recommendations for the management of rheumatoid arthritis with synthetic and biological disease-modifying antirheumatic drugs: 2013 update. Ann Rheum Dis. 2014;73:492–509.
6. Galvao TF, Zimmermann IR, da Mota LM, Silva MT, Pereira MG. Withdrawal of biologic agents in rheumatoid arthritis: a systematic review and meta-analysis. Clin Rheumatol. 2016;35:1659–68.
7. Kuijper TM, Lamers-Karnebeek FB, Jacobs JW, Hazes JM, Luime JJ. Flare rate in patients with rheumatoid arthritis in low disease activity or remission when tapering or stopping synthetic or biologic DMARD: a systematic review. J Rheumatol. 2015;42:2012–22.
8. Schett G, Emery P, Tanaka Y, Burmester G, Pisetsky DS, Naredo E, et al. Tapering biologic and conventional DMARD therapy in rheumatoid arthritis: current evidence and future directions. Ann Rheum Dis. 2016;75:1428–37.
9. Gvozdenovic E, Allaart CF, van der Heijde D, Ferraccioli G, Smolen JS, Huizinga TW, et al. When rheumatologists report that they agree with a guideline, does this mean that they practise the guideline in clinical practice? Results of the International Recommendation Implementation Study (IRIS). RMD Open. 2016;2:e000221.
10. Neogi T, Aletaha D, Silman AJ, Naden RL, Felson DT, Aggarwal R, et al. The 2010 American College of Rheumatology/European League Against Rheumatism classification criteria for rheumatoid arthritis: Phase 2 methodological report. Arthritis Rheum. 2010;62:2582–91.
11. de Bekker-Grob EW, Rose JM, Donkers B, Essink-Bot ML, Bangma CH, Steyerberg EW. Men's preferences for prostate cancer screening: a discrete choice experiment. Br J Cancer. 2013;108:533–41.
12. Ryan M. Discrete choice experiments in health care. BMJ. 2004;328:360–1.
13. Kjaer T, Bech M, Gyrd-Hansen D, Hart-Hansen K. Ordering effect and price sensitivity in discrete choice experiments: need we worry? Health Econ. 2006;15:1217–28.
14. Haschka J, Englbrecht M, Hueber AJ, Manger B, Kleyer A, Reiser M, et al. Relapse rates in patients with rheumatoid arthritis in stable remission tapering or stopping antirheumatic therapy: interim results from the prospective randomised controlled RETRO study. Ann Rheum Dis. 2016;75:45–51.
15. Tanaka Y, Hirata S, Kubo S, Fukuyo S, Hanami K, Sawamukai N, et al. Discontinuation of adalimumab after achieving remission in patients with established rheumatoid arthritis: 1-year outcome of the HONOR study. Ann Rheum Dis. 2015;74:389–95.
16. van der Woude D, Young A, Jayakumar K, Mertens BJ, Toes RE, van der Heijde D, et al. Prevalence of and predictive factors for sustained disease-modifying antirheumatic drug-free remission in rheumatoid arthritis: results from two large early arthritis cohorts. Arthritis Rheum. 2009;60:2262–71.
17. Kavanaugh A, Lee SJ, Curtis JR, Greenberg JD, Kremer JM, Soto L, et al. Discontinuation of tumour necrosis factor inhibitors in patients with rheumatoid arthritis in low-disease activity: persistent benefits. Data from the Corrona registry. Ann Rheum Dis. 2015;74:1150–5.
18. Alivernini S, Peluso G, Fedele AL, Tolusso B, Gremese E, Ferraccioli G. Tapering and discontinuation of TNF-alpha blockers without disease relapse using ultrasonography as a tool to identify patients with rheumatoid arthritis in clinical and histological remission. Arthritis Res Ther. 2016;18:39.
19. Iwamoto T, Ikeda K, Hosokawa J, Yamagata M, Tanaka S, Norimoto A, et al. Prediction of relapse after discontinuation of biologic agents by ultrasonographic assessment in patients with rheumatoid arthritis in clinical remission: high predictive values of total gray-scale and power Doppler scores that represent residual synovial inflammation before discontinuation. Arthritis Care Res. 2014;66:1576–81.
20. Naredo E, Valor L, De la Torre I, Montoro M, Bello N, Martinez-Barrio J, et al. Predictive value of Doppler ultrasound-detected synovitis in relation to failed tapering of biologic therapy in patients with rheumatoid arthritis. Rheumatology (Oxford). 2015;54:1408–14.
21. Rech J, Hueber AJ, Finzel S, Englbrecht M, Haschka J, Manger B, et al. Prediction of disease relapses by multibiomarker disease activity and autoantibody status in patients with rheumatoid arthritis on tapering DMARD treatment. Ann Rheum Dis. 2016;75:1637–44.
22. Deighton C, O'Mahony R, Tosh J, Turner C, Rudolf M. Management of rheumatoid arthritis: summary of NICE guidance. BMJ. 2009;338:b702.

11

Clinical and demographic factors associated with change and maintenance of disease severity in a large registry of patients with rheumatoid arthritis

George W. Reed[1,4*], David H. Collier[2], Andrew S. Koenig[3], Katherine C. Saunders[4], Dimitrios A. Pappas[4,5], Heather J. Litman[4], Joel M. Kremer[4,6] and Sameer Kotak[3]

Abstract

Background: We examined models to predict disease activity transitions from moderate to low or severe and associated factors in patients with rheumatoid arthritis (RA).

Methods: Data from RA patients enrolled in the Corrona registry (October 2001 to August 2014) were analyzed. Clinical Disease Activity Index (CDAI) definitions were used for low (≤10), moderate (>10 and ≤22), and severe (>22) disease activity states. A Markov model for repeated measures allowing for covariate dependence was used to model transitions between three (low, moderate, severe) states and estimate population transition probabilities. Mean sojourn times were calculated to compare length of time in particular states. Logistic regression models were used to examine impacts of covariates (time between visits, chronological year, disease duration, age) on disease states.

Results: Data from 29,853 patients (251,375 visits) and a sub-cohort of 9812 patients (46,534 visits) with regular visits (every 3–9 months) were analyzed. The probability of moving from moderate to low or severe disease by next visit was 47% and 18%, respectively. Patients stayed in moderate disease for mean 4.25 months (95% confidence interval: 4.18–4.32). Transition probabilities showed 20% of patients with low disease activity moved to moderate or severe disease within 6 months; >35% of patients with moderate disease remained in moderate disease after 6 months. Results were similar for the regular-visit sub-cohort. Significant interactions with prior disease state were seen with chronological year and disease duration.

Conclusion: A substantial proportion of patients remain in moderate disease, emphasizing the need for treat-to-target strategies for RA patients.

Keywords: Rheumatoid arthritis, Disease activity, Prediction, Markov model, Clinical Disease Activity Index

Background

Rheumatoid arthritis (RA) is a chronic, systemic inflammatory disease, which can lead to progressive joint destruction and accumulating disability from autoimmune processes that target the synovium [1]. Several effective and safe medications can decrease the level of inflammation and achieve a low disease activity state or even remission [2]. Treat-to-target principles emphasize the need for achievement of remission or low disease activity [3]. However, reaching a state of continuous and stable remission or low disease activity is not observed in all patients despite aggressive therapy [4–7], and a number of studies have shown that moderate or high disease activity is not uncommon in treated patients [8–12]. RA disease activity in treated patients frequently fluctuates over time. Continuous surveillance by the treating physician is therefore needed to maintain disease activity at low levels and diminish the probability of joint damage and associated disability. Medications may fail to control the disease activity for long

* Correspondence: George.Reed@umassmed.edu
[1]University of Massachusetts Medical School, 55 Lake Ave North, Worcester, MA 01605, USA
[4]Corrona LLC, Southborough, MA, USA
Full list of author information is available at the end of the article

periods of time because of development of resistance, the autoimmune process maintaining the RA-related inflammation may become more active, and the disease activity may flare.

The current therapy guidelines provide a therapy algorithm, which recommends all patients should be treated with conventional synthetic disease-modifying antirheumatic drugs (csDMARDs) as first-line therapy, or if they fail to achieve low disease activity or remission with a tumor necrosis factor inhibitor (TNFi). If there is primary or secondary treatment failure and the patient returns to a state of moderate disease activity, a different TNFi can be tried, followed by switch to a non-TNFi biologic DMARD (bDMARD) after failure of a second TNFi [3]. However, this model of therapy does not take into account characteristics that may affect the probability of a patient to return to low disease activity or remission regardless of therapy. It is possible that the previous history of disease activity fluctuation, coupled with other patient and disease characteristics, may be able to predict the future "behavior" of the disease and thus decisions about the aggressiveness of therapy could be tailored according to these probabilities.

For patients with moderate disease activity, the evolution of disease activity over time is particularly difficult to predict currently. Understanding the patterns of fluctuation as patients transition out of moderate disease activity provides an assessment of the unmet needs in the RA patient population regardless of treatment or duration of disease.

The most common modeling techniques that have been used to predict evolution of disease activity in RA include decision trees, Markov models, individual sampling methods, and discrete event simulation [13]. These have mainly been applied to perform cost effectiveness and cost utility analyses using real or simulated populations [13–16]. Few studies have used the models to examine clinical trends in RA development and factors associated with these transitions. In the current study we examined the feasibility of using Markov models and clinical registry data to estimate transition probabilities and the impact of covariates on these transitions. We focused on the group of patients with moderate disease activity and compared mean times that these patients remained in their current disease state to patients in other disease states. We used the Corrona registry database as the clinical patient population to provide a proof of principle that these models can potentially be used to evaluate clinically relevant associations with disease state transitions.

Methods

Patients

Patients evaluated in the current analyses were enrolled in the Corrona registry. The Corrona registry has been described in detail elsewhere [17]. Briefly, the Corrona registry comprises a prospective US observational cohort of patients with arthritis who are enrolled by participating rheumatologists [17, 18]. The Corrona registry was founded in 2001. The Corrona Rheumatology Practice Network is composed of more than 100 private and academic practices across 42 states within the USA, with more than 350 rheumatologists contributing data. All geographic regions in the continental USA are represented and there are no restrictions on age, disease activity, or disease duration or other restrictions to patient participation in the registry.

Data are collected from both patients and their treating rheumatologists, who gather information on disease duration, prognosis, disease severity and activity, medical comorbidities, use of medications including csDMARDs and bDMARDs, and adverse events. Follow-up assessments are requested at least as often as every 6 months and completed during routine clinical encounters. At each Corrona registry visit patients and physicians record data on disease severity and activity, RA and other medications, adverse events, quality of life, selected laboratory and imaging results, and sociodemographic information. Visits have occurred at a median interval of 4.4 months.

The study population used for analysis of the impact of intervals between visits consisted of 29,853 RA patients with 251,375 visits with Clinical Disease Activity Index (CDAI) components measured at all visits in Corrona from October 2001 to August 2014. Only 1.2% of patients (n = 371) were dropped because of a visit with no CDAI assessment. A subset of patients with all visit intervals between 3 and 9 months (regular-visit sub-cohort) was used for covariate analyses beyond visit length, and included 9812 RA patients with 46,534 visits.

Measurement of disease activity

Disease activity was measured using the CDAI, an established composite measure of disease activity [19]. CDAI is calculated based on the number of swollen and tender joints, the patient's self assessment of overall RA disease activity (scale of 1–10), and the physician's (or evaluator's) assessment of overall RA disease activity (scale of 1–10 where 10 is maximal activity). CDAI uses the 28-joint scale to evaluate the number of swollen and tender joints - thus ankles and feet are excluded. Inflammation markers are not included in CDAI calculation. CDAI cutoffs have been established to define different disease activity states; remission is defined by a CDAI ≤2.8, low disease activity is defined by a CDAI >2.8 and ≤10, moderate disease activity is defined by a CDAI >10 and ≤22 and high disease activity is defined by a CDAI >22 [19]. A patient with moderate disease activity was identified when the patient's CDAI score changed from low disease activity or remission to moderate disease activity. This patient was then followed for any disease activity transitions from that initial transition to a moderate state.

Model disease activity states

Model

RA patients are considered to transition over time among disease states defined by CDAI. While the disease activity score is a continuous scale, the discrete states are used for clinical guidance. Markov models provide a convenient probability model for examining discrete states and estimating the likelihood of patient transitions among states. They can be estimated with simple models based on a patient's current state or more complex models that account for patient transition history. The models provide population-based estimates on transitions and with the inclusion of patient covariates can and would provide clinically relevant information.

Figure 1 illustrates a model using three states (remission/low, moderate, and high) where transition probabilities (π_{ij}) are defined as the probability of moving from one state to another ($i \neq j$), or remaining in the same state ($i = j$). For example, π_{LM} represents the probability of transitioning from low disease to moderate disease while π_{LL} represents the probability of remaining in low disease state.

A full description of the Markov chain methodology is provided in the Additional file 1.

Model fit and variable time intervals

Within the model framework the impact of a range of covariates on patient movement among disease states can be examined. With clinical registry data collected at a patient's usual clinical visit, the time between visits will vary and it is important to first assess the potential confounding of the time between visits on transition probabilities to understand adjustments to the model that may be needed for visit interval variation.

The 3-state model was fit using multinomial logistic regression models with a robust variance estimator to account for remaining intragroup (within patient) correlation across visits. The 3-state model was also fit using a multi-state model to describe how an individual moves between states and fitting the transition probability matrix over an interval of 6 months. Mean months to switching states were estimated based on the probabilities of the next move of the process [20]. The current disease activity state was modeled as a function of the prior state and the time between visits divided into quintiles. The interaction of prior state and time between visits was included in the model to examine the impact of time interval on estimated transition probabilities. In addition, predicted transition probabilities from the multinomial model were estimated for the full population and for those patients with all visit intervals between 3 and 9 months (regular-visit sub-cohort) to examine the impact of variability of visits on the model estimates.

Additional fits used the 2-state model to illustrate the model fitting and interpretation. A logistic regression model for the current disease state was fitted with a robust variance estimator. The interaction of select covariates and the prior state were used in the model. We examined three factors (in addition to controlling for visit interval): year (to examine trends over time based on evolving treatment guidelines and availability of new treatments),

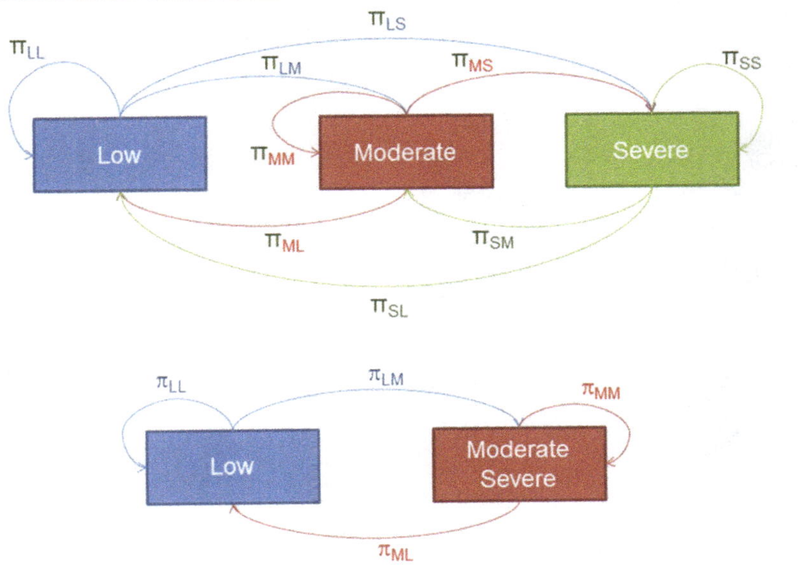

Fig. 1 Transition probabilities for the 3-state model of disease severity. π probability, *LL* transition from low to low activity, *LS* transition from low to severe activity, *LM* transition from low to moderate activity, *MM* transition from moderate to moderate activity, *ML* transition from moderate to low activity, *MS* transition from moderate to severe activity, *SM* transition from severe to moderate activity, *SL* transition from severe to low activity, *SS* transition from severe to severe activity

disease duration (stability of disease with duration), and age (impact of aging on disease variability). Covariates were measured at each time point (visit). All models were adjusted for the length of time between visits (3–4, 4–5, 5–6, 6–7, 7–8, 8–9 months). Covariates examined were chronological year (2001–2004, 2005–2006, 2007–2008, 2009–2010, 2011–2012, 2013–2014), duration of disease (0–3, 3–10, >10 years) and age (<50, 50–64, ≥65 years).

Results

Patient demographic and clinical characteristics are shown in Table 1. The regular-visit sub-cohort was similar to the full population except for slightly lower disease activity, functionality, and duration of RA. The interquartile range (IQR) for visit intervals in the full population was 3.5–6.2 months (mean 5.4 months; standard deviation (SD) 3.1). In the regular-visit sub-cohort the IQR was 4.0–6.2 months (mean 5.3 months; SD 1.5). There were 8304 patients among the full population that were in moderate disease activity at their first visit as defined in "Methods."

Table 2 shows the estimated transition probabilities using the full population from the 3-state model based on the multinomial model. Probabilities using the regular-visit cohort were similar, with differences in the estimates ranging from 0.0 to 0.05 for the 3-state model. Table 2 also presents the estimated transition probabilities from the 3-state model considering a multi-state model over an interval of 6 months; these estimates are similar to the original 3-state model. Among patients in moderate disease activity, mean time to another state was 4.25 months (standard error (SE) 0.04 months), meaning that the mean time that a patient remained in moderate disease activity was 4.25 months. This estimate was greatly increased among patients in low disease activity (mean 19.38 (SE 0.15) months) and similar among patients in severe disease activity (mean 5.30 (SE 0.06) months).

We further assessed the impact of the length of visit intervals on transition probabilities using the interaction of visit interval and prior state in the regular-visit sub-cohort. Additional file 1: Tables S1 and S2 show the estimated odds ratios (ORs) of the estimated model with interaction terms and the estimated increased (or decreased) risk of moderate/severe disease if the prior state was low or moderate/severe. A large OR (12.4) suggested an increased risk of the current state being moderate/severe if the prior state was moderate/severe vs low for the reference visit interval of 3–4 months.

The estimated ORs for the risk of transitioning from low disease to moderate disease were all >1, indicating higher odds of transitioning from a prior state of low to a current state of moderate/severe if the visit interval was longer but not all were significant. The estimated ORs for the risk of transitioning from moderate disease to moderate disease were all < 1, indicating lower odds of remaining in moderate disease with longer intervals. Again, the estimated ORs were close to 1 and not all statistically significant. The impact of the length of visit intervals was not large, but suggested that models should be adjusted for this potential confounder.

To illustrate how the model can examine covariate associations with transition probabilities we examined three

Table 1 Patient demographic and clinical characteristics

	Full population (excluding those with regular visits) (n = 20,041)	Regular visits sub-cohort (n = 9812)
Age, mean years (SD)	57.9 (13.4)	59.3 (13.5)
Sex, *n* female (%)	15,193 (76.3)	7360 (75.8)
Duration of RA, mean years (SD)	9.1 (9.7)	8.7 (9.7)
Disabled, *n* (%)	2439 (12.3)	1072 (11.1)
Patient pain[a], mean score (SD)	34.6 (27.7)	33.6 (27.8)
TJC28, mean *n* (SD)	4.6 (6.2)	4.1 (5.8)
SJC28, mean *n* (SD)	4.5 (5.6)	3.6 (5.0)
PtGA, mean score (SD)	32.0 (26.7)	30.9 (26.6)
PGA, mean score (SD)	25.7 (21.9)	23.5 (21.5)
CDAI, mean score (SD)	14.8 (13.3)	13.0 (12.6)
CDAI category, *n* (%)		
Low (score >2.8 to ≤10)	9435 (47.1)	5269 (53.7)
Moderate (score >10 to ≤22)	5674 (28.3)	2634 (26.8)
Severe (score >22)	4929 (24.6)	1909 (19.5)
History of biologic DMARD use, *n* (%)	9411 (47.0)	4485 (45.7)

SD standard deviation, *RA* rheumatoid arthritis, *TJC28* tender joint count based on 28 joints, *SJC28* swollen joint count based on 28 joints, *PtGA* patient global assessment, *PGA* physician global assessment, *CDAI* Clinical Disease Activity Index, *DMARD* disease-modifying antirheumatic drug

[a]Patient pain was rated on a visual analog scale of 0–100

Table 2 Estimated transition probabilities

	Prior state	Current state		
		Low	Moderate	Severe
3-State model				
Full population	Low	0.82	0.15	0.03
	Moderate	0.47	0.35	0.18
	Severe	0.13	0.39	0.48
Regular-visit sub-cohort	Low	0.84	0.13	0.03
	Moderate	0.52	0.33	0.15
	Severe	0.16	0.41	0.43
3-State model assuming a 6-month interval				
Full population	Low	0.81	0.15	0.05
	Moderate	0.46	0.37	0.17
	Severe	0.26	0.33	0.41
Regular-visit sub-cohort	Low	0.84	0.13	0.03
	Moderate	0.48	0.38	0.14
	Severe	0.28	0.34	0.38

factors: year, disease duration, and age. Separate models adjusted only for visit intervals (not shown) estimated a significant interaction of the prior disease state and year and disease duration but no significant interaction with age. Table 3 shows the results from the multivariable logistic model using all four factors.

Effects over time were seen in the probability of transitioning from a low disease state to moderate/severe disease with ORs <1 for 2007 onward, indicating a lower likelihood of moving to moderate/severe disease from a low disease state. There was little to no impact on the transition probabilities of remaining in moderate disease with ORs close to 1. Longer disease duration had lower odds for transition from low to moderate/severe disease but higher odds for remaining in moderate/severe disease. Age effects were similar regardless of prior disease state (interaction not significant) so were added to the model only as a main effect. ORs were close to 1, with the OR for age 50–64 years estimated at 1.2, indicating this age group was at a slightly higher risk of ending in moderate/severe disease (whether transitioning from low disease or remaining in moderate/severe disease).

Table 3 Covariate associations with transition probabilities

Covariate	OR (95% CI)
Year (reference: 2001–2004)	
Effect on transition from low to moderate/severe disease	
2005–2006	0.865 (0.700 to 1.068)
2007–2008	0.593 (0.471 to 0.746)
2009–2010	0.583 (0.474 to 0.716)
2011–2012	0.615 (0.506 to 0.748)
2013–2014	0.605 (0.497 to 0.735)
Effect on transition from moderate/severe to moderate/severe disease	
2005–2006	1.055 (0.853 to 1.304)
2007–2008	0.911 (0.733 to 1.133)
2009–2010	0.824 (0.679 to 0.999)
2011–2012	0.888 (0.740 to 1.066)
2013–2014	1.004 (0.837 to 1.205)
Duration of RA (reference: 0 to 3 years)	
Effect on transition from low to moderate/severe disease	
3 to 10 years	0.777 (0.698 to 0.865)
>10 years	0.840 (0.752 to 0.939)
Effect on transition from moderate/severe to moderate/severe disease	
3 to 10 years	1.167 (1.045 to 1.303)
>10 years	1.379 (1.236 to 1.539)
Age (reference: <50 years)[a]	
50 to 64 years	1.176 (1.082 to 1.279)
≥65 years	1.024 (0.939 to 1.117)
Visit interval (reference: 3 to < 4 months)	
Effect on transition from low to moderate/severe disease	
4 to <5 months	1.057 (0.940 to 1.187)
5 to <6 months	1.085 (0.961 to 1.226)
6 to <7 months	1.201 (1.057 to 1.364)
7 to <8 months	1.349 (1.160 to 1.568)
8 to 9 months	1.171 (0.977 to 1.403)
Effect on transition from moderate/severe to moderate/severe disease	
4 to <5 months	0.931 (0.831 to 1.042)
5 to <6 months	0.801 (0.712 to 0.902)
6 to <7 months	0.779 (0.686 to 0.886)
7 to <8 months	0.799 (0.683 to 0.935)
8 to 9 months	0.866 (0.729 to 1.028)

CI confidence interval, *RA* rheumatoid arthritis
[a]No interaction with prior state and age was noted so the effect was the same for the transition from low to moderate/severe and from moderate/severe to moderate/severe disease

Discussion

The severity of RA symptoms is currently unpredictable with clinical tools or with laboratory or imaging biomarkers, making management of this chronic disease a challenge for both patients and physicians [21]. Only a fraction of patients will reach constant and longstanding remission while on one or more therapies. More frequently, disease activity fluctuates over time despite therapy, due to a variety of reasons, such as development of resistance to medications, increases in the activity of the RA-related autoimmune process, or other factors that may interfere with medication effectiveness. Several studies of separate populations have shown that a considerable fraction of patients with RA have moderate or high disease activity [8–10]. In our study of a subset of biologic-agent-naïve patients in the Corrona database with disease duration >1 year, rates of low, moderate, and high disease activity were approximately 58%, 30%, and 12%, respectively [22]. The Markov models used in these analyses provide insight into patients with moderate disease and estimated transitions among disease levels in the real world, and provide a proof of concept of using these models to understand covariates associated with transition probabilities even when clinic visits are not at fixed intervals.

Markov models based on real-world data from patients with RA were used in this study to estimate disease state transition probabilities from clinical visit to clinical visit. We analyzed data from all RA patients in the Corrona database and the subset of patients with relatively regular visits with a range of intervals from 3 to 9 months. The transition probabilities remained stable even with longer times between visits, demonstrating the robustness of this methodology when applied to data from real-world practice.

Our results showed that for a patient in low disease activity, the probability of moving to moderate disease was 15% and to severe disease was 3% over an interval of 6 months. Thus over a 6-month period a patient has a 20% chance of moving out of low disease activity. In patients with moderate disease, while there was a 47% probability of moving to low disease, there was still 53% probability of remaining in moderate disease or even moving to severe disease. Patients with severe disease had 48% probability of remaining in the severe state, 39% probability of moving to moderate disease, and only 13% probability of achieving low disease activity. Patients in moderate disease activity remained in that state for an average of only 4 months, whereas patients in low disease activity remain there for an average of approximately 19 months. This illustrates the need to better understand the treatment of patients in moderate disease activity so that their disease can be managed so as to increase the likelihood that a patient will proceed to low rather than high disease activity. A renewed emphasis on the treat-to-target strategy and its timing specifically in patients with moderate disease might be considered.

Modeling approaches like the one used in this study may help us better understand the natural history of the disease in the era of biologic and targeted synthetic medications. Such approaches may be used to evaluate the effectiveness of therapies on a population level, and perhaps identify areas for improvement in therapy and the need for more aggressive treatment. These models indicate an unmet need for an expanded array of treatment options for patients with moderate or severe disease. Notably, these models and observations could have only been obtained from very large data sets, such as the Corrona registry.

The models were able to illustrate changing trends in disease state movement across the years and as duration of disease increased in patients. The lower odds in the later years for transitioning from low to moderate disease illustrate how treatment strategies have developed over time that have enabled patients to remain in low disease activity. However, the impact has not extended to moving at least some patients from moderate to low disease as illustrated by the similar time to transition over the years, another indication of unmet need in the RA population. Longer duration of disease showed lower odds of transitioning from low to moderate disease, which may be an indication of more disease fluctuations at disease onset as best treatments are determined. However, there were greater odds of remaining in moderate disease with longer duration, which may also indicate stability of RA severity in patients with long-standing disease and more difficulty in changing the disease state.

Prior use of Markov models in RA [13–16] have concentrated on health economic models. The proposed models reported here were used as a tool to assess factors that impact the transition probabilities, which would assist in understanding population trends and eventually individual modifiable factors. Markov models assume that a patient is always in one of a finite number of discrete health states, called Markov states. All events are represented as transitions from one state to another. Disease activity is a continuous measure and the discrete Markov states are therefore artifacts that are used to summarize changes in disease activity. However, the spectrum of RA disease severity fits within a clinical paradigm related to treatment changes and "treat-to-target" goals, and provides a simplified model of patient disease fluctuations.

Limitations to the study include restriction to the single index of CDAI (potentially inflated by chronic damage in patients with longstanding disease) and the limited covariates used in proof-of-concept work. Additional disease measures and states and additional covariates can be examined in future work.

Conclusion

In summary, this work provides a proof of concept of the Markov model for assessing associations with disease state transitions in patients with RA and insights into how treatment trends over time have impacted these transition times. Even with variable visit intervals the model provided robust estimates, and further studies to examine effects of other variables on changes in the severity of RA disease activity are warranted. In addition, our results indicate that while the mean time in moderate disease is short, indicating effective treatment in many patients, there is still a substantial proportion that remain in moderate disease after 6 months (or worse, have an increase in severity to severe disease), indicating an unmet need in the treatment of patients with RA. Future research should aim at determining specific modifiable covariates that can impact disease transitions and allow development of algorithms that could possibly be applied to individual patients to predict fluctuations of disease activity and assist in decisions regarding the aggressiveness of therapy.

Abbreviations

bDMARD: Biologic Disease-modifying antirheumatic drug; CDAI: Clinical Disease Activity Index; DMARD: Disease-modifying antirheumatic drug; OR: Odds ratio; RA: Rheumatoid arthritis; SD: Standard deviation; SE: Standard error

Acknowledgements

Dikran Toroser (Amgen Inc.) and Julia R. Gage (on behalf of Amgen Inc.) assisted with editing the manuscript.

Funding

This study was sponsored by Corrona, LLC. The Corrona RA registry has been supported through contracted subscriptions in the last two years by AbbVie Inc., Amgen Inc., Astra Zeneca, Bristol-Myers Squibb Co., Crescendo Pharmaceuticals Corp., Genentech Inc., Horizon Pharma USA, Janssen Pharmaceuticals, Inc., Eli Lilly and Co., Novartis International AG, Pfizer Inc., and UCB, Inc. Financial support for this study was provided by Immunex, a wholly owned subsidiary of Amgen Inc. and by Wyeth, which was acquired by Pfizer in October 2009.

Authors' contributions

GWR contributed to the conception and design of the study, acquisition of data, analysis of the data, interpretation of the results, and drafting and critically revising the manuscript. DHC contributed to the conception and design of the study, analysis of data, interpretation of results, and drafting and critically revising the manuscript. ASK contributed to the conception and design of the study, analysis of data, interpretation of results, and drafting and critically revising the manuscript. KCS contributed to the conception and design of the study, analysis of data, interpretation of results, and critically revising the manuscript. DAP contributed to the interpretation of the data and critically revising the manuscript. HJL contributed to the analysis of the data, interpretation of the results, and critically revising the manuscript. JMK contributed to acquisition of data, analysis of data, interpretation of the results, and drafting and critically revising the manuscript. SK contributed to the interpretation of the results and critically revising the manuscript. All authors approved the final submitted draft of the manuscript.

Competing interests

GWR is an employee and shareholder of Corrona, LLC, and holds an appointment at University of Massachusetts. DHC is an employee and shareholder of Amgen Inc. ASK is an employee and shareholder of Pfizer Inc. SK is a former employee and shareholder of Pfizer Inc. KCS and HJL are employees of Corrona, LLC. DAP is an employee of Corrona, LLC and instructor for Novartis. JMK serves on advisory boards for AbbVie, Inc., Bristol-Myers Squibb Company, Genentech, Inc., Eli Lilly and Company, and Pfizer, Inc.; serves on the board of directors for Corrona, LLC; is an investigator for AbbVie, Inc., Bristol-Myers Squibb Company, Genentech, Inc., Eli Lilly and Company, and Pfizer, Inc.; is on the speaker's bureau for Amgen Inc., and is a shareholder of Corrona, LLC. No non-financial conflicts of interest exist for any of the authors.

Ethics approval and consent to participate

Due to the non-interventional, observational study design, use of a limited dataset (i.e., contains no direct identifiers) is exempt from institutional review board (IRB) and ethics committee (EC) review. The Corrona RA US protocol was reviewed and approved by a central IRB, New England Independent Review Board (NEIRB). For academic investigative sites that did not receive a waiver to use the central IRB, full board approval was obtained from the respective governing IRBs and documentation of approval was submitted to the Sponsor prior to initiating any study procedures. All registry subjects were required to provide written informed consent prior to participating.

Author details

[1]University of Massachusetts Medical School, 55 Lake Ave North, Worcester, MA 01605, USA. [2]Amgen Inc., Thousand Oaks, CA, USA. [3]Pfizer Inc., Collegeville, PA, USA. [4]Corrona LLC, Southborough, MA, USA. [5]Columbia University College of Physicians and Surgeons, New York, NY, USA. [6]Albany Medical College and The Center for Rheumatology, Albany, NY, USA.

References

1. Choy E. Understanding the dynamics: pathways involved in the pathogenesis of rheumatoid arthritis. Rheumatology (Oxford). 2012;51 Suppl 5:v3–11.
2. Upchurch KS, Kay J. Evolution of treatment for rheumatoid arthritis. Rheumatology (Oxford). 2012;51 Suppl 6:vi28–36.
3. Singh JA, Saag KG, Bridges Jr SL, Akl EA, Bannuru RR, Sullivan MC, Vaysbrot E, McNaughton C, Osani M, Shmerling RH, et al. 2015 American College of Rheumatology guideline for the treatment of rheumatoid arthritis. Arthritis Rheumatol. 2016;68(1):1–26.
4. Kievit W, Fransen J, Adang EM, den Broeder AA, Bernelot Moens HJ, Visser H, van de Laar MA, van Riel PL. Long-term effectiveness and safety of TNF-blocking agents in daily clinical practice: results from the Dutch Rheumatoid Arthritis Monitoring register. Rheumatology (Oxford). 2011;50(1):196–203.
5. Uhlig T, Lie E, Norvang V, Lexberg AS, Rodevand E, Kroll F, Kalstad S, Olsen IC, Kvien TK. Achievement of remission and low disease activity definitions in patients with rheumatoid arthritis in clinical practice: Results from the NOR-DMARD Study. J Rheumatol. 2016;43(4):716–23.
6. Conigliaro P, Chimenti MS, Triggianese P, Ballanti E, Sunzini F, Duca I, Perricone R. Remission and low disease activity in a cohort of real-life patients with rheumatoid arthritis treated with first-line antitumour necrosis factor. J Int Med Res. 2016;44(1 suppl):90–4.
7. Einarsson JT, Geborek P, Saxne T, Kristensen LE, Kapetanovic MC. Sustained remission improves physical function in patients with established rheumatoid arthritis, and should be a treatment goal: a prospective observational cohort study from southern Sweden. J Rheumatol. 2016;43(6):1017–23.
8. Carpenter L, Nikiphorou E, Norton S, Jayakumar K, Dixey J, Young A. Patients with moderate disease activity in the first 5 years of rheumatoid arthritis still progress radiographically despite conventional disease modifying therapy (abstract 2135). Arthritis Rheum. 2014;66(10 Suppl):S933–4.
9. Nikiphorou E, Norton S, Young A, Carpenter L, Dixey J, Walsh DA, Kiely P, Davies P, Hill L, Gough A, et al. Association between rheumatoid arthritis disease activity, progression of functional limitation and long-term risk of orthopaedic surgery: combined analysis of two prospective cohorts supports EULAR treat to target DAS thresholds. Ann Rheum Dis. 2016;75(12): 2080–6.
10. Nikiphorou E, Carpenter L, Norton S, Kiely P, Dixey J, Young A. Different levels of moderate disease in rheumatoid arthritis (RA) are associated with varying risk for joint destruction and failure. Time to update DAS cut-offs for biologic DMARD use? (abstract OP0179). Ann Rheum Dis. 2015;74 Suppl 2:139.
11. Pappas DA, Kent JD, Greenberg JD, Mason MA, Kremer JM, Holt RJ. Delays in initiation of disease-modifying therapy in rheumatoid arthritis patients: Data from a US-based registry. Rheumatol Ther. 2015;2(2):153–64.
12. Solomon DH, Reed GW, Kremer JM, Curtis JR, Farkouh ME, Harrold LR, Hochberg MC, Tsao P, Greenberg JD. Disease activity in rheumatoid arthritis and the risk of cardiovascular events. Arthritis Rheumatol. 2015;67(6):1449–55.
13. Scholz S, Mittendorf R. Modeling rheumatoid arthritis using different techniques - a review of model construction and results. Health Econ Rev. 2014;4:18.
14. Beresniak A, Dupont DM, Becker JC, Merkesdal S. Interest of modelling in rheumatoid arthritis. Clin Exp Rheumatol. 2012;30(4 Suppl 73):S96–101.
15. Kobelt G, Lindgren P, Young A. Modelling the costs and effects of leflunomide in rheumatoid arthritis. Eur J Health Econ. 2002;3(3):180–7.
16. Kobelt G, Lindgren P, Lindroth Y, Jacobson L, Eberhardt K. Modelling the effect of function and disease activity on costs and quality of life in rheumatoid arthritis. Rheumatology (Oxford). 2005;44(9):1169–75.
17. Kremer J. The CORRONA database. Ann Rheum Dis. 2005;64 Suppl 4:iv37–41.
18. Greenberg JD, Bingham 3rd CO, Abramson SB, Reed G, Sebaldt RJ, Kremer J. Effect of cardiovascular comorbidities and concomitant aspirin use on selection of cyclooxygenase inhibitor among rheumatologists. Arthritis Rheum. 2005;53(1):12–7.
19. Aletaha D, Martinez-Avila J, Kvien TK, Smolen JS. Definition of treatment response in rheumatoid arthritis based on the simplified and the clinical disease activity index. Ann Rheum Dis. 2012;71(7):1190–6.
20. Jackson C. Multi-state models for panel data: The msm package for R. J Statistical Software. 2011;38(8):1–28.

12

Increased serum concentrations of IL-1 beta, IL-21 and Th17 cells in overweight patients with rheumatoid arthritis

Hirofumi Shoda, Yasuo Nagafuchi, Yumi Tsuchida, Keiichi Sakurai, Shuji Sumitomo, Keishi Fujio*
and Kazuhiko Yamamoto

Abstract

Backgrounds: Obesity is associated with worse disease activity and drug responses in patients with rheumatoid arthritis (RA). However, the immunological mechanisms responsible for the relationship between RA and obesity have not yet been clarified in detail. This study aimed to elucidate the immunological mechanisms contributing to the pathogenesis of RA in overweight patients.

Methods: The frequencies of $CD4^+$ T cell, B cell and monocyte subsets were analyzed in RA (n = 81) and healthy donors (n = 99) by flow cytometry, and were compared between three groups (body mass index (BMI) <20, ≥20 to 25, >25). Serum cytokines were measured using multiplex ELISA. Gene expression was analyzed by quantitative PCR. Clinical information was extracted from medical records.

Results: The frequencies of T helper (Th)17 ($CD4^+$CD45RA-CXCR5-CXCR3-$CCR6^+$) cells and plasmablasts (PB) were significantly increased in patients with RA with BMI >25. Significant correlation was observed between BMI and Th17 cells in patients with RA. No significant differences in cell frequencies between the three BMI groups were observed in the healthy donors. Serum interleukin (IL)-1β and IL-21 significantly correlated with BMI in RA patients. Gene expression patterns in Th17 cells from overweight patients with RA showed the characteristics of pathogenic Th17 cells.

Conclusions: Quantitative and qualitative changes in Th17 cells were characteristic in overweight patients with RA.

Keywords: Rheumatoid arthritis, Body mass index, Th17, IL-1β, IL-21

Background

Rheumatoid arthritis (RA) is caused by genetic and environmental factors. In addition, some environmental factors, such as smoking, markedly affect the prognosis of patients with RA. Obesity has also been proposed as one of the environmental risk factors for RA. Obesity modifies the disease course of RA, and also results in poor responses to biological therapy [1, 2]. Cohort studies have demonstrated worse disease activity in obese patients with early RA [3]. Patients with RA who have a high body mass index (BMI) were recently reported to have worse long-term outcomes in disease activity, function, and comorbidities [4]. However, other studies have provided paradoxical findings in which the radiographic evidence of progression of bone damage was slower in obese patients with RA [5, 6]. Therefore, the influence of obesity on RA remains controversial.

Several immune cells orchestrate and play important roles in the pathogenesis of RA. We previously performed immunological cell typing in patients with RA and healthy donors (HDs) [7]. Using flow cytometry, the frequencies of peripheral T cell and B cell subsets and monocytes were measured and analyzed based on associations with several clinical parameters, including disease activity. In the previous study, the frequencies of the peripheral immune cells were compared, and some differences were identified, such as an increase of $CD14^+CD16^+$ monocytes and decreases of T helper (Th)17.1 cells, memory B cells in patients with RA [7]. In the present study, we analyzed this database in view of their relationship with BMI in

* Correspondence: kfujio-tky@umin.ac.jp
Department of Allergy and Rheumatology, Graduate School of Medicine, the University of Tokyo, 7-3-1 Hongo, Bunkyo-ku, Tokyo, Japan

order to identify the immunological features in overweight patients with RA.

Methods

Patients with RA and healthy donors

We recruited 81 patients with RA between April 2013 and March 2015, who fulfilled the 2010 American College of Rheumatology/European League Against Rheumatism classification criteria [8], and 99 HDs. The comparison of age, sex distribution, and BMI between patients with RA and HDs are indicated in Additional file 1: Table S1. All the donors were without active infection or malignancy. The following clinical data were collected: age, sex, disease duration, BMI, methotrexate (MTX) usage, biological disease-modifying anti-rheumatic drug (bDMARD) usage, rheumatoid factor (RF) titer, anti-cyclic citrullinated peptide (CCP) antibody titer, Disease Activity Score 28 joint-erythrocyte sedimentation rate (DAS28esr), the clinical disease activity index (CDAI) and Health Assessment Questionnaire (HAQ) Disability Index. RF titers were measured using latex coagulating nephelometry (cutoff value of 15 IU/ml). Anti-CCP antibody titers were measured using a chemiluminescence enzyme immunoassay (cutoff value of 4.5 U/ml, Medical and Biological Laboratories, Japan). All donors provided written informed consent, and the use of human peripheral blood samples was approved by the Ethical Committee of the University of Tokyo Hospital (number 10154 and G3582). The methods of the present study were performed in accordance with the approved guidelines.

Fluorescence-activated cell sorting (FACS) and immunophenotyping

All collected blood samples were freshly analyzed by flow cytometry. Human peripheral blood mononuclear cells were isolated by Ficoll-Paque Plus density gradient centrifugation (GE Healthcare). The following antibodies were used: Human Fc Receptor Binding Inhibitor Purified (eBioscience), CD3-PE-Cy7 (UCHT1, BioLegend), CD3-PerCP-Cy5.5 (UCHT1, BioLegend), CD4-PerCP-Cy5.5 (OKT4, BioLegend), CD4-V500 (RPA-T4, BD Biosciences), CD14-FITC (M5E2, BioLegend), CD16-PerCP-Cy5.5 (3G8, BioLegend), CD19-APC-Cy7 (HIB19, BioLegend), CD19-V500 (HIB19, BD Biosciences), CD25-Brilliant Violet 421 (BC96, BioLegend), CD25-PE-Cy7 (BC96, eBioscience), CD27-FITC (O323, eBioscience), CD38-PE-Cy7 (HIT2, BioLegend), CD45RA-APC-Cy7 (HI100, BioLegend), CXCR3-Brilliant Violet 421 (1C6, BD Biosciences), CXCR5-Alexa Fluor 488 (RF8B2, BD Biosciences), and CCR6-PE (11A9, BD Biosciences). Flow cytometric analysis and cell sorting were performed on an 8-color MoFlo XDP (Beckman Coulter).

Subset definitions were described in a previous study. We classified $CD4^+$ T cell and B cell subsets and monocytes based on the Human Immunology Project classification [9] and also added modifications for subsets already reported to be important in RA [7]. According to the Human Immunology Project classification [9], Th17 cells were defined as $CD3^+$ $CD4^+$ CD25- CD45RA- CXCR5- CXCR3- $CCR6^+$ cell population. Th17.1 cells were defined as $CD3^+$ $CD4^+$ CD25- CD45RA- CXCR5- $CXCR3^+$ $CCR6^+$ cell population, which were reported as one of the Th populations which exhibited both Th1 and Th17 features [10, 11]. Detailed gating strategies were indicated in the previous article [8].

Multiplex cytokine analysis

Serum concentrations of interleukin (IL)-1β, IL-6, IL-10, IL-17A, IL-21, interferon(IFN)-γ, granulocyte macrophage-colony stimulating factor (GM-CSF) and tumor necrosis factor (TNF)-α were measured using the Milliplex MAP kit (the Human Soluble Cytokine Receptor Magnetic Bead Panel and Human High Sensitivity T Cell Magnetic Panel, Merck Millipore) and BioPlex 3D system (Bio-Rad), according to the manufacturer's instructions. In order to reduce false amplification by heterophilic antibodies, HeteroBlock (Omega Biologicals) was added to all serum samples in order to achieve a final concentration of 150 μg/ml [8]. Serum samples for cytokine measurement were obtained from 19 patients with RA.

Quantitative PCR

RNA was extracted from FACS-sorted Th17 ($CD3^+$ $CD4^+$ CD25- CD45RA- CXCR5- CXCR3- $CCR6^+$) cells using the RNeasy Micro Kit (Qiagen). RNA was reverse-transcribed to cDNA with random primers (Invitrogen) and Superscript III according to the manufacturer's protocol (Invitrogen). Quantitative real-time PCR analysis was performed using SYBR Green Master Mix (Qiagen) and the CFX Connect Real-Time PCR (Bio-Rad). The results of real-time PCR are shown in terms of relative expression to glyceraldehyde-3-phosphate dehydrogenase (GAPDH). Analyzed genes were selected on the basis of a previous study [12]. The primers used in real-time PCR are listed in Additional file 1: Table S2.

Statistical analysis

Differences between groups were tested with one-way analysis of variance (ANOVA) and the unpaired *t* test with post-hoc Bonferroni correction. Relationships between cell frequencies and BMI were evaluated by Pearson's correlation coefficient. Relationships between cytokines and BMI were evaluated by Spearman's correlation coefficient. Multiple variable regression was performed to predict the frequencies of Th17 cells based on the indicated variables. *P* values <0.05 were considered to be significant.

Results

Immunological cell typing and BMI in patients with RA and healthy donors

Subjects were categorized into three groups according to BMI <20, ≥20 to 25, >25), as previously defined [1–4]. A summary of patient profiles is listed in Table 1. No significant differences were observed in clinical background, including age, disease duration, anti-CCP antibody positivity, and therapies among the three BMI groups, except for the serum titers of RF (Table 1). Disease activity scores and HAQ scores were not significantly different between the three BMI groups. The frequencies of the $CD4^+$ T cell and B cell subsets and monocytes were compared between the three BMI groups among healthy donors and patients with RA (Table 2). The frequencies of Th17 cells ($CD3^+CD4^+$CD45RA-CD25-CXCR5-CXCR3-$CCR6^+$) and plasmablasts (PB) were significantly different in the three BMI groups among patients with RA, and were significantly increased in the RA group with BMI >25 (Table 2 and Fig. 1a). In contrast, no significant difference was observed in immune cell frequencies in the three BMI groups among healthy donors (Table 3 and Additional file 2: Figure S1). We then investigated the relationship between BMI and immune cell frequencies. The frequency of Th17 cells positively correlated with BMI in patients with RA ($r^2 = 0.25$, $p < 0.0001$) (Fig. 1b). No correlations were found between PB and BMI in patients with RA ($r^2 = 0.013$ (PB)). The frequencies of Th17 cells were compared between patients with RA and HDs in each BMI category, and there was no significant difference (BMI <20: RA 5.40 ± 2.89, HDs 7.05 ± 2.83, $p = 0.084$, 20 < BMI <25: RA 6.44 ± 3.47, HDs 8.51 ± 2.75, $p = 0.061$, BMI >25: RA 10.68 ± 5.36, HDs 8.41 ± 1.92, $p = 0.26$). Moreover, multivariate analysis demonstrated that BMI was an independent predictor of the frequencies of Th17 cells in patients with RA (Table 4). Taken together, these results revealed immunological characteristics of overweight patients with RA, particularly a significant increase in Th17 cells.

Serum IL-1β concentrations correlated with BMI in patients with RA

Pro-inflammatory cytokines, such as IL-1β, IL-6 and TNF-α, which are the targets of bDMARDs, play pivotal roles in RA pathogenesis. Serum pro-inflammatory cytokines were measured in patients with RA and were analyzed for correlation with BMI (Fig. 2). Serum IL-1β and IL-21 were positively correlated with BMI. In addition, serum IL-17A and GM-CSF were weakly positively correlated with BMI. In contrast, serum IFN-γ was negatively correlated with BMI. Notably, serum IL-6, IL-10 and TNF-α were not correlated with BMI (Fig. 2).

Gene expression patterns in Th17 cells in overweight patients with RA

Gene expression patterns in Th17 cells were analyzed in overweight and non-overweight patients with RA (Fig. 3). The characteristic gene expression patterns in pathogenic Th17 cells, including pro-inflammatory cytokines and chemokines (CSF-2 (GM-CSF), IL-17A, IL-17 F, IL-22, CCL3, CCL4, and CCL5) [12], were significantly increased in the Th17 cells of overweight patients with RA. In contrast, the characteristic gene expression patterns in non-pathogenic Th17 cells, such as IL-10, AHR, and, MAF [12], were slightly

Table 1 Summary of the clinical information on the patients with rheumatoid arthritis

	BMI <20	20 < BMI <25	BMI >25	*P* value
Clinical data				
Number	16	46	19	
Female (%)	81.3%	73.9%	84.2%	
Age (years)	56.9 ± 17.3	64.2 ± 11.0	59.3 ± 11.5	ns
Disease duration (months)	66.0 ± 110.1	72.4 ± 140.5	72.4 ± 171.1	ns
DAS28esr	4.67 ± 1.79	4.53 ± 1.33	4.93 ± 1.62	ns
CDAI	19.5 ± 12.9	17.4 ± 10.7	21.6 ± 16.1	ns
HAQ	0.87 ± 0.77	1.22 ± 0.92	1.39 ± 0.99	ns
Anti-CCP antibody (%)	87.5%	84.7%	89.4%	ns
RF (U/ml)	145.3 ± 295.8	164.9 ± 311.3	445.1 ± 649.7	0.035*
MTX (mg/week)	9.5 ± 2.5	9.0 ± 2.9	8.0 ± 3.11	ns
PSL dose (mg/day)	3.5 ± 4.1	3.6 ± 6.7	3.68 ± 3.89	ns
bDMARDs (%)	12.5%	13.0%	15.7%	ns

Data are shown as mean +/− SD, unless stated otherwise. Differences were analyzed by one-way analysis of variance. *Abbreviations*: *BMI* body mass index, *DAS* disease activity score, *CDAI* Clinical Disease Activity Index, *HAQ* Health Assessment Questionnaire, *CCP* cyclic-citrullinated peptide, *RF* rheumatoid factor, *MTX* methotrexate, *PSL* prednisolone, *bDMARD* biological disease-modifying anti-rheumatic drug, *ns* not significant. *$P < 0.05$

Table 2 Summary of peripheral immune cell frequencies in patients with rheumatoid arthritis

	BMI <20	20 < BMI <25	BMI >25	*P* value
CD4+ T cells (%)				
Total	44.2 ± 8.71	42.6 ± 13.1	40.3 ± 11.93	0.51
Naive T cells	32.1 ± 25.6	29.8 ± 23.7	35.7 ± 16.1	0.32
Memory T cells	26.7 ± 14.3	29.9 ± 13.2	36.7 ± 12.4	0.18
CD25 + Treg cells	6.26 ± 10.9	9.79 ± 16.4	6.19 ± 11.8	0.69
Follicular helper T cells	9.73 ± 6.05	9.95 ± 5.40	11.88 ± 6.17	0.69
Th1 cells	5.48 ± 3.18	5.50 ± 3.09	5.76 ± 2.65	0.13
Th2 cells	9.36 ± 6.81	14.52 ± 9.88	15.79 ± 5.77	0.53
Th17 cells	5.40 ± 2.89	6.44 ± 3.47	10.68 ± 5.36	0.0029**
Th17.1 cells	4.30 ± 3.38	3.71 ± 2.31	5.61 ± 4.30	0.96
B cells (%)				
Total	6.36 ± 5.75	7.70 ± 6.03	5.11 ± 3.74	0.29
Naive B cells	65.3 ± 15.0	66.3 ± 21.2	63.1 ± 17.7	0.86
Switch- memory B cells	5.36 ± 3.63	4.53 ± 3.46	3.79 ± 21.8	0.064
Switch + memory B cells	16.9 ± 8.21	16.8 ± 11.7	19.9 ± 13.6	0.50
Double negative B cells	12.5 ± 8.55	12.5 ± 11.3	12.0 ± 9.33	0.99
Plasmablast	1.59 ± 1.88	1.79 ± 2.90	3.35 ± 3.51	0.020*
Monocytes (%)				
$CD14^{+}$ CD16-	82.3 ± 17.5	85.3 ± 10.5	86.3 ± 8.58	0.66
$CD14^{+}CD16^{+}$	4.77 ± 3.71	4.57 ± 3.16	3.49 ± 2.11	0.48
$CD14^{mid}CD16^{+}$	11.7 ± 13.9	8.85 ± 6.99	9.26 ± 6.64	0.59

The percentages of total $CD4^{+}$ T cells and B cells are shown as a ratio to the total number of lymphocytes. The percentages of cell subsets are shown as a ratio to total $CD4^{+}$ T cells, B cells, and monocytes. The definitions of cell subsets were based on the Human Immunology Project classification [9]. Data are shown as mean +/− SD. *BMI* body mass index, *Treg* T regulatory cells, *Th* T helper. Differences were analyzed by one-way analysis of variance: $^{*}p < 0.05$, $^{**}p < 0.01$

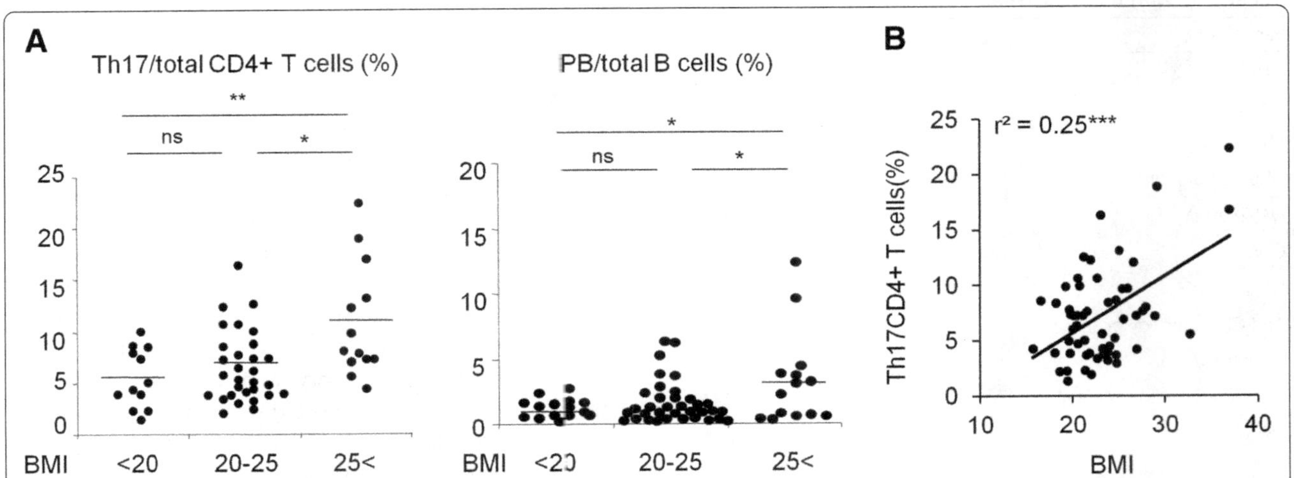

Fig. 1 Frequencies of peripheral immune cells according to body mass index (*BMI*). **a** Comparison of the frequencies of T helper 17 (*Th17*) cells and plasmablasts (*PB*) between the three different BMI groups among patients with rheumatoid arthritis (RA). **b** The relationship between BMI and the frequencies of Th17 cells in patients with RA. Relationships were evaluated by Pearson's correlation coefficient: $^{*}p < 0.05$, $^{**}p < 0.01$, $^{***}p < 0.001$, *ns* not significant

Table 3 Summary of peripheral immune cell frequencies in healthy donors

	BMI <20 (n = 40)	20 < BMI <25 (n = 51)	BMI >25 (n = 8)	*P* value
$CD4^+$ T cells (%)				
Total	40.1 ± 9.55	40.0 ± 9.17	35.7 ± 5.32	0.46
Naive T cells	57.9 ± 12.4	51.6 ± 10.3	48.3 ± 15.1	0.056
Memory T cells	30.6 ± 10.0	34.0 ± 7.97	36.5 ± 9.77	0.077
$CD25^+$Treg cells	2.83 ± 1.16	3.51 ± 1.41	3.75 ± 1.92	0.069
Follicular helper T cells	9.43 ± 3.63	11.9 ± 3.91	12.7 ± 6.35	0.083
Th1 cells	7.25 ± 3.03	7.79 ± 2.86	8.85 ± 3.37	0.34
Th2 cells	8.12 ± 3.61	8.80 ± 3.72	9.47 ± 4.72	0.54
Th17 cells	7.05 ± 2.83	8.51 ± 2.75	8.41 ± 1.92	0.066
Th17.1 cells	7.94 ± 4.72	8.87 ± 4.01	9.79 ± 6.88	0.46
B cells (%)				
Total	4.73 ± 2.91	5.15 ± 2.69	6.15 ± 2.14	0.39
Naive B cells	54.9 ± 14.6	53.5 ± 17.0	66.0 ± 11.4	0.12
Switch- memory B cells	10.4 ± 5.12	10.1 ± 4.11	8.01 ± 2.21	0.38
$Switch^+$memory B cells	27.1 ± 11.6	27.5 ± 11.6	19.5 ± 7.69	0.18
Double negative B cells	7.64 ± 4.33	8.17 ± 6.65	6.48 ± 2.75	0.70
Plasmablast	4.11 ± 7.73	3.19 ± 3.78	2.16 ± 1.73	0.59
Monocytes (%)				
$CD14^+CD16-$	90.7 ± 4.93	89.7 ± 4.75	88.2 ± 5.93	0.39
$CD14^+CD16+$	2.02 ± 1.23	2.31 ± 1.26	3.05 ± 2.57	0.15
$CD14^{mid}CD16+$	6.78 ± 3.69	7.33 ± 3.87	7.90 ± 3.39	0.67

The percentages of total $CD4^+$ T cells and B cells are shown as a ratio to the total number of lymphocytes. The percentages of cell subsets are shown as a ratio to total $CD4^+$ T cells, B cells, and monocytes. Data are shown as mean +/− SD. *BMI* body mass index, *Treg* T regulatory cells, *Th* T helper. Differences were analyzed by one-way analysis of variance: $^*p < 0.05$

Table 4 Multiple variable regression was calculated to predict the frequencies of Th17 cells based on the indicated variables in patients with rheumatoid arthritis (n = 81)

Variables	β regression coefficient	*P* value
Sex	0.244	0.32
Age	−0.158	0.089
BMI	0.495	0.0011**
Disease duration	0.155	0.36
DAS28esr	−0.048	0.89
CDAI	0.120	0.73
HAQ	0.110	0.51
Anti-CCP antibody positivity	0.243	0.67
RF titer (U/mL)	−0.097	0.52
MTX user	0.218	0.11
PSL user	0.177	0.26
bDMARDs user	−0.132	0.38

BMI body mass index, *DAS28esr* Disease Activity Score 28 joints-erythrocyte sedimentation rate, *CDAI* Clinical Disease Activity Index, *HAQ* Health Assessment Questionnaire, *Anti-CCP* anti-citrullinated peptide, *RF* rheumatoid factor, *MTX* methotrexate, *PSL* prednisolone, *bDMARDS* biological disease-modifying anti-rheumatic drugs. $^{**}P < 0.01$

decreased in the Th17 cells of the overweight patients with RA. These results demonstrated that not only the quantity, but also the quality of Th17 cells had pathogenically changed in the overweight patients with RA.

Discussion

The pathological role of obesity in RA remains unclear. Some studies have reported radiographic evidence of protective effects of obesity, while others have demonstrated worse clinical disease course and drug responses to anti-TNF therapy in obese patients with RA [1–4]. Few studies have investigated the mechanisms responsible for the relationship between BMI and the RA disease course. In our study, there was no significant correlation between BMI and ongoing disease activity and the HAQ score in patients with RA. As we reported previously, disease activities were correlated with T cell activation via T cell receptor signaling [7], and we thought that these factors mainly contributed to the ongoing inflammation. RA is thought to be a heterogeneous disease and the immunological abnormalities also differ from patients to patients [13]. For example, TNF-inhibitor-resistant patients with RA

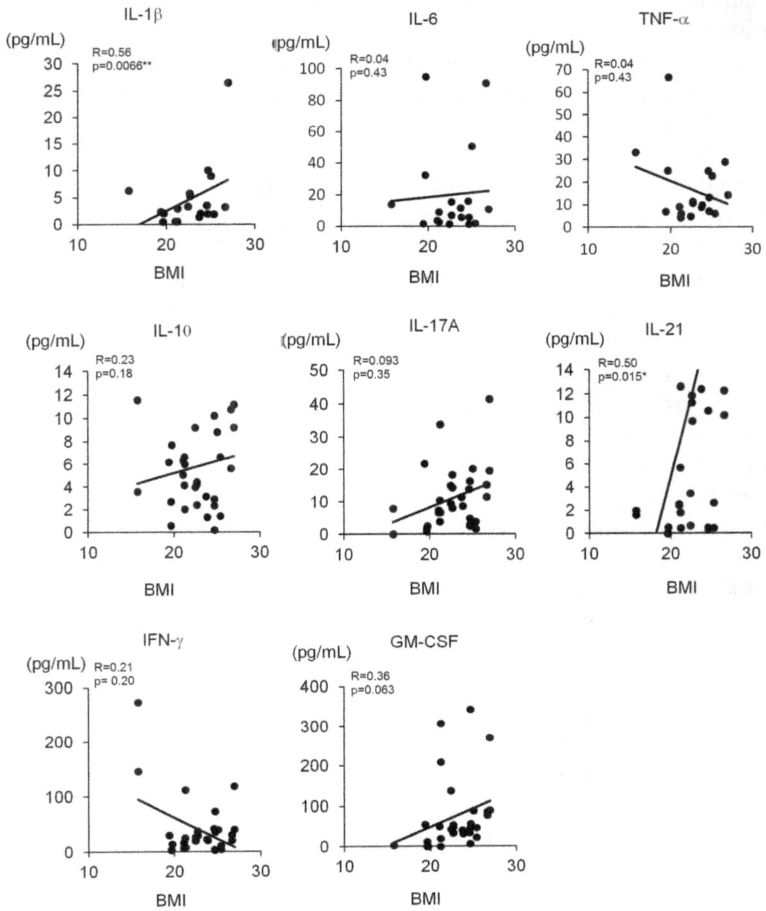

Fig. 2 Relationship between body mass index (*BMI*) and serum cytokines in patients with rheumatoid arthritis (RA). Relationships were evaluated by Spearman's correlation coefficient. Serum samples for cytokine measurement were obtained from 19 patients with RA. *$P < 0.05$. *IFN* interferon, *GM-CSF* granulocyte macrophage-colony stimulating factor

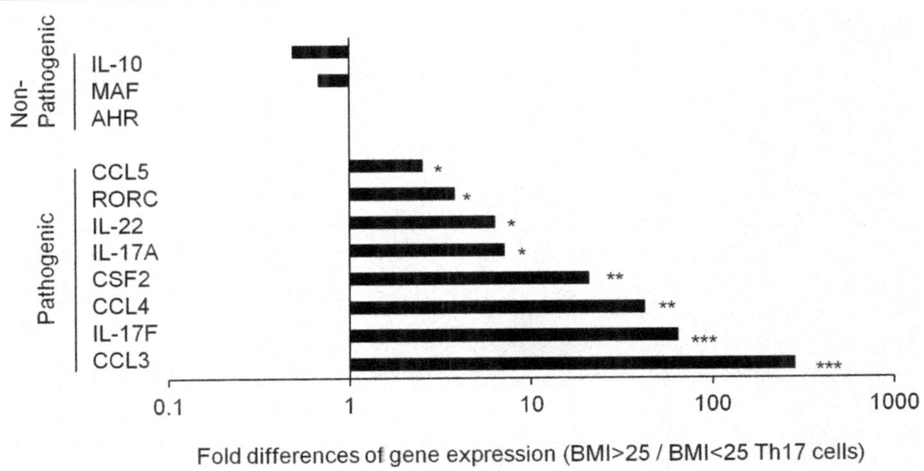

Fig. 3 Gene expression patterns in Th17 cells from patients with rheumatoid arthritis (RA). Fold differences of gene expression patterns in Th17 cells were indicated between patients with body mass index (*BMI*) < 25 and BMI >25 among patients with RA (n = 3, respectively). *$P < 0.05$, **$P < 0.01$, ***$P < 0.001$

sometimes respond to anti-IL-6 therapy or anti-T-cell therapy [14]. These clinical observations support the idea that the immunological abnormalities were heterogeneous in patients with RA. We demonstrated the upregulation of serum IL-1β, IL-21 and Th17 cells in overweight patients with RA. In this study, we defined Th17 cells according to the Human Immunology Project classification [9], and it was reported that IL-17-producing cells were markedly enriched in this population [15]. Notably, the significant correlation between Th17 cells and BMI was only observed in patients with RA, not in HDs. This fact suggested a possibility that the RA-specific inflammatory process would amplify the fat-oriented inflammatory process in the overweight patients with RA. Therefore, the overweight patients with RA were supposed to be a subgroup of patients with RA with the characteristic immunological phenotypes. IL-1β, IL-21 and Th17 cells play important roles in the pathogenesis of RA in several aspects. IL-1β is one of the representative pro-inflammatory cytokines in RA and blockade of IL-1 is one of the therapeutic choices [16]. IL-21 was reported as an inducer of Th17 cells in RA synovium [17]. Especially, the pathological roles of Th17 cells in RA were reported, such as secreting pro-inflammatory cytokines [17, 18]. In this way, the upregulation of Th17 cells could contribute to the pathogenesis of RA in the overweight patients. As the relationship between obesity and progression of bone damage is controversial [1–6], the relationship between BMI and radiological prognos is needs to be elucidated in several different cohorts.

Obesity has recently been thought to be a chronic inflammation process. Adipose tissue is an endocrine/paracrine organ and secretes pro-inflammatory cytokines. Adipose tissue also secretes adipokines, which have been reported to be increased in patients with RA and have been associated with joint damage [19]. For example, leptin has been identified as an inducer of Th17 cells, and hit as been shown to exacerbate collagen-induced arthritis (CIA) by enhancing Th17 cell responses [20]. Resistin-like molecule α is an adipokine that induces Th17 cells in the colitis model [21]. Visfatin strongly induces IL-6, IL-8, and matrix metalloproteinases by synovial fibroblasts [22]. Although we did not include these adipokines in this study, they could relate to the pathogenesis of the overweight patients with RA. Furthermore, free fatty acid also sensitizes dendritic cells to induce Th17 response, and could be a possible mediator in RA pathogenesis [23]. These points will be addressed in the future.

A recent report suggested that nucleotide-binding domain, leucine-rich containing family, pyrin domain-containig-3 (Nlrp3) inflammasome plays a pivotal role in obesity-induced chronic inflammation, and Nlrp3 inflammasome activates caspase-1, which induces the secretion of IL-1β [24]. These findings support the idea that being overweight is associated with chronic systemic inflammation and pro-inflammatory phenotypes in patients with RA, such as an increase in serum IL-1β, and may affect the clinical disease course and drug responses in obese patients with RA. To address this point further, body fat measurement is more appropriate than BMI, and the association between body fat mass and the immunological parameters will be elucidated. In addition, obesity plays several roles in inflammatory processes in the joints. For example, mechanical joint damage is more evident in obese people, and this kind of minor trauma is thought to induce the inflammation in the joints [6], which would cause excess cytokine secretions and Th17 differentiations in RA.

In the present study, Th17 cells were increased in the overweightp with RA. In mouse models, obesity was shown to aggravate CIA by promoting Th17 cell differentiation [25]. Moreover, gene expression patterns in Th17 cells had the characteristics of pathogenic Th17 cells in the overweight patients with RA. The importance of Th17 cells in the pathogenesis of RA has already been demonstrated [18, 26, 27]. Pathogenic Th17 cells secrete pro-inflammatory cytokines, such as IL-21, which play pivotal roles in the synovial inflammation [18]. IL-1β is crucially involved in the differentiation and pathogenicity of human Th17 cells [28]. These findings suggest that the chronic inflammation in the adipose tissue contributed to the increases in serum IL-1β and induced the differentiation of pathogenic Th17 cells in the overweight patients with RA. The obese patients with RA have exhibited worse responses to TNF-α inhibitors [1, 2]. These findings have contributed to the individualized selection of bDMARDs for patients with RA, and an anti-IL-1β, anti-IL-21 and anti-Th17 cell strategy may represent a better option for the obese patients with RA. In the case of obese psoriatic arthritis, weight reduction was associated with greater response to TNF-inhibitor [29], and weight reduction will also be a reasonable approach to recover the response to the therapies in patients with RA.

Limitations of this study were as follows: (1) the analysis of Th17 subset was based on CCR expression, but not on the production of IL-17; (2) the sample sizes were relatively small in some studies, including the gene expression study, which was only based on BMI <25/>25; (3) serum cytokines were not measured in the whole patient group; (4) the study subjects were the Japanese population; (5) the other adipokines, such as adiponectin and leptin, were not measured;and (6) age-matched healthy controls were missing. These points will be elucidated in future.

Conclusions

In conclusion, BMI was closely associated with chronic systemic inflammation in patients with RA, and quantitative and qualitative changes in Th17 cells were observed in overweight patients with RA. We assumed that the overweight patients with RA were a subgroup of patients with RA who had the characteristic immunological phenotypes. These results provide insights into the immunological mechanisms underlying worse clinical courses and drug responses in obese patients. Individualized therapy will be addressed on the basis of these observations.

Abbreviations

bDMARD: biological disease-modifying anti-rheumatic drug; BMI: Body mass index; CCP: Cyclic citrullinated peptide; CDAI: Clinical Disease Activity Index; CIA: Collagen-induecd arthritis; DAS: Disease Activity Score; DAS28esr: Disease Activity Score 28 joint-erythrocyte sedimentation rate; ESR: Erythrocyte sedimentation rate; FACS: fluorescence-activated cell sorting; GM-CSF: Granulocyte macrophage-colony stimulating factor; HAQ: Health Assessment Questionnaire Disability Index; HD: Healthy donor; IFN: Interferon; IL: Interleukin; MTX: Methotrexate; Nlrp3: Nucleotide-binding domein, leucine-rich containing family, pyrin domain-containing-3; PB: plasmablasts; PSL: prednisolone; RA: Rheumatoid arthritis; RF: Rheumatoid factor; Th: T helper; TNF: Tumor necrosis factor

Acknowledgements

This study was supported by the Ministry of Health, Labor and Welfare, Ministry of Education, Culture, Sports, Science and Technology KAKENHI Grant-in-Aid for Scientific Research (C) (26461462).

Funding

None.

Authors' contributions

HS, YN, YT, KS, and SS obtained and analyzed the patient data. HS interpreted the patient data and prepared the manuscript. KF and KY supervised the study. All the authors read and approved the final manuscript.

Competing interests

KY received financial support or fees from AbbVie, Astellas, BMS, Daiichi-Sankyo, MitsubishiTanabe, Pfizer, Sanofi, Santen, Takeda, Teijin., Boehringer Ingelheim, Chugai, Eisai, Ono, Taisho Toyama, UCB., ImmunoFuture, Asahi Kasei, and Janssen. KF received financial support or fees from Astellas, BMS, Daiichi-Sankyo, MitsubishiTanabe, Pfizer, Santen, Takeda, Chugai, Eisai, Taisho Toyama and UCB., and Janssen. All other authors declare no competing financial interests. All the authors declare no non-financial conflicts of interest.

Consent for publication

Written consent for publication was obtained from all the participants in this study.

References

1. Klaasen R, Wijbrandts CA, Gerlag DM, Tak PP. Body mass index and clinical response to infliximab in rheumatoid arthritis. Arthritis Rheum. 2011;63:359–64.
2. Gremese E, Carletto A, Padovan M, Atzeni F, Raffeiner B, Giardina AR, et al. Obesity and reduction of the response rate to anti-tumor necrosis factor alpha in rheumatoid arthritis: an approach to a personalizaed medicine. Arthritis Care Res. 2013;65:94–100.
3. Sandberg ME, Bengtsson C, Kallberg H, Kallberg H, Wesley A, Klareskog L, et al. Overweight decreases the chance of achieving good response and low disease activity in early rheumatoid arthritis. Ann Rheum Dis. 2014;73: 2029–33.
4. Ajeganova S, Andersson ML, Hafstrom I, BARFOT Study Group. Association of obesity with worse disease severity in rheumatoid arthritis as well as with comorbidities: a long-term follow up from disease onset. Arthritis Care Res. 2013;65:78–87.
5. van der Helm-wan Mil AHM, van der Kooij SM, Allaart CF, et al. A high body mass index has a protective effect on the amount of joint destruction in small joints in early rheumatoid arthritis. Ann Rheum Dis. 2008;67:769–74.
6. Iannone F, Lopalco G, Rigante D, Orlando I, Cantarini L, Lapadula G. Impact of obesity on the clinical outcome of rheumatological patients in biotherapy. Autoimmune Rev. 2016;15:447–50.
7. Nagafuchi Y, Shoda H, Sumitomo S, Nakachi S, Kato R, Tsuchida Y, et al. Immunophenotyping of rheumatoid arthritis reveals a linkage between HLA-DRB1 genotype, CXCR4 expression on memory CD4$^+$ T cells, and disease activity. Sci Rep. 2016;6:29338.
8. Aletaha D, Neogi T, Silman AJ, Funovits J, Felson DT, Bingham CO, et al. 2010 rheumatoid arthritis classification criteria: an American College of Rheumatology/European League Against Rheumatism collaborative initiative. Ann Rheum Dis. 2010;69:1580–8.
9. Maecker HT, McCoy JP, Nussenblatt R. Standardizing immunophenotyping for the Human Immunology Project. Nat Rev Immunol. 2012;12:191–200.
10. Nistala K, Adams S, Cambrook H, Urse S, Olivito B, de Jager W, et al. Th17 plasticity in human autoimmune arthritis is derived by the inflammatory environment. Proc Natl Acad Sci U S A. 2010;107:14751–6.
11. Paulissen SMJ, van Hamburg JP, Davelaar N, Vroman H, Hazes JMW, de Jong PHP, et al. CCR6$^+$Th cell populations distinguish ACPA positive and ACPA negative rheumatoid arthritis. Arthritis Res Ther. 2015;17:344.
12. Lee Y, Awasthi A, Yosef N, Quintana FJ, Xiao S, Peters A, et al. Induction and molecular signature of pathogenic Th17 cells. Nat Immunol. 2012;13:991–9.
13. Weyand CM, McCarthy TG, Goronzy JJ. Correlation between disease phenotype and genetic heterogeneity in rheumatoid arthritis. J Clin Invest. 1995;95:2120–6.
14. Moots RJ, Naisbett-Groet B. The efficacy of biologic agents in patients with rheumatoid arthritis and an inadequate response to tumor necrosis factor inhibitors: a systematic review. Rheumatoogy. 2012;51:2252–61.
15. Shen H, Goodall JC, Gaston JSH. Frequency and phenotype of peripheral blood Th17 cells in ankylosing spondylitis and rheumatoid arthritis. Arthritis Rheum. 2009;60:1647–56.
16. Cavalli G, Dinarello CA. Treating rheumatological diseases and co-morbidities with interleukin-1 blocking therapies. Rheumatology (Oxford). 2015;54:2134–44.
17. Niu X, He D, Zhang X, Yue T, Li N, Zhang JZ, et al. IL-21 regulates Th17 cells in rheumatoid arthritis. Hum Immunol. 2010;71:334–41.
18. van den Berg WB, McInnes IB. Th17 cells and IL-17 focus on immunopathogenesis and immunotherapeutics. Semin Arthritis Rheum. 2013;43:158–70.
19. Rho YH, Solus J, Sokka T, Oeser A, Chung CP, Gebretsadik T, et al. Adipocytokines are associated with radiographic joint damage in rheumatoid arthritis. Arthritis Rhuem. 2009;60:1906–14.
20. Deng J, Liu Y, Yang M, Wang S, Zhang M, Wang X, et al. Leptin exacerbates collagen-induced arthritis via enhancement of Th17 cell response. Arthritis Rheum. 2012;64:3564–73.
21. Osborne LC, Joyce KL, Alenghat T, Sonnenberg GF, Giacomin PR, Du Y, et al. Resistin-like molecule α promotes pathogenic Th17 cell responses and bacterial-induced intestinal inflammation. J Immunol. 2013;190:2292–300.
22. Gómez R, Conde J, Scotece M, Gómez-Reino JJ, Lago F, Gualillo O. What's new in our understanding of the role of adipokines in rheumatic diseases? Nat Rev Rheumatol. 2011;7:528–36.
23. Stelzner K, Herbert D, Popkova Y, Lorz A, Schiller J, Gericke M, et al. Free fatty acids sensitize dendritic cells to amplify TH1/TH17-immune responses. Eur J Immunol. 2016;46:2043–53.
24. Vandanmagsar B, Youm YH, Ravssin A, Galgani JE, Stadler K, Mynatt RL, et al. The NALP3 inflammasome instigates obesity-induced inflammation and insulin resistance. Nat Med. 2011;17:179–88.
25. Jhun JY, Yoon BY, Park MK, Oh HJ, Byun JK, Lee SY, et al. Obesity aggravates the joint inflammation in a collagen-induced arthritis model through deviation to Th17 differentiation. Exp Mol Med. 2012;44:424–31.

13

Interleukin-10-producing LAG3^{+} regulatory T cells are associated with disease activity and abatacept treatment in rheumatoid arthritis

Shinichiro Nakachi[1], Shuji Sumitomo[1], Yumi Tsuchida[1], Haruka Tsuchiya[1], Masanori Kono[1], Rika Kato[1], Keiichi Sakurai[1], Norio Hanata[1], Yasuo Nagafuchi[1], Shoko Tateishi[1,2], Hiroko Kanda[1,2], Tomohisa Okamura[1,3], Kazuhiko Yamamoto[1] and Keishi Fujio[1*]

Abstract

Background: Regulatory T cells (Tregs) play a role in the suppression of inflammation in autoimmune diseases, and lymphocyte activation gene 3 (LAG3) was reported as a marker of interleukin (IL)-10-producing Tregs. We aimed to clarify the function of human IL-10-producing $CD4^{+}CD25^{-}LAG3^{+}$ T cells (LAG3^{+} Tregs) and their association with rheumatoid arthritis (RA).

Methods: LAG3^{+} Tregs of human peripheral blood mononuclear cells (PBMCs) were cultured with B cells and follicular helper T cells to examine antibody suppression effects. The frequency of LAG3^{+} Tregs was evaluated in peripheral blood samples from 101 healthy donors and 85 patients with RA. In patients treated with abatacept, PBMC samples were analyzed before and after treatment. Naive CD4^{+} T cells were sorted and cultured in the presence of abatacept, followed by flow cytometric analysis and function assays.

Results: LAG3^{+} Tregs produced high amounts of IL-10 and interferon-γ, and they suppressed B-cell antibody production more strongly than CD25^{+} Tregs. Cell-to-cell contact was required for the suppressive function of LAG3^{+} Tregs. The frequency of LAG3^{+} Tregs was lower in patients with RA, especially those with higher Clinical Disease Activity Index scores. LAG3^{+} Tregs significantly increased after 6 months of abatacept treatment, whereas CD25^{+} Tregs generally decreased. Abatacept treatment in vitro conferred LAG3 and EGR2 expression on naive CD4^{+} T cells, and abatacept-treated CD4^{+} T cells exhibited suppressive activity.

Conclusions: IL-10-producing LAG3^{+} Tregs are associated with the immunopathology and therapeutic response in RA. LAG3^{+} Tregs may participate in a mechanism for the anti-inflammatory and immune-modulating effects of targeted therapy for costimulation.

Keywords: LAG3, Regulatory T cell, IL-10, Abatacept, Rheumatoid arthritis, Antibody production

* Correspondence: kfujio-tky@umin.ac.jp
[1]Department of Allergy and Rheumatology, Graduate School of Medicine, the University of Tokyo, 7-3-1 Hongo, Bunkyo-ku, Tokyo 113-8655, Japan
Full list of author information is available at the end of the article

Background

Rheumatoid arthritis (RA) is the most common type of autoimmune disease. It is characterized by synovial inflammation, production of autoantibodies including anticitrullinated protein antibody (ACPA), and destruction of cartilage and bone. With regard to the pathogenesis of RA, dendritic cells and macrophages are initially activated, and they present autoantigens to T cells, leading to the expansion of autoreactive T cells [1]. Autoreactive B cells also play a central role through their differentiation into long-lived memory B cells and autoantibody-producing plasma cells [2]. Activation of autoreactive T cells and B cells further stimulates macrophages to produce proinflammatory cytokines such as tumor necrosis factor-α, interleukin (IL)-1β, and IL-6. Therefore, adaptive immunity mediated by autoreactive T cells and B cells can be one of the most important targets in the therapy of RA [3].

Regulatory T cells (Tregs) constitute a subpopulation of T cells that plays an indispensable role in maintaining tolerance to self-antigens and immunological homeostasis. A lack of Tregs or their dysfunction leads to a breakdown of immunological tolerance to self-antigens and can result in autoimmune diseases [4, 5]. A number of Treg subsets have been identified over the years [6–10], and cluster of differentiation $CD4^{+}CD25^{+}FOXP3^{+}$ regulatory T cells ($CD25^{+}$ Treg) [6] and $CD4^{+}$ IL-10-producing regulatory T cells (IL-10-producing Tregs) [7] are the best characterized among them.

$CD25^{+}$ Tregs develop mainly in the thymus to specifically express the Forkhead box P3 (*Foxp3*) gene [11]. Scurfy mice, which have a frameshift mutation in the *Foxp3* gene, exhibit severe inflammatory infiltration of the skin and liver [12]. However, many organs, including the central nervous system, joints, and small intestine, remain unaffected in scurfy mice [13]. These results suggest the existence of additional important mechanisms other than $CD25^{+}$ Tregs that support self-tolerance against many organs including joints [14].

IL-10-producing Tregs are characterized by the production of high amounts of IL-10 without FOXP3 expression. IL-10-producing Tregs have been reported to ameliorate experimental autoimmune encephalitis [15] and colitis [7] in mouse models. Thus far, IL-10-producing Tregs have primarily been reported as induced populations in the presence of vitamin D_3 [16], anti-CD46 antibody [17], rapamycin [18], or IL-27 [19, 20]. This is due in part to the difficulty in identifying naturally occurring IL-10-producing Tregs because of the lack of definitive surface markers. However, recent reports have shown that lymphocyte activation gene 3 (LAG3) protein, a major histocompatibility complex class II-binding CD4 homologue, is expressed on IL-10-producing $CD4^{+}$ T cells and is a candidate phenotypic surface marker for IL-10-producing Tregs [21–23].

We have previously identified murine $CD4^{+}CD25^{-}LAG3^{+}$ regulatory T cells that produce high amounts of IL-10 and interferon (IFN)-γ, lack Foxp3 expression, and suppress B-cell antibody production [21, 23]. They are regulated by early growth response gene 2 (Egr2), which is important for the maintenance of T-cell anergy by negatively regulating T-cell activation [24]. We therefore hypothesized that human $CD4^{+}CD25^{-}LAG3^{+}$ T cells might have the same functions as those in mice and that they might be associated with human autoimmune diseases. We aimed to characterize $CD4^{+}CD25^{-}LAG3^{+}$ T cells in healthy and autoimmune states and to determine the impact of abatacept treatment that targets T-cell responses.

Methods

Blood samples and clinical data

All clinical investigations conformed to the Declaration of Helsinki principles and were approved (10154 and G3582) by the ethics committee of the University of Tokyo. Peripheral blood mononuclear cells (PBMCs) were obtained from 101 self-reported screened healthy donors and 85 patients with RA who fulfilled the 1987 American College of Rheumatology revised criteria or the 2010 American College of Rheumatology/European League Against Rheumatism classification criteria. Moreover, PBMCs were taken from four healthy donors vaccinated with a seasonal inactivated influenza virus in 2013. Clinical characteristics and laboratory data were documented on the day of sample collection. All subjects provided written informed consent.

Cell isolation and flow cytometry

PBMCs were isolated from whole blood by Ficoll-Paque Plus (GE Healthcare Life Sciences, Pittsburgh, PA, USA) gradient separation. Fc receptor binding inhibitor (eBioscience, San Diego, CA, USA) was added to the isolated PBMCs. They were stained with the following monoclonal antibodies (mAbs) for 20 minutes: Alexa Fluor 488 anti-C-X-C chemokine receptor type 5 (anti-CXCR5; RF8B2), phycoerythrin (PE) anti-C-C chemokine receptor type 6 (anti-CCR6; 11A9), Brilliant Violet 412 anti-CXCR3 (1C6), and V500 anti-CD4 (RPA-T4) from BD Biosciences (San Jose, CA, USA); Alexa Fluor 488 anti-CD49b (AK7), peridinin-chlorophyll protein (PerCP)-Cy5.5 anti-CD3 (UCHT1), PerCP-Cy5.5 anti-CCR7 (G043H7), allophycocyanin anti-CD19 (HIB19), allophycocyanin-Cy7 anti-CD45RA (HI100), and Brilliant Violet 421 anti-CD25 (BC96) from BioLegend (San Diego, CA, USA); PE-Cy7 anti-CD127 (eBioRDR5) from eBioscience; and PE anti-LAG3 polyclonal antibody (FAB2319P, 4:100) from R&D Systems (Minneapolis, MN, USA). All cell subsets were analyzed and sorted by eight-color MoFlo XDP (Beckman Coulter Life Sciences, Indianapolis, IN, USA). Each subset was defined as having the following immunophenotype: naive CD4$^+$ T cells were CD4$^+$CD45RA$^+$CD25$^-$LAG3$^-$CCR7$^+$ (Fig. 1) or CD4$^+$CD45RA$^+$ (Fig. 4); follicular helper T (T_{FH}) cells were CD4$^+$CD45RA$^-$CXCR5$^+$CD25$^-$LAG3$^-$; CD25$^+$ Tregs were CD4$^+$CD45RA$^-$CD25$^+$LAG3$^-$CD127^{dim}; type 1 helper T (Th1) cells were CD4$^+$CD45RA$^-$CXCR3$^+$CCR6$^-$; Th2 cells were CD4$^+$CD45RA$^-$CXCR3$^-$CCR6$^-$; Th17 cells were CD4$^+$CD45RA$^-$CXCR3$^-$CCR6$^+$; LAG3$^+$ Tregs were CD4$^+$CD45RA$^-$CD25$^-$LAG3$^+$; and B cells were CD3$^-$CD19$^+$. Data were analyzed using FlowJo software (FlowJo, Ashland, OR, USA).

Measurement of cytokines by enzyme-linked immunosorbent assay

CD4$^+$ T cells (2×10^4 cells/well) were stimulated with plate-bound anti-CD3 mAb (5.0 μg/ml, UCHT1; R&D Systems) and anti-CD28 mAb (1.0 μg/ml, 37407; R&D Systems) in flat-bottomed 96-well plates for 3 days. Concentrations of IL-10, IFN-γ, and IL-17A in the supernatants were measured using enzyme-linked immunosorbent assay (ELISA) kits according to the manufacturer's protocol (OptEIA Human IL-10 ELISA Kit II; BD Biosciences; Human IFN-γ ELISA Ready-SET-Go! and Human IL-17A ELISA Ready-SET-Go!; eBioscience). Cells were cultured in Gibco RPMI 1640 medium (Invitrogen, Paisley, UK) supplemented with 10% FBS (Equitech-Bio, Kerrville, TX, USA), 100 μg/ml L-glutamine, 100 U/ml penicillin, 100 μg/ml streptomycin, and 50 μM 2-mercaptoethanol (Life Technologies, Carlsbad, CA, USA).

B-cell and T-cell coculture

Each CD4$^+$ T cell subset (1×10^5 cells/well) was cocultured with B cells (1×10^5 cells/well) and T_{FH} cells (5×10^4 cells/well) in round-bottomed 96-well plates. Recombinant staphylococcal enterotoxin B (SEB) (2 μg/ml; Toxin Technology, Sarasota, FL, USA) was added to stimulate B cells. Blocking antihuman IL-10 mAb (25209; R&D Systems), blocking antihuman Fas ligand mAb (100410; R&D Systems), or mouse immunoglobulin G1κ (IgG1κ) isotype control (eBioscience) was added at a concentration of 10 μg/ml on the first day of the coculture in the same experimental system as above. To assess cell-cell contact, a coculture experiment was performed using a Transwell plate (HTS Transwell-96 System [3381]; Corning Life Sciences, Acton, MA, USA) with the following cells: B cells, 3×10^5 cells/well; T_{FH} cells, 2×10^5 cells/well; and CD4$^+$CD25$^-$LAG3$^+$CD45RA$^-$ T cells, 1×10^5 cells/well. The concentrations of IgG, IgA, and IgM in

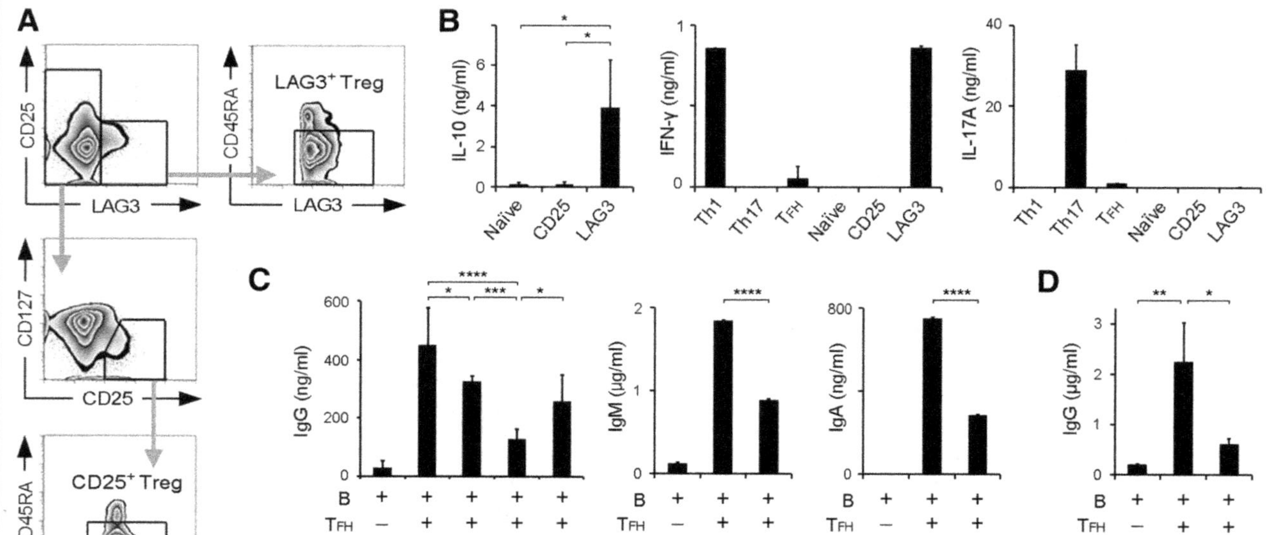

Fig. 1 Human CD4$^+$CD25$^-$LAG3$^+$ T cells suppressed antibody production. **a** Gating strategy of fluorescence-activated cell sorting analysis for CD4$^+$CD25$^-$LAG3$^+$CD45RA$^-$ T cells (LAG3$^+$ Tregs) and CD4$^+$CD25$^+$CD127^{dim}CD45RA$^-$ T cells (CD25$^+$ Tregs). **b** IL-10, IFN-γ, and IL-17A protein levels in the culture supernatants after 3 days of incubation of the indicated T-cell subsets was determined by ELISA ($n = 6$). **c** B cells and T_{FH} cells were cocultured with the indicated subsets for 12 days in the presence of SEB stimulation, and total IgG, IgM, and IgA production was determined by ELISA ($n = 6$). **d** B cells and T_{FH} cells were cocultured with CD4$^+$CD25$^-$LAG3$^+$CD49b$^-$ T cells for 12 days in the presence of SEB stimulation, and total IgG was determined by ELISA ($n = 3$). All error bars represent SD. * $P < 0.05$; ** $P < 0.01$; *** $P < 0.001$; **** $P < 0.0001$. All P values were calculated by one-way analysis of variance and Tukey's multiple-comparisons test. *CD* Cluster of differentiation, *ELISA* Enzyme-linked immunosorbent assay, *IFN-γ* Interferon-γ, *Ig* Immunoglobulin, *IL* Interleukin, *LAG3* Lymphocyte activation gene 3, *RA* Rheumatoid arthritis, *SEB* Staphylococcal enterotoxin B, T_{FH} Follicular helper T cell, *Treg* Regulatory T cell

the 12-day culture supernatant were measured by ELISA (Human IgG ELISA Quantitation Set, Human IgA ELISA Quantitation Set, and Human IgM ELISA Quantitation Set; Bethyl Laboratories, Montgomery, TX, USA).

Culture in the presence of abatacept

Antigen-presenting cells (APCs) were sorted as $CD3^-$ cells and irradiated with 30 Gy. Abatacept was purchased from Bristol-Myers Squibb (Princeton, NJ, USA) and used at a final concentration of 10 μg/ml. Human IgG1 Fc (R&D Systems) was added as a control. Cultured cells were analyzed and sorted as 7-amino actinomycin D (7-AAD)-negative cells at day 4 (BioLegend). Sorted 7-AAD-negative $CD4^+$ T cells were cultured with B cells and T_{FH} cells in the aforementioned system to investigate the suppressive function of the cells induced by abatacept.

Quantitative real-time polymerase chain reaction

Total RNA was isolated using RNeasy Micro Kit (QIAGEN, Valencia, CA, USA) according to the manufacturer's protocol. Complementary DNA was synthesized with SuperScript III Reverse Transcriptase (Life Technologies) and oligo(dT) primers, and it was mixed with SYBR Green Master Mix (Life Technologies). The real-time polymerase chain reaction (PCR) primer pairs were as follows: human EGR2 sense: 5′-TGGAGAGAACAGG TCGTTGG-3′ and antisense: 5′-CTGGATGAGGCTGT GGTTG-3′; FAS sense: 5′-TGCAGAAGATGTAGATT GTGTGATGA-3′ and antisense: 5′-GGGTCCGCGTG CAGTTTATT-3′, and CD247 sense: 5′-GGGAGAATG ATGGATGTGAA-3′ and antisense: 5′-CCGATGAA CCCCTAAACCA-3′. Quantitative PCR was conducted using an iCycler PCR system (Bio-Rad Laboratories, Hercules, CA, USA). The expression of each gene was normalized to the glyceraldehyde 3-phosphate dehydrogenase housekeeping gene (*GAPDH*) (forward: 5′-GAAGGTGAAGGTCGGAGTC-3′ and reverse: 5′-GAAGATGGTGATGGGATTTC-3′).

Statistical analysis

Data are presented as mean ± SD. Statistical differences between groups were evaluated using an unpaired two-tailed Student's t test, the Mann-Whitney U test, or the Wilcoxon signed-rank test for comparing two groups, and one-way analysis of variance or the Kruskal-Wallis test was used to compared three or more groups. P values less than 0.05 were considered statistically significant (* $P < 0.05$; ** $P < 0.01$; *** $P < 0.001$; **** $P < 0.0001$). Calculations were conducted using Prism version 5.03 software (GraphPad Software Inc., La Jolla, CA, USA). To compare the frequency of Tregs in patients, a statistical analysis was conducted using R version 3.1.2 software (R Foundation for Statistical Computing, Vienna, Austria).

Results

Human $CD4^+CD25^-LAG3^+CD45RA^-$ T cells produce IL-10 and suppress antibody production

In human PBMCs, we identified $CD4^+CD25^-LAG3^+$ T cells that were negative for Foxp3. Confirmation of Foxp3 expression and suppressive activity of control $CD4^+CD25^+$ Tregs indicated the adequacy of gating strategies (Fig. 1a and Additional file 1: Figures S1 and S2). Upon T-cell receptor (TCR) stimulation, $CD4^+CD25^-LAG3^+$ T cells produced high amounts of IL-10, amounts of IFN-γ as much as Th1 cells, and no IL-17A (Fig. 1b), consistent with the results for murine $CD4^+CD25^-LAG3^+$ Tregs [21]. Intracellular staining revealed that more $LAG3^+$ T cells (mean 14.2%) expressed IL-10 than naive $CD4^+$ T cells (mean 4.8%) (Additional file 1: Figure S3). Given that murine $CD4^+CD25^-LAG3^+$ Tregs efficiently control B-cell functions, we cocultured these cells with B cells and T_{FH} cells and measured IgG in the supernatants. When SEB was used to imitate the antigen-specific interaction between B cells and T_{FH} cells, we found that $CD4^+CD25^-LAG3^+$ T cells significantly suppressed IgG production by B cells (Fig. 1c). Moreover, $CD4^+CD25^-LAG3^+$ T cells also suppressed IgM and IgA (Fig. 1c), which indicated that $CD4^+CD25^-LAG3^+$ T cells inhibited immunoglobulin production instead of inhibiting class switching. In a previous study, $LAG3^+CD49b^+$ T cells were reported to have the suppressive function of T cells among IL-10-producing Tregs [22]. Therefore, we assessed whether CD49b was required for antibody suppression by $CD4^+CD25^-LAG3^+$ T cells and found that $CD49b^-CD4^+CD25^-LAG3^+$ T cells significantly suppressed antibody production (Fig. 1d). Taken together, these results showed that $CD4^+CD25^-LAG3^+$ T cells in human PBMCs produced high levels of IL-10 and suppressed B-cell antibody production, regardless of CD49b expression.

The suppressive function of $CD4^+CD25^-LAG3^+$ T cells requires cell-to-cell contact

We conducted experiments using Transwell plates and found that the suppressive function of $CD4^+CD25^-LAG3^+$ T cells was abrogated in the absence of direct contact with B cells or T_{FH} cells (Fig. 2a). Among interactions between cell surface molecules, Fas–Fas ligand interaction is associated with antibody suppression of murine $LAG3^+$ Tregs [23]. In a blocking experiment, the addition of anti-Fas ligand antibody abrogated the suppressive function of these cells, whereas anti-IL-10 antibody did not affect this suppression (Fig. 2b). This suggests that $CD4^+CD25^-LAG3^+$ T cells exerted their suppressive function in a manner requiring Fas–Fas ligand interaction rather than IL-10.

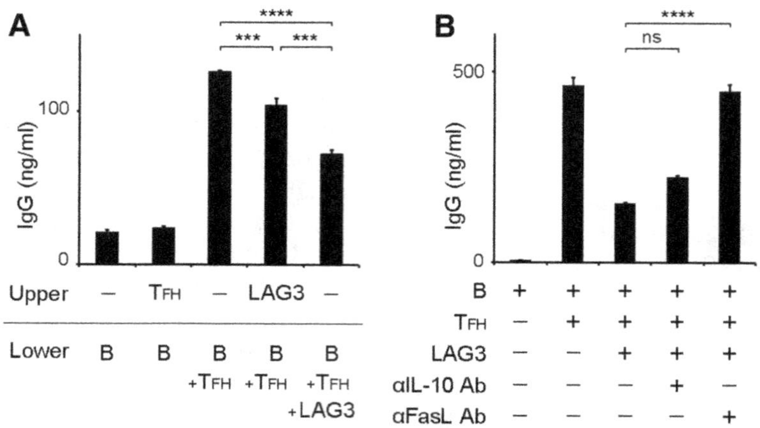

Fig. 2 LAG3$^+$ Tregs suppressed B-cell antibody production independent of IL-10. **a** B cells and T_{FH} cells were cocultured with LAG3$^+$ Tregs under staphylococcal enterotoxin B stimulation in Transwells for 12 days. The indicated subsets were placed in upper and lower chambers as described. Total IgG production was determined by ELISA ($n = 3$). **b** Anti-IL-10 antibody and anti-FasL antibody were added to the same coculture system as in (**a**). Total IgG production was determined by ELISA ($n = 3$). All error bars represent SD. *** $P < 0.001$; **** $P < 0.0001$. All P values were calculated by one-way analysis of variance and Tukey's multiple-comparison test. *Ab* Antibody, *ELISA* Enzyme-linked immunosorbent assay, *FasL* Fas ligand, *Ig* Immunoglobulin, *IL* Interleukin, *LAG3* Lymphocyte activation gene 3, T_{FH} Follicular helper T cell, *Treg* Regulatory T cell

The frequency of LAG3$^+$ Tregs was decreased in patients with rheumatoid arthritis and significantly increased with abatacept treatment

We analyzed 101 healthy subjects and 85 patients with RA to assess LAG3$^+$ Treg frequency (Table 1). The frequency of LAG3$^+$ Tregs was significantly lower in patients with RA than in healthy donors (3.76 ± 2.72% in RA vs 5.07 ± 2.78% in healthy donors, $P < 0.001$) (Fig. 3a). Moreover, the frequency of LAG3$^+$ Tregs in untreated patients with RA was significantly lower than that of healthy donors ($P < 0.05$) (Fig. 3b). Whereas the frequency of CD25$^+$ Tregs in patients with RA was significantly lower than that in healthy donors ($P < 0.05$) (Fig. 3a), in the patients with untreated RA, the frequency of CD25$^+$ Tregs was not different from that in healthy donors (Fig. 3b). Moreover, LAG3$^+$ Tregs demonstrated a significant decrease in patients with higher disease activity ($P < 0.05$) (Fig. 3c), whereas the frequencies of CD25$^+$ Tregs were similar regardless of disease states. However, there were not significant correlations

Table 1 Baseline demographics and clinical characteristics

	RA ($n = 85$)	Naive RA ($n = 16$)	RA before abatacept ($n = 18$)
Female sex, *n* (%)	67 (79)	10 (63)	15 (83)
Age, years	58.9 (13.1)	55.9 (12.2)	62.7 (13.2)
Disease duration, months	139.4 (153.9)	6.7 (8.3)	187.5 (144.2)
DAS28-CRP	3.7 (1.5)	4.1 (1.6)	4.2 (1.3)
DAS28-ESR	4.4 (1.6)	4.9 (1.6)	4.9 (1.2)
CDAI	16.6 (12.1)	21.6 (14.5)	21.4 (11.7)
Rheumatoid factor, % positive	74 (87)	15 (94)	15 (83)
Anti-CCP antibody, % positive	72 (85)	13 (81)	18 (100)
Levels of CRP, mg/dl	1.81 (3.24)	3.40 (5.30)	1.54 (2.85)
Treatment naive, *n* (%)	16 (19)	16 (100)	0 (0)
Treatment with MTX, *n* (%)	41 (48)	0 (0)	10 (56)
Treatment with biologics, *n* (%)	19 (22)	0 (0)	5 (28)
TNF-α inhibitor	8 (9)	0 (0)	3 (17)
Tocilizumab	5 (6)	0 (0)	2 (11)
Abatacept	6 (7)	0 (0)	0 (0)

Abbreviations: RA Rheumatoid arthritis, *DAS28* Disease Activity Score in 28 joints, *CRP* C-reactive protein, *ESR* Erythrocyte sedimentation rate, *CDAI* Clinical Disease Activity Index, *CCP* Cyclic citrullinated peptide, *MTX* Methotrexate, *TNF* Tumor necrosis factor
Data are presented as mean (SD), unless otherwise specified

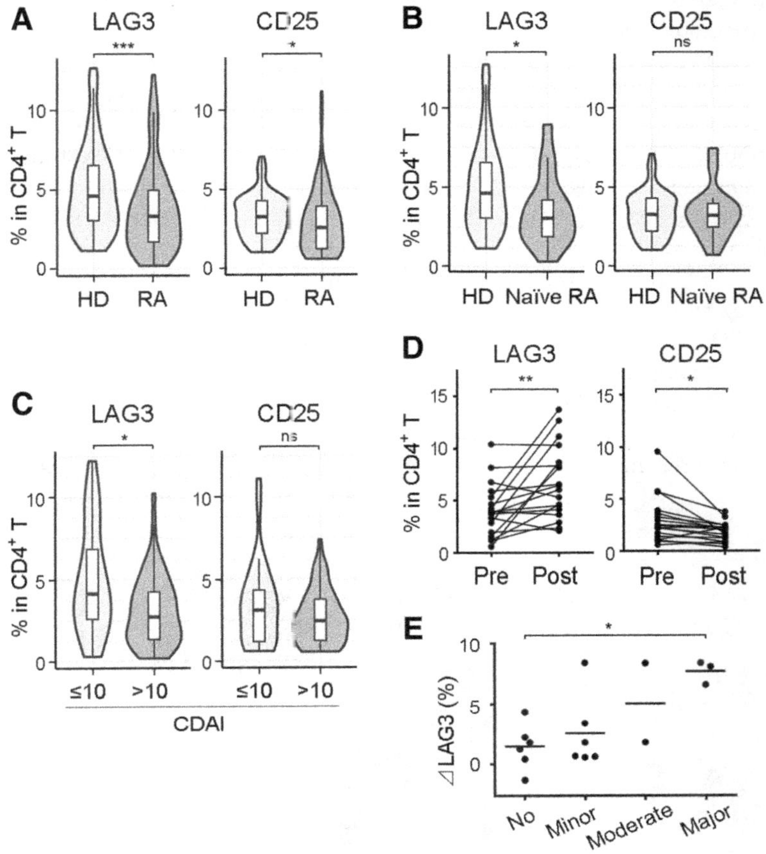

Fig. 3 Frequencies of LAG3$^+$ Tregs and CD25$^+$ Tregs in patients with RA and in healthy volunteers, as well as the effect of abatacept treatment. **a** and **b** PBMCs were taken from healthy donors (HD; $n = 101$) and patients with RA ($n = 85$, including 16 nontreated patients [naive RA]), and Treg subsets were assessed. **c** Patients with RA were divided into two groups according to Clinical Disease Activity Index (CDAI). Treg subsets were assessed (CDAI ≤10, $n = 30$; CDAI >10, $n = 55$). **d** Treg subsets were analyzed immediately before and 6 months after abatacept treatment ($n = 18$). **e** Changes of percentages of LAG3$^+$ Tregs in CD4$^+$ T cells (ΔLAG3) were evaluated in accordance with treatment response to abatacept ($n = 18$). No response was defined as less than 50% improvement from baseline CDAI. Minor response was defined as at least a 50% improvement from baseline CDAI. Moderate response was defined as at least a 70% improvement from baseline CDAI. Major response was defined as at least an 85% improvement from baseline CDAI. *, $P < 0.05$; **, $P < 0.01$; ***, $P < 0.001$. Statistics: (**a**–**c**) unpaired two-tailed Student's *t* tests, (**d**) Wilcoxon signed-rank test, (**e**) Kruskal-Wallis test and Dunn's multiple-comparisons test. *CD* Cluster of differentiation, *LAG3* Lymphocyte activation gene 3, *ns* Not significant, *PBMC* Peripheral blood mononuclear cell, *RA* Rheumatoid arthritis, *Treg* Regulatory T cell

between ACPA or rheumatoid factor (RF) titers and frequencies of CD25$^+$ Tregs or LAG3$^+$ Tregs (Additional file 1: Figure S4). To investigate the effect of RA treatment for LAG3$^+$ Tregs, we focused on patients undergoing treatment with abatacept (Table 1). Abatacept treatment significantly increased the frequency of LAG3$^+$ Tregs and significantly decreased the frequency of CD25$^+$ Tregs (Fig. 3d). Moreover, we divided abatacept-treated patients into four groups (no response, minor response, moderate response, and major response) following the definition of treatment response based on Clinical Disease Activity Index [25, 26]. We analyzed the correlation between treatment response and increase in LAG3$^+$ Tregs and found that LAG3$^+$ Tregs significantly increased in the patients with a major response to abatacept compared with the patients with no response (Fig. 3e). The same result was obtained from the analysis using the definition of treatment response based on Disease Activity Score in 28 joints based on erythrocyte sedimentation rate (Additional file 1: Figure S5). Taken together, LAG3$^+$ Tregs were present at a lower frequency in patients with RA than in healthy donors. Among patients with RA, the frequency of LAG3$^+$ Tregs was inversely correlated with disease activity. Moreover, abatacept increased the frequency of LAG3$^+$ Tregs in patients with RA.

Abatacept facilitates the differentiation of LAG3$^+$ Treg-like cells

Naive CD4$^+$ T cells from healthy donors were cultured in the absence or presence of abatacept with irradiated APCs and anti-CD3 antibody for 4 days. When naive CD4$^+$ T cells were cultured with abatacept, CD4$^+$CD25

$^{-}$LAG3^{+} T cells were more strongly induced than naive CD4^{+} T cells cultured without abatacept ($P < 0.0001$) (Fig. 4a). In contrast, the CD4^{+} T cells expressing CD25 decreased in the presence of abatacept (Fig. 4a). Moreover, the expression levels of *EGR2* and *FAS* were increased in the abatacept-treated group ($P < 0.01$) (Fig. 4b). The expression of *CD274* (programmed death-ligand 1 [*PD-L1*]) had a tendency to increase in the abatacept-treated group. Egr2 is a key transcription factor that regulates LAG3^{+} Tregs [21]. Both Fas [23] and PD-L1 [27] were reported to be involved in LAG3^{+} Treg suppression ability. Furthermore, abatacept-induced CD4^{+} T cells significantly suppressed antibody production compared with the positive control ($P < 0.0001$) (Fig. 4c). Taken together, these results indicated that abatacept facilitated the differentiation of Egr2-expressing LAG3^{+} Treg-like cells from naive CD4^{+} T cells.

Active immunization increases Th1 cells and decreases LAG3^{+} Tregs

At this point, it was possible that immunological stimulation in RA may have contributed to the decrease of LAG3^{+} Tregs. We addressed whether LAG3^{+} Tregs exhibited numerical alteration in response to active immunization. Vaccination triggers an immune response in human bodies, preparing Th1 cells and memory B cells to respond quickly to previously encountered antigens. To investigate whether LAG3^{+} Tregs were affected by an immune response against foreign antigens, we inoculated four healthy subjects with seasonal influenza vaccine, which is a hemagglutinin fraction of influenza virus mixed strains grown in fertilized chicken eggs without adjuvant, and evaluated T-cell subsets in PBMCs at days 0, 7, and 14. All four subjects showed an increase in the frequency of Th1 cells and a reciprocal decrease

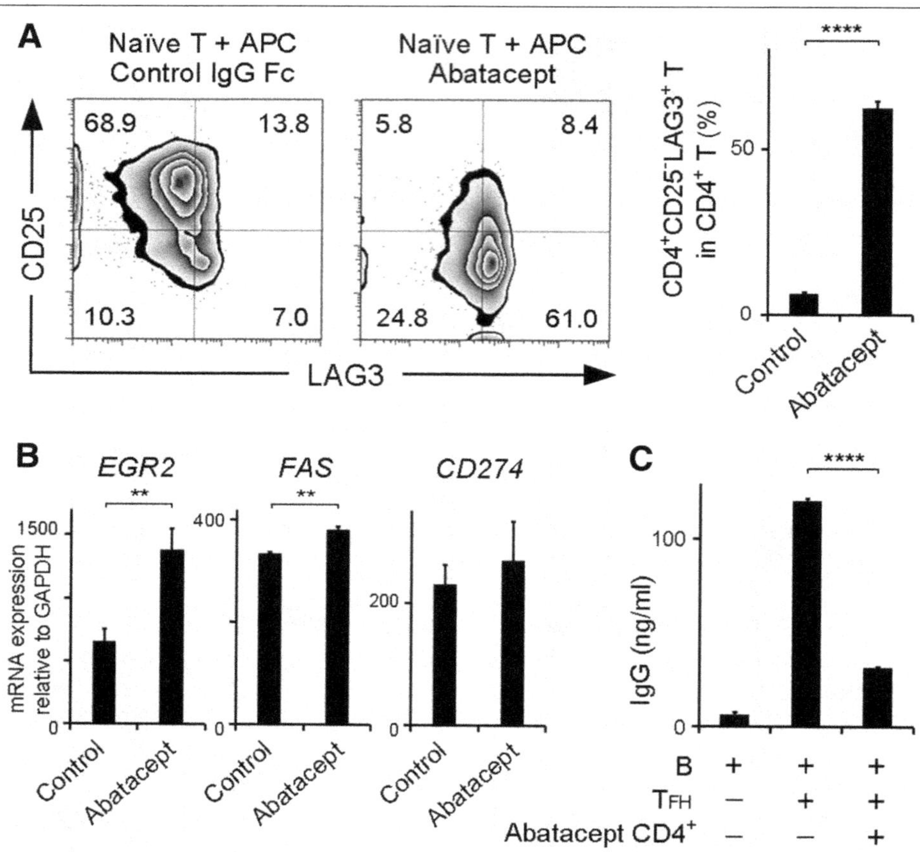

Fig. 4 Effect of abatacept on the CD4^{+}CD25^{-}LAG3^{+} T-cell subset in vitro. **a** Naive CD4^{+} T cells and antigen-presenting cells (APCs) taken from healthy donors were cultured with anti-CD3 antibody in the presence of abatacept, and FACS was conducted on day 4. Representative FACS data from three independent experiments are shown. Percentages of CD4^{+}CD25^{-}LAG3^{+} T cells in CD4^{+} T cells are presented in the bar graph ($n = 3$). **b** Quantitative real-time polymerase chain reaction analysis of *EGR2*, *FAS*, and *CD274* (*PDL1*) mRNA expression in the cells that were induced from naive CD4^{+} T cells in the presence of abatacept ($n = 3$). **c** Sorted 7-amino actinomycin D-negative CD4^{+} T cells were cultured with B cells and T_{FH} cells under staphylococcal enterotoxin B stimulation for 12 days, and total IgG production was determined by ELISA ($n = 3$). All error bars represent SD. ** $P < 0.001$; **** $P < 0.0001$. All *P* values were calculated by unpaired two-tailed Student's *t* test. *CD* Cluster of differentiation 4, *EGR2* Early growth response gene 2, *FACS* Fluorescence-activated cell sorting, *GAPDH* Glyceraldehyde 3-phosphate dehydrogenase, *IgG* Immunoglobulin G, *LAG3* Lymphocyte activation gene 3, *mRNA* Messenger RNA, *PDL1* Programmed death-ligand 1, T_{FH} Follicular helper T cell

in that of LAG3$^+$ Tregs at day 7. Both Th1 cells and LAG3$^+$ Tregs recovered their baseline percentages at day 14 (Fig. 5). In a former report, influenza vaccine administration did not influence the number of total CD4$^+$ CD25$^+$ T cells, and it was supposed that the response to vaccine depends on the activation of different subsets of CD4$^+$CD25$^+$ T cells [28]. Active immunization may reduce the frequency of LAG3$^+$ Tregs and increase that of Th1 cells to enhance immune responses.

Discussion

We detected the human counterpart of murine LAG3$^+$ Tregs [23] that produce high amounts of IL-10 and IFN-γ and strongly suppress B-cell antibody production. Although there are several reports stating that T cells suppress B-cell antibody production, most of them are related to CD25$^+$ Tregs [29–31]. We found that human LAG3$^+$ Tregs suppress B-cell antibody production more strongly than CD25$^+$ Tregs. On one hand, an experiment using Transwell plates revealed that cell-to-cell contact played a great role in B-cell suppression by LAG3$^+$ Tregs and that Fas–Fas ligand interaction might be involved in the mechanism. On the other hand, because LAG3$^+$ Tregs suppressed B-cell antibody production to a certain extent even if they were separated from B and T_{FH} cells, it is difficult to deny the effect of some cytokines. One possible cytokine is transforming growth factor (TGF)-β3 because it is highly expressed in human LAG3$^+$ Tregs, and murine LAG3$^+$ Tregs directly suppress B-cell activation through TGF-β3 [23].

Regardless of CD49b expression, LAG3$^+$ cells produced high amounts of IL-10 and suppressed B-cell antibody production, although Gagliani et al. concluded that coexpression of LAG3 and CD49b was necessary to identify human IL-10-producing T cells [22]. The difference may be due to the very low frequency of CD4$^+$ CD25$^-$LAG3$^+$CD49b$^+$ T cells observed in our study. Although the role of CD49b should be investigated further, our results confirmed that LAG3 is a unique marker for IL-10-producing CD4$^+$ T cells.

On one hand, in the patients with untreated RA, the frequency of CD25$^+$ Tregs was not different from that observed in healthy donors, consistent with previous reports [32–34]. On the other hand, the frequency of LAG3$^+$ Tregs was significantly lower in patients with RA than in healthy donors, and it was particularly low in patients with RA with higher disease activity. These results imply that LAG3$^+$ Tregs are involved in regulating the pathophysiology of RA. Among several possible mechanisms, one is suppression of B-cell functions. Autoreactive B cells not only produce autoantibody that can potentiate immune responses but also can directly interact with T cells by antigen presentation, leading to cytokine production and germinal center formation [1, 35]. A pathogenic role for B cells other than antibody production was confirmed by the efficacy of rituximab with limited reduction of ACPA titers in RA [36]. The other possibility is that LAG3$^+$ Tregs regulate RA via IL-10 production. IL-10-producing Tregs ameliorate collagen-induced arthritis in mice [37]. Moreover, Th17 cells play

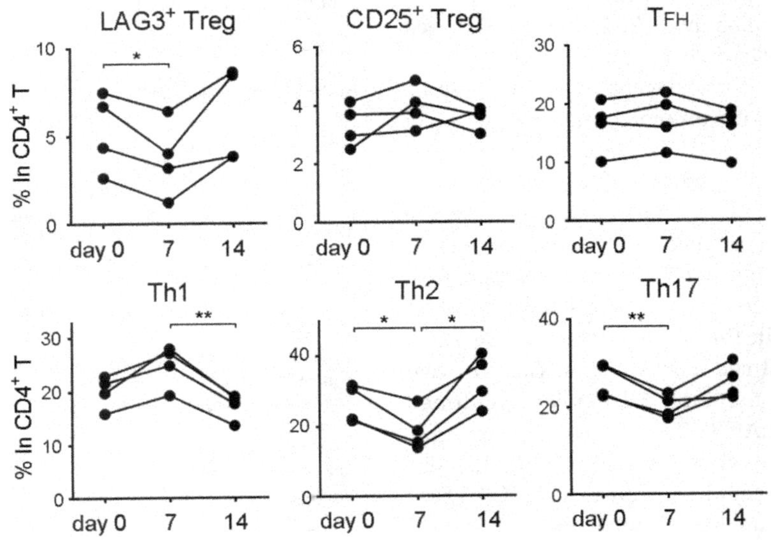

Fig. 5 Successive changes of CD4$^+$ T-cell subsets after vaccination. Four healthy donors were inoculated with influenza vaccine. The indicated T-cell subsets were evaluated on day 0 (before vaccination), day 7, and day 14. * $P < 0.05$; ** $P < 0.01$. *P* values were calculated by one-way analysis of variance and Tukey's multiple-comparisons test. *CD* Cluster of differentiation, *LAG3* Lymphocyte activation gene 3, *ns* Not significant, T_{FH} Follicular helper T cell, *Th* Helper T cell, *Treg* Regulatory T cell

crucial roles in the development of RA [38], and IL-10-producing Tregs control inflammation by Th17 cells in an IL-10-dependent manner [39].

Administration of the costimulatory inhibitor abatacept significantly increased the frequency of LAG3$^+$ Tregs in patients with RA. Moreover, naive CD4$^+$ T cells stimulated in the presence of abatacept developed into CD4$^+$ T cells with LAG3$^+$ Treg-like manifestations. Although it is difficult to confirm the relationship between abatacept and LAG3$^+$ Tregs, the expression of EGR2 strongly suggests the induction of LAG3$^+$ Treg-like cells. The transcription factor EGR2 is identified as a T-cell anergy-associated gene [24] that is induced by TCR stimulation in the absence of costimulation. Moreover, EGR2 is highly expressed in both murine and human LAG3$^+$ Tregs [21, 23]. Because abatacept binds to B7 molecules on APCs and inhibits T-cell costimulation [40], there is a possibility that abatacept enhances EGR2 expression by CD4$^+$ T cells and increases the number of LAG3$^+$ Tregs. Moreover, there was a significant increase in *FAS* expression and the tendency of *CD274* (*PDL1*) expression to increase in the abatacept-treated cells. Because Fas [23] and PD-L1 [27] were reported to play a role in the suppression ability of LAG3$^+$ Tregs, there is a possibility that abatacept-treated cells exert suppressive ability using FAS or PD-L1 in the same way as naturally occurring LAG3$^+$ Tregs.

Immunological stimulation such as autoimmunity and vaccination may reduce the number of LAG3$^+$ Tregs via costimulation. LAG3$^+$ Tregs could participate in the anti-inflammatory and immune-modulating effects achieved by a targeting therapy for costimulation. Actually, abatacept administration in patients with RA reduced the serum levels of immunoglobulins, ACPA, and RF as well as the percentage of postswitch memory B cells [41]. Increases in LAG3$^+$ Tregs by abatacept treatment may be associated with control of humoral immunity. The fact that abatacept induces a general decrease of CD25$^+$ Tregs is not consistent with the clinical efficacy of abatacept [42]. Increases of LAG3$^+$ Tregs may compensate for the reduction of CD25$^+$ Tregs in abatacept-treated patients.

With regard to the mechanisms of the suppressive ability of LAG3$^+$ Tregs, multiple systems have been reported to be involved. In the present study, we revealed the importance of cell-cell contact and Fas. In vivo experiments using Fas-mutant B6/*lpr* mice confirmed that Fas expressed on LAG3$^+$ Tregs plays a critical role in suppressing B-cell antibody production [23], and our results suggest that Fas could contribute to LAG3$^+$ Treg suppressive ability in humans. However, our Transwell experiment also suggested that soluble factors have some effect because LAG3$^+$ Treg suppression was still observed even if cell-to-cell contact was lost. One candidate is TGF-β3, which is highly expressed by both murine and human LAG3$^+$ Tregs [43]. In vivo experiments confirmed that TGF-β3 strongly ameliorates B-cell-mediated pathology [23] and that TGF-β3 suppresses human B-cell differentiation into plasmablasts and antibody secretion [44]. We suppose that multiple mechanisms, including soluble factors (IL-10, TGF-β3) and cell-to-cell contact (PD-L1 and Fas), work together in bringing about LAG3$^+$ Treg suppression.

In a previous report, Egr2-transduced LAG3$^+$ Treg-like CD4$^+$ T cells exhibited antigen-specific immunosuppressive capacity in vivo. On the basis of these findings, human LAG3$^+$ Tregs are supposed to be specific to self-antigens associated with autoimmune disease; however, proving antigen specificity in human Tregs is difficult and remains to be elucidated.

Collectively, the results of our study suggest that human IL-10-producing-LAG3$^+$ Tregs regulate immune responses related to the pathogenesis of RA. The induction of LAG3$^+$ Tregs by abatacept implies a previously unrecognized role of IL-10-producing Tregs in the mode of action of abatacept.

Conclusions

IL-10-producing LAG3$^+$ Tregs in human PBMCs suppress the antibody production of B cells independent of IL-10. The frequency of LAG3$^+$ Tregs is decreased in patients with RA and significantly increased with abatacept treatment. Abatacept-treated CD4$^+$ T cells exhibit LAG3$^+$ Treg-like function.

Additional file

Additional file 1: Supplementary methods and figures. **Figure S1** Expression of FOXP3 in LAG3$^+$ Tregs and CD25$^+$ Tregs. Freshly isolated human CD4$^+$ T cells were stained for FOXP3 and LAG3. Representative FACS data from three independent experiments are shown. **Figure S2** In vitro T-cell proliferation assay. Carboxyfluorescein succinimidyl ester-labeled naive T cells were cultured with irradiated APCs and CD25$^+$ Tregs for 72 h. Representative FACS data from three independent experiments are shown. **Figure S3** Frequencies of IL-10$^+$ cells in 7-AAD$^-$ cells detected in intracellular staining of naive CD4$^+$ T cells and LAG3$^+$ Tregs ($n = 4$). * $P < 0.05$ by Mann-Whitney *U* test. **Figure S4** Scatterplot of frequencies of CD25$^+$ Tregs or LAG3$^+$ Tregs vs ACPA titer or RF ($n = 83$). *P* value is for Spearman's rank correlation coefficient. *rho* Spearman's rho. Linear regression line is drawn as a *blue line*, and 95% CI region is presented as a *gray area*. **a** Scatterplot of frequencies of CD25$^+$ Tregs vs ACPA titer. **b** Scatterplot of frequencies of CD25$^+$ Tregs vs RF titer. **c** Scatterplot of frequencies of LAG3$^+$ Tregs vs ACPA titer. **d** Scatterplot of frequencies of LAG3$^+$ Tregs vs RF titer. **Figure S5** Changes in percentages of LAG3$^+$ Tregs in CD4$^+$ T cells (**Δ**LAG3) were evaluated in accordance with treatment response to abatacept ($n = 18$). Patients were divided into three groups (no response, moderate response, and good response) following European League Against Rheumatism response criteria based on DAS28-ESR. * $P < 0.05$ by Kruskal-Wallis test and Dunn's multiple-comparisons test. (ZIP 963 kb)

Abbreviations

7-AAD: 7-Amino actinomycin D; Ab: Antibody; ACPA: Anticitrullinated protein antibody; APC: Antigen-presenting cell; CCP: Cyclic citrullinated peptide; CCR6: C-C chemokine receptor type 6; CCR7: C-C chemokine receptor type 7; CD: Cluster of differentiation; CDAI: Clinical Disease Activity Index;

CRP: C-reactive protein; CXCR3: C-X-C chemokine receptor type 3; CXCR5: C-X-C chemokine receptor type 5; DAS28: Disease Activity Score in 28 joints; Egr2: Early growth response gene 2; ELISA: Enzyme-linked immunosorbent assay; ESR: Erythrocyte sedimentation rate; FACS: Fluorescence-activated cell sorting; FasL: Fas ligand; Foxp3: Forkhead box P3; *GAPDH*: Glyceraldehyde 3-phosphate dehydrogenase; HD: Healthy donor; IFN-γ: Interferon-γ; Ig: Immunoglobulin; IL: Interleukin; LAG3: Lymphocyte activation gene 3; mAb: Monoclonal antibody; mRNA: Messenger RNA; MTX: Methotrexate; PBMC: Peripheral blood mononuclear cell; PCR: Polymerase chain reaction; PD-L1: Programmed death-ligand 1; PE: Phycoerythrin; PerCP: Peridinin-chlorophyll protein; RA: Rheumatoid arthritis; RF: Rheumatoid factor; RPMI: Roswell Park Memorial Institute medium; SEB: Staphylococcal enterotoxin B; TCR: T-cell receptor; T_{FH}: Follicular helper T cell; TGF-β: Transforming growth factor-β; Th1: Type 1 helper T cell; Th17: T helper 17 cell; TNF-α: Tumor necrosis factor-α; Treg: Regulatory T cell

Acknowledgements
We thank the patients and healthy volunteers who participated in this research. We thank K. Watada, J. Takezawa, A. Inoue, and M. Anraku for their excellent technical assistance. We thank K. Kubo, H. Harada, M. Shibuya, Y. Iwasaki, K. Michishita, T. Eri, Y. Seri, and M. Ohshima for their help in collecting patients' data.

Funding
This work was supported by the Ministry of Health, Labour and Welfare, Ministry of Education, Culture, Sports, Science and Technology under a Grant-in-Aid for Scientific Research (KAKENHI) (S) (23229007), a Grant-in-Aid for challenging Exploratory Research (25670459), and a Grant-in-Aid for Young Scientists (B) (15 K19566) from the Japan Society for the Promotion of Science. Part of this work was supported by a grant from Bristol-Myers Squibb (BMKK130307).

Authors' contributions
SN, SS, YT, HT, MK, RK, TO, KY, and KF conceived of, designed, and analyzed the experiments and contributed to writing the manuscript. SN, SS, and KF carried out all experiments. KS, NH, YN, ST, and HK helped with obtaining human samples and clinical data. All authors read and approved the final manuscript.

Competing interests
KY received financial support or fees from AbbVie, Astellas Pharma, Bristol-Myers Squibb, Daiichi-Sankyo, MitsubishiTanabe Pharma, Pfizer, Sanofi, Santen, Takeda, Teijin, Boehringer Ingelheim, Chugai, Eisai, Ono, Taisho Toyama, UCB, ImmunoFuture, Asahi Kasei, and Janssen. KF received financial support or fees from Astellas Pharma, Bristol-Myers Squibb, Daiichi-Sankyo, MitsubishiTanabe Pharma, Pfizer, Santen, Takeda, Chugai, Eisai, Taisho Toyama, UCB, and Janssen. SS received financial support or fees from AbbVie, Eisai, Chugai, Takeda, Bristol-Myers Squibb, and UCB. All other authors declare that they have no competing interests.

Author details
[1]Department of Allergy and Rheumatology, Graduate School of Medicine, the University of Tokyo, 7-3-1 Hongo, Bunkyo-ku, Tokyo 113-8655, Japan. [2]Department of Immunotherapy Management, Graduate School of Medicine, the University of Tokyo, 7-3-1 Hongo, Bunkyo-ku, Tokyo 113-8655, Japan. [3]Max Planck-The University of Tokyo Center for Integrative Inflammology, The University of Tokyo, 4-6-1 Komaba, Meguro-ku, Tokyo 153-8505, Japan.

References
1. Smolen JS, Aletaha D, Redlich K. The pathogenesis of rheumatoid arthritis: new insights from old clinical data? Nat Rev Rheumatol. 2012;8:235–43.
2. McInnes IB, Schett G. The pathogenesis of rheumatoid arthritis. N Engl J Med. 2011;365:2205–19.
3. Esensten JH, Wofsy D, Bluestone JA. Regulatory T cells as therapeutic targets in rheumatoid arthritis. Nat Rev Rheumatol. 2009;5:560–5.
4. Roncarolo MG, Battaglia M. Regulatory T-cell immunotherapy for tolerance to self antigens and alloantigens in humans. Nat Rev Immunol. 2007;7:585–98.
5. Sakaguchi S, Yamaguchi T, Nomura T, Ono M. Regulatory T cells and immune tolerance. Cell. 2008;133:775–87.
6. Sakaguchi S, Sakaguchi N, Asano M, Itoh M, Toda M. Immunologic self-tolerance maintained by activated T cells expressing IL-2 receptor α-chains (CD25): breakdown of a single mechanism of self-tolerance causes various autoimmune diseases. J Immunol. 1995;155:1151–64.
7. Groux H, O'Garra A, Bigler M, Rouleau M, Antonenko S, de Vries JE, et al. A $CD4^+$ T-cell subset inhibits antigen-specific T-cell responses and prevents colitis. Nature. 1997;389:737–42.
8. Linterman MA, Pierson W, Lee SK, Kallies A, Kawamoto S, Rayner TF, et al. $Foxp3^+$ follicular regulatory T cells control the germinal center response. Nat Med. 2011;17:975–82.
9. Lim HW, Hillsamer P, Banham AH, Kim CH. Cutting edge: direct suppression of B cells by $CD4^+CD25^+$ regulatory T cells. J Immunol. 2005;175:4180–3.
10. Kim HJ, Verbinnen B, Tang X, Lu L, Cantor H. Inhibition of follicular T-helper cells by $CD8^+$ regulatory T cells is essential for self tolerance. Nature. 2010;467:328–32.
11. Hori S, Nomura T, Sakaguchi S. Control of regulatory T cell development by the transcription factor Foxp3. Science. 2003;299:1057–61.
12. Brunkow ME, Jeffery EW, Hjerrild KA, Paeper B, Clark LB, Yasayko SA, et al. Disruption of a new forkhead/winged-helix protein, scurfin, results in the fatal lymphoproliferative disorder of the scurfy mouse. Nat Genet. 2001;27:68–73.
13. Chen Z, Benoist C, Mathis D. How defects in central tolerance impinge on a deficiency in regulatory T cells. Proc Natl Acad Sci U S A. 2005;102:14735–40.
14. Fujio K, Okamura T, Yamamoto K. The family of IL-10-secreting $CD4^+$ T cells. Adv Immunol. 2010;105:99–130.
15. Fitzgerald DC, Zhang GX, El-Behi M, Fonseca-Kelly Z, Li H, Yu S, et al. Suppression of autoimmune inflammation of the central nervous system by interleukin 10 secreted by interleukin 27-stimulated T cells. Nat Immunol. 2007;8:1372–9.
16. Barrat FJ, Cua DJ, Boonstra A, Richards DF, Crain C, Savelkoul HF, et al. In vitro generation of interleukin 10-producing regulatory $CD4^+$ T cells is induced by immunosuppressive drugs and inhibited by T helper type 1 (Th1)- and Th2-inducing cytokines. J Exp Med. 2002;195:603–16.
17. Kemper C, Chan AC, Green JM, Brett KA, Murphy KM, Atkinson JP. Activation of human $CD4^+$ cells with CD3 and CD46 induces a T-regulatory cell 1 phenotype. Nature. 2003;421:388–92.
18. Battaglia M, Stabilini A, Draghici E, Gregori S, Mocchetti C, Bonifacio E, et al. Rapamycin and interleukin-10 treatment induces T regulatory type 1 cells that mediate antigen-specific transplantation tolerance. Diabetes. 2006;55:40–9.
19. Awasthi A, Carrier Y, Peron JP, Bettelli E, Kamanaka M, Flavell RA, et al. A dominant function for interleukin 27 in generating interleukin 10-producing anti-inflammatory T cells. Nat Immunol. 2007;8:1380–9.
20. Apetoh L, Quintana FJ, Pot C, Joller N, Xiao S, Kumar D, et al. The aryl hydrocarbon receptor interacts with c-Maf to promote the differentiation of type 1 regulatory T cells induced by IL-27. Nat Immunol. 2010;11:854–61.
21. Okamura T, Fujio K, Shibuya M, Sumitomo S, Shoda H, Sakaguchi S, Yamamoto K. $CD4^+CD25^-LAG3^+$ regulatory T cells controlled by the transcription factor Egr-2. Proc Natl Acad Sci U S A. 2009;106:13974–9.
22. Gagliani N, Magnani CF, Huber S, Gianolini ME, Pala M, Licona-Limon P, et al. Coexpression of CD49b and LAG-3 identifies human and mouse T regulatory type 1 cells. Nat Med. 2013;19:739–46.
23. Okamura T, Sumitomo S, Morita K, Iwasaki Y, Inoue M, Nakachi S, et al. TGF-β3-expressing $CD4^+CD25^-LAG3^+$ regulatory T cells control humoral immune responses. Nat Commun. 2015;6:6329.
24. Safford M, Collins S, Lutz MA, Allen A, Huang CT, Kowalski J, et al. Egr-2 and Egr-3 are negative regulators of T cell activation. Nat Immunol. 2005;6:472–80.
25. Aletaha D, Martinez-Avila J, Kvien TK, Smolen JS. Definition of treatment response in rheumatoid arthritis based on the simplified and the clinical disease activity index. Ann Rheum Dis. 2012;71:1190–6.
26. Smolen JS, Aletaha D. Scores for all seasons: SDAI and CDAI. Clin Exp Rheumatol. 2014;32(5 Suppl 85):S75–9.
27. Sumitomo S, Nakachi S, Okamura T, Tsuchida Y, Kato R, Shoda H, et al. Identification of tonsillar $CD4^+CD25^-LAG3^+$ T cells as naturally occurring IL-10-producing regulatory T cells in human lymphoid tissue. J Autoimmun. 2017;76:75–84.
28. Del Porto F, Lagana B, Biselli R, Donatelli I, Campitelli L, Nisini R, et al. Influenza vaccine administration in patients with systemic lupus

erythematosus and rheumatoid arthritis: safety and immunogenicity. Vaccine. 2006;24:3217–23.

29. Gotot J, Gottschalk C, Leopold S, Knolle PA, Yagita H, Kurts C, et al. Regulatory T cells use programmed death 1 ligands to directly suppress autoreactive B cells in vivo. Proc Natl Acad Sci U S A. 2012;109:10468–73.
30. Iikuni N, Lourenco EV, Hahn BH, La Cava A. Cutting edge: regulatory T cells directly suppress B cells in systemic lupus erythematosus. J Immunol. 2009;183:1518–22.
31. Zhao DM, Thornton AM, DiPaolo RJ, Shevach EM. Activated $CD4^+CD25^+$ T cells selectively kill B lymphocytes. Blood. 2006;107:3925–32.
32. Mottonen M, Heikkinen J, Mustonen L, Isomaki P, Luukkainen R, Lassila O. $CD4^+CD25^+$ T cells with the phenotypic and functional characteristics of regulatory T cells are enriched in the synovial fluid of patients with rheumatoid arthritis. Clin Exp Immunol. 2005;140:360–7.
33. Ehrenstein MR, Evans JG, Singh A, Moore S, Warnes G, Isenberg DA, et al. Compromised function of regulatory T cells in rheumatoid arthritis and reversal by anti-TNFα therapy. J Exp Med. 2004;200:277–85.
34. Cao D, Malmstrom V, Baecher-Allan C, Hafler D, Klareskog L, Trollmo C. Isolation and functional characterization of regulatory $CD25^{bright}CD4^+$ T cells from the target organ of patients with rheumatoid arthritis. Eur J Immunol. 2003;33:215–23.
35. Byng-Maddick R, Ehrenstein MR. The impact of biological therapy on regulatory T cells in rheumatoid arthritis. Rheumatology (Oxford). 2015;54:768–75.
36. Edwards JC, Szczepanski L, Szechinski J, Filipowicz-Sosnowska A, Emery P, Close DR, et al. Efficacy of B-cell-targeted therapy with rituximab in patients with rheumatoid arthritis. N Engl J Med. 2004;350:2572–81.
37. Asnagli H, Martire D, Belmonte N, Quentin J, Bastian H, Boucard-Jourdin M, et al. Type 1 regulatory T cells specific for collagen type II as an efficient cell-based therapy in arthritis. Arthritis Res Ther. 2014;16:R115.
38. Leipe J, Grunke M, Dechant C, Reindl C, Kerzendorf U, Schulze-Koops H, et al. Role of Th17 cells in human autoimmune arthritis. Arthritis Rheum. 2010;62:2876–85.
39. Huber S, Gagliani N, Esplugues E, O'Connor Jr W, Huber FJ, Chaudhry A, et al. Th17 cells express interleukin-10 receptor and are controlled by $Foxp3^-$ and $Foxp3^+$ regulatory $CD4^+$ T cells in an interleukin-10-dependent manner. Immunity. 2011;34:554–65.
40. Fiocco U, Sfriso P, Oliviero F, Pagnin E, Scagliori E, Campana C, et al. Co-stimulatory modulation in rheumatoid arthritis: the role of (CTLA4-Ig) abatacept. Autoimmun Rev. 2008;8:76–82.
41. Scarsi M, Paolini L, Ricotta D, Pedrini A, Piantoni S, Caimi L, et al. Abatacept reduces levels of switched memory B cells, autoantibodies, and immunoglobulins in patients with rheumatoid arthritis. J Rheumatol. 2014;41:666–72.
42. Pieper J, Herrath J, Raghavan S, Muhammad K, Vollenhoven R, Malmstrom V. CTLA4-Ig (abatacept) therapy modulates T cell effector functions in autoantibody-positive rheumatoid arthritis patients. BMC Immunol. 2013;14:34.
43. Morita K, Okamura T, Inoue M, Komai T, Teruya S, Iwasaki Y, et al. Egr2 and Egr3 in regulatory T cells cooperatively control systemic autoimmunity through Ltbp3-mediated TGF-β3 production. Proc Natl Acad Sci U S A. 2016;113:E8131–40.
44. Tsuchida Y, Sumitomo S, Ishigaki K, Suzuki A, Kochi Y, Tsuchiya H, et al. TGF-β3 inhibits antibody production by human B cells. PLoS One. 2017;12, e0169646.

14

Ultrasonography and magnetic resonance imaging changes in patients with polymyalgia rheumatica treated by tocilizumab

Anaïs Huwart[1,5*], Florent Garrigues[1], Sandrine Jousse-Joulin[2,3], Thierry Marhadour[2], Dewi Guellec[2], Divi Cornec[2], Maelenn Gouillou[4], Alain Saraux[2,3] and Valérie Devauchelle-Pensec[2,3]

Abstract

Background: This study assessed inflammatory changes using ultrasound (US) and magnetic resonance imaging (MRI) in patients taking tocilizumab for polymyalgia rheumatica (PMR).

Methods: Eighteen patients were included in the prospective open-label TENOR study and received three tocilizumab infusions, without corticosteroids. B-mode and power Doppler US and MRI (T1 and T2-short time inversion recuperation weighted sequences) of the hips and shoulders were performed at weeks 0, 2, and 12. Subacromial, trochanteric, and iliopsoas bursitis and intraarticular glenohumeral and coxofemoral effusions/synovitis were scored from 0 to 3. Changes over time and US–MRI correlations were evaluated.

Results: At baseline, the proportions of shoulders and hips with bursitis were 93 and 100% by MRI and 61 and 13% by US; and the corresponding proportions for intraarticular effusions/synovitis were 100 and 100% by MRI and 57 and 53% by US. Imaging findings did not improve during the first two treatment weeks. From baseline to week 12, bursitis improved significantly at all four joints by MRI ($P = 0.005$) and US ($P = 0.029$) and intraarticular effusions/synovitis by US only ($P = 0.001$). The proportion of abnormalities that improved by week 12 was 42% by MRI and 37% by US. MRI detected bursitis in a larger proportion of hips (73% versus 13%) and US in a larger proportion of shoulders (57% versus 28%), whereas no difference was found for intraarticular effusions/synovitis. At baseline, agreement between US and MRI findings was poor.

Conclusions: US and MRI showed significant improvements in inflammatory lesions during tocilizumab treatment of PMR.

Keywords: Polymyalgia rheumatica, Magnetic resonance imaging, Ultrasonography, Tocilizumab

Background

Polymyalgia rheumatica (PMR) is an inflammatory condition of unknown origin affecting people aged 50 years or older [1]. The main symptoms are inflammatory pain and prolonged morning stiffness of the shoulder and/or pelvic girdles [2]. Laboratory tests show severe systemic inflammation, and systemic corticosteroid therapy is rapidly effective [3–5].

Corticosteroids, however, induce numerous adverse events [6]. Tocilizumab (TCZ) is a humanized monoclonal antibody whose ability to block the IL-6 receptor inhibits the proinflammatory pathway. TCZ holds promise for the treatment of PMR [7–9].

Magnetic resonance imaging (MRI) and ultrasonography (US) are the main imaging techniques for detecting inflammation in and about the proximal joints [10–12] and, consequently, play a major role in evaluating PMR [13]. Subacromial-subdeltoid (SASD) bursitis, although not specific, is the imaging hallmark of PMR [14–16]. Hip joint bursitis and synovitis may explain the hip girdle symptoms experienced by patients with PMR [10, 17].

* Correspondence: Anais.huwart@gmail.com
[1]Radiology Department, Cavale Blanche Hospital and Brest Occidentale University, Brest, France
[5]Radiology Unit, Hôpital de Cornouaille, 14 avenue Yves Thépot, F 29000 Quimper, France
Full list of author information is available at the end of the article

Another sign of proximal joint inflammation described in PMR is the presence of effusions in the glenohumeral and coxofemoral joints.

The follow-up of patients with PMR relies chiefly on serial determinations of the clinical PMR activity score (PMR-AS) and on laboratory markers for inflammation (C-reactive protein (CRP) and erythrocyte sedimentation rate) [18]. MRI and US are useful, however, to assess the treatment response. Both TCZ and corticosteroids effectively suppress the inflammatory process and would therefore be expected to normalize joint imaging findings. Studies using MRI [4, 16] and US [10, 19] found improvements during corticosteroid therapy. No similar studies are available with TCZ. Furthermore, the level of agreement between MRI and US findings is unknown.

We reported recently that TCZ monotherapy was effective in recent-onset PMR [20]. In 20 patients, the PMR-AS consistently fell below 10 by week 12, and no relapses occurred during follow-up (24 weeks). Similar results were obtained with a TCZ–corticosteroid combination [21]. The effect of treatment on MRI and US signs of inflammation was not assessed in these studies.

Here, our primary objective was to assess MRI and US changes during TCZ monotherapy for recent-onset PMR. Bursitis was assessed at the subacromial, trochanteric, and iliopsoas sites and intraarticular effusion/synovitis at the glenohumeral and coxofemoral joints. Our secondary objective was to assess agreement between MRI and US findings at baseline.

Methods

Patients

We conducted a prospective, cross-sectional, multicenter study in patients with PMR included in the TENOR study (Tocilizumab Effect iN pOlymyalgia Rheumatica) [20] (ClinicalTrials.gov NCT01713842) between September 2012 and May 2014. As described previously, TENOR was a double-blind study of TCZ, without corticosteroids, used to treat recent-onset active PMR. All patients met Chuang et al.'s criteria for PMR [22]. TCZ therapy was considered effective if 75% of patients had PMR-AS ≤ 10 by week 12. Three TCZ infusions were given, at weeks 0, 4, and 8. At one of the study centers (Brest), US and MRI of the shoulders and hips were performed at weeks 0, 2, and 12, using a standardized protocol. These imaging data form the basis for the study reported here.

Imaging procedure

US was performed using an ESAOTE MyLab™ 60 machine (Esaote Medical, Saint-Germain-en-Laye, France) with an LA 523 4-13 MHz probe. B-mode and power Doppler were performed at each site. Bursitis was assessed at the SASD, trochanteric, and iliopsoas sites. The glenohumeral and coxofemoral joints were evaluated for synovitis and intraarticular effusion. Tenosynovitis of the long head of the biceps was sought. US abnormalities by B-mode or power Doppler imaging were graded using the OMERACT [23] semi-quantitative scale (0, no abnormalities; 1, mild; 2, moderate; and 3, marked) [24].

MRI was performed using a Philips Achieva 3 T machine (update dStream; Philips, Amsterdam, the Netherlands) with a 32-channel surface antenna. The following sequences were acquired at the shoulder and hip girdles: axial T1 turbo spin echo (T1 TSE), axial T2 short time inversion recuperation (T2 STIR), and coronal T2 STIR. For the T1 TSE sequence, the matrix was 828 × 420 and the field of view 53 × 32 cm at the shoulders; corresponding values were 720 × 404 and 46 × 31 cm, respectively, at the hips. Repetition time was 659 ms, echo time 20 ms, and slice thickness 4 mm. Fifty images were acquired in each plane. For the T2 STIR sequence at the shoulder, the matrix was 328 × 382 in the coronal plane and 524 × 210 in the axial plane; corresponding values at the hip were 356 × 420 and 468 × 264, respectively. Fields of view were 32 × 48 cm and 47 × 28 cm for coronal and axial imaging of the shoulder, respectively; corresponding values at the hip were 35 × 52 cm and 46 × 35 cm, respectively. Repetition and echo times at the shoulder were 4828 ms and 65 ms in the coronal plane and 2721 ms and 75 ms in the axial plane, respectively; corresponding values at the hip were 4979 ms and 60 ms in the coronal plane and 4677 ms and 65 ms in the axial plan. In the coronal plane, 22 slices were obtained with a thickness of 5 mm at the shoulders and 24 slices with a slice thickness of 4 mm at the hips. In the axial plane, 50 slices 4 mm in thickness were acquired at all sites.

Bursitis was defined as a high T2 signal and was assessed at the same three sites investigated by US. Effusion was also defined as a high T2 signal and was assessed at the glenohumeral joint, bicipital groove, and coxofemoral joint. For practical reasons, MRI was performed without contrast injection and a high T2 signal could therefore indicate synovitis and/or effusion. Abnormalities were scored using the already described OMERACT [23] semi-quantitative 0–3 scale (Fig. 1) [12, 16, 25, 26].

Image analysis

US images were performed by two experienced observers (TM and SJ-J) specialized in osteoarticular US. MRIs were read by a senior radiologist (FG). All observers were blinded to patient data, and the MRI images for a given patient were read together but in random order. Before the study, intraobserver reliability was assessed by having the senior radiologist read 40 MRIs twice at an interval of 1 month. The kappa coefficient was 0.85 (0.72; 0.97).

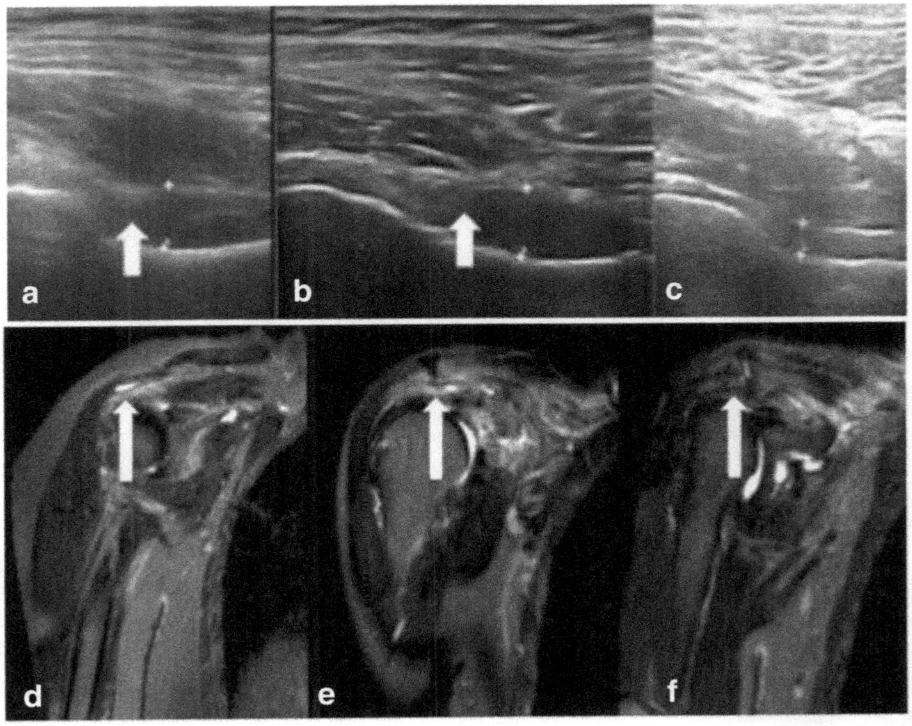

Fig. 1 Improvements in ultrasound (US) and magnetic resonance imaging (MRI) abnormalities during tocilizumab therapy. (**1**) US: coxofemoral effusion at baseline (**a**), week 2 (**b**), and week 12 (**c**). Synovitis with synovial hypertrophy (arrows) scored 3 at baseline, 2 at week 2, and 0 at week 12. (**2**) MRI: subacromial bursitis at baseline (**d**, score = 3), week 2 (**e**, score = 2), and week 12 (**f**, score = 0)

The reference for imaging abnormalities was considered at joint level.

Statistical analysis

Continuous variables were described as median and interquartile range (IQR) and categorical variables as n (%). Values at two time points were compared by applying the Wilcoxon signed-rank test for paired data. To evaluate sensitivity to change, we considered the sums of the two shoulder scores, of the two hip scores, and of the scores at both shoulders and hips.

Agreement between US and MRI findings at baseline was evaluated by computing Cohen's kappa coefficient. Kappa values were interpreted as follows: < 0, no agreement; < 0.20, slight agreement; 0.21–0.40, fair agreement; 0.41–0.60, moderate agreement; 0.61–0.80, substantial agreement; and 0.81–1.00, almost perfect agreement.

Results

Setting and participants

Eighteen patients were included at the Brest center, seven women and 11 men, with a mean age of 71 years (range 58–83 years) and a mean body mass index of 28 ± 1 kg/m^2. Mean serum CRP was 82 ± 16 mg/L (range 12–251) at baseline and 3 ± 2 mg/L (range 0.2–25.9) at week 12; corresponding values for the mean pain visual analog scale (VAS) score were 6.0 ± 0.5 (range 2.8–9.3) and 2.2 ± 0.4 (range 0.1–7.0). At baseline, 16 (89%) patients had shoulder-girdle pain and 16 (89%) had hip-girdle pain; corresponding numbers at week 12 were five (28%) and three (17%) patients, respectively. Mean PMR-AS was 38 ± 2 at baseline and 7 ± 1 at week 12. All patients improved clinically and achieved the TENOR end point of PMR-AS ≤ 10 by week 12.

US and MRI evaluation

Technical problems precluded MRI in three patients. Another patient had MRI of the hips but not at the shoulders, due to severe pain. This left 28 shoulders and 30 hips with US and MRI data at baseline and at week 12 (Table 1). Bursitis defined as a score ≥ 1 was identified by MRI at the shoulders in 26 joints (93%) and at the hips in 30 joints (100%). Bursitis was less often detected by US, particularly at the hips (four joints, 13%). MRI was also more sensitive for detecting joint effusion/synovitis defined as a score ≥ 1 at both the shoulders and the hips. When bursitis or effusion/synovitis was defined as a score ≥ 2, the proportion of patients with the abnormality was smaller, but MRI remained more sensitive than US.

Sensitivity to change

Figure 2 and Table 2 report the changes in the median US and MRI scores with TCZ therapy. The only

Table 1 Percentage of patients with abnormalities by MRI and US at baseline and at week 12

			Abnormality defined as a score[a] ≥ 1		Abnormality defined as a score[a] ≥ 2	
			Bursitis[b]	Effusion/synovitis[c]	Bursitis[b]	Effusion/synovitis[c]
Inclusion	MRI	Shoulders	93% (26/28)	100% (28/28)	64% (18/28)	71% (20/28)
		Hips	100% (30/30)	100% (30/30)	80% (24/30)	67% (20/30)
	US	Shoulders	61% (17/28)	57% (16/28)	21% (6/28)	21% (6/28)
		Hips	13% (4/30)	53% (16/30)	3% (1/30)	30% (9/30)
Week 12	MRI	Shoulders	93% (26/28)	100% (28/28)	46% (13/28)	64% (18/28)
		Hips	80% (24/30)	100% (30/30)	23% (7/30)	47% (14/30)
	US	Shoulders	36% (10/28)	50% (14/28)	0% (0/28)	18% (5/28)
		Hips	10% (3/30)	30% (9/30)	3% (1/30)	3% (1/30)

MRI magnetic resonance imaging *US* ultrasonography
[a]OMERACT Outcome Measures in Rheumatology score on a 0–3 scale, where 0 is normal
[b]Bursitis: subacromial bursitis at the shoulders and trochanteric and iliopsoas bursitis at the hips
[c]Shoulders: glenohumeral joint and long head of biceps; hips: coxofemoral joints

significant improvement from baseline to week 2 was for bursitis by MRI. In contrast, significant improvements occurred from baseline to week 12 for US bursitis ($P = 0.029$), US effusions ($P = 0.001$), and MRI bursitis ($P = 0.005$). Effusion/synovitis by MRI did not improve significantly from baseline to week 12 ($P = 0.231$). Improvements in SASD bursitis were better shown by US than by MRI.

Changes in severity of imaging study abnormalities during TCZ therapy

Table 3 presents the proportions of US and MRI abnormalities whose score improved by at least 1 point from baseline to week 12. Overall, improvement ≥ 1 point occurred for 43/116 (37%) US abnormalities and 49/116 (42%) MRI abnormalities. The score remained unchanged for 59/116 (51%) US abnormalities and 58/116 (50%) MRI abnormalities. Worsening was uncommon, both for bursitis (5% by MRI and 17.5% by US) and for effusion/synovitis (10% by MRI and 7% by US). Improvements in hip bursitis were more often detected by MRI (22/30, 73%) than by US (4/30, 13%). At the shoulders, in contrast, improvements in bursitis were detected more often by US (16/28, 57%) than by MRI (8/28, 29%).

Table 4 presents the proportions of US and MRI abnormalities that resolved fully; that is, whose score fell from ≥ 2 at baseline to ≤ 1 at week 12. The proportion of abnormalities that resolved was larger by US than by MRI.

MRI–US agreement at baseline

Agreement was first studied with abnormalities defined as a score ≥ 1 by MRI, B-mode US, or power Doppler US (Table 5). Then, because MRI proved highly sensitive for detecting small abnormalities, we repeated the assessment using scores ≥ 2 by MRI and ≥ 1 by B-mode or power Doppler US. Agreement was slight at the hips but substantial at the shoulders.

Discussion

This is the first study of US and MRI changes in patients given TCZ without corticosteroids to treat recent-onset PMR. TCZ is being evaluated as a promising treatment for PMR. Using 18 F-FDG positron emission tomography–computed tomography, we demonstrated

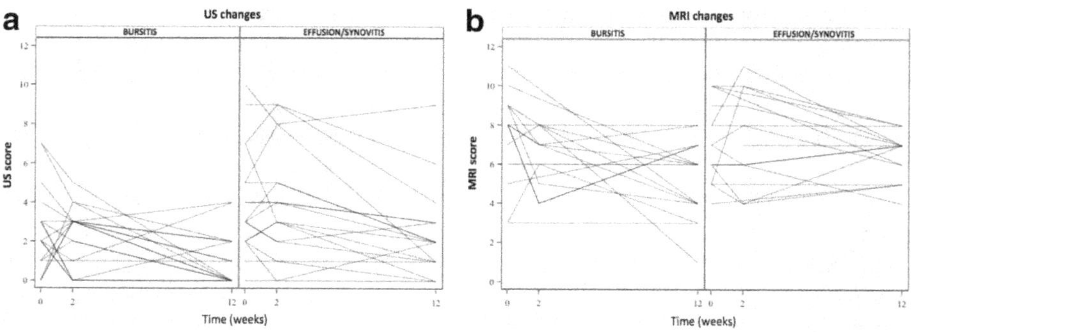

Fig. 2 Changes in median ultrasound (US) and magnetic resonance imaging (MRI) scores during tocilizumab therapy. The bursitis and effusion/synovitis scores were computed by summing the scores for both shoulders and both hips. **a** MRI: bursitis (left) and effusion/synovitis (right). **b** US: bursitis (left) and effusion/synovitis (right). Individual patients are shown

Table 2 MRI and US findings at baseline and 2 and 12 weeks after starting tocilizumab therapy

	Week 0	Week 2	Week 12	Wilcoxon test *P* value	
				Week 0 vs week 2	Week 0 vs week 12
MRI (all four joints)					
Bursitis	8 (6–9)	7 (5–8)	6 (4–7)	0.109	0.005*
Effusion/synovitis	7 (5–9)	7 (6–9)	7 (5.5–7)	0.719	0.231
MRI (both shoulders)					
Bursitis	4 (2–4)	4 (3–4)	3.5 (2–4)	1.000	0.406
Effusion/synovitis	4 (3–5)	4 (3–5)	3.5 (3–4)	0.625	0.176
MRI (both hips)					
Bursitis	4 (3–6)	3 (2–4)	2 (1.5–3)	0.031*	< 0.001*
Effusion/synovitis	4 (2–4)	4 (3–4)	3 (2–4)	1.000	0.117
US (all four joints)					
Bursitis	2 (1–3)	3 (1–3)	0.5 (0–2)	0.575	0.029*
Effusion/synovitis	3 (2–5)	3.5 (2–5)	2 (1–3)	1.000	0.001*
US (both shoulders)					
Bursitis	2 (1–3)	2 (0–3)	0.5 (0–1)	0.542	0.018*
Effusion/synovitis	2 (1–3)	2.5 (1–4)	1 (1–2)	0.781	0.059
US (both hips)					
Bursitis	0 (0–1)	0 (0–0)	0 (0–0)	1.000	0.625
Effusion/synovitis	2 (0–3)	1 (0–2)	0 (0–2)	0.560	0.002*

Data are median (interquartile range)
MRI magnetic resonance imaging *US* ultrasonography
*Significant differences, Wilcoxon signed-rank test ($P < 0.05$)

Table 3 Changes in severity of ultrasound (US) and magnetic resonance imaging (MRI) abnormalities from baseline to week 12

		Hips	Shoulders	Four joints
Bursitis[a]				
US	Improvement	13% (4/30)	57% (16/28)	34% (20/58)
	No change	77% (23/30)	18% (5/28)	48% (28/58)
	Worsening	10% (3/30)	25% (7/28)	17% (10/58)
MRI	Improvement	73% (22/30)	29% (8/28)	52% (30/58)
	No change	27% (8/30)	61% (17/28)	43% (25/58)
	Worsening	0% (0/30)	11% (3/28)	5% (3/58)
Effusion/synovitis[b]				
US	Improvement	47% (14/30)	32% (9/28)	40% (23/58)
	No change	50% (15/30)	57% (16/28)	53% (31/58)
	Worsening	3% (1/30)	11% (3/28)	7% (4/58)
MRI	Improvement	33% (10/30)	32% (9/28)	32% (19/58)
	No change	57% (17/30)	57% (16/28)	57% (33/58)
	Worsening	10% (3/30)	11% (3/28)	10% (6/58)

[a]Bursitis: subacromial bursitis at the shoulders and trochanteric and iliopsoas bursitis at the hips
[b]Shoulders: glenohumeral joint and long head of biceps; hips: coxofemoral joints

previously a significant but moderate decrease in the maximal standardized uptake value after 12 weeks of TCZ therapy [27].

In this study, patients underwent US and MRI at baseline and then 2 and 12 weeks into TCZ therapy. At baseline, MRI proved highly sensitive for detecting inflammatory lesions at the shoulders and hips. Thus, most patients had shoulder inflammation and all had hip inflammation. However, the clinical relevance of the

Table 4 Number of findings of bursitis and effusion/synovitis, defined as a score[a] ≥ 2, at baseline and at week 12, and percentages of abnormalities whose scores fell below 2 between baseline and week 12

		Baseline	Week 12	Grade < 2
MRI	Four joints	82/116	45/82	45% (37/82)
	Bursitis[b]	42/58	17/42	60% (25/42)
	Effusion/synovitis[c]	40/58	28/40	30% (12/40)
US	Four joints	24/116	5/24	71% (17/24)
	Bursitis[b]	9/58	0/9	100% (9/9)
	Effusion/synovitis[c]	15/58	5/15	67% (10/15)

MRI magnetic resonance imaging *US* ultrasonography
[a]OMERACT Outcome Measures in Rheumatology score on a 0–3 scale, where 0 is normal
[b]Bursitis: subacromial bursitis at the shoulders and trochanteric and iliopsoas bursitis at the hips
[c]Shoulders: glenohumeral joint and long head of biceps; hips: coxofemoral joints

Table 5 Agreement (kappa coefficient) between ultrasonography (US) and magnetic resonance imaging (MRI) at baseline

US/MRI	Bursitis[a]	Effusion/synovitis[b]	Bursitis[a]	Effusion/synovitis[b]
Right hip	0.03 (−0.04; 0.11)	0.31 (−0.002; 0.62)	0.12 (−0.05; 0.29)	0.29 (−0.21; 0.78)
Left hip	0	0.16 (−0.22; 0.54)	0.03 (−0.04; 0.11)	0.09 (−0.37; 0.55)
Right shoulder	0.28 (−0.04; 0.11)	0.20 (−0.05; 0.45)	0.19 (−0.23; 0.61)	0.51 (0.04; 0.99)
Left shoulder	−0.08 (−0.52; 0.37)	0.20 (−0.05; 0.45)	−0.40 (−0.74; −0.06)	**0.70** (0.32; 1)
Both hips	0.02 (−0.02; 0.05)	0.23 (−0.01; 0.42)	0.07 (−0.01; 0.16)	0.18 (−0.16; 0.52)
Both shoulders	0.11 (−0.16; 0.38)	0.20 (0.02; 0.37)	−0.14 (−0.50; 0.22)	**0.61** (0.30; 0.91)
Four joints	0.02 (−0.01; 0.15)	0.21 (0.06; 0.37)	−0.07 (−0.28; 0.13)	0.38 (0.15; 0.62)

Two left-hand columns: MRI and US abnormalities defined as a score ≥ 1. Two right-hand columns: MRI abnormalities defined as a score ≥ 2 and US abnormalities as a score ≥ 1

[a]Bursitis: subacromial bursitis at the shoulders and trochanteric and iliopsoas bursitis at the hips

[b]Shoulders: glenohumeral joint and long head of biceps; hips: coxofemoral joints

minimal abnormalities that can be detected by MRI deserves discussion. High sensitivity may explain the persistence of effusions/synovitis after TCZ therapy by MRI but not by US. The US technique was less sensitive than MRI, showing SASD bursitis in 61% and hip bursitis in 13% of patients. Although SASD bursitis is recognized as a good diagnostic criterion for PMR [3], its frequency is controversial. Previous US studies found SASD in only18% [10] and 10% [28] of patients, in part because some patients were treated during the study and in part because US lacks sensitivity for detecting deep or thin abnormalities. In a previous study, of 57 untreated patients, 55 had abnormalities by US [12]. Finally, in a study of 50 patients with new-onset PMR, synovitis and/or effusion was consistently found in at least one joint [24].

Except for hip bursitis, the imaging study abnormalities failed to improve during the first 2 weeks of TCZ therapy. In rheumatoid arthritis, in contrast, early improvements have been reported with TCZ. However, in our study, TCZ was used alone, without corticosteroids, and at week 2 the patients had received a single infusion. A different treatment protocol might induce earlier improvements. Another possible explanation is that the inflammatory lesions in PMR may take time to respond to treatment. By week 12, the US and MRI abnormalities were significantly improved, in keeping with results in RA [29]. Thus, US and/or MRI may deserve consideration for objectively assessing the treatment response to 12 weeks of TCZ therapy. The serum CRP level is not a good monitoring tool, as it declines dramatically due to the mechanism of action of TCZ [30].

MRI and US proved sensitive to change during TCZ therapy for PMR. Nevertheless, the imaging study findings remained unchanged in a substantial proportion of patients, despite clinical improvements. Thus, the imaging study abnormalities may improve more slowly than the clinical manifestations. If imaging studies are used for follow-up, their timing should be given careful consideration. In a prospective 12-week study of 53 patients given corticosteroids to treat PMR, US was as sensitive, or more sensitive, to change compared to the clinical and laboratory markers of disease activity [19]. In a small minority of patients, the US and MRI findings worsened, despite clinical improvements. Worsening of imaging study findings may be related to intercurrent events (e.g., osteoarthritis flares) or may indicate limited reproducibility of image acquisition or interpretation.

At baseline, there was little agreement between US and MRI. Many patients had numerous inflammatory lesions by MRI but not by US. We therefore evaluated agreement between the two methods using a score ≥ 2 to define MRI abnormalities and a score ≥ 1 to define US abnormalities. In this analysis, agreement was substantial to nearly perfect (kappa = 0.61; 0.30–0.91) at the shoulders and poor at the hips. This difference is consistent with the larger number of US abnormalities detected at the shoulders than at the hips, which is probably due to the deeper position and, consequently, decreased accessibility of hip structures.

The main limitation of our study is its low statistical power due to the small sample size. We included patients enrolled at only one of the centers participating in a small, proof-of-concept study. Moreover, given the absence of a placebo arm, changes due to TCZ therapy cannot be differentiated from those due to the natural course of PMR. For practical reasons, the US studies were performed by two sonographers, but both were highly experienced and used to working together. TCZ is an emerging treatment for PMR, and our study provides the first data about its effects on imaging study abnormalities. Moreover, most of the earlier studies of imaging in PMR assessed MRI or US but not both [19, 31].

So, regarding our results, MRI could be useful in PMR for patients with atypical symptoms due to the high frequency of hip and shoulder abnormalities revealed by this procedure. Imaging can help to follow patients with residual pain after treatment.

Conclusion

In patients given TCZ to treat recent-onset PMR, MRI and US showed improvements in bursitis and in effusions/synovitis in a substantial proportion of patients. These improvements were significant by week 12. In many patients, however, the imaging study abnormalities remained unchanged despite clinical improvements. US may be a good imaging technique for assessing the treatment response in PMR because it can show a complete regression of the lesions and also as it is noninvasive and widely available.

Abbreviations

18 F-FDG: Fluorodeoxyglucose; 3 T: 3 Tesla; CRP: C-reactive protein; IQR: Interquartile range; MRI: Magnetic resonance imaging; PMR: Polymyalgia rheumatica; PMR-AS: Polymyalgia rheumatica activity score; SASD: Subacromial-subdeltoid; STIR: Short time inversion recuperation; TCZ: Tocilizumab; TENOR: Tocilizumab Effect iN pOlymyalgia Rheumatica; TSE: Turbo spin echo; US: Ultrasonography

Acknowledgements

The authors thank the rheumatologists and general practitioners who referred their patients to the TENOR study. They are grateful to Marie Jezequel and Nathalie Bihannic (CIC) for centralizing the material and to Audrey Le Goff-Coquet and Valentine Guiton (DRCI). The authors also thank the staff for their time and commitment to this work.

Funding

Roche-Chugai provided an unconditional grant for the study and donated the Tocilizumab. Roche-Chugai had no role in the design or conduct of the study; data collection, analysis, or interpretation; or preparation, revision, or approval of the manuscript.

Authors' contributions

VD-P, AS, FG, and AH made substantial contributions to the conception and design of the study. FG, TM, SJ-J, and AH made substantial contributions to the acquisition of data. MG and AH analyzed and interpreted the patient data. VD-P and AH were the major contributors to writing of the manuscript. DG, DC, VD-P, AS, TM, SJ-J, MG, and FG helped to revise the manuscript. All authors read and approved the final manuscript.

Authors' information

Not applicable.

Competing interests

The authors declare that they have no competing interests.

Author details

[1]Radiology Department, Cavale Blanche Hospital and Brest Occidentale University, Brest, France. [2]Rheumatology Department, Cavale Blanche Hospital and Brest Occidentale University, Brest, France. [3]INSERM UMR 1227, Laboratoire d'Immunothérapie et Pathologies lymphocytaires B, Labex "Immunotherapy, Graft, Oncology", Brest Occidentale University, 29609 Brest Cedex, France. [4]Clinical Investigation Centre (CIC) 1412, Institut National de la Santé et de la Recherche Médicale (INSERM), Brest, France. [5]Radiology Unit, Hôpital de Cornouaille, 14 avenue Yves Thépot, F 29000 Quimper, France.

References

1. Kermani TA, Warrington KJ. Polymyalgia rheumatica. Lancet. 2013;331(9860):63–72. https://doi.org/10.1016/S0140-6736(12)60680-1.
2. Muller S, Hider SL, Helliwell T, et al. Characterising those with incident polymyalgia rheumatica in primary care: results from the PMR Cohort Study. Arthritis Res Ther. 2016;18(1):200. https://doi.org/10.1186/s13075-016-1097-8.
3. Dasgupta B, Salvarani C, Schirmer M, et al. Developing classification criteria for polymyalgia rheumatica: comparison of views from an expert panel and wider survey. J Rheumatol. 2008;35:270–77.
4. Salvarani C, Cantini F, Olivieri I, Barozzi L, Macchioni L, Boiardi L, Niccoli L, Padula A, Pulsatelli LMR. Corticosteroid injections in polymyalgia rheumatica: a double-blind, prospective, randomized, placebo controlled study. J Rheumatol. 2000;27(6):1470–6.
5. Hernández-Rodríguez J1, Cid MC, López-Soto A, et al. Treatment of polymyalgia rheumatica: a systematic review. Arch Intern Med. 2009; 169(20):1839–50. https://doi.org/10.1001/archinternmed.2009.352.
6. Li CDB. Corticosteroids in polymyalgia rheumatica—a review of different treatment schedules. Clin Exp Rheumatol. 2000;18(4 Suppl 20):S56–7.
7. Macchioni P, Boiardi L, Catanoso M, et al. Tocilizumab for polymyalgia rheumatica: report of two cases and review of the literature. Semin Arthritis Rheum. 2013;43(1):113–8. https://doi.org/10.1016/j.semarthrit.2013.01.003.
8. Izumi K, Kuda H, Ushikubo M, Kuwana M, Takeuchi T, Oshima H. Tocilizumab is effective against polymyalgia rheumatica: experience in 13 intractable cases. RMD Open. 2015;1(1):e000162. https://doi.org/10.1136/rmdopen-2015-000162.
9. Devauchelle-Pensec V. Has the time come for biotherapies in giant cell arteritis and polymyalgia rheumatica? Joint Bone Spine. 2016;83(5):471.
10. Koski JM. Ultrasonographic evidence of synovitis in axial joints in patients with polymyalgia rheumatica. Br J Rheumatol. 1992;31(3):201–3.
11. Pavlica P, Barozzi L, Salvarani C, Cantini FOI. Magnetic resonance imaging in the diagnosis of PMR. Clin Exp Rheumatol. 2000;18(4 Suppl 20):S38–9.
12. Cantini F, Salvarani C, Olivieri I, et al. Shoulder ultrasonography in the diagnosis of polymyalgia rheumatica: a case-control study. J Rheumatol. 2001;28(5):1049–55.
13. Macchioni P, Boiardi L, Catanoso M, Pazzola G, Salvarani C. Performance of the new 2012 EULAR/ACR classification criteria for polymyalgia rheumatica: comparison with the previous criteria in a single-centre study. Ann Rheum Dis. 2014;73(6):1190–3. https://doi.org/10.1136/annrheumdis-2013-204167.
14. Mackie SL, Koduri G, Hill CL, et al. Accuracy of musculoskeletal imaging for the diagnosis of polymyalgia rheumatica: systematic review. RMD Open. 2015;1(1):e000100. https://doi.org/10.1136/rmdopen-2015-000100.
15. Zaccaria A, Latinakis G, Oliveri M, Maio T, Frisone G, Versace F. The support of the ultrasonography of the shoulder in the diagnosis of polymyalgia rheumatica with normal erythrocyte sedimentation rate. Reumatismo. 2009;61(4):290–7.
16. Salvarani C, Cantini F, Olivieri I, Barozzi L, Macchioni L, Niccoli L, Padula A, De Matteis MPP. Proximal bursitis in active polymyalgia rheumatica. Ann Intern Med. 1997;127(1):27–31.
17. O'Duffy JD, Wahner HWHG. Joint imaging in polymyalgia rheumatica. Mayo Clin Proc. 1976;51(8):519–24.
18. Salvarani C, Cantini F, Boiardi L, Hunder GG. Polymyalgia rheumatica. Best Pract Res Clin Rheumatol. 2004;18(5):705–22. https://doi.org/10.1016/j.berh.2004.06.003.
19. Jiménez-Palop M, Naredo E, Humbrado L, et al. Ultrasonographic monitoring of response to therapy in polymyalgia rheumatica. Ann Rheum Dis. 2010;69(5):879–82. https://doi.org/10.1136/ard.2009.113555.
20. Devauchelle-Pensec V, Berthelot JM, Cornec D, et al. Efficacy of first-line tocilizumab therapy in early polymyalgia rheumatica: a prospective longitudinal study. Ann Rheum Dis. 2016;75(8):1506–10. https://doi.org/10.1136/annrheumdis-2015-208742.
21. Lally L, Forbess L, Hatzis C, Spiera R. Brief Report: A prospective open-label phase IIa trial of tocilizumab in the treatment of polymyalgia rheumatica. Arthritis Rheumatol. 2016;68(10):2550–4.
22. Chuang T, Hunder G, Ilstrup D. Polymyalgia rheumatica: a 10-year epidemiologic and clinical study. Ann Intern Med. 1982;97:672–80.
23. Boers M, Kirwan JR, Wells G, et al. Developing core outcome measurement sets for clinical trials: OMERACT filter 2.0. J Clin Epidemiol. 2014;67(7):745–53. https://doi.org/10.1016/j.jclinepi.2013.11.013.
24. Frediani B, Falsetti P, Storri L, et al. Evidence for synovitis in active polymyalgia rheumatica: sonographic study in a large series of patients. J Rheumatol. 2002;29(1):123–30.
25. Cantini F, Niccoli L, Nannini C, et al. Inflammatory changes of hip synovial structures in polymyalgia rheumatica. Clin Exp Rheumatol. 2005;23(4):462–8.
26. Salvarani C, Barozzi L, Cantini F, Niccoli L, Boiardi L, Valentino M, Pipitone N, Bajocchi G, Macchioni P, Catanoso MG, Olivieri GGHI. Cervical interspinous bursitis in active polymyalgia rheumatica. Clin Exp Rheumatol. 2013;31(4):526–31. https://doi.org/10.1136/ard.2007.084723.

27. Palard-Novello X, Querellou S, Gouillou M, et al. Value of 18 F-FDG PET/CT for therapeutic assessment of patients with polymyalgia rheumatica receiving tocilizumab as first-line treatment. Eur J Nucl Med Mol Imaging. 2016;43(4):773–9. https://doi.org/10.1007/s00259-015-3287-z.
28. Coari G, Paoletti FIA. Shoulder involvement in rheumatic diseases. Sonographic findings. J Rheumatol. 1999;26(3):668–73.
29. Grosse U, Henes J, Grozinger G, et al. Anatomic-functional (perfusion-based) magnetic resonance imaging follow-up in patients with rheumatoid arthritis treated with anti-interleukin 6 antibodies: a comparison with clinical scores and serologic data. J Comput Assist Tomogr. 2015;39(1):75–82. https://doi.org/10.1097/RCT.0000000000000152.
30. Kneepkens EL, van den Oever I, Plasencia CH, Pascual-Salcedo D, de Vries A, Hart M, Nurmohamed MT, Balsa A, Rispens T WG. Serum tocilizumab trough concentration can be used to monitor systemic IL-6 receptor blockade in pat. Scand J Rheumatol. 2017;46(2):87–94. https://doi.org/10.1080/03009742.2016.1183039.
31. Ochi J, Nozaki T, Okada M, et al. MR findings of the shoulder and hip joint in patients with polymyalgia rheumatica. Mod Rheumatol. 2015;7595(5):1–37. https://doi.org/10.3109/14397595.2015.1008725.

Effect of filgotinib, a selective JAK 1 inhibitor, with and without methotrexate in patients with rheumatoid arthritis: patient-reported outcomes

Mark Genovese[1,5*], Rene Westhovens[2], Luc Meuleners[3], Annegret Van der Aa[3], Pille Harrison[3], Chantal Tasset[3] and Arthur Kavanaugh[4]

Abstract

Background: The aim was to assess patient-reported outcomes (PROs) in patients with rheumatoid arthritis (RA) treated with filgotinib during two phase 2b, 24-week, randomized, placebo-controlled studies.

Methods: Patients with moderate-to-severe active RA and an inadequate response to methotrexate (MTX) were randomized to daily placebo or filgotinib 50 mg, 100 mg, or 200 mg as add-on therapy to MTX (NCT01888874) or as monotherapy (NCT01894516). At week 12, nonresponders receiving filgotinib 50 mg in both studies or placebo in the add-on study, and all patients receiving placebo as monotherapy, were re-assigned to filgotinib 100 mg. PROs were measured using the Health Assessment Questionnaire - Disability Index (HAQ-DI) including Patient Pain assessed by visual analog scale, and the Patient Global Assessment of Disease Activity (Patient Global), the Functional Assessment of Chronic Illness Therapy (FACIT)-Fatigue Scale (Version 4), and the 36-Item Short Form Health Survey (SF-36).

Results: At week 12, improvements in all PROs, apart from the SF-36 mental component in the add-on study, were statistically better with filgotinib than placebo; some improvements were noted as early as the first assessment time point (week 1 or week 4). Filgotinib improved HAQ-DI by 0.58–0.84 points, FACIT-Fatigue by 6.9–11.4 points, Patient Global by 25.2–35.6 mm, and Pain by 24.2–37.9 mm; scores were maintained or improved to week 24. Across all PROs, more patients achieved minimal clinically important differences and normative values with filgotinib 200 mg than placebo. Patients re-assigned to filgotinib 100 mg at week 12 experienced improvements in PROs between weeks 12 to 24.

Conclusions: Filgotinib as MTX add-on therapy or as monotherapy demonstrated rapid and sustained (to 24 weeks) improvements in health-related quality of life and functional status in patients with active RA.

Keywords: Rheumatoid Arthritis, Filgotinib, Patient-Reported Outcome Measures, JAK inhibitor

* Correspondence: genovese@stanford.edu
[1]Division of Immunology and Rheumatology, Stanford School of Medicine, Stanford, CA, USA
[5]Division of Immunology and Rheumatology, Stanford School of Medicine, 1000 Welch RD #203, Palo Alto, CA 94304, USA
Full list of author information is available at the end of the article

Background

Rheumatoid arthritis (RA) is a chronic, inflammatory disease, characterized by painful, swollen joints during periods of active inflammation [1]. With suboptimum management, joint damage may occur, leading to loss of function and disability, accompanied by systemic features such as anemia and weight loss during periods of disease activity [2, 3]. The clinical manifestations of RA challenge patients' coping skills: quality of life (QoL) can become severely impaired both in terms of physical and mental health [3, 4]. Although therapeutic advances have been made over recent decades, patients still face serious challenges: side effects occur and treatment responses may be slow, incomplete, and unsustained.

Janus kinase (JAK) inhibitors offer promise as targeted synthetic disease-modifying antirheumatic drugs (tsDMARDs) by blocking JAK-mediated signaling pathways that are implicated in the pathology of RA [5–8]. Filgotinib (GLPG0634/GS-6034) is an oral, selective inhibitor of JAK1, based on both biochemical and whole-blood assays [9, 10].

Two 24-week, placebo-controlled, phase 2b studies demonstrated that filgotinib was well-tolerated and efficacious in treating the signs and symptoms of RA in patients with moderate-to-severe active RA and an inadequate response to methotrexate (MTX) [11, 12]. The DARWIN 1 study evaluated filgotinib as add-on therapy to MTX and the DARWIN 2 study assessed filgotinib as monotherapy. In both studies, significantly more patients achieved the primary endpoint, an American College of Rheumatology (ACR)20 response, after 12 weeks of treatment with filgotinib 200 mg or 100 mg (or with 50 mg in the monotherapy study) versus placebo, and responses were maintained or improved until the end of the 24-week treatment period. Importantly, ACR20 responses were achieved quickly – by 2 weeks for the higher doses [11, 12].

Patient-reported outcomes (PROs) provide insight into patient QoL and the impact of disease on functional capacity – they are important assessors of the value of new therapeutics for RA, alongside evaluations of clinical effects and safety. Both clinical studies measured PROs as prespecified secondary endpoints to ascertain the effect of filgotinib on health-related QoL (HRQoL). Here, we report in detail the findings from PROs measured in both the MTX add-on (DARWIN 1) and monotherapy (DARWIN 2) studies, including the speed of response, whether responses were clinically meaningful, the proportion of patients who achieved normalized PRO scores, and the influence of clinical response on PROs.

Methods

Full methods have been published previously [11, 12]. In brief, both studies were 24-week, multicenter, randomized, double-blind, placebo-controlled, phase 2b, dose-finding studies of oral filgotinib.

Study design and treatments

In the MTX add-on study (ClinicalTrials.gov identifier NCT01888874), filgotinib was administered orally in combination with a stable dose of MTX. Patients were randomized to receive placebo or one of three daily doses of filgotinib – 50 mg, 100 mg, or 200 mg – either once daily (q.d.) or as 25-mg, 50-mg, or 100-mg doses twice daily (b.i.d.), in a 1:1:1:1:1:1:1 ratio. In the monotherapy study (NCT01894516), patients were randomized to receive placebo or one of three filgotinib daily doses (50 mg, 100 mg, or 200 mg q.d.), in a 1:1:1:1 ratio. In both studies, randomization was stratified by geographical region and previous use of biologic DMARDs (bDMARDs) (to which < 10% of the total study population had been previously exposed).

At week 12, patients were assessed for response, defined as a 20% improvement in swollen joint count (SJC) based on 66 joints and tender joint count (TJC) based on 68 joints. Nonresponders in the placebo, 25 mg b.i.d., and 50 mg q.d. groups of the MTX add-on study were reassigned to the filgotinib 100 mg q.d. or 50-mg b.i.d. groups. In the monotherapy study, all patients in the placebo group and nonresponders in the filgotinib 50-mg q.d. group were reassigned to the filgotinib 100-mg q.d. group (Additional file 1: Figure S1). Responders continued in their allocated treatment group for the remainder of the study.

Written approval was obtained before initiation of the study from the Medical Ethical Committee of University Hospitals KU Leuven (reference ML9437; study site of the Principal Investigator for the DARWIN 1 study) and the University of California San Diego Human Research Protections Program (reference 140642; study site of the Principal Investigator for the DARWIN 2 study), and from the appropriate independent ethics committee or institutional review board for each of the 106 study centers in the DARWIN 1 and 59 study centers in the DARWIN 2 studies (Additional file 2: Document 1 and Additional file 3: Document 2, respectively). Both studies were conducted in accordance with the ethical principles of the Declaration of Helsinki, International Council on Harmonisation good clinical practice guidelines, and all applicable national and local laws and regulatory requirements. All patients provided written, informed consent prior to study participation.

Patients

In both studies, enrolled patients were ≥ 18 years of age with a diagnosis of RA for ≥ 6 months prior to screening, met the 2010 ACR/European League Against Rheumatism criteria for RA and ACR functional classes

I–III, had ≥ 6/66 SJC and ≥ 8/68 TJC and a screening serum C-reactive protein ≥ 0.7 times the upper limit of the laboratory normal range. Patients receiving oral glucocorticoids (≤ 10 mg/day) or nonsteroidal anti-inflammatory drugs had to be on a stable dose for ≥ 4 and ≥ 2 weeks, respectively, before baseline.

In the MTX add-on study, patients had been receiving MTX for ≥ 6 months and were on a stable dose (15–25 mg/week, oral or parenteral) 4 weeks before screening. In the monotherapy study, patients had shown an inadequate response to MTX (in the opinion of the treating physician) and were washed out from MTX at least 4 weeks prior to baseline.

Outcomes and assessments

PROs were measured using the Health Assessment Questionnaire-Disability Index (HAQ-DI), including Patient Pain assessed on a visual analog scale (VAS) [13], Patient Global Assessment of Disease Activity (Patient Global) VAS [14], Functional Assessment of Chronic Illness Therapy (FACIT)-Fatigue Scale (Version 4), and 36-Item Short Form Health Survey (SF-36) [15, 16]. The three constituent PROs of the ACR response criteria, HAQ-DI, Patient Global and Patient Pain, were measured at baseline (day − 1) and at weeks 1, 2, 4, 8, 12, 16, 20, and 24. Two additional PRO measures, the FACIT-Fatigue Scale and SF-36, were measured at baseline and at weeks 4, 12, and 24. Changes from baseline in PRO parameters were examined, along with active group versus placebo comparisons. Minimal clinically important differences (MCIDs) were assessed as change from baseline, defined as a 0.22-point decrease on a scale of 0–3 for HAQ-DI scores [17], a 10-mm decrease on a scale of 0–100 mm for Patient Pain and Patient Global [18], a 4-point increase on a scale of 0–52 in FACIT-Fatigue score, [19] and a 2.5-point increase on a scale of 0–100 for SF-36 physical component summary (PCS) and mental component summary (MCS) scores [17]. At week 12, the proportions of patients who reached normalized PRO values were measured for HAQ-DI, FACIT-Fatigue, and PCS and MCS, based on normative values ≤0.5 for HAQ-DI (minimal disease activity) [20], ≥40 for FACIT-Fatigue [21], and ≥50 for PCS and MCS scores [22, 23]. The PRO instruments, MCIDs and normalized values used in this study are summarized in Additional file 4: Table S1.

Sample sizes and statistical analyses

All randomized patients who received at least one dose of study drug were included in the intent-to-treat (ITT) population. Patients who switched treatments at week 12 were handled as discontinuations and data were imputed from week 12 onwards. Missing data were accounted for using a last observation carried forward computation. Between-group comparisons were done for each filgotinib dose group versus the placebo group. Hommel's closed testing correction procedure was applied to adjust for multiplicity. Corrected p values <0.05 were considered indicative of a statistically significant comparison.

MCIDs and normative analyses were exploratory and were not tested for significance. Similarly, this study was not powered for any formal comparisons among the dose groups, or between the q.d. and b.i.d. regimens, which were examined in an exploratory fashion via a model containing both variables. No adjustment for multiplicity was made for these exploratory comparisons.

Results

Patient characteristics

A total of 594 patients in the MTX add-on study and 283 patients in the monotherapy study received at least one dose of study drug and were included in the ITT population. Additional file 1: Figure S1A and B illustrate patient flow through the studies.

Baseline patient demographics and disease characteristics by treatment group for both studies have been reported previously and were similar between the two overall study populations (Additional file 4: Table S2) and were balanced between the treatment groups within each study [11, 12].

Scores for PROs at baseline indicated a population with a high disease burden in line with moderate-to-severe RA activity scores; levels of disability reported were similar across the treatment groups in both studies (Table 1).

HAQ-DI

Changes from baseline in the HAQ-DI have been reported previously [11, 12]. To recapitulate, all treatment groups in both studies had a reduction in HAQ-DI scores over the course of the study (Table 2). At week 24 in the MTX add-on study, scores were better improved in the filgotinib-100 mg and 200-mg groups than in the placebo group (decrease of 0.66–0.90 points vs 0.37 points, respectively; $p < 0.01$). At week 12 in the monotherapy study, scores showed better improvement in the filgotinib 50-mg, 100-mg, and 200-mg groups than in the placebo group (decrease of 0.66 to 0.74 points vs 0.23 points, respectively; $p < 0.001$).

Patient Global

In both studies, all treatment groups had a reduction in Patient Global scores over the 24-week period (Fig. 1a, b and Table 2). In the MTX add-on study, at week 24, scores had decreased by 17.9 mm in the placebo group and by 27.3–39.1 mm in the filgotinib groups. A statistically significantly greater improvement in Patient Global

Table 1 Patient-reported outcomes at baseline (ITT populations)

	Methotrexate add-on study							Monotherapy study				
	Placebo (*N* = 86)	50 mg q.d. (*N* = 82)	100 mg q.d. (*N* = 85)	200 mg q.d. (*N* = 86)	25 mg b.i.d. (*N* = 86)	50 mg b.i.d. (*N* = 85)	100 mg b.i.d. (*N* = 84)	Placebo (*N* = 72)	50 mg q.d. (*N* = 72)	100 mg q.d. (N = 70)	200 mg q.d. (*N* = 69)	Score interpretation
HAQ-DI, mean (SE)	1.69 (0.06)	1.71 (0.07)	1.70 (0.07)	1.76 (0.06)	1.70 (0.05)	1.78 (0.06)	1.78 (0.07)	1.80 (0.06)	1.84 (0.07)	1.80 (0.07)	1.79 (0.06)	0–3; higher score indicates higher disability
Patient Global, mean (SE)	64.2 (1.96)	68.2 (2.23)	67.6 (2.09)	68.7 (2.09)	64.3 (1.95)	65.7 (1.92)	66.6 (2.20)	71.1 (2.02)	68.6 (2.41)	71.5 (2.23)	68.9 (2.07)	VAS score 0–100; higher score indicates lower health state
Patient Pain, mean (SE)	65.7 (2.16)	66.9 (2.20)	65.4 (2.41)	67.0 (2.16)	65.7 (2.23)	67.8 (2.12)	67.2 (2.19)	71.6 (2.37)	71.0 (2.38)	72.6 (1.85)	68.1 (2.35)	VAS score 0–100; higher score indicates more severe pain
FACIT-Fatigue, mean (SE)	26.2 (1.09)	26.2 (1.10)	26.6 (1.06)	25.2 (1.25)	28.1 (1.18)	26.2 (1.04)	25.6 (1.25)	25.1 (1.12)	25.1 (1.28)	24.8 (1.13)	24.8 (1.16)	0–52; higher score indicates better QoL
SF-36 PCS, mean (SE)	33.0 (0.71)	32.7 (0.75)	31.6 (0.79)	31.6 (0.64)	31.6 (0.69)	31.3 (0.73)	32.2 (0.78)	31.1 (0.70)	31.1 (0.82)	30.9 (0.76)	31.8 (0.90)	0–100; higher score indicates better QoL
SF-36 MCS, mean (SE)	42.8 (1.09)	42.2 (1.26)	44.0 (1.11)	41.4 (1.14)	45.5 (1.29)	44.7 (1.23)	42.1 (1.29)	40.5 (1.31)	42.8 (1.32)	41.2 (1.23)	42.6 (1.17)	0–100; higher score indicates better QoL

b.i.d. twice daily; *HAQ-DI* Health Assessment Questionnaire-Disability Index, *FACIT* Functional Assessment of Chronic Illness Therapy, *ITT* intent-to-treat, *MCS* mental component summary score, *PCS* physical component summary score, *Patient Global* Patient Global Assessment of Disease Activity, *q.d.* once daily, *QoL* quality of life, *SE* standard error, *SF-36*, 36-Item Short Form Health Survey, *VAS* visual analog scale

Table 2 Change from baseline in patient reported outcome scores at week 12 and week 24

Time-point	Methotrexate add-on study dosing group							Monotherapy study dosing group			
		Once daily (q.d.)			Twice daily (b.i.d.)			Once daily (q.d.)			
	Placebo	50	100	200	25	50	100	Placebo	50	100	200
Health Assessment Questionnaire-Disability Index (HAQ-DI), points											
Week 12	−0.38	−0.58	−0.65*	−0.75***	−0.59	−0.58	−0.84***	−0.23	−0.66***	−0.68***	−0.74***
Week 24	−0.37	−0.63	−0.78***	−0.82***	−0.62**	−0.66**	−0.90***	NA[a]	−0.69	−0.79	−0.85
Functional Assessment of Chronic Illness Therapy (FACIT)-Fatigue scale, points											
Week 12	5.6	7.6	9.5*	11.4***	6.9	8.4	11.3***	3.9	9.5***	10.2***	11.2***
Week 24	6.0	7.9	11.1***	11.6**	7.7	9.0	12.8***	NA[a]	10.0	11.3	13.7
Patient global assessment of disease activity (Patient Global), mm											
Week 12	−16.7	−25.2	−29.1*	−34.2***	−25.2*	−27.0*	−35.6***	−11.5	−27.5***	−30.0***	−28.2***
Week 24	−17.9	−29.4*	−34.4*	−34.9*	−27.3*	−28.1*	−39.1***	NA[a]	−29.1	−32.2	−35.1
Pain, mm											
Week 12	−16.9	−24.8	−27.4*	−31.4**	−24.2	− 28.3*	−37.9***	−13.3	−29.2***	−31.5***	−31.3***
Week 24	−17.0	−27.1*	−32.7***	−34.6***	−26.9*	−27.7*	−37.9***	NA[a]	−29.1	−35.1	−37.7
Short Form-36: Physical component score (PCS), points											
Week 12	3.2	6.7**	8.4***	8.9***	7.5**	7.1**	10.5***	3.0	7.1**	7.8***	8.6***
Week 24	2.8	7.3***	9.9***	9.7***	7.8***	7.9***	11.6***	NA[a]	6.9	10.0	9.7
Short Form-36: Mental component score (MCS), points											
Week 12	4.3	4.4	5.1	8.1	3.5	3.1	6.2	2.7	4.9*	6.9**	6.8**
Week 24	4.7	4.3	6.7	7.2	3.8	3.5	7.1	NA[a]	5.1	7.7	8.5

b.i.d. twice daily; *HAQ-DI* Health Assessment Questionnaire-Disability Index, *FACIT* Functional Assessment of Chronic Illness Therapy, *MCS* mental component summary score, *PCS* physical component summary score, *Patient Global* Patient Global Assessment of Disease Activity, *q.d.* once daily

[a]At week 12, patients receiving placebo in the add-on study and patients receiving placebo and filgotinib 50 mg q.d. in the monotherapy study who had not achieved a 20% improvement in swollen joint count and tender joint count were reassigned to receive filgotinib 100 mg q.d. (both studies) or 50 mg b.i.d. (methotrexate add-on study only). Patients who switched treatments at week 12 were handled as discontinuations and data were imputed from week 12 onwards using last observation carried forward

P values given for pair-wise comparison with placebo: $*p < 0.05$; $**p < 0.01$; $***p < 0.001$

scores was noted as early as week 1 in the filgotinib 100-mg b.i.d. group versus placebo. By week 12, statistically significant improvements were seen in all but the 50-mg q.d. group versus placebo, and these improvements were sustained to week 24.

In the monotherapy study, scores at week 12 had decreased by 11.5 mm in the placebo group and by 27.5–30.0 mm in the filgotinib groups; at week 24, scores in the filgotinib groups were 29.1–35.1 mm lower than at baseline. Improvements in scores were statistically significant in all filgotinib groups versus placebo at week 1.

Patient Pain

In both studies, all placebo and filgotinib dosing groups had a reduction in Patient Pain scores over the course of the study (Fig. 2c, d and Table 2).

At week 24 in the MTX add-on study, scores had decreased by 17.0 mm in the placebo group and by 26.9–37.9 mm in the filgotinib groups. Statistically significantly greater improvements in pain versus placebo were noted as early as week 1 in the filgotinib 100-mg b.i.d. group, from week 2 in the filgotinib 200-mg q.d. group, and from week 4 in the 100-mg q.d. group (Fig. 2c).

In the monotherapy study, scores at week 12 had decreased by 13.3 mm in the placebo group and by 29.2–31.5 mm in the filgotinib groups; at week 24, scores in the filgotinib groups were 29.1–37.7 mm lower than at baseline. Statistically significantly greater improvements in Patient Pain scores were seen as early as week 1 in the filgotinib 200-mg q.d. group, by week 2 in the 50-mg q.d. group, and in all groups from week 4 to week 12 (Fig. 2d). Reductions in pain were maintained to week 24 in both studies.

FACIT-Fatigue scale

In both studies, all treatment groups demonstrated numerical increases in FACIT-Fatigue scores over the course of the 24-week treatment period (Fig. 2 and Table 2), indicating reduced fatigue. At week 24 in the MTX add-on study, scores had increased by 6.0 points in the placebo group and by 7.7–12.8 points in the filgotinib groups. Statistically significantly greater improvements versus placebo were observed from the first measured time point—week 4—for

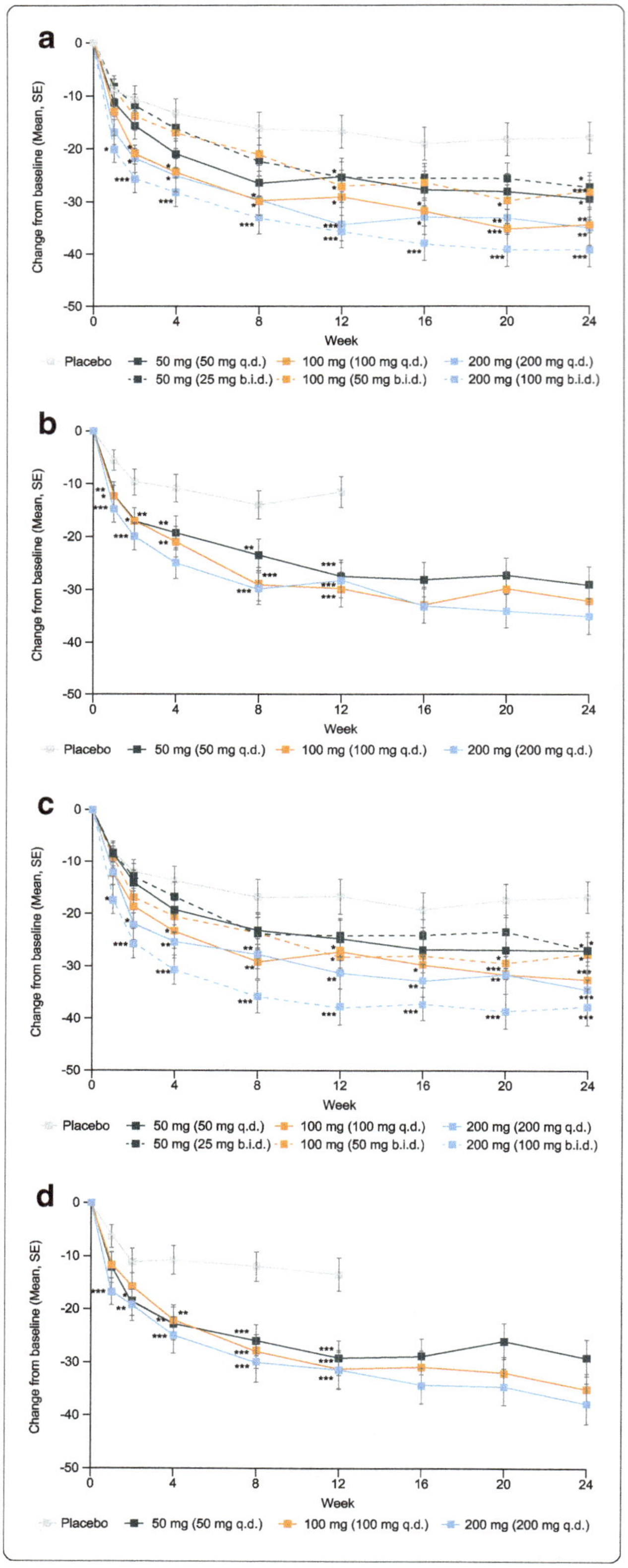

Fig. 1 Patient Global scores, methotrexate (MTX) add-on (**a**) and monotherapy (**b**); Patient Pain scores, MTX add-on (**c**) and monotherapy (**d**). *P* values given for pair-wise comparison with placebo: $^*p < 0.05$; $^{**}p < 0.01$; $^{***}p < 0.001$. At week 12, patients receiving placebo in the MTX add-on study and patients receiving placebo and filgotinib 50 mg once daily (q.d.) in the monotherapy study, who had not achieved a 20% improvement in swollen joint count (SJC) and tender joint count (TJC) were reassigned to receive filgotinib 100 mg q.d. (both studies) or 50 mg twice daily (b.i.d.) (MTX add-on study). Patients who switched treatments at week 12 were handled as discontinuations and data were imputed from week 12 onwards using last observation carried forward. SE, standard error

filgotinib 100 mg q.d. and 100 mg b.i.d.. By week 12, improvements in the filgotinib 200-mg q.d. group were also statistically significantly greater than in the placebo group and remained so until week 24. There was no significant improvement in FACIT-Fatigue scores versus placebo at any time point in the filgotinib 50-mg b.i.d., 50-mg q.d., or 25-mg b.i.d. treatment groups (Fig. 2a).

In the monotherapy study, scores at week 12 were increased by 3.9 points in the placebo group and by 9.5–11.2 points in the filgotinib groups; at week 24, scores in the filgotinib groups were 10.0–13.7 points higher than at baseline. Statistically significantly greater improvements versus placebo were observed at week 4 in the monotherapy study in all filgotinib groups; these improvements versus placebo were maintained until week 12 and FACIT-Fatigue scores continued to increase to week 24 (Fig. 2b).

SF-36

In both studies, improvements in both PCS and MCS scores were observed in all treatment groups (Fig. 3 and Table 2).

PCS

At week 24 in the MTX add-on study, PCS scores had increased by 2.8 points in the placebo group and by 7.3–11.6 points in the filgotinib groups. Statistically significant improvements versus placebo were observed at week 4 in the filgotinib 100-mg b.i.d. and 200-mg q.d. groups. By week 12, statistically significantly greater improvements were observed in all the filgotinib dosing groups compared with placebo, which continued to week 24 (Fig. 3a).

In the monotherapy study, PCS scores at week 12 were increased by 3.0 points in the placebo group and by 7.1–8.6 points in the filgotinib groups; at week 24, scores in the filgotinib groups were 6.9–10.0 points higher than at baseline. Statistically significantly greater improvements versus placebo were observed at week 4 in all filgotinib groups until week 12, and scores were maintained or improved further until week 24 (Fig. 3b).

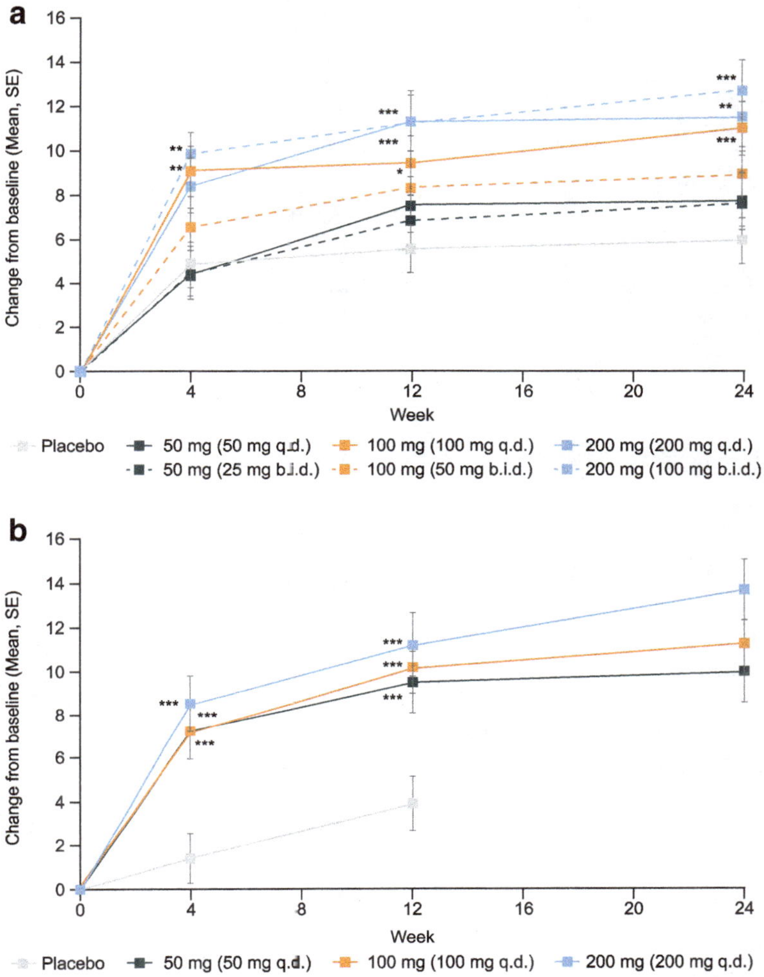

Fig. 2 Functional Assessment of Chronic Illness Therapy (FACIT)-Fatigue, methotrexate (MTX) add-on (**a**) and monotherapy (**b**) studies. *P* values given for pair-wise comparison with placebo: $^{*}p < 0.05$; $^{**}p < 0.01$; $^{***}p < 0.001$. At week 12, patients receiving placebo in the MTX add-on study and patients receiving placebo and filgotinib 50 mg once daily (q.d.) in the monotherapy study who had not achieved a 20% improvement in swollen joint count (SJC) and tender joint count (TJC) were reassigned to receive filgotinib 100 mg q.d. (both studies) or 50 mg twice daily (b.i.d.) (MTX add-on study only). Patients who switched treatments at week 12 were handled as discontinuations and data were imputed from week 12 onwards using last observation carried forward. SE, standard error

MCS

In the add-on study, SF-36 MCS scores at week 24 had increased by 4.7 points in the placebo group and by 3.5–7.2 points in the filgotinib groups; however, these changes were not statistically significant in any filgotinib group (Fig. 3c).

Contrastingly, in the monotherapy study, there was a statistically significant difference in MCS in the filgotinib 100-mg q.d. group versus placebo at week 4 and in all filgotinib groups by week 12; SF-36 MCS scores remained stable or continued to improve until week 24 (Fig. 3d).

MCIDs

As detailed in Table 3, the placebo groups experienced MCIDs across PROs, ranging between 42% and 61% of patients at week 12; however, a numerically larger proportion of patients in the filgotinib groups achieved MCIDs at week 12 compared with placebo across all PROs for the vast majority of doses tested (range 45–86%; significance not determined). The three exceptions to this trend were patients in the MTX add-on study in the 50-mg q.d. group with respect to FACIT-Fatigue score and the 25-mg b.i.d. and 50-mg b.i.d. groups with respect to SF-36 MCS. The highest-dose groups in both studies were generally associated with the largest proportions of patients reporting MCIDs.

Normative values

In an exploratory analysis of both studies, a numerically larger proportion of patients in each of the filgotinib groups achieved normalized PRO values at week 12 versus

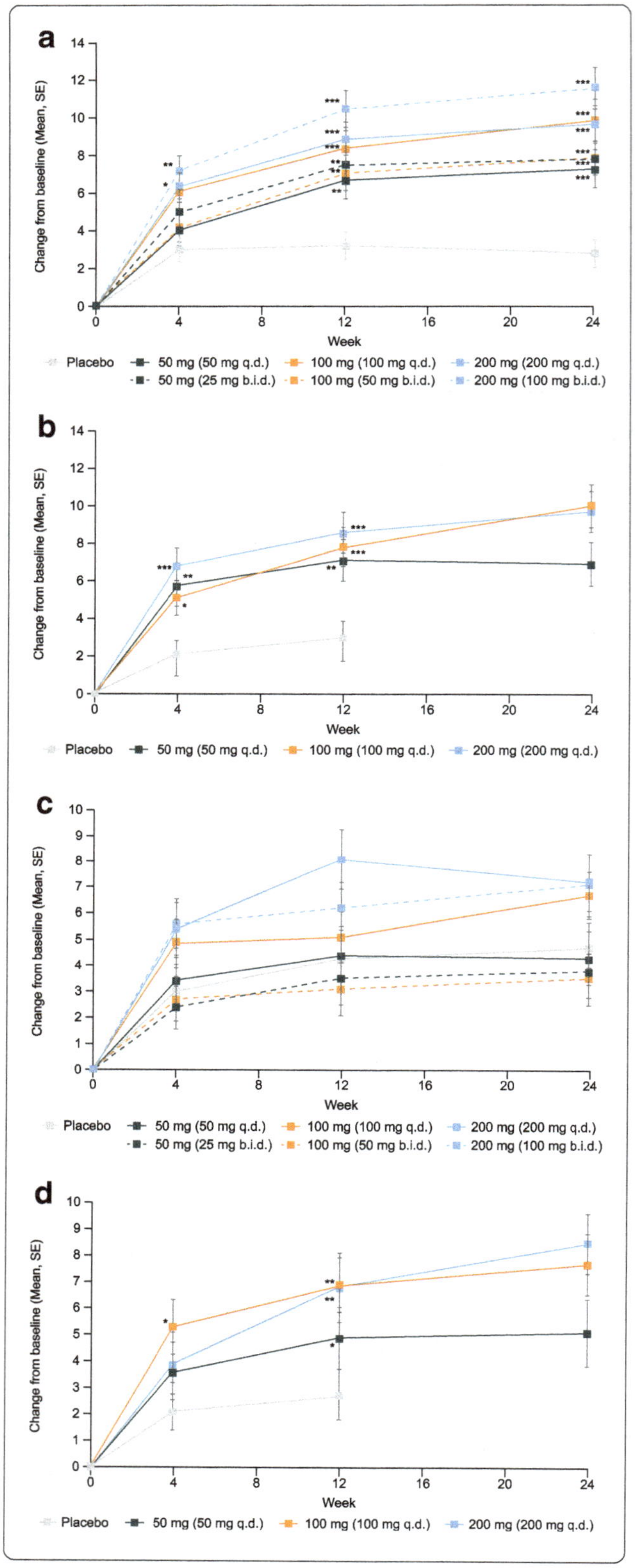

Fig. 3 SF-36 physical component score (PCS), methotrexate (MTX) add-on (**a**) and monotherapy (**b**); SF-36 mental component score (MCS), MTX add-on (**c**), and monotherapy (**d**). *P* values given for pair-wise comparison with placebo: *$p < 0.05$; **$p < 0.01$; ***$p < 0.001$. At week 12, patients receiving placebo in the MTX add-on study and patients receiving placebo and filgotinib 50 mg once daily (q.d.) in the monotherapy study who had not achieved a 20% improvement in swollen joint count (SJC) and tender joint count (TJC) were reassigned to receive filgotinib 100 mg q.d. (both studies) or 50 mg twice daily (b.i.d.) (MTX add-on study only). Patients who switched treatments at week 12 were handled as discontinuations and data were imputed from week 12 onwards using last observation carried forward. SE, standard error; SF-36, 36-Item Short Form Health Survey

the placebo groups (Additional file 4: Table S3). The single exception was seen for SF-36 MCS, in which 38% of subjects in the placebo group of the MTX add-on study achieved scores ≥50 compared with 37% of patients in the 50-mg q.d. group.

PRO responses by clinical response status

Patients who had not achieved a clinical response (ACR20) to treatment at week 12 and who were randomized from placebo or 50 mg filgotinib to 100 mg filgotinib daily experienced improvements in PRO scores from week 12 to week 24. At week 24, many of the scores reported by initial nonresponders were similar to those achieved by responders in the 100 mg filgotinib groups at week 12.

At week 12, patients who had demonstrated a clinical response to treatment in terms of ACR20 and ACR50 were numerically more likely to achieve normative PRO scores than nonresponders (Additional file 5: Figure S2; Additional file 6: Figure S3 and Additional file 7: Figure S4 for ACR20 responses (data not shown for ACR50 responses)). This pattern was observed consistently in both studies and across dose groups. Nonresponders in the placebo groups were numerically less likely to achieve normative PRO values compared with nonresponders in the filgotinib 100-mg and 200-mg groups for all PRO measures except SF-36 PCS.

Dosing schedules

In both studies an overall dose effect was observed on all PROs (Table 2). In the MTX add-on study, after 24 weeks of treatment, there appeared to be a numerically better response with filgotinib 100 mg q.d. compared with 50 mg b.i.d. across all PROs (Figs. 1, 2 and 3). In contrast, numerically greater improvements were observed with filgotinib 100 mg b.i.d. compared with 200 mg q.d. across all PROs, with the exception of SF-36 MCS scores. Only the SF-36 MCS scores were significantly different between the 100-mg q.d. and 50-mg b.i.d. groups (least squares mean difference, 2.9; 95% confidence interval, 0.4 to 5.4; $p = 0.0249$ (uncorrected p value)). There were no apparent differences between dosing regimens with the 50-mg daily dose.

Table 3 Patients achieving MCIDs for each PRO at week 12

	Methotrexate add-on study							Monotherapy study (all q.d. doses)			
	Placebo (*N* = 86)	50 mg q.d. (*N* = 82)	100 mg q.d. (*N* = 85)	200 mg q.d. (*N* = 86)	25 mg b.i.d. (*N* = 86)	50 mg b.i.d. (*N* = 85)	100 mg b.i.d. (*N* = 84)	Placebo (*N* = 72)	50 mg (*N* = 72)	100 mg (*N* = 70)	200 mg (*N* = 69)
HAQ-DI, *n* (%)	49 (57)	60 (73)	64 (75)	74 (86)	61 (71)	57 (67)	70 (83)	37 (52)	51 (73)	55 (79)	55 (80)
Patient Global, *n* (%)	52 (61)	56 (68)	60 (71)	67 (78)	58 (67)	62 (73)	65 (77)	35 (49)	56 (78)	50 (71)	52 (75)
Patient Pain, *n* (%)	50 (58)	54 (66)	55 (66)	66 (77)	59 (69)	58 (68)	67 (80)	39 (55)	54 (77)	51 (73)	56 (81)
FACIT-Fatigue scale, *n* (%)	51 (59)	47 (57)	60 (71)	64 (74)	54 (63)	55 (65)	59 (71)	32 (45)	48 (69)	52 (74)	51 (74)
SF-36 PCS, *n* (%)	43 (50)	55 (67)	60 (71)	68 (79)	58 (67)	62 (73)	66 (80)	30 (42)	48 (69)	49 (70)	54 (78)
SF-36 MCS, *n* (%)	49 (57)	44 (54)	48 (57)	64 (74)	43 (50)	38 (45)	53 (64)	34 (48)	39 (56)	52 (74)	46 (67)

Minimal clinically important differences (MCIDs) were defined as follows: 0.22-point decrease from baseline in the Health Assessment Questionnaire–Disability Index (HAQ-DI); 10% (10 mm) decrease from baseline in the 'Patient' Global Assessment of Disease Activity and Patient Pain visual analog scale (VAS) scores; 4-point increase in the Functional Assessment of Chronic Illness Therapy (FACIT)-Fatigue score; 2.5-point increase from baseline in the 36-Item Short Form Health Survey (SF-36) physical component score (PCS) and mental component score (MCS)
b.i.d. twice daily, *PRO* patient-reported outcome, *q.d.* once daily

Discussion

Two placebo-controlled studies assessed the efficacy and safety of filgotinib in combination with MTX or as monotherapy. Over 24 weeks of treatment, filgotinib provided statistically significant improvements versus placebo across measured PROs, covering a range of aspects of patient HRQoL, including pain, functional status, physical wellbeing, and fatigue. There was also a trend towards improvements in mental health, which was statistically significant compared to placebo in the monotherapy study. A rapid onset of effect was observed for improvements in HRQoL with the active treatment. Onset of effect was generally faster in the higher dose groups: a significantly greater improvement in Patient Global and Patient Pain scores was seen at week 2 in the filgotinib 200-mg groups versus placebo in both studies, and in the FACIT-Fatigue and SF-36 PCS at the first measured time point (week 4). Furthermore, patients in the 200-mg filgotinib groups in both studies were numerically more likely to achieve MCIDs across PROs versus patients on placebo. Similarly, the active treatment was associated with a numerically larger proportion of patients achieving normative PRO scores than placebo patients in all but one outcome. PRO scores appeared to mirror measures of clinical efficacy as ACR20 and ACR50 responders were numerically more likely to achieve normative PRO scores than nonresponders.

This analysis was not powered to compare filgotinib dose groups; however, an exploratory analysis was performed to better inform regimen choices in future studies. In the MTX add-on study, in which both q.d and b.i.d. dosing regimens were tested, there were numerically better responses with a daily dose of filgotinib 100 mg when given as a 100-mg q.d. dose versus a 50-mg b.i.d. dose across all PROs, although this only reached statistical significance in one outcome (SF-36 MCS). Conversely, with a daily dose of filgotinib 200 mg, treatment response appeared to be higher with a 100-mg b.i.d. dose versus a 200-mg q.d. dose across all PROs, with the exception of the SF-36 MCS.

The strong placebo effect cannot be overlooked. For example, at week 12, 61% of patients in the MTX add-on study and 49% of patients in the monotherapy study receiving placebo reported a MCID in terms of Patient Global scores. As well as being striking in itself, the placebo effect may have influenced differences in results between the two studies. For example, whereas all filgotinib groups in the monotherapy study had statistically significant improvements in SF-36 MCS scores versus placebo, in the MTX add-on study, there were no such significant improvements in any active treatment group. These divergent findings may be explained by the administration of MTX in the add-on study, thus the "placebo" group continued to receive an active treatment, which may underlie the rapid increase in SF-36 scores in this group (versus more modest gains in the placebo group of the monotherapy study). This also highlights the complex nature of the psychological burden of RA, suggesting that patient emotional wellbeing is affected by factors beyond the treatment itself. It is notable that the placebo response in this study is in line with that observed during studies of other RA therapies [24–29].

The limitations of these studies include the inherent subjectivity of PRO measures, although PROs do give valuable information on the treatment effect. Patients may have experienced inflated improvements in their health status as a result of the more attentive care and close monitoring received in clinical trials or as a result of high expectations of novel treatments, as suggested by the placebo effect noted above. The switching of all patients in the placebo group in the monotherapy study, and nonresponders in the placebo and filgotinib 50-mg groups in the MTX add-on study, means that placebo control was maintained for the first 12 weeks only (owing to the ethical implications of leaving patients without effective treatment). Furthermore, as the overall studies were of 6-month duration, the longer-term impact of filgotinib treatment remains to be determined.

Conclusions

In both studies, rapid and sustained improvements in PROs during 24 weeks of treatment were observed when filgotinib was given in combination with MTX or as monotherapy, and as a q.d. or b.i.d. dosing regimen, to patients with moderate-to-severe active RA. The clinical benefits of filgotinib previously reported [11, 12] gain added value when combined with patient insights such as these, which confirm the potential ability of filgotinib to improve patients' HRQoL as well as the signs and symptoms of disease.

Additional files

Additional file 1: Figure S1. Patient disposition during the methotrexate (MTX) add-on study (A) and the monotherapy study (B). (ZIP 1513 kb)

Additional file 2: Document 1. List of ethical bodies that approved the DARWIN 1 study for each of the 106 study centers. (PDF 129 kb)

Additional file 3: Document 2. List of ethical bodies that approved the DARWIN 2 study for each of the 59 study centers. (PDF 68 kb)

Additional file 4: Table S1. Patient-reported outcomes: summary of instruments used and minimally important clinical differences used in this study. **Table S2.** Baseline patient characteristics. **Table S3.** Proportion of patients who achieved normative scores at week 12 in the methotrexate add-on and monotherapy studies. (DOCX 34 kb)

Additional file 5: Figure S2. Proportion of subjects achieving normative HAQ-DI score (≤0.5) at week 12 according to ACR20 responder status in the methotrexate (MTX) add-on study (A) and monotherapy study (B). (EPS 1981 kb)

Additional file 6: Figure S3. Proportion of subjects achieving normative FACIT-Fatigue score (≥40) at week 12 according to ACR20 responder status in the MTX add-on study (A) and monotherapy study (B). (EPS 1984 kb)

Additional file 7: Figure S4. Proportion of subjects achieving normative SF-36 PCS and MCS scores (≥50) at week 12 according to ACR20 responder status. A PCS, MTX add-on, B PCS, monotherapy, C MCS, MTX add-on, D MCS, monotherapy. (EPS 2249 kb)

Abbreviations

ACR: American College of Rheumatology; bDMARDs: Biologic DMARDs; b.i.d: Twice daily; FACIT: Functional Assessment of Chronic Illness Therapy; HAQ-DI: Health Assessment Questionnaire-Disability Index; HRQoL: Health-related quality of life; ITT: Intent-to-treat; JAK: Janus kinase; MCIDs: Minimal clinically important differences; MCS: Mental component summary; MTX: Methotrexate; PCS: Physical component summary; PRO: Patient-reported outcome; q.d.: Once daily; QoL: Quality of life; RA: Rheumatoid arthritis; SE: Standard error; SF-36: 36-Item Short Form Health Survey; SJC: Swollen joint count; TJC: Tender joint count; tsDMARDs: Targeted synthetic disease-modifying antirheumatic drugs; VAS: Visual analog scale

Acknowledgements

The authors would like to thank the participants, principal investigators and study staff. Additional statistical support was provided by Corinne Jamoul. Editorial assistance was provided by Fishawack Communications Ltd., funded by Galapagos NV.

Funding

The DARWIN 1 and 2 studies were funded by Galapagos NV.

Authors' contributions

MG, RW, AV, PH, CT, and AK were involved in analyzing the study data and writing the manuscript. LM performed the statistical analyses. All authors read and approved the final manuscript.

Authors' information

RW and AK were the principal investigators of the MTX-add on study and monotherapy study, respectively. PH was the medical lead, and AV the clinical study lead, for both studies.

Ethics approval and consent to participate

Written approval was obtained before initiation of the study from the Medical Ethical Committee of University Hospitals KU Leuven (reference ML9437; study site of the Principal Investigator for DARWIN 1) and the University of California San Diego Human Research Protections Program (reference 140642; study site of the Principal Investigator for DARWIN 2), and from the appropriate independent ethics committee or institutional review board for each of the 106 study centers in DARWIN 1 and 59 study centers in DARWIN 2. Both phase 2b studies were conducted in accordance with the ethical principles of the Declaration of Helsinki, International Council on Harmonisation good clinical practice guidelines, and all applicable national and local laws and regulatory requirements. All patients provided written, informed consent prior to study participation.

Competing interests

L.M., A.V., P.H., and C.T. are employees of Galapagos NV, Belgium. M.G. has received grants from Pfizer, Gilead, Astellas, Vertex, and Eli Lilly and has consulted for Pfizer, Gilead, Astellas, Vertex, Eli Lilly, and Galapagos NV. R.W. received unrestricted research grant from Roche to his institution and was advisor for Jansen (Golimumab) and part of the speakers' bureau of BMS. A.K. has received compensation for consultancy work, or has been involved in the conduct of clinical research studies, for AbbVie, Amgen, Celgene, Eli Lilly, Janssen, Novartis, Pfizer, and UCB and has consulted for Galapagos NV.

Author details

[1]Division of Immunology and Rheumatology, Stanford School of Medicine, Stanford, CA, USA. [2]Department of Development and Regeneration KU Leuven, Skeletal Biology and Engineering Research Center; Rheumatology, University Hospitals Leuven, Leuven, Belgium. [3]Galapagos NV, Mechelen, Belgium. [4]University of California San Diego, La Jolla, CA, USA. [5]Division of Immunology and Rheumatology, Stanford School of Medicine, 1000 Welch RD #203, Palo Alto, CA 94304, USA.

References

1. American College of Rheumatology. Rheumatoid Arthritis. In: Disease & Conditions. American College of Rheumatology website; 2016. http://www.rheumatology.org/I-Am-A/Patient-Caregiver/Diseases-Conditions/Rheumatoid-Arthritis. Accessed 2 Mar 2018.
2. Arshad A, Rashid R, Benjamin K. The effect of disease activity on fat-free mass and resting energy expenditure in patients with rheumatoid arthritis versus noninflammatory arthropathies/soft tissue rheumatism. Mod Rheumatol. 2007;17:470–5.
3. Gerhold K, Richter A, Schneider M, Bergerhausen HJ, Demary W, Liebhaber A, et al. Health-related quality of life in patients with long-standing rheumatoid arthritis in the era of biologics: data from the German biologics register RABBIT. Rheumatology (Oxford). 2015;54:1858–66.
4. Wang SL, Chang CH, Hu LY, Tsai SJ, Yang AC, You ZH. Risk of developing depressive disorders following rheumatoid arthritis: a nationwide population-based study. PLoS One. 2014;9:e107791.
5. Heinrich PC, Behrmann I, Muller-Newen G, Schaper F, Graeve L. Interleukin-6-type cytokine signalling through the gp130/Jak/STAT pathway. Biochem J. 1998;334(Pt 2):297–314.

6. Choy E. Understanding the dynamics: pathways involved in the pathogenesis of rheumatoid arthritis. Rheumatology (Oxford). 2012; 51(Suppl 5):v3–11.
7. Dayer JM, Choy E. Therapeutic targets in rheumatoid arthritis: the interleukin-6 receptor. Rheumatology (Oxford). 2010;49:15–24.
8. Norman P. Selective JAK inhibitors in development for rheumatoid arthritis. Expert Opin Investig Drugs. 2014;23:1067–77.
9. Van Rompaey L, Galien R, van der Aar EM, Clement-Lacroix P, Nelles L, Smets B, et al. Preclinical characterization of GLPG0634, a selective inhibitor of JAK1, for the treatment of inflammatory diseases. J Immunol. 2013;191:3568–77.
10. Galien R, Brys R, Van der Aa A, Harrison P, Tasset C. Absence of Effects of Filgotinib on Erythrocytes, CD8+ and NK Cells in Rheumatoid Arthritis Patients Brings Further Evidence for the JAK1 Selectivity of Filgotinib [abstract]. Arthritis Rheumatol. 2015;67(suppl 10). http://acrabstracts.org/abstract/absence-of-effects-of-filgotinib-on-erythrocytes-cd8-and-nk-cells-in-rheumatoid-arthritis-patients-brings-further-evidence-for-the-jak1-selectivity-of-filgotinib/. Accessed 2 Mar 2018.
11. Westhovens R, Taylor PC, Alten R, Pavlova D, Enríquez-Sosa F, Mazur M, Greenwald M, Van der Aa A, Vanhoutte F, Tasset C, Harrison P. Filgotinib (GLPG0634/GS-6034), an oral JAK1 selective inhibitor, is effective in combination with methotrexate (MTX) in patients with active rheumatoid arthritis and insufficient response to MTX: results from a randomised, dose-finding study. Ann Rheum Dis. 2016;76:998–1008.
12. Kavanaugh A, Kremer J, Ponce L, Cseuz R, Reshetko OV, Stanislavchuk M, Greenwald M, Van der Aa A, Vanhoutte F, Tasset C, Harrison P. Filgotinib (GLPG0634/GS-6034), an oral selective JAK1 inhibitor, is effective as monotherapy in patients with active rheumatoid arthritis: results from a randomised, dose-finding study. Ann Rheum Dis. 2017;76:1009–19.
13. Fries JF, Spitz P, Kraines RG, Holman HR. Measurement of patient outcome in arthritis. Arthritis Rheum. 1980;23:137–45.
14. Nikiphorou E, Radner H, Chatzidionysiou K, Desthieux C, Zabalan C, van Eijk-Hustings Y, et al. Patient global assessment in measuring disease activity in rheumatoid arthritis: a review of the literature. Arthritis Res Ther. 2016;18:251.
15. Ware JE Jr, Sherbourne CD. The MOS 36-item short-form health survey (SF-36). I. Conceptual framework and item selection. Med Care. 1992;30: 473–83.
16. McHorney CA, Ware JE Jr, Raczek AE. The MOS 36-Item Short-Form Health Survey (SF-36): II. Psychometric and clinical tests of validity in measuring physical and mental health constructs. Med Care. 1993;31:247–63.
17. Wolfe F, Michaud K, Strand V. Expanding the definition of clinical differences: from minimally clinically important differences to really important differences. Analyses in 8931 patients with rheumatoid arthritis. J Rheumatol. 2005;32:583–9.
18. Strand V, Boers M, Idzerda L, Kirwan JR, Kvien TK, Tugwell PS, et al. It's good to feel better but it's better to feel good and even better to feel good as soon as possible for as long as possible. Response criteria and the importance of change at OMERACT 10. J Rheumatol. 2011;38:1720–7.
19. Cella D, Yount S, Sorensen M, Chartash E, Sengupta N, Grober J. Validation of the Functional Assessment of Chronic Illness Therapy Fatigue Scale relative to other instrumentation in patients with rheumatoid arthritis. J Rheumatol. 2005;32:811–9.
20. Wells GA, Boers M, Shea B, Brooks PM, Simon LS, Strand CV, et al. Minimal disease activity for rheumatoid arthritis: a preliminary definition. J Rheumatol. 2005;32:2016–24.
21. Cella D, Lai JS, Chang CH, Peterman A, Slavin M. Fatigue in cancer patients compared with fatigue in the general United States population. Cancer. 2002;94:528–38.
22. Maglinte GA, Hays RD, Kaplan RM. US general population norms for telephone administration of the SF-36v2. J Clin Epidemiol. 2012;65:497–502.
23. Maruish ME. (Ed.). User's manual for the SF-36v2 Health Survey (3rd ed.). Lincoln, RI: QualityMetric Incorporated. ISBN: 1-891810-28-6.
24. Strand V, Kosinski M, Chen CI, Joseph G, Rendas-Baum R, Graham NM, et al. Sarilumab plus methotrexate improves patient-reported outcomes in patients with active rheumatoid arthritis and inadequate responses to methotrexate: results of a phase III trial. Arthritis Res Ther. 2016;18:198.
25. Strand V, van Vollenhoven RF, Lee EB, Fleischmann R, Zwillich SH, Gruben D, et al. Tofacitinib or adalimumab versus placebo: patient-reported outcomes from a phase 3 study of active rheumatoid arthritis. Rheumatology (Oxford). 2016;55:1031–41.
26. Hazes JM, Taylor P, Strand V, Purcaru O, Coteur G, Mease P. Physical function improvements and relief from fatigue and pain are associated with increased productivity at work and at home in rheumatoid arthritis patients treated with certolizumab pegol. Rheumatology (Oxford). 2010;49:1900–10.
27. Genovese MC, Smolen JS, Weinblatt ME, Burmester GR, Meerwein S, Camp HS, et al. Efficacy and safety of ABT-494, a selective JAK-1 inhibitor, in a phase IIb study in patients with rheumatoid arthritis and an inadequate response to methotrexate. Arthritis Rheumatol. 2016;68:2857–66.
28. Emery P, Blanco R, Maldonado Cocco J, Chen YC, Gaich CL, DeLozier AM, et al. Patient-reported outcomes from a phase III study of baricitinib in patients with conventional synthetic DMARD-refractory rheumatoid arthritis. RMD Open. 2017;3:e000410.
29. Wallenstein GV, Kanik KS, Wilkinson B, Cohen S, Cutolo M, Fleishmann R, et al. Effects of the oral Janus kinase inhibitor tofacitinib on patient-reported outcomes in patients with active rheumatoid arthritis: results of two phase 2 randomised controlled trials. Clin Exp Rheumatol. 2016;34:430–42.

16

Does the presence of magnetic resonance imaging-detected osteitis at diagnosis with rheumatoid arthritis lower the risk for achieving disease-modifying antirheumatic drug-free sustained remission

L. E. Burgers[1*], D. M. Boeters[1], M. Reijnierse[2] and A. H. M. van der Helm-van Mil[1,3]

Abstract

Background: Although infrequent, some rheumatoid arthritis (RA) patients achieve disease-modifying antirheumatic drug (DMARD)-free sustained remission. The absence of RA-specific autoantibodies, such as anticitrullinated protein antibodies (ACPA), is known to be associated with this outcome but further mechanisms underlying the chronic nature of RA are largely unknown. Magnetic resonance imaging (MRI)-detected bone marrow edema (BME), or osteitis, strongly predicts erosive progression and is associated with ACPA positivity. Therefore, we hypothesized that the presence of MRI-detected osteitis is also predictive of not achieving DMARD-free sustained remission and that the presence of osteitis mediates the association between ACPA and DMARD-free sustained remission.

Methods: A 1.5 T unilateral hand and foot MRI was performed at disease presentation in 238 RA patients, evaluating BME, synovitis, and tenosynovitis (summed as MRI inflammation score). DMARD-free sustained remission, defined as the absence of clinical synovitis after DMARD cessation that persisted during the total follow-up, was assessed (median follow-up 3.8 years). Associations between the different MRI-detected inflammatory features and this outcome were studied. A mediation analysis was performed to study whether the presence of BME mediated the association between ACPA and DMARD-free sustained remission. Finally, patterns of MRI-detected inflammation with regard to DMARD-free sustained remission were studied using partial least squares (PLS) regression.

Results: Forty-six (19.3%) patients achieved DMARD-free sustained remission. ACPA positivity associated independently with remission (hazard ratio (HR) 0.16, 95% confidence interval (CI) 0.06–0.39). In contrast, no associations were observed between MRI-detected BME (HR 0.99, 95% CI 0.94–1.03), or other MRI inflammatory features, and achieving DMARD-free sustained remission. Thus, the presence of BME did not mediate the association between ACPA and DMARD-free sustained remission. Furthermore, a PLS analysis revealed that patients who did or did not achieve remission could not be distinguished by patterns of MRI-detected inflammation.

Conclusions: At disease presentation, osteitis, as well as other MRI-detected inflammatory features, was not associated with achieving DMARD-free sustained remission over time. Thus, imaging predictors for joint damage and disease persistence differ. The processes mediating RA chronicity remain largely unsolved.

Keywords: Magnetic resonance imaging, Rheumatoid arthritis, Early rheumatoid arthritis, Outcomes research

* Correspondence: l.e.burgers@lumc.nl
[1]Department of Rheumatology, Leiden University Medical Center, C-01-046, PO Box 9600, 2300 RC Leiden, The Netherlands
Full list of author information is available at the end of the article

Background

As joint damage is becoming less prevalent in patients with rheumatoid arthritis (RA), the focus is shifting to other disease outcomes such as disease-modifying antirheumatic drug (DMARD)-free sustained remission [1]. DMARD-free sustained remission means that DMARDs can be discontinued without the recurrence of clinical synovitis [1, 2]. Thanks to improved treatment strategies, DMARD-free sustained remission is more feasible and corresponds with perceived normalization of physical functioning and pain, fatigue, and stiffness levels for patients [1, 3].

Pathophysiological mechanisms behind RA chronicity or, the opposite, DMARD-free sustained remission are largely unknown [4]. Short symptom duration at disease presentation has been shown to be predictive suggesting that the timing of disease modification is important [1, 2, 5]. The strongest predictor for DMARD-free sustained remission is the absence of RA-specific autoantibodies, such as anticitrullinated protein antibodies (ACPA) [1, 2]. This suggests that patients who can achieve this outcome are inherently different.

Joint destruction and not achieving DMARD-free sustained remission are both characteristics of a severe disease course. Therefore, hypothetically, predictors for both outcomes are similar. ACPA are such an example. However, local joint inflammation, measured using the swollen joint count (SJC), while predictive for erosive progression [6, 7], was not predictive for DMARD-free sustained remission [1, 2]. A more sensitive method to detect local inflammation is magnetic resonance imaging (MRI). In addition to synovitis and tenosynovitis, MRI can detect bone marrow edema (BME), also called osteitis. Osteitis is not specific for RA as it has also been observed in other conditions such as psoriatic arthritis and in symptom-free controls [8–10]. In RA, the presence of osteitis is strongly predictive for erosive progression, with odds ratios reported up to 60 [8, 11–13]. The process of joint destruction is likely to be ACPA-driven since ACPA-positive RA patients have higher osteitis scores [14, 15]. Furthermore, ACPA have been shown to be able to induce osteoclastogenesis leading to subsequent bone loss [16] and a histologic study of bone samples in which MRI-detected osteitis is present revealed an increased presence of osteoclasts compared with control samples [17]. Thus, osteitis appears to be a mediator in the link between ACPA and erosive progression.

Our ultimate aim is to increase the understanding of processes involved in achieving DMARD-free sustained remission or disease chronicity. With the underlying assumption that predictors for erosive progression and not achieving DMARD-free sustained remission are similar, we hypothesized that the presence of osteitis at disease presentation also associates with a decreased chance of achieving DMARD-free sustained remission. Furthermore, we hypothesized that the association between ACPA and DMARD-free sustained remission is mediated by osteitis. To evaluate these hypotheses, associations between MRI-detected inflammation and DMARD-free sustained remission were evaluated and a mediation analysis was performed. Finally, to study not only the presence of osteitis itself, but also its relationship with other types of MRI-detected inflammation, and its location, and achieving DMARD-free sustained remission, we looked at whether a pattern of MRI-detected inflammation (covering the type of MRI inflammatory feature, severity, and location) could distinguish patients who did and did not achieve this outcome over time.

Methods

Patients

The Leiden Early Arthritis Clinic (EAC) is a population-based inception cohort that includes patients with clinically confirmed synovitis of ≥1 joint and a symptom duration of <2 years [18]. Between August 2010 and September 2014 an MRI was performed at baseline in 598 consecutive patients. Of these patients, 275 fulfilled the 1987 and/or 2010 criteria for RA and were treated with DMARDs during the first year. Thirty-seven patients were excluded (22 because they never received DMARD therapy despite fulfilling classification criteria, 4 because the MRI was performed without contrast, and 11 because of participation in a trial with initial biologic therapy that differed from routine care) [19, 20]. Thus, in total 238 RA patients were studied (Fig. 1). According to local and national guidelines, RA patients were initially treated with methotrexate (started at or after the 2-week visit); after failure, another conventional DMARD was initiated or added. Biologicals were allowed after failure of >2 conventional DMARDs and were used in 22 patients (9%) of whom none achieved DMARD-free sustained remission. Treatment was steered by disease activity score (DAS). All patients had scheduled EAC visits at 4 months, 8 months, 12 months, 18 months, 24 months, and then yearly. Besides these visits, regular visits were planned when deemed necessary by either the patient or rheumatologist (usually every 3–4 months). All patients provided written informed consent. The study was approved by the local medical ethical committee.

MRI

A unilateral 1.5 T MRI of the metacarpophalangeal (MCP; 2–5) joints, wrist, and metatarsophalangeal (MTP; 1–5) joints of the most painful side or, in case of equally severe symptoms, of the dominant side was made <2 weeks after inclusion. MRIs were scored on BME and synovitis in line with the RA MRI scoring

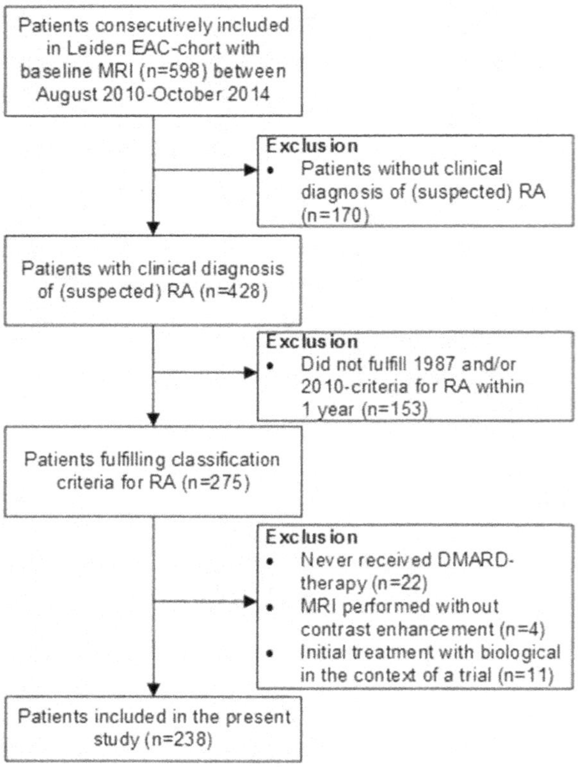

Fig. 1 Flowchart of patient selection. DMARD disease modifying antirheumatic drug, EAC early arthritis clinic, MRI magnetic resonance imaging, RA rheumatoid arthritis

(RAMRIS) method [21] and on tenosynovitis according to Haavardsholm et al. [22]. The total MRI inflammation score was the sum of total BME, synovitis, and tenosynovitis scores. MRIs were scored by two experienced readers (intraclass correlation coefficient (ICC) 0.94) who were blinded to clinical data. The mean scores of the two readers were taken. More information about the MRI scanning protocol and scoring method has been described previously [10, 23, 24] and is provided in Additional file 1 (Supplementary methods).

DMARD-free sustained remission

Medical records of all patients were reviewed in April 2017 for the presence of DMARD-free sustained remission, defined as the absence of clinical synovitis that persisted after cessation of DMARDs during the total subsequent follow-up. The follow-up duration after DMARD cessation had to be ≥ 1 year to fulfill the definition. The date of remission was the date 1 year after DMARD cessation. For patients not achieving remission, the date of censoring was the date of reviewing the medical records or an earlier date in case patients were lost to follow-up.

Statistical analysis

Associations between baseline characteristics, including MRI-detected inflammatory features and DMARD-free sustained remission, were assessed using univariable and multivariable Cox regression analyses. Partial least squares (PLS) regression was used to study whether certain patterns of MRI-detected inflammation discriminated between patients who did and did not achieve remission. This was done since not only the single presence of BME but also information on its presence in combination with other MRI-detected inflammatory features, or the location of BME, could be discriminative. Previous studies observed that BME is often present in certain carpal bones of symptom-free controls (such as the lunate) which may be caused by mechanical factors, and suggests that the location of BME can be relevant for the interpretation [10]. PLS regression clusters features and locations of MRI-detected inflammation that frequently occur together into factors, and presents for each factor the variance in the outcome that is explained by this factor. These factors can then be plotted against each other to look for clustering. A mediation analysis was performed according to Baron and Kenny [25]. Detailed statistical information is provided in Additional file 1. SPSS V.23.0 software was used.

Results

Patient characteristics

Of the 238 studied patients, 46 (19.3%) achieved DMARD-free sustained remission after a median duration of 2.8 (interquartile range (IQR) 2.0–3.5) years. For patients who did not achieve DMARD-free sustained remission, the median follow-up duration was 3.8 (IQR 3.0–5.0) years. Table 1 presents the baseline characteristics. The majority of patients were female and the mean age was 57 years. Associations between clinical characteristics and achieving DMARD-free sustained remission are shown in Table 2. Only the presence of ACPA was independently associated (hazard ratio (HR) 0.16, 95% confidence interval (CI) 0.06–0.39) with DMARD-free sustained remission.

Association between MRI-detected inflammatory features and DMARD-free sustained remission

The MRI-detected BME score was not associated with achieving DMARD-free sustained remission (HR 0.99, 95% CI 0.94–1.03). This was the same for MRI-detected synovitis (HR 1.03, 95% CI 0.97–1.09), tenosynovitis (HR 1.04, 95% CI 0.99–1.10), and the total MRI inflammation score (HR 1.01, 95% CI 0.99–1.03) (Table 3). Also, in multivariable models where corrections were made for the simultaneous presence of other inflammatory features and ACPA, BME was not associated with remission (Table 3).

Table 1 Baseline clinical and MRI characteristics of all patients and separately for patients that have and have not achieved DMARD-free sustained remission

	All patients (n = 238)	DMARD-free sustained remission (n = 46)	No remission (n = 192)
Clinical characteristics			
Age in years, mean (SD)	57 (14)	62 (13)	55 (14)
Female gender, n (%)	157 (66)	28 (61)	129 (67)
Symptom duration in weeks	15 (7–32)	14 (5–21)	17 (7–34)
Symptom duration > 12 weeks, n (%)	100 (42)	20 (44)	80 (42)
HAQ score, mean (SD)	0.9 (0.6)	1.1 (0.5)	1.0 (0.9)
68-TJC	8 (4–14)	9 (5–17)	8 (4–13)
66-SJC	5 (2–10)	8 (3–13)	5 (2–10)
CRP mg/L	9 (3–21)	17 (9–27)	8 (3–20)
ESR mm/h, mean (SD)	30 (24)	33 (25)	29 (24)
ACPA-positive, n (%)	120 (50)	6 (13)	114 (59)
RF-positive, n (%)	140 (59)	16 (35)	124 (65)
MRI characteristics			
BME score	3.5 (1.0–8.0)	4.0 (1.4–7.3)	3.5 (1.0–8.5)
Synovitis score	5.0 (2.5–9.5)	7.3 (3.0–10.0)	4.5 (2.5–9.5)
Tenosynovitis score	4.0 (1.5–7.5)	4.5 (1.8–9.3)	4.0 (1.5–7.0)
Total MRI inflammation score	13.5 (6.5–26.0)	16.5 (6.4–27.6)	12.5 (6.5–25.5)

All values are shown as median (interquartile range) unless indicated otherwise
Values are missing as follows (n): symptom duration (2), HAQ (13), TJC (11), SJC (12), and ESR (2)
ACPA anticitrullinated protein antibodies, *BME* bone marrow edema, *CRP* C-reactive protein, *DMARD* disease-modifying antirheumatic drug, *ESR* erythrocyte sedimentation rate, *HAQ* health assessment questionnaire, *MRI* magnetic resonance imaging, *RF* rheumatoid factor, *SD* standard deviation; *SJC* swollen joint count, *TJC* tender joint count

Table 2 Results of univariable and multivariable Cox regression analyses of clinical baseline characteristics in relation to achievement of DMARD-free sustained remission

	Univariable HR (95% CI)	Multivariable HR (95% CI)[a]
Clinical characteristics		
Age in years	1.04 (1.02–1.07)*	1.02 (0.99–1.04)
Female gender	0.81 (0.45–1.47)	
Symptom duration > 12 weeks	0.83 (0.46–1.50)	
HAQ score	1.11 (0.69–1.78)	
68-TJC	1.02 (0.98–1.05)	
66-SJC	1.06 (1.02–1.10)*	1.03 (0.99–1.08)
CRP mg/L	1.01 (1.0–1.02)*	1.00 (0.99–1.01)
ESR mm/h	1.01 (1.0–1.02)	
ACPA-positive	0.12 (0.05–0.27)*	0.16 (0.06–0.39)*
RF-positive	0.33 (0.18–0.61)*	0.80 (0.4[illegible]–1.6)

ACPA anticitrullinated protein antibodies, *CI* confidence interval, *CRP* C-reactive protein, *DMARD* disease-modifying antirheumatic drug, *ESR* erythrocyte sedimentation rate, *HAQ* health assessment questionnaire, *HR* hazard ratio, *RF* rheumatoid factor, *SJC* swollen joint count, *TJC* tender joint count
*$p < 0.05$
[a]The multivariable model includes all variables that showed a significant association with sustained DMARD-free remission in univariable Cox regression analyses. A total of 224 patients were included in the multivariable model since data on the tested variables were incomplete for 14 patients. No statistically significant differences were present between patients with missing data and the patient included in the multivariable model (data not shown)

Mediation analysis revealed that BME did not mediate the association between ACPA and DMARD-free sustained remission (Fig. 2).

Patterns of MRI-detected inflammation

Finally, we questioned whether a combination of features (covering the inflammatory features, the severity, and the location of MRI-detected inflammation), not a single inflammatory feature, was able to distinguish between patients who did and did not achieve DMARD-free sustained remission. Using PLS, two factors were identified that together explained 15.0% of the variance. When these factors were plotted against each other, no clear clusters were observed. Thus, no patterns of MRI-detected inflammation were identified that were associated with achieving DMARD-free remission (Fig. 3).

Discussion

Mechanisms underlying (the resolution of) the chronic nature of RA are scarcely understood. Moreover, there are few known predictors for DMARD-free sustained remission. Although MRI-detected inflammation, and osteitis in particular, is a potent predictor for erosive progression [8, 11, 13], this imaging marker was not predictive for DMARD-free sustained remission.

Table 3 Associations between MRI-detected inflammation and achieving DMARD-free sustained remission over time

Type of MRI-detected inflammation	Univariable model HR (95% CI)	Multivariable model 1[a] HR (95% CI)	Multivariable model 2[b] HR (95% CI)
BME	0.99 (0.94–1.03)	0.96 (0.99–1.02)	1.00 (0.94–1.07)
Synovitis	1.03 (0.97–1.09)	1.04 (0.95–1.15)	1.00 (0.90–1.10)
Tenosynovitis	1.04 (0.99–1.10)	1.03 (0.95–1.11)	1.01 (0.94–1.08)
Total inflammation	1.01 (0.99–1.03)	–	–

All HRs are per point increase of MRI-detected inflammation

BME bone marrow edema, *CI* confidence interval, *DMARD* disease-modifying antirheumatic drug, *HR* hazard ratio, *MRI* magnetic resonance imaging

[a]Multivariable model 1 includes MRI-detected BME, synovitis and tenosynovitis

[b]Multivariable model 2 includes MRI-detected BME, synovitis and tenosynovitis as well as ACPA

The absence of this association was surprising since ACPA has been associated with higher osteitis scores [14, 15] and less DMARD-free sustained remission [2]. Although our data showed an association between ACPA and osteitis, there was no association between osteitis and achieving DMARD-free sustained remission. Therefore, osteitis did not mediate the association of ACPA with DMARD-free sustained remission (Fig. 2).

Thus, the studied imaging predictors for erosive progression and RA chronicity differed. Previous studies on genetic factors also showed that, although *IL2RA* and *HLA-DRB1*-encoding shared epitope alleles were risk factors for both outcomes, the majority of genetic factors associated with erosive progression were not associated with RA persistence [26, 27]. Together, this suggests that pathophysiological mechanisms underlying erosive progression and RA persistence are different. Thus, our main hypothesis, namely that imaging predictors for both outcomes are similar, is likely unjust. So far, only the absence of autoantibodies and short symptom duration have been shown to be predictive for DMARD-free sustained remission. Besides these factors, there are probably other, yet unknown, host and environmental factors that play pivotal roles in processes underlying disease resolution.

This study evaluated MRI-detected inflammation at diagnosis in relation to achieving DMARD-free sustained remission over time. Thus, the hypothesis that was tested presumed that patients that achieved remission were already different in respect to joint inflammation in an early, DMARD-naive disease phase. Our study did not contain longitudinal MRI data. Although we previously observed that osteitis is often a persisting feature [6], we did not perform an MRI at the time of remission. Others observed, in DMARD-treated patients in DAS remission, that residual inflammation was present in the majority of patients (up to 96% for synovitis) [28–30]. The clinical relevance of residual inflammation is unclear, although it is suggested that its presence in patients that still receive DMARD treatment is associated with ongoing erosive progression [30]. While our

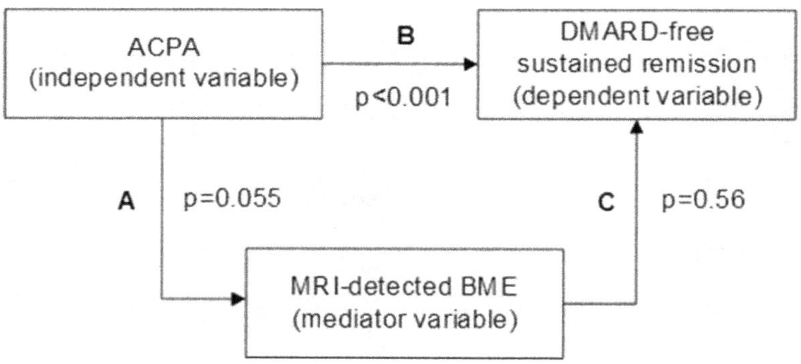

Fig. 2 Schematic overview of the causal path between ACPA and DMARD-free sustained remission that was studied using a mediation model as described by Baron and Kenny [25]. According to the Baron and Kenny model there are three requirements for a true mediation relationship. The first step is to regress the dependent variable on the independent variable to confirm that the independent variable is predictive for the dependent variable. In our data, the absence of anticitrullinated protein antibodies (ACPA) was indeed predictive for disease-modifying antirheumatic drug (DMARD)-free sustained remission (HR 0.16, $p < 0.001$). The second step is to regress the mediator variable on the independent variable to confirm that the independent variable is a predictor of the mediator. The association between ACPA and bone marrow edema (BME) was not statistically significant although there was a strong tendency towards significance ($\beta = 1.58$, $p = 0.055$). The final step would be to regress the dependent variable on both the mediator and independent variable to confirm that the mediator is a significant predictor of the dependent variable and the effect of the independent variable from the first step is greatly reduced. This was not the case (HR for ACPA corrected for BME 0.12, $p < 0.001$). As shown in Table 2, BME scores were not associated with DMARD-free sustained remission (HR 0.99, $p = 0.56$). Thus, this mediation analysis revealed that magnetic resonance imaging (MRI)-detected BME does not mediate the association of ACPA with not achieving DMARD-free sustained remission

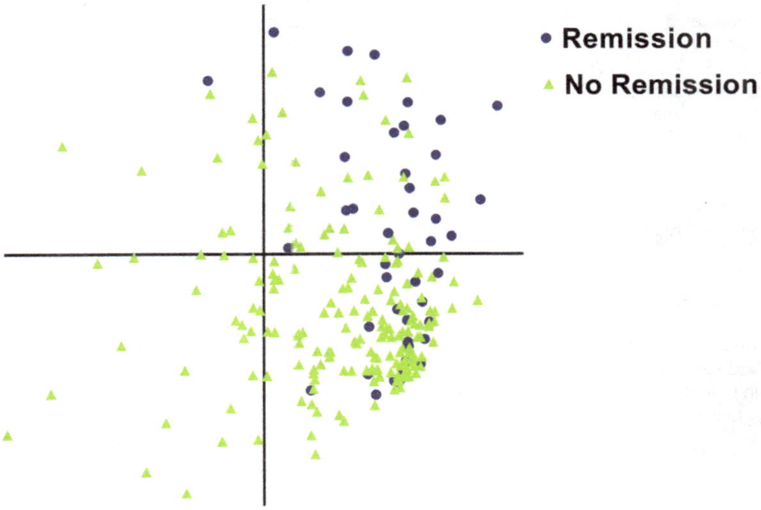

Fig. 3 A combination of MRI features (covering type, location, and severity of inflammation) did not cluster RA patients who did or did not achieve DMARD-free sustained remission over time. This figure depicts the results of a PLS regression analysis. Two factors were identified that together explained 15.0% of the explained variance between patients who did and did not achieve DMARD-free sustained remission over time. Individual patient scores on factor 1 (*y* axis) and factor 2 (*x* axis) are plotted against each other. The figure reveals that there is overlap, which means that there are no clear patterns of MRI-detected inflammation that discriminated between patients who did and did not achieve DMARD-free sustained remission

definition of remission was stricter than those used in the cited studies, we do not know whether MRI-detected synovitis is present in patients that achieved DMARD-free sustained remission. Low-grade synovitis has also been observed in symptom-free patients [10] and, as our defined status of sustained DMARD-free remission corresponds with normalized levels of function, fatigue, and pain [1, 3], it is questionable if remaining MRI-detected synovitis, if present after having achieved DMARD-free sustained remission, is clinically relevant.

Patients included in this study fulfilled either the 1987 and/or 2010 criteria for RA. If not used correctly, the 2010 criteria could lead to misclassification of patients with RA, thereby influencing the study results [31]. To prevent misclassification, the classification criteria were used as intended, namely only in patients with a clinical (suspected) diagnosis of RA. Furthermore, patients who never received DMARD therapy were excluded (Fig. 1). When analyses were repeated in patients fulfilling the 1987 criteria for RA (n = 186), results remained similar (data not shown).

However, this association was not significant in multivariable analysis was surprising as this was not observed in two previous studies [1, 2]. However, this association was significant in multivariable analysis. Since local inflammation measured by sensitive imaging was also not associated with DMARD-free remission, the overall conclusion is that the extent of local inflammation at first presentation is not related to the likelihood of achieving DMARD-free remission.

One limitation of our study is that, despite applying a stringent definition of remission where clinical synovitis had to be absent ≥ 1 year after DMARD cessation, the available follow-up might be insufficient to detect flares after several years of follow-up. Another limitation is the sample size; although large for an MRI study, it is unknown if results would have been different in an even larger dataset. However, there was not even a tendency towards an association between BME and remission.

A strength of this study is that the data were obtained in a center in which DAS-steered treatment regimens imply that in case of DAS < 2.4 DMARDs are tapered and subsequently stopped. This strategy contributed to the relative high percentage of patients (19%) that achieved DMARD-free sustained remission. Other studies with varying follow-up durations reported ranges of DMARD-free remission between 3.6% and 22% [4]. Nonetheless, despite local protocols, rheumatologists had the freedom not to taper medication in patients in DAS remission. Therefore, it is possible that the current percentage is an underestimation.

Conclusions

In conclusion, the presence of MRI-detected osteitis at the time of presentation with RA, although shown to be strongly predictive for erosive progression, was not associated with lower hazards on achieving DMARD-free sustained remission. Additionally, the current data demonstrate that MRI is not helpful in identifying patients who can achieve DMARD-free sustained remission over time. Finally, although acknowledging that the processes involved in joint damage are different from those mediating RA chronicity, the pathophysiology of the latter remains elusive.

Abbreviations
ACPA: Anticitrullinated protein antibodies; BME: Bone marrow edema; CI: Confidence interval; DAS: Disease activity score; DMARD: Disease-modifying antirheumatic drug; EAC: Early Arthritis Clinic; HR: Hazard ratio; IQR: Interquartile range; MCP: Metacarpophalangeal; MRI: Magnetic resonance imaging; MTP: Metatarsophalangeal; PLS: Partial least squares; RA: Rheumatoid arthritis; RAMRIS method: RA MRI scoring; SJC: Swollen joint count

Acknowledgements
The authors thank W.P. Nieuwenhuis and E.C. Newsum for scoring all MRIs used in this study.

Funding
This work was supported by a Vidi-grant of the Netherlands Organisation for Scientific Research and has received funding from the European Research Council (ERC) under the European Union's Horizon 2020 research and innovation programme (Starting grant, agreement No 714312).

Authors' contributions
All authors made contributions to conception of the study, were involved in revising the manuscript and gave final approval to the version to be published. LEB and AHMvdHvM designed the study, interpreted the data, and drafted the manuscript. LEB and DMB acquired the data. LEB analyzed the data. MR is a radiologist involved in the development of the MRI scanning protocol used in this study. All authors read and approved the final manuscript.

Competing interests
The authors declare that they have no competing interests.

Author details
[1]Department of Rheumatology, Leiden University Medical Center, C-01-046, PO Box 9600, 2300 RC Leiden, The Netherlands. [2]Department of Radiology, Leiden University Medical Center, Leiden, the Netherlands. [3]Department of Rheumatology, Erasmus Medical Center, Rotterdam, the Netherlands.

References
1. Ajeganova S, van Steenbergen HW, van Nies JAB, Burgers LE, Huizinga TWJ, van der Helm-van Mil AHM. Disease-modifying antirheumatic drug-free sustained remission in rheumatoid arthritis: an increasingly achievable outcome with subsidence of disease symptoms. Ann Rheum Dis. 2015; https://doi.org/10.1136/annrheumdis-2014-207080.
2. van der Woude D, Young A, Jayakumar K, Mertens BJ, Toes REM, van der Heijde D, et al. Prevalence of and predictive factors for sustained disease-modifying antirheumatic drug-free remission in rheumatoid arthritis: results from two large early arthritis cohorts. Arthritis Rheum. 2009;60:2262–71.
3. van Tuyl LH, Smolen JS, Wells GA, Scholte-Voshaar M, Hoogland W, Boers M. Patient perspective on remission in rheumatoid arthritis. J Rheumatol. 2011;38:1735–8.
4. Nagy G, van Vollenhoven RF. Sustained biologic-free and drug-free remission in rheumatoid arthritis, where are we now? Arthritis Res Ther. 2015;17:181.
5. van der Kooij SM, Goekoop-Ruiterman YPM, de Vries-Bouwstra JK, Güler-Yüksel M, Zwinderman AH, Kerstens PJSM, et al. Drug-free remission, functioning and radiographic damage after 4 years of response-driven treatment in patients with recent-onset rheumatoid arthritis. Ann Rheum Dis. 2009;68:914–21.
6. van Leeuwen MA, van der Heijde DM, van Rijswijk MH, Houtman PM, van Riel PL, van de Putte LB, et al. Interrelationship of outcome measures and process variables in early rheumatoid arthritis. A comparison of radiologic damage, physical disability, joint counts, and acute phase reactants. J Rheumatol. 1994;21:425–9.
7. Möttönen TT. Prediction of erosiveness and rate of development of new erosions in early rheumatoid arthritis. Ann Rheum Dis. 1988;47:648–53.
8. McQueen FM. Bone marrow edema and osteitis in rheumatoid arthritis: the imaging perspective. Arthritis Res Ther. 2012;14:224.
9. McQueen F, Lassere M, Østergaard M. Magnetic resonance imaging in psoriatic arthritis: a review of the literature. Arthritis Res Ther. 2006;8:207.
10. Mangnus L, van Steenbergen HW, Reijnierse M, van der Helm-van Mil AHM. Magnetic resonance imaging-detected features of inflammation and erosions in symptom-free persons from the general population. Arthritis Rheumatol. 2016;68:2593–602.
11. Nieuwenhuis WP, van Steenbergen HW, Stomp W, Stijnen T, Huizinga TWJ, Bloem JL, et al. The course of bone marrow edema in early undifferentiated and rheumatoid arthritis; a longitudinal MRI study on bone level. Arthritis Rheumatol. 2016;68(5):1080–8.
12. Krabben A, Stomp W, van Nies JAB, Huizinga TWJ, van der Heijde D, Bloem JL, et al. MRI-detected subclinical joint inflammation is associated with radiographic progression. Ann Rheum Dis. 2014;73:2034–7.
13. Bøyesen P, Haavardsholm EA, van der Heijde D, Østergaard M, Hammer HB, Sesseng S, et al. Prediction of MRI erosive progression: a comparison of modern imaging modalities in early rheumatoid arthritis patients. Ann Rheum Dis. 2011;70:176–9.
14. Boeters DM, Nieuwenhuis WP, Verheul MK, Newsum EC, Reijnierse M, Toes REM, et al. MRI-detected osteitis is not associated with the presence or level of ACPA alone, but with the combined presence of ACPA and RF. Arthritis Res Ther. 2016;18:179.
15. Tamai M, Kawakami A, Uetani M, Takao S, Tanaka F, Nakamura H, et al. The presence of anti-cyclic citrullinated peptide antibody is associated with magnetic resonance imaging detection of bone marrow oedema in early stage rheumatoid arthritis. Ann Rheum Dis. 2006;65:133–4.
16. Harre U, Georgess D, Bang H, Bozec A, Axmann R, Ossipova E, et al. Induction of osteoclastogenesis and bone loss by human autoantibodies against citrullinated vimentin. J Clin Invest. 2012;122:1791–802.
17. Dalbeth N, Smith T, Gray S, Doyle A, Antill P, Lobo M, et al. Cellular characterisation of magnetic resonance imaging bone oedema in rheumatoid arthritis; implications for pathogenesis of erosive disease. Ann Rheum Dis. 2009;68:279–82.
18. de Rooy DPC, van der Linden MPM, Knevel R, Huizinga TWJ, van der Helm-van Mil AHM. Predicting arthritis outcomes—what can be learned from the Leiden Early Arthritis Clinic? Rheumatology. 2011;50:93–100.
19. Bijlsma JWJ, Welsing PMJ, Woodworth TG, Middelink LM, Pethö-Schramm A, Bernasconi C, et al. Early rheumatoid arthritis treated with tocilizumab, methotrexate, or their combination (U-Act-Early): a multicentre, randomised, double-blind, double-dummy, strategy trial. Lancet. 2016;388:343–55.
20. Emery P, Bingham CO, Burmester GR, Bykerk VP, Furst DE, Mariette X, et al. Certolizumab pegol in combination with dose-optimised methotrexate in DMARD-naïve patients with early, active rheumatoid arthritis with poor prognostic factors: 1-year results from C-EARLY, a randomised, double-blind, placebo-controlled phase III study. Ann Rheum Dis. 2017;76:96–104.
21. Østergaard M, Edmonds J, McQueen F, Peterfy C, Lassere M, Ejbjerg B, et al. An introduction to the EULAR–OMERACT rheumatoid arthritis MRI reference image atlas. Ann Rheum Dis. 2005;64:i3–7.
22. Haavardsholm EA, Østergaard M, Ejbjerg BJ, Kvan NP, Kvien TK. Introduction of a novel magnetic resonance imaging tenosynovitis score for rheumatoid arthritis: reliability in a multireader longitudinal study. Ann Rheum Dis. 2007;66:1216–20.
23. van Steenbergen HW, Mangnus L, Reijnierse M, Huizinga TWJ, van der Helm-van Mil AHM. Clinical factors, anticitrullinated peptide antibodies and MRI-detected subclinical inflammation in relation to progression from clinically suspect arthralgia to arthritis. Ann Rheum Dis. 2016; https://doi.org/10.1136/annrheumdis-2015-208138.
24. Nieuwenhuis WP, Mangnus L, van Steenbergen HW, Newsum EC, Huizinga TWJ, Reijnierse M, et al. Older age is associated with more MRI-detected inflammation in hand and foot joints. Rheumatology (Oxford). 2016;55:2212–9.
25. Baron RM, Kenny DA. The moderator-mediator variable distinction in social psychological research: conceptual, strategic, and statistical considerations. J Pers Soc Psychol. 1986;51:1173–82.
26. Knevel R, de Rooy DPC, Zhernakova A, Gröndal G, Krabben A, Steinsson K, et al. Association of variants in IL2RA with progression of joint destruction in rheumatoid arthritis. Arthritis Rheum. 2013;65:1684–93.
27. van Steenbergen HW, van Nies JAB, Ruyssen-Witrand A, Huizinga TWJ, Cantagrel A, Berenbaum F, et al. IL2RA is associated with persistence of rheumatoid arthritis. Arthritis Res Ther. 2015;17:244.
28. Anandarajah A, Thiele R, Giampoli E, Monu J, Seo G-S, Feng C, et al. Patients with rheumatoid arthritis in clinical remission manifest persistent joint inflammation on histology and imaging studies. J Rheumatol. 2014;41:2153–60.

Fatigue independently predicts different work disability dimensions in etanercept-treated rheumatoid arthritis and ankylosing spondylitis patients

Katie L. Druce[1], Laraine Aikman[2], Maria Dilleen[3], Annie Burden[4], Piotr Szczypa[2] and Neil Basu[5,6,7*]

Abstract

Background: Work disability remains a significant problem in ankylosing spondylitis (AS) and rheumatoid arthritis (RA), despite biological therapy. This study aimed to test the hypothesis that the prevalent symptom of fatigue longitudinally predicts work disability among RA and AS patients commencing etanercept.

Methods: Two observational studies, comprising RA and AS etanercept commencers, respectively, were analysed. Both provided data on work disability over 1 year and a comprehensive set of putative predictors, including fatigue. A series of repeated measures models were conducted, including baseline variables, visit (6/12 months), and the interaction between visit and each of the explanatory variables.

Results: A total of 1003 AS and 1747 RA patients were assessed. For AS, fatigue was significantly associated with presenteeism (linear mixed model coefficient 3.75, 95% confidence interval (CI) 2.14 to 5.36) and activity impairment (2.62, 1.26 to 3.98), but not with work productivity loss (1.81, −0.40 to 4.02) or absenteeism (generalised linear mixed model odds ratio (OR) 1.18, 95% CI 0.92 to 1.51). In RA, fatigue was associated with presenteeism (coefficient 3.44, 95% CI 2.17 to 4.70), activity impairment (1.52, 0.79 to 2.26), work productivity loss (4.16, 2.47 to 5.85), and absenteeism (OR 1.23, 95% CI 1.02 to 1.49). The lack of significant interactions between fatigue and visit supported a consistent effect of baseline fatigue over time.

Conclusions: Among patients beginning etanercept therapy, fatigue has a significant and independent effect on absenteeism, presenteeism, productivity loss, and activity impairment for RA patients and a significant but dimension-selective effect on work disability among AS patients.

Keywords: Fatigue, Work disability, Rheumatoid arthritis, Spondyloarthritis

Background

Inflammatory rheumatic diseases, such as rheumatoid arthritis (RA) and ankylosing spondylitis (AS), are a substantial cause of work disability [1], a key outcome for both the patient and society. Estimates indicate that within 10 years of symptom onset up to 70% of patients become work disabled [2], rising to approximately 90% as disease duration increases [3].

Biological therapies have significantly minimised the physical sequelae of poorly controlled inflammation, such as joint destruction [4–6]. This in turn has been associated with an improvement in patient outcomes including those relating to work capacities [4–8]. Despite these gains, work disability remains an issue for the majority of RA and AS patients and it has become increasingly clear that the determinants of work disability

* Correspondence: neilbasu@abdn.ac.uk
[5]Epidemiology Group, School of Medicine, Medical Sciences and Nutrition, University of Aberdeen, Aberdeen, UK
[6]Aberdeen Centre for Arthritis and Musculoskeletal Health, University of Aberdeen, Aberdeen, UK
Full list of author information is available at the end of the article

in inflammatory diseases are not necessarily inflammatory in origin [9–11].

Fatigue, a patient priority inconsistently associated with inflammation [12], is possibly one such determinant. This symptom represents a persistent, unmanageable, and unpredictable issue [13–15] which is reported by up to 80% of patients with AS and RA. The impact of fatigue is multi-dimensional. For example, levels of physical activity are reduced and relationships are harmed [13, 14]. Yet the symptom is poorly managed, and many patients feel this subject is ignored by their clinicians. Subsequent attempts to self-manage by trial and error are typically unsuccessful [14, 16].

Anecdotally, patients have identified fatigue as a principal barrier to employment and productivity [13, 16]. The subsequent need to reduce work hours, relinquish roles, or even retire from work altogether have been attributed to the emotional, physical, and cognitive consequences of the symptom [3, 13, 16, 17]. However, the empirical evidence supporting these attributions is limited.

To date, analyses of the relationship between fatigue and work disability have generally examined cross-sectional data in small sample sizes [3, 18] and knowledge regarding the long-term nature of the relationship is sparse. Indeed, a previous systematic review of work disability predictors in RA surprisingly failed to identify any studies that have evaluated fatigue as a putative factor [19]. Furthermore, no study designs examining the impact of fatigue have employed a comprehensive measure of work disability which is necessary to adequately capture this complex multi-dimensional construct. To evaluate the different components, which include presenteeism (reduced performance at work due to ill health) and productivity in addition to the traditionally applied measure of absenteeism, suitably designed and detailed tools should be applied [20]. Finally, to our knowledge, no investigation has compared the fatigue-work disability relationship between distinct rheumatic disorders.

We have previously observed that patients commonly report continuing high levels of fatigue despite successfully attaining clinical remission (Disease Activity Score (DAS28) < 2.6) 6 months after commencing biologic therapy [21]. We now hypothesise that, in this current era of biological therapies, fatigue is independently associated with continuing levels of work disability among patients with inflammatory rheumatic diseases. Specifically, this study aimed to examine whether fatigue independently predicts different work disability dimensions, adjusting for clinical and psychosocial factors, over 1 year in working patient populations commencing etanercept, a commonly prescribed biologic. Furthermore, we obtained data from two near-identical studies on AS and RA to compare the relative impact of fatigue on work disability between these two common, but pathologically distinct, inflammatory rheumatic diseases.

Methods

Data were obtained from 6518 patients recruited to one of two observational studies on patients with clinician-confirmed AS ($n = 1663$; clinical study number NCT00544557) or RA ($n = 4855$; clinical study number NCT00488475) who were commencing etanercept as part of routine clinical practice in Germany. Ethical approval for the original studies was obtained from the Ethics Committee of the State Chamber of Physicians (Landesaertzekammer; NCT00544557, 21 September 2007; NCT00488475, 15 September 2006).

Both cohorts were followed-up for 1 year. Data collected at baseline, 6 months, and 1 year contributed to this study. Of the variables captured, data obtained for these analyses comprised fatigue, work disability, demographics, clinical, and psychosocial status.

Fatigue

Fatigue was measured using visual analogue scales (VAS) anchored from 'no fatigue' to 'worst possible fatigue'. Although limited to providing a global assessment of fatigue, VAS have been extensively used and validated across most of the rheumatic disease spectrum. In the AS cohort, the VAS was extracted from the self-reported Bath Ankylosing Spondylitis Disease Activity Index (BASDAI) questionnaire and was thus scored 0–10 cm. In the RA cohort, the VAS was originally scored 0–100 mm but was converted into a 0–10 cm scale to facilitate comparability.

Work disability

Work disability was measured using the six-item self-report Work Productivity and Activity Impairment—Special Health Problems (WPAI:SHP). The WPAI:SHP assesses the impact of the participant's condition on work and daily activities for the past 7 days. The WPAI:SHP has been validated for use in both AS [22] and RA [23], and can be modified for any health problem by specifying the disease/condition of interest in the questions.

The questionnaire comprises four subscales: absenteeism, presenteeism, overall work impairment (absenteeism plus presenteeism), and daily activity impairment. Scores are transformed into impairment percentages ranging from 0 to 100%, with high scores indicating greater impairment and reduced productivity.

The absenteeism subscale was heavily skewed, with over 80% of patients reporting no absenteeism. This variable was therefore dichotomised (as 0 or > 0) for the analysis; all other subscales were treated as continuous variables.

Demographics

Of the information captured at baseline, participant age, sex, and current working status (currently employed or not) were of interest.

Clinical status

Physicians assessed disease activity using an 11-point Likert scale, from 0 'no disease activity' to 10 'high disease activity' in the AS cohort, and a 0–100 mm VAS from 0 mm 'no disease activity' to 100 mm 'maximum possible disease activity' in the RA cohort. C-reactive protein (CRP) was measured from blood samples taken at baseline.

Psychosocial status

Self-reported pain and anxiety/depression were considered potential confounders. Pain was recorded by an 11-point Likert scale, from 0 'least possible pain' to 10 'worst possible pain' in the AS cohort, and by a 0–100 mm VAS from 0 mm 'minimum possible pain' to 100 mm 'maximum possible pain' in the RA cohort. Anxiety/depression was recorded using the anxiety and depression field of the European Quality of Life 5 Dimensions (EQ-5D) questionnaire. The EQ-5D has been validated for use in RA and AS populations [24, 25] and has three possible ordinal outcomes: no problems, some problems, and extreme problems.

Analysis

In those participants who were employed at baseline (irrespective of proportion of work impairment due to absenteeism), repeated measures models (repeated by visit within subject) using a compound symmetry covariance structure were used to investigate the longitudinal relationship between each work disability score at 6 and/or 12 months and baseline fatigue. For absenteeism (dichotomised as 0 or >0), a generalised linear mixed model was used with binomial distribution and logit link, while a linear mixed model was used for the remaining subscales.

Initial models included baseline fatigue and other potential baseline predictors as explanatory variables, visit (6/12 months), and the interaction between visit and each of the explanatory variables. The model was then manually stepwise reduced, removing the most non-significant interactions at each step and then the most non-significant main effects (unless there was a significant interaction with visit, in which case the main effect was retained to allow the total effect at each visit to be quantified). A nominal 5% level of significance was used, but terms were retained at the 10% level if they modified the fatigue effect.

All continuous variables included in the models were standardised to aid non-statistical comparison between the diseases. Such that the resultant regression coefficients should be interpreted as the number of standard deviations the dependent variable would change per one standard deviation increase in the predictor.

All analyses were carried out using SAS© version 9.3.

Results

Of 1663 AS patients, 1003 (60%) were working at baseline and could be included in this analysis. The majority (63%, $n = 635$) were male, with a mean age of 40.7 years (standard deviation 10.6). Of 4855 RA patients, 1747 (36%) were working at baseline and were eligible for this analysis. Just under three-quarters (72%) were female, with a mean age of 47.3 years (9.9) (Table 1).

Apart from the expected greater proportion of male AS versus RA patients, the cohorts were comparable at baseline. No relevant differences in clinical, psychosocial, or work disability domains were observed.

Fatigue as a predictor of work and activity impairment in AS

Of the variables entered into the model, only baseline absenteeism (odds ratio (OR) 4.59, 95% confidence interval (CI) 2.91 to 7.25) and having some, versus no, problems with anxiety or depression (OR 1.77, 95% CI 1.12 to 2.80) were associated with a statistically significant increase in the odds of absenteeism at 6 and 12 months (Table 2). Although fatigue at baseline was associated with a small increase in the odds of absenteeism, the result was not significant (OR 1.18, 95% CI 0.92 to 1.51).

Fatigue at baseline was a statistically significant predictor of presenteeism at 6 and 12 months (standardized beta co-efficient (β) 3.75, 95% CI 2.14 to 5.36) unit increase in impairment. Age (β 4.48, 95% CI 3.07 to 5.89) and presenteeism at baseline (β:6.25, 95% CI 4.67 to 7.82) were also associated with a statistically significant increase in presenteeism. Being male was associated with reduced impairment of presenteeism over time (β −4.65, 95% CI −7.62 to −1.68) as was baseline CRP level (β −1.83, 95% CI −3.53 to −0.13).

Increased work productivity loss over time was predicted by age (β 5.22, 95% CI 3.52 to 6.93) and work productivity loss at baseline (β 6.62, 95% CI 4.53 to 8.71), as well as having some (β 3.76, 95% CI 0.09 to 7.42) or extreme (β 12.32, 95% CI 1.38 to 23.26) problems with anxiety or depression, compared with no problems. Fatigue at baseline was not associated with work productivity loss (β 1.81, 95% CI −0.40 to 4.02) and, although pain was at 6 months (β 2.77, 95% CI 0.34 to 5.20), the significant interaction between visit and pain score at baseline suggests a negligible effect of baseline pain by 12 months.

Table 1 Baseline characteristics of the 1003 AS patients and 1747 RA patients who were working at baseline

Parameter		AS	*n*	RA	*n*
Age (years), mean (SD)		40.7 (10.6)	1003	47.3 (9.9)	1747
Female, %		36.7	1003	72.4	1747
Disease duration (years), mean (SD)		7.3 (7.8)	979	7.9 (7.6)	1654
Disease activity	0–10 Likert, mean (SD)	6.3 (1.7)	1000	–	
	0–100 mm VAS, mean (SD)	–		59.1 (18.0)	1724
CRP (mg/dL), median (min, max)		1.0 (0.0, 42.7)	906	0.9 (0.0, 20.0)	1534
Fatigue	0–10 cm VAS, mean (SD)	5.6 (2.4)	997	–	
	0–100 mm VAS, mean (SD)	–		57.4 (24.9)	1735
Pain	0–10 Likert, mean (SD)	6.3 (2.2)	990	–	
	0–100 mm VAS, mean (SD)	–		61.6 (21.4)	1736
Anxiety/depression (EQ-5D)	No problems, %	53.6	998	52.1	1738
	Some problems, %	42.7		44.4	
	Extreme problems, %	3.7		3.6	
WPAI:SHP					
% work time missed due to AS/RA[a]	No timed missed	61.9	776	61.3	1293
	Some time missed	38.1		38.7	
% impairment while working due to AS/RA[b], mean (SD)		48.3 (26.9)	889	49.5 (27.1)	1530
% overall work impairment due to AS/RA[c], mean (SD)		52.9 (29.8)	716	54.1 (29.0)	1171
% activity impairment due to AS/RA[d], mean (SD)		53.4 (24.6)	990	54.0 (24.9)	1718

[a]Absenteeism
[b]Presenteeism
[c]Work productivity loss
[d]Activity impairment
AS, ankylosing spondylitis; CRP, C-reactive protein; EQ-5D, European Quality of Life 5 Dimensions; RA, rheumatoid arthritis; SD, standard deviation; VAS, visual analogue scale; WPAI:SHP, Work Productivity and Activity Impairment—Special Health Problems

Finally, increased activity impairment during the course of the study was associated with age (β 5.07, 95% CI 3.96 to 6.19), having some (β 3.27, 95% CI 0.85 to 5.68) or extreme (β 10.74, 95% CI 5.35 to 16.14) problems with anxiety or depression compared with no problems, having increased fatigue at baseline (β 2.62, 95% CI 1.26 to 3.98), and higher impairment at baseline (β 8.51, 95% CI 7.14 to 9.87). Higher baseline inflammation, as measured by CRP, was associated with a reduction in activity impairment at 6 and 12 months (β −2.76, 95% CI −3.85 to −1.67).

Fatigue as a predictor of work and activity impairment in RA

In patients with RA, the likelihood of absenteeism at 6 and 12 months was significantly higher in those with more fatigue at baseline (OR 1.23, 95% CI 1.02 to 1.49), who were older (OR 1.20, 1.00 to 1.44), and who reported absenteeism at baseline (OR 4.75, 3.35 to 6.75). Greater inflammation at baseline was associated with a decreased likelihood of reporting absenteeism over the course of the study (OR 0.82, 95% CI 0.68 to 0.98) (Table 3).

Increased presenteeism over time was significantly predicted by baseline fatigue (β 3.44, 95% CI 2.17 to 4.71) and age (β 1.44, 95% CI 0.26 to 2.63). Presenteeism at baseline was associated with a statistically significant increase in presenteeism at 6 and 12 months (Table 3).

Of all the putative predictors entered into the models, only fatigue (β 4.16, 95% CI 2.47 to 5.85) and baseline work productivity loss (β 9.43, 95% CI 7.74 to 11.12) were associated with increased work productivity loss over time. Increased activity impairment at 6 and 12 months was significantly associated with fatigue (β 1.52, 95% CI 0.79 to 2.26), older age (β 3.25, 95% CI 2.61 to 3.90), and having some (β 2.80, 95% CI 1.40 to 4.20) or extreme (β 5.81, 95% CI 2.82 to 8.79) problems with anxiety or depression, compared with no problems. Baseline activity impairment was associated with greater impairment over time (β 9.41, 95% CI 8.59 to 10.23 at 6 months), but the significant interaction between baseline activity impairment and visit suggested a reduced effect was present by 12 months.

Comparison of fatigue as a predictor of work disability between RA and AS

The most consistent predictive factor for both populations was the baseline level of the predicted work outcome. Otherwise, although overall fatigue was a commonly

Table 2 Baseline variables predictive of WPAI:SHP subscales at 6 and 12 months in 1003 AS patients

Predictor		Odds ratio (95% CI)
Outcome: absenteeism		
Fatigue		1.18 (0.92 to 1.51)
% work time missed due to AS (> 0 vs 0)		4.59 (2.91 to 7.25)
Anxiety/depression	Some vs none	1.77 (1.12 to 2.80)
	Extreme vs none	0.87 (0.26 to 2.86)
	Extreme vs some	0.49 (0.15 to 1.57)
Visit 12 months vs 6 months		1.001 (0.70 to 1.44)
Predictor		Standardized beta-coefficient (β) (95% CI)
Outcome: presenteeism		
Fatigue		3.75 (2.14 to 5.36)
Male vs female		−4.65 (−7.62 to −1.68)
Age (years)		4.48 (3.07 to 5.89)
CRP		−1.83 (−3.53 to −0.13)
% impairment while working due to AS		6.25 (4.67 to 7.82)
Visit 12 months vs 6 months		−0.99 (−2.57 to 0.60)
Outcome: Work productivity loss		
Fatigue		1.81 (−0.40 to 4.02)
Male vs female		−3.57 (−7.29 to 0.15)
Age (years)		5.22 (3.52 to 6.93)
Pain		2.77 (0.34 to 5.20)
Pain at 12 months vs pain at 6 months		−2.49 (−4.49 to −0.49)
% overall work impairment due to AS		6.62 (4.53 to 8.71)
Anxiety/depression	Some vs none	3.76 (0.09 to 7.42)
	Extreme vs none	12.32 (1.38 to 23.26)
Visit 12 months vs 6 months		−1.42 (−3.42 to 0.59)
Outcome: Activity impairment		
Fatigue		2.62 (1.26 to 3.98)
Age (years)		5.07 (3.96 to 6.19)
CRP		−2.76 (−3.85 to −1.67)
% activity impairment due to AS		8.51 (7.14 to 9.87)
Anxiety/depression	Some vs none	3.27 (0.85 to 5.68)
	Extreme vs none	10.74 (5.35 to 16.14)
Visit 12 months vs 6 months		−1.10 (−2.35 to 0.15)

AS, ankylosing spondylitis; CI, confidence interval; CRP, C-reactive protein; RA, rheumatoid arthritis; VAS, visual analogue scale; WPAI:SHP, Work Productivity and Activity Impairment—Special Health Problems

identified independently significant predictor of work disability in both RA and AS patients, its effect appears more prominent among RA patients in relation to other putative predictors while, in AS patients, the effect of anxiety/depression was relatively stronger. In contrast, other variables such as disease activity and pain did not appear to be important in these study samples.

When considering the associations between fatigue and the different work disability components, both similarities and differences existed across RA and AS patients. For both diseases, fatigue was associated with presenteeism (AS: β 3.75, 95% CI 2.14 to 5.36; RA: β 3.44, 95% CI 2.17 to 4.71) and activity impairment (AS: β 2.62, 95% CI 1.26 to 3.98; RA: β 1.52, 95% CI 0.79 to 2.26). However, fatigue was identified as a significant predictor of all four work disability components under investigation in our RA population, while fatigue was not identified as an independent predictor of absenteeism or work productivity loss among AS patients. In both studies, no interactions between fatigue and

Table 3 Baseline variables predictive of WPAI:SHP subscales at 6 and 12 months in 1747 RA patients

Predictor		Odds ratio (95% CI)
Outcome: absenteeism		
Fatigue		1.23 (1.02 to 1.49)
Age (years)		1.20 (1.00 to 1.44)
CRP		0.82 (0.68 to 0.98)
% work time missed due to RA (> 0 vs 0)		4.75 (3.35 to 6.75)
Visit 12 months vs 6 months		1.10 (0.83 to 1.46)
Predictor		Standardized beta-coefficient (β) (95% CI)
Outcome: presenteeism		
Fatigue		3.44 (2.17 to 4.71)
Age (years)		1.44 (0.26 to 2.63)
% impairment while working due to RA		9.36 (7.96 to 10.76)
% impairment at 12 months vs % impairment at 6 months		−1.98 (−3.39 to −0.58)
Visit 12 months vs 6 months		−1.16 (−2.57 to 0.24)
Outcome: Work productivity loss		
Fatigue		4.16 (2.47 to 5.85)
% overall work impairment due to RA		9.43 (7.74 to 11.12)
Visit 12 months vs 6 months		−0.60 (−2.64 to 1.44)
Outcome: Activity impairment		
Fatigue		1.52 (0.79 to 2.26)
Male vs female		−1.83 (−3.33 to −0.33)
Age (years)		3.25 (2.61 to 3.90)
% activity impairment due to RA		9.41 (8.59 to 10.23)
% activity impairment at 12 months vs % activity impairment at 6 months		−1.92 (−2.67 to −1.18)
Anxiety/depression	Some vs none	2.80 (1.40 to 4.20)
	Extreme vs none	5.81 (2.82 to 8.79)
Visit 12 months vs 6 months		−2.36 (−3.10 to −1.61)

CI, confidence interval; CRP, C-reactive protein; RA, rheumatoid arthritis; WPAI:SHP, Work Productivity and Activity Impairment—Special Health Problems

visit were significant, suggesting a consistent effect of fatigue over the following 12-month period.

Discussion

In this large study, fatigue had a significant and independent effect on all work disability dimensions at 6 and 12 months for patients with RA commencing etanercept. For AS patients who commenced etanercept, fatigue was identified as having a significant effect on presenteeism and overall activity impairment only. Across both studies, the lack of significant interactions between fatigue and visit suggests a consistent effect of baseline fatigue over the following 12-month period.

This study adds to the growing body of evidence highlighting the great importance of this previously ignored symptom among patients with inflammatory rheumatic diseases, and particularly emphasizes the economic impact of fatigue for both the individual and society as a whole. The existence of this relationship in the context of expensive biological treatment serves to enhance the economic issues further—despite their prescription, work disability remains an issue. The data presented herein support the case for targeting fatigue in parallel (employing, for example, non-pharmacological approaches) with a view to optimizing work-related outcomes and so providing even greater societal returns to the considerable pharmacological investments that global health systems have made in recent years. Furthermore, the study uniquely indicates that fatigue is importantly associated with work disability across two disparate disease populations, although the apparent differential effect on work disability dimensions should encourage some consideration of disease-specific issues during the development of appropriate interventions.

The few previous studies to quantitatively examine the relationship between RA and AS fatigue and work disability have been mostly cross-sectional and have all reported a significant association between these two factors [3, 18, 26, 27]. Of the longitudinal assessments, Zirkzee and colleagues found fatigue to be only weakly associated ($p = .131$) with deteriorating work status at 1 year among a small, likely underpowered, sample ($n = 69$) of Dutch patients newly diagnosed with inflammatory arthritis [28]. Similarly, fatigue was identified as a significant univariable, but not multivariable, predictor of receiving a work disability pension in a Norwegian study ($n = 159$) that aimed long-term work disability (the follow-up time point was 7 years) [29]. However, for patients, the predictors of shorter-term work disability are likely to be more informative in the context of preventative intervention development. Such future therapies may rescue patients from more immediate personal financial concerns related to their employment.

Pre-existing deficiencies in work disability measures were consistently the strongest predictors of the same outcome at 1 year. While this is intuitive, more surprising was the absence of independent associations between disease activity or pain and work disability.

This observation may reflect the success of biological therapies in targeting these factors during the follow-up of these cohorts and subsequently attenuating any association. Although fatigue may also be a mediator of the relationship between pain or disease activity and work disability, it is also plausible that no strong relationship may actually exist between these variables. Certainly, a previous systematic review only reported inconsistent evidence for a relationship between these traditional clinical factors [19].

In keeping with a previous report [30], we have shown that levels of fatigue and work disability are comparable between RA and AS working age populations. However, in this study, fatigue appears to differentially impact the domains of work impairment in RA and AS. One possible explanation for this difference may be the (expected) higher prevalence of males within the AS cohort. Work disability has previously been found to be dependent on the work status of the spouse [9], i.e. those married to a working partner are more likely to reduce/stop their own work when compromised by disease. In many cultures, including in Germany, it remains common for males to adopt the traditional role as the principal economic provider for the family unit. Thus, the threshold for work disability in response to fatigue could be higher as a result of their greater financial responsibilities. Another explanation is that the impact of fatigue may be greater for females compared with males. In rheumatic disease, fatigue is consistently reported to be greater among females for reasons as yet undetermined [31]. Finally, the nature of fatigue (and subsequent impact) may be distinct between AS and RA resulting from separate pathways.

Certainly, in terms of developing preventative interventions, the differential impact of fatigue as well as the more prominent association between anxiety/depression and work disability for AS compared with RA patients supports the delivery of disease-specific rather than generic interventions to prevent work disability.

A number of potential limitations should be considered when interpreting these results. Firstly, participants were new commencers of biological therapies and so were not representative of all AS and RA patients. The majority of RA and AS patients do not receive biological therapies [32, 33]. Such patients are typically characterised by high levels of disease activity and past disease-modifying anti-rheumatic drug failure. Data from both the German and UK biologics registers, which also recruit disease controls, indicate that RA patients not receiving biologicals are demographically similar, but AS patients tend to be younger [34–36]. Although it is possible that these results may not be generalisable, the population frame (which enables the selection of those patients with significant work disability despite a trial of biological therapy) is ideal to help us elucidate those determinants of work disability that are not necessarily fully related to inflammation (such as fatigue). We also acknowledge that generalisability of our identified associations may be influenced by cultural differences. For example, attitudes towards work [37], resilience factors [38], and availability of social security [26] support may influence the levels of work disability and all may vary between countries (although this may not necessarily confound the relationship with fatigue).

Secondly, in the absence of a control group, we cannot quantify the effect of etanercept on either fatigue or work productivity. Nevertheless, additional analyses showed that, among those still taking etanercept at 12 months (RA $n = 1091$, AS $n = 689$), average reductions of 20% were seen in presenteeism, work productivity loss, and activity impairment in both cohorts while absenteeism reduced by an average of 8–15% in RA and AS, respectively (data not shown).

Furthermore, work impairment is likely multifactorial in origin. While we were able to access data on a number of factors which are commonly implicated with this outcome, a number of other potentially interesting variables, for example sleep disturbance, co-medications, and disease severity, were not captured by the study and could not be incorporated into this analysis. Thirdly, given the observational design of this study, causality cannot be inferred although it seems quite possible given what we already know from patient reports. Finally, the psychosocial measures available to us for this secondary analysis provided only non-specific global measures of the underlying constructs of interest. For example, the EQ-5D does not enable the relative contributions of anxiety and depression to be separately determined.

Similarly, we acknowledge that our use of a VAS to capture fatigue may not have fully captured this complex construct relative to multi-dimensional measures, such as the Bristol Rheumatoid Arthritis Fatigue Multi-Dimensional Questionnaire (BRAF MDQ) or Chalder Fatigue Questionnaire (CFQ) [39]. Fatigue VAS scales are, however, considered suitable for use for those seeking to obtain a global measurement of fatigue, and are sensitive to change and are commonly used, aiding comparison with other diseases [39].

Future studies should seek to validate these finding using different fatigue instruments in different sampling frames. The development of interventions to reduce work disability among patients with arthritis is a key priority for patients and researchers alike. The targets for such interventions are likely to be multiple, but this study provides evidence that fatigue-specific measures should be a key component in the development of any future interventions. Existing evidence supports the efficacy of non-pharmacological interventions such as exercise and cognitive behavioural therapies for fatigue in the context of inflammatory rheumatic diseases [40]. A better understanding of the biology of fatigue will be important for the development of alternative therapies in the future.

Conclusions

This is the largest study to examine the longitudinal association between fatigue and work impairment and, by selecting two cohorts which underwent near-identical interventions and data collection procedures, the first to enable the comparison of this relationship between two different rheumatic diseases. We have demonstrated that, among patients beginning etanercept therapy, fatigue has a significant effect on the absenteeism, presenteeism, productivity loss, and activity impairment of patients with RA, and a significant but dimension-selective effect on work disability among AS patients. In addition to pharmacological treatment of inflammation, fatigue-alleviating interventions such as cognitive behavioural therapy and exercise should be tested in both RA and AS patients with a view to modifying the course of this crucial outcome.

Abbreviations

AS: Ankylosing spondylitis; BASDAI: Bath Ankylosing Spondylitis Disease Activity Index; BRAF MDQ: Bristol Rheumatoid Arthritis Fatigue Multi-Dimensional Questionnaire; CFQ: Chalder Fatigue Questionnaire; CI: Confidence interval; CRP: C-reactive protein; DAS28: Disease Activity Score for 28 joints; EQ-5D: European Quality of Life 5 Dimensions; OR: Odds ratio; RA: Rheumatoid arthritis; VAS: Visual analogue scales; WPAI:SHP: Work Productivity and Activity Impairment—Special Health Problems

Acknowledgements

Assistance with proofreading the manuscript and journal formatting was provided by Paul Oakley of Engage Scientific and was funded by Pfizer. The authors would like to thank Dr. Joachim Sieper. The authors would also like to thank all of the German investigators who contributed to data collection.

Funding

This study was supported by Pfizer. The sponsor was involved in the study design, collection, analysis, and interpretation of data, as well as revising the manuscript for intellectual content.

Availability of data and materials

Pfizer's policies on the provision of clinical trial data are set out on our website: http://www.pfizer.com/research/clinical_trials/trial_data_and_results.
In addition to posting clinical trial results on the clinicaltrials.gov registry, Pfizer provides secure access to anonymized patient-level data to qualified researchers in response to scientifically valid research proposals. Further details can be found at:
http://www.pfizer.com/research/clinical_trials/trial_data_and_results/data_requests.
Data from Pfizer-sponsored global interventional clinical studies are available from:
• Trials conducted for medicines, vaccines, and medical devices for indications that have been approved in the US and/or EU.
• Trials conducted for medicines, vaccines, and medical devices that have been terminated (i.e. development for all indications has been discontinued).
Data from these trials will be made available 24 months after study completion.
Pfizer's practices adhere to the principles for responsible data sharing laid out by the European Federation of Pharmaceutical Industries and Associations (EFPIA) and the Pharmaceutical Research and Manufacturers of America (PhRMA; http://phrma.org/sites/default/files/pdf/PhRMAPrinciplesForResponsibleClinicalTrialDataSharing.pdf

Authors' contributions

All authors (KLD, LA, MD, AB, PS, and NB) contributed substantially to the conception of the work and interpretation of the data. AB was responsible for conducting the statistical analysis. KLD was responsible for drafting the original version of the manuscript, which all other authors (LA, MD, AB, PS, and NB) revised critically. All authors (KLD, LA, MD, AB, PS, and NB) approved the final version of the document to be published and agree to be accountable for all aspects of the work in ensuring that questions related to the accuracy or integrity of any part of the work are appropriately investigated and resolved.

Competing interests

NB has received research funding and lecture fees from Pfizer. MD, LA, and PS are employees of Pfizer and hold company stock or shares. AB is an employee of Quanticate and is a paid contractor to Pfizer. KLD declares that she has no competing interests.

Author details

[1]Arthritis Research UK Centre for Epidemiology, Faculty of Biology Medicine and Health, the University of Manchester, Manchester M13 9PT, UK. [2]Medical Affairs, Pfizer, Sandwich, UK. [3]Statistics, Global Product Development, Pfizer, Sandwich, UK. [4]Quanticate, Hitchin, UK. [5]Epidemiology Group, School of Medicine, Medical Sciences and Nutrition, University of Aberdeen, Aberdeen, UK. [6]Aberdeen Centre for Arthritis and Musculoskeletal Health, University of Aberdeen, Aberdeen, UK. [7]Arthritis Research UK/MRC Centre for Musculoskeletal Health and Work, University of Aberdeen, Aberdeen, UK.

References

1. Mau W, Listing J, Huscher D, Seidler H, Zink A. Employment across chronic inflammatory rheumatic diseases and comparison with the general population. J Rheumatol. 2005;32(4):721–8.

2. Verstappen SMM. Rheumatoid arthritis and work: the impact of rheumatoid arthritis on absenteeism and presenteeism. Best Pract Res Clin Rheumatol. 2015;29(3):495–511.
3. Barlow JH, Wright CC, WIlliams B, Keat A. Work disability among people with ankylosing spondylitis. Arthtitis Care & Research. 2001;45(5):424–9.
4. Hoving JL, Bartelds GM, Sluiter JK, Sadiraj K, Groot I, Lems WF, et al. Perceived work ability, quality of life, and fatigue in patients with rheumatoid arthritis after a 6-month course of TNF inhibitors: prospective intervention study and partial economic evaluation. Scandanavian. J Rheumatol. 2009;38(4):246–50.
5. Hazes JM, Taylor P, Strand V, Purcaru O, Coteur G, Mease P. Physical function improvements and relief from fatigue and pain are associated with increased productivity at work and at home in rheumatoid arthritis patients treated with certolizumab pegol. Rheumatology. 2010;49(10):1900–10.
6. Keat AC, Gaffney K, Gilbert AK, Harris C, Leeder J. Influence of biologic therapy on return to work in people with work disability due to ankylosing spondylitis. Rheumatology. 2008;47(4):481–3.
7. Yelin EH, Trupin L, Katz P, Lubeck D, Rush S, Wanke L. Association between etanercept use and employment outcomes among patients with rheumatoid arthritis. Arthritis & Rheumatology. 2003;48(11):3046–54.
8. ter Wee MM, Lems WF, Usan H, Gulpen A, Boonen A. The effect of biological agents on work participation in rheumatoid arthritis patients: a systematic review. Ann Rheum Dis. 2012;71(2):161–71.
9. Verstappen SMM, Bijlsma JWJ, Verkleij H, Buskens E, Blaauw AAM, Ter Borg EJ, et al. Overview of work disability in rheumatoid arthritis patients as observed in cross-sectional and longitudinal surveys. Arthritis Care & Research. 2004;51(3):488–97.
10. Martindale J, Shukla R, Goodacre J. The impact of ankylosing spondylitis/axial spondyloarthritis on work productivity. Best Pract Res Clin Rheumatol. 2015;29(3):512–23.
11. National Rheumatoid Arthritis Society N. 'I Want to Work' Survey. 2014. https://www.nras.org.uk/data/files/Publications/I%20want%20to%20work%20survey%202007.pdf.
12. Druce KL, Basu N. Fatigue in rheumatology: what can we target for treatment? International Journal of Rheumatology. 2014;9:574–49.
13. Mancuso CA, Paget SA, Charlson ME. Adaptations made by rheumatoid arthritis patients to continue working: a pilot study of workplace challenges and successful adaptations. Arthritis Care & Research. 2000;13(2):89–99.
14. Hewlett S, Cockshott Z, Byron M, Kitchen K, Tipler S, Pope D, et al. Patients' perceptions of fatigue in rheumatoid arthritis: overwhelming, uncontrollable, ignored. Arthritis Care & Research. 2005;53(5):697–702.
15. Mengshoel AM. Life strain-related tiredness and illness-related fatigue in individuals with ankylosing spondylitis. Arthritis Care & Research. 2010;62(9):1272–7.
16. Connolly D, Fitzpatrick C, O'Toole L, Doran M, O'Shea F. Impact of fatigue in rheumatic diseases in the work environment: a qualitative study. Int J Environ Res Public Health. 2015;12(11):13807–22.
17. Repping-Wuts H, Uitterhoeve R, Van Riel P, van Achterberg T. Fatigue as experienced by patients with rheumatoid arthritis (RA): a qualitative study. Int J Nurs Stud. 2008;45(7):995–1002.
18. Chung CP, Sokka T, Arbogast PG, Pincus T. Work disability in early rheumatoid arthritis: higher rates but better clinical status in Finland compared with the US. Ann Rheum Dis. 2017;65(12):1653–7.
19. de Croon EM, Sluiter JK, Nijssen TF, Dijkmans BAC, Lankhorst GJ, Frings-Dresen MHW. Predictive factors of work disability in rheumatoid arthritis: a systematic literature review. Ann Rheum Dis. 2004;63:1362–7.
20. Institute of Medicine and National Research Council (Council IoMaNR). Survey Measurement of Work Disability: Summary of a Workshop. Washington, DC: The National Academies Press; 2000.
21. Druce KL, Bhattacharya Y, Jones GT, Macfarlane GJ, Basu N. Most patients who reach disease remission following anti-TNF therapy continue to report fatigue: results from the British Society for Rheumatology Biologics Register for Rheumatoid Arthritis. Rheumatology. 2016;55(10):1786–90.
22. Reilly MC, Gooch KL, Wong RL, Kupper H, van der Heijde D. Validity, reliability and responsiveness of the Work Productivity and Activity Impairment Questionnaire in ankylosing spondylitis. Rheumatology. 2010; 49(4):812–9.
23. Tang K, Beaton DE, Boonen A, Gignac MA, Bombardier C. Measures of Work Disability and Productivity: Rheumatoid Arthritis Specific Work Productivity Survey (WPS-RA), Workplace Activity Limitations Scale (WALS), Work Instability Scale for Rheumatoid Arthritis (RA-WIS), Work Limitations Questionnaire (WLQ), and Work Productivity and Activity Impairment Questionnaire (WPAI). Arthritis Care & Research. 2011;63(S11):S337–49.
24. Hurst NP, Kind P, Ruta D, Hunter M, Stubbings A. Measuring health-related quality of life in rheumatoid arthritis: validity, responsiveness and reliability of EuroQol (EQ-5D). Rheumatology. 1997;36(5):551–9.
25. Haywood KL, Garratt AM, Dziedzic K, Dawes PT. Generic measures of health-related quality of life in ankylosing spondylitis: reliability, validity and responsiveness. Rheumatology. 2002;41(12):1380–7.
26. Sokka T, Kautiainen H, Pincus T, Verstappen SMM, Aggarwal A, Alten R, et al. Work disability remains a major problem in rheumatoid arthritis in the 2000s: data from 32 countries in the QUEST-RA Study. Arthritis Res Ther. 2010;12(2):R42.
27. Boonen A, Chorus AM, Miedema HS, van der Heijde D, Landewe R, Schouten H, et al. Withdrawal from labour force due to work disability in patients with ankylosing spondylitis. Ann Rheum Dis. 2001;60(11):1033–9.
28. Zirkee EJM, Sneep AC, de Buck PDM, Allaart CF, Peeters AJ, Ronday HK, et al. Sick leave and work disability in patients with early arthritis. Clin Rheumatol. 2008;27:11–9.
29. Odegård S, Finset A, Kvien T, Mowinckel P, Uhlig T. Work disability in rheumatoid arthritis is predicted by physical and psychological health status: a 7-year study from the Oslo RA register. Scandanavian. J Rheumatol. 2005;34(6):441–7.
30. Chorus AM, Miedema HS, Boonen A, Van Der Linden S. Quality of life and work in patients with rheumatoid arthritis and ankylosing spondylitis of working age. Ann Rheum Dis. 2003;62(12):1178–84.
31. Nikolaus S, Bode C, Taal E, de Laar MA. Fatigue and factors related to fatigue in rheumatoid arthritis: a systematic review. Arthritis Care & Research. 2013;65(7):1128–46.
32. Zhang J, Xie F, Delzell E, Chen L, Kilgore ML, Yun H, et al. Trends in the use of biologic agents among rheumatoid arthritis patients enrolled in the US medicare program. Arthtitis Care & Research. 2013;65:1743–51.
33. Dean LE, Macfarlane GJ, MacDonald AG, Jones GT. The natural history of ankylosing spondylitis: results from the Scotland and Ireland Registry for Ankylosing Spondylitis. Rheumatology. 2014;53:i143–4.
34. Hyrich K, Symmons D, Watson K, Silman A. BSRBR Control Centre Consortium. Baseline comorbidity levels in biologic and standard DMARD treated patients with rheumatoid arthritis: results from a national patient register. Ann Rheum Dis. 2006;65:895–8.
35. Jones GT, Dean LE, Basu N, Kay L, Pathan E, Sturrock RD, et al. The British Society for Rheumatology Biologics Register for Ankylosing Spondylitis: characteristics of study participants. Rheumatology. 2015;54:i36.
36. Curtis JR, Jain A, Askling J, Bridges L, Carmona L, Dixon WGA. Comparison of patient characteristics and outcomes in selected European and US Rheumatoid Arthritis Registries. Semin Arthritis Rheum. 2010;40:2–14e1.
37. Saari LM, Judge TA. Employee attitudes and job satisfaction. Hum Resour Manag. 2004;43(4):395–407.
38. Gunnestad A. Resilience in a cross-cultural perspective: how resilience is generated in different cultures. J Intercult Commun. 2006;11:1–20.
39. Hewlett S, Dures E, Almeida C. Measures of fatigue: Bristol Rheumatoid Arthritis Fatigue Multi-Dimensional Questionnaire (BRAF MDQ), Bristol Rheumatoid Arthritis Fatigue Numerical Rating Scales (BRAF NRS) for Severity, Effect, and Coping, Chalder Fatigue Questionnaire (CFQ), Checklist Individual Strength (CIS20R and CIS8R), Fatigue Severity Scale (FSS), Functional Assessment Chronic Illness Therapy (Fatigue)(FACIT-F), Multi-Dimensional Assessment of Fatigue (MAF), Multi-Dimensional Fatigue Inventory (MFI), Pediatric Quality Of Life (PedsQL) Mult-Dimensional Fatigue Scale, Profile of Fatigue (ProF), Short Form 36 Vitality Subscale (SF-36 VT), and Visual Analog Scales (VAS). Arthritis Care & Research. 2011;63(S11):S263–86.
40. Cramp F, Hewlett S, Almeida C, et al. Non-pharmacological interventions for fatigue in rheumatoid arthritis. Cochrane Database Syst Rev 2013;8: CD008322.

18

A comparative clinical study of PF- 06410293, a candidate adalimumab biosimilar, and adalimumab reference product (Humira®) in the treatment of active rheumatoid arthritis

Roy M. Fleischmann[1*], Rieke Alten[2], Margarita Pileckyte[3], Kasia Lobello[4], Steven Y. Hua[5], Carol Cronenberger[4], Daniel Alvarez[4], Amy E. Bock[6] and K. Lea Sewell[6]

Abstract

Background: This double-blind, randomized, 78-week study evaluated the efficacy, safety, immunogenicity, pharmacokinetics, and pharmacodynamics of PF-06410293, a candidate adalimumab biosimilar, versus adalimumab reference product (Humira®) sourced from the EU (adalimumab-EU) in biologic-naïve patients with active rheumatoid arthritis (RA) despite methotrexate (MTX) (10–25 mg/week). We report results for the first 26 weeks of treatment.

Methods: Patients with active RA (N = 597) were randomly assigned (1:1) to PF-06410293 or adalimumab-EU, while continuing with MTX treatment. The primary endpoint was American College of Rheumatology 20% improvement (ACR20) at week 12. Therapeutic equivalence was concluded if the two-sided 95% confidence interval (CI) for the ACR20 difference between the two arms was entirely contained within the symmetric equivalence margin (±14%). Additionally, a two-sided 90% CI was calculated by using an asymmetric equivalence margin (−12%, 15%). Secondary efficacy endpoints to week 26 included ACR20/50/70, change from baseline Disease Activity Score based on high-sensitivity C-reactive protein [DAS28–4(CRP)], European League Against Rheumatism (EULAR) response, DAS28–4(CRP) of less than 2.6, and ACR/EULAR remission. QuantiFERON-TB testing was performed at screening and week 26.

Results: Patients (78.7% of whom were female and whose mean age was 52.5 years) had a mean baseline RA duration of 6.8 years. The mean baseline DAS28–4(CRP) values were 5.9 (PF-06410293) and 6.1 (adalimumab-EU). The observed week-12 ACR20 values were 68.7% (PF-06410293) and 72.7% (adalimumab-EU) in the intention-to-treat population. With non-responder imputation, the treatment difference in week-12 ACR20 was −2.98% and corresponding CIs—95% CI (−10.38%, 4.44%) and 90% CI (−9.25%, 3.28%)—were entirely contained within the equivalence margins (symmetric and asymmetric, respectively). The secondary efficacy endpoints were similar between arms. Over 26 weeks, injection-site reactions occurred in 1.7% versus 2.0%, hypersensitivity events in 4.4% versus 8.4%, pneumonia in 0.7% versus 2.0%, and opportunistic infections in 2.4% versus 1.7% in the PF-06410293 and adalimumab-EU arms, respectively. One death due to myocardial infarction occurred (adalimumab-EU arm). Rates of anti-drug antibody incidence were 44.4% (PF-06410293) and 50.5% (adalimumab-EU).

(Continued on next page)

* Correspondence: rfleischmann@arthdocs.com
[1]Southwestern Medical Center, Metroplex Clinical Research Center, University of Texas, 8144 Walnut Hill Lane, Suite 810, Dallas, TX 75231, USA
Full list of author information is available at the end of the article

(Continued from previous page)

Conclusions: The study results demonstrate that efficacy, safety, and immunogenicity of PF-06410293 and adalimumab-EU were similar during the first 26 weeks of treatment in patients with active RA on background MTX.

Keywords: Rheumatoid arthritis, Adalimumab, Biosimilar, Comparative clinical study

Background

The introduction of biologic disease-modifying antirheumatic drugs (bDMARDs) has been a major advance in the treatment of patients with rheumatoid arthritis (RA), providing an important addition to the previously available therapy options [1]. Adalimumab, a recombinant fully human immunoglobulin G1 monoclonal antibody, inhibits the interaction of tumor necrosis factor (TNF) with surface TNF receptors by specifically binding to TNF-α and has been shown to reduce clinical symptoms and inhibit radiographic progression in patients with RA [2–4]. Adalimumab is approved for multiple indications in addition to RA [5, 6].

The US Food and Drug Administration (FDA) defines a biosimilar as "a biopharmaceutical that is highly similar to an already licensed biologic product (the reference product), notwithstanding minor differences in clinically inactive components, and for which there are no clinically meaningful differences in purity, potency, and safety between the two products" [7]. The European Medicines Agency requires that a biosimilar show "similarity to the reference biologic with respect to quality, biologic activity, safety, and efficacy" [8]. Biosimilars may expand patient access to bDMARDs because of potentially lower drug prices as a result of price competition within the product market, resulting in savings for health-care systems and patients [9–11].

PF-06410293 is in development as a candidate adalimumab biosimilar. Peptide mapping data demonstrate that PF-06410293 has a primary amino acid sequence identical to that of adalimumab reference product and is similar in comparative analytical, functional, and binding assessments [12]. Pharmacokinetic (PK) similarity was demonstrated following single-dose administration of PF-06410293 and adalimumab to healthy volunteers (Pfizer unpublished observation) [13]. The current comparative clinical study compared the efficacy, safety, immunogenicity, PK, and pharmacodynamics (PD) of PF-06410293 with adalimumab reference product (Humira®) sourced from the EU (adalimumab-EU) in patients with active RA and an inadequate response to methotrexate (MTX).

Methods

Study population

Patients with active RA and an inadequate response to MTX represent a sensitive and appropriate population for biosimilar comparability trials. Adults (at least 18 years old) with a diagnosis of active RA at least 4 months, based on the 2010 American College of Rheumatology/European League Against Rheumatism (ACR/EULAR) criteria [14], were eligible for inclusion. Active RA was defined as at least six tender and at least six swollen joints (at screening and baseline) with a high-sensitivity C-reactive protein (hs-CRP) of at least 8 mg/L at screening (Additional file 1).

Patients were ineligible if they met any of the following criteria: prior treatment with adalimumab, lymphocyte-depleting therapy, or more than two doses of one biologic therapy; inadequate washout of any second DMARD, pregnancy or breastfeeding, clinically significant laboratory abnormalities, current infection, congestive heart failure (New York Heart Association grade 3/4), untreated or inadequately treated latent or active tuberculosis (TB), malignancy within the previous 5 years, or a positive test for human immunodeficiency virus or hepatitis B or C virus (Additional file 2).

Study design and treatments

This was a multinational, two-arm, double-blind, randomized, comparative clinical study in patients with active RA and was conducted at 173 centers in Australia, Brazil, Bulgaria, Colombia, the Czech Republic, Estonia, Georgia, Germany, Hungary, Japan, Lithuania, Mexico, New Zealand, Peru, Poland, the Republic of Korea, Serbia, South Africa, Spain, Taiwan, Ukraine, the Russian Federation, UK, and the US. Patients were randomly assigned (1:1) on day 1 (stratified by geographic region) to receive either PF-06410293 or adalimumab-EU. There were three 26-week treatment periods and a 16-week follow-up after last dose of study drug (Fig. 1). Prior to dosing at week 26, patients in the adalimumab-EU arm were blindly re-randomized (1:1) to continue on adalimumab-EU or switch to PF-06410293. At week 52, all patients remaining on adalimumab-EU were switched to PF-06410293 for open-label treatment during the third treatment period. Herein, we report data from the first 26 weeks of the study. The number of tender (68) and swollen (66) joints was determined by an independent blinded joint assessor.

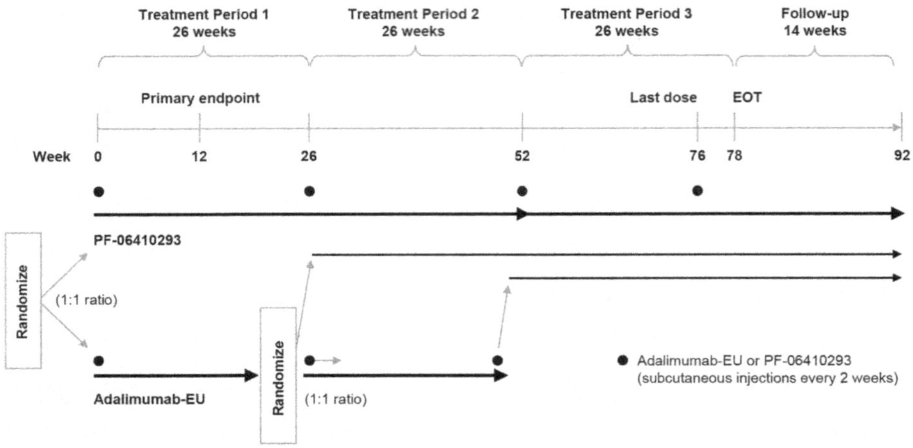

Fig. 1 Study design. Abbreviations: *Adalimumab-EU* adalimumab sourced from the European Union, *EOT* end of treatment

PF-06410293 or adalimumab-EU was administered as a subcutaneous injection (40 mg every other week using a prefilled syringe) in addition to a stable background dose of oral or intramuscular MTX (10–25 mg/week) and oral folic/folinic acid; lower doses of MTX (6 mg/week) were allowed if indicated in local guidance or standards of care. Patients could receive concomitant low-dose oral corticosteroids (≤10 mg prednisone or equivalent per day), one non-steroidal anti-inflammatory drug, and non-opioid or specific opioid analgesics or both. Treatment could be delayed by up to 24 h prior to the next injection for illness or scheduling issues. Dosing could be temporarily held at the discretion of the investigator for an adverse event (AE) and resumed after the AE resolved, unless the patient missed three sequential injections.

Primary study endpoint

The primary efficacy endpoint was the proportion of patients achieving an ACR20 response [15] at week 12. Week 12 is considered the beginning of the plateau of the time-response curve for ACR20 and, as such, is a more sensitive time point for the assessment of rapidity of response in biosimilar comparability trials in RA as suggested by regulatory authorities. Therefore, this trial evaluated the primary endpoint at week 12 rather than week 26, as used in the historical registration trials for adalimumab in patients with RA.

Secondary endpoints and assessments

Secondary efficacy endpoints through week 26 included ACR20 (at time points in addition to week 12), ACR50, ACR70, change from baseline in Disease Activity Score 28 joints: four components based on hs-CRP [DAS28–4(CRP)], EULAR response, DAS28–4(CRP) of less than 2.6, ACR/EULAR remission, and change from baseline in individual ACR components, including Health Assessment Questionnaire Disability Index (HAQ-DI). The sponsor selected DAS28–4(CRP) rather than DAS28–4(erythrocyte sedimentation rate [ESR]) to determine clinical response, as CRP is performed in a central laboratory. A cutoff of less than 2.6 was used to define DAS28(CRP) "remission" and not more than 3.2 as "low disease activity" rather than the lower numbers that have been shown to best correlate with the DAS28(ESR) formula [16].

Safety endpoints included type, incidence, severity, timing, seriousness, and investigator-determined relatedness of AEs—using the National Cancer Institute Common Terminology Criteria for Adverse Events (Version 4.03)—and laboratory abnormalities (Covance, Indianapolis, IN, USA). Safety evaluations during study treatment included physical examinations, electrocardiograms, and QuantiFERON-TB Gold testing (at screening and week 26).

Prespecified treatment-emergent adverse events (TEAEs) of special interest were injection-site reactions (ISRs), opportunistic infections (defined for this study to include zoster, cytomegalovirus, latent/active TB, atypical mycobacteria, systemic fungal infections and oral thrush, pneumocystis, legionella, salmonellosis, shigellosis, vibrio, and other infections), and anaphylaxis/angioedema/urticaria. Additional prespecified TEAE categories of interest included blood and lymphatic events, cardiovascular events, demyelinating conditions, gastric/hepatic events, hypersensitivity events, infections and infestations, and neoplasms.

Anti-drug antibodies (ADAs) and neutralizing antibodies (NAbs) were tested at baseline and weeks 2, 6, 12, and 26. Serum samples were analyzed by using a tiered approach of laboratory screening, confirmation, and titer determination. Serum samples were analyzed for ADA at QPS, LLC (Newark, DE, USA) by using a single validated electrochemiluminescent immunoassay. ADA-positive samples were then tested for neutralizing activity with a validated cell-based assay using PF-06410293 as the capture agent.

PK serum samples were obtained at baseline and weeks 1, 2, 6, 12, and 26 and evaluated for PF-06410293 or adalimumab-EU concentrations by using a validated, sensitive, and specific enzyme-linked immunosorbent assay with a lower limit of quantification of 250 ng/mL (QPS). The prespecified PD marker was hs-CRP.

Statistical methods

With the assumption of a week-12 ACR20 response rate of 60% for both PF-06410293 and adalimumab-EU, a sample size of 560 patients was determined to provide about 85% power to demonstrate therapeutic equivalence between the treatment arms, and the symmetric margin of ±14% was used for the primary endpoint. This equivalence margin was derived from a meta-analysis of published data from registration studies for adalimumab in patients with RA [2, 3, 17, 18] and was endorsed by both the European Medicines Agency and the Pharmaceuticals and Medical Devices Agency. Exact methods were used to calculate the confidence interval (CI) for the treatment difference in primary efficacy endpoint of week-12 ACR20, using non-responder imputation (NRI) for missing data and for patients with permanent discontinuation of study drug prior to week 12. Therapeutic equivalence was concluded if the two-sided 95% CI for the treatment difference was entirely contained within ±14% margin and additionally if the two-sided 90% CI for the same treatment difference was within the asymmetric margin of −12% to 15% (as requested by the FDA).

The intention-to-treat (ITT) population, defined as all randomly assigned patients, was the primary analysis population. Sensitivity analyses of the primary and secondary endpoints used the per protocol (PP) population, defined as all patients who received study treatment up to week 12, had a week-12 evaluation, and had no major protocol deviations. The DAS28−4(CRP) change from baseline was analyzed by using an analysis of covariance for repeated-measures data approach.

Safety and immunogenicity analyses were performed for the safety population (defined as randomly assigned patients who received any study treatment) on the prespecified TEAEs of special interest and categories of special interest with risk differences (RDs) and 95% CIs by using the asymptotic approach of Miettinen and Nurminen [19]. Transient ADA response after treatment (including the follow-up period) was defined as either a single positive ADA result or two positive sampling time points where the first and last ADA-positive samples (irrespective of any negative samples in between) were separated by less than 16 weeks and the patient's last ADA sampling time result was negative [20]. PK analysis was conducted for all dosed patients who provided at least one post-dose drug concentration measurement and was summarized by treatment and ADA status by using descriptive statistics (mean, standard deviation [SD], median, and minimum and maximum). PD analysis using hs-CRP concentration over time was summarized by descriptive statistics according to treatment.

Results

Patient disposition and demographics

In total, 1231 patients were screened and 597 eligible patients—297 to PF-06410293 and 300 to adalimumab-EU—were randomly assigned to receive study treatment (Additional file 3). Low hs-CRP level was the main reason for screen failure. The safety population included 596 patients, and one adalimumab-EU patient was randomly assigned and not dosed. In both treatment arms, the median duration of study treatment was 24.1 weeks. The first treatment period to week 26 was completed by 286 (96.3%) out of 297 patients in the PF-06410293 arm and 273 (91.0%) out of 300 in the adalimumab-EU arm. Overall, 30 (10.1%) out of 297 patients in the PF-06410293 arm and 46 (15.3%) out of 300 in the adalimumab-EU arm were excluded from the PP population. In most cases, exclusion was due to incomplete study drug dosing up to week 12 for 16 (5.4%) out of 297 patients in the PF-06410293 arm and 34 (11.3%) out of 300 in the adalimumab-EU arm. In the PF-06410293 arm, 29 (9.8%) out of 297 patients, compared with 51 (17.1%) out of 299 in the adalimumab-EU arm, missed one or more doses. This included 18 (6.1%) out of 297 and 34 (11.4%) out of 299 patients who missed one or more doses because of an AE in the PF-06410293 and adalimumab-EU arms, respectively.

Patient demographic and baseline RA characteristics were similar between the treatment arms (Table 1). At baseline, patients had a mean age of 52.5 years, 78.7% were female, and the mean RA duration was 6.8 years. Mean baseline swollen joint counts were 15.4 versus 17.0 and tender joint counts were 24.3 versus 26.7 in the PF-06410293 and adalimumab-EU arms, respectively. Mean baseline DAS28−4(CRP) values were 5.9 (PF-06410293) and 6.1 (adalimumab-EU). Across the two arms, the mean MTX dose was 15.2 mg/week and 55.9% of patients were receiving oral corticosteroids (Table 1).

Efficacy

Primary endpoint

Based on the primary efficacy endpoint of ACR20 response rate at week 12, therapeutic equivalence between PF-06410293 and adalimumab-EU was demonstrated by using both prespecified equivalence margins. With

Table 1 Baseline patient demographic and clinical characteristics (ITT population)

	PF-06410293 *n* = 297	Adalimumab-EU *n* = 300
Demographics[a]		
Gender, n (%)		
Female	241 (81.1)	229 (76.3)
Male	56 (18.9)	71 (23.7)
Age, mean (SD), years	51.5 (13.6)	53.5 (12.9)
Weight, mean (SD), kg	74.7 (17.5)	76.2 (20.8)
Body mass index, mean (SD), kg/m^2	27.5 (6.1)	28.1 (7.3)
Race, n (%)		
White	261 (87.9)	256 (85.3)
Black	6 (2.0)	9 (3.0)
Asian	16 (5.4)	17 (5.7)
Other	14 (4.7)	18 (6.0)
Ethnicity, n (%)		
Hispanic/Latino	25 (8.4)	29 (9.7)
Not Hispanic/Latino	272 (91.6)	271 (90.3)
Clinical characteristics		
RA duration, mean (SD), years	6.8 (7.2)	6.8 (6.9)
Positive RF or anti-CCP antibody or both, n (%)	242 (81.5)	245 (81.7)
Swollen joint count, mean (SD)	15.4 (7.8)	17.0 (9.8)
Tender joint count, mean (SD)	24.3 (12.3)	26.7 (14.8)
hs-CRP, mg/L		
Mean (SD)	21.3 (22.7)	22.8 (25.2)
Median (range)	14.7 (0.2–169)	16.0 (0.2–192)
DAS28–4(CRP), mean (SD)	5.9 (0.9)	6.1 (0.9)
HAQ-DI, mean (SD)	1.5 (0.6)	1.7 (0.6)
Prior use of one biologic drug, n (%)	8 (2.7)	5 (1.7)
Number of prior and current non-biologic DMARDs (in addition to MTX), mean (SD)	1.5 (0.9)	1.5 (0.9)
MTX dose, mean (SD), mg/week	15.2 (4.4)	15.2 (4.5)
Corticosteroid use, n (%)	164 (55.2)	170 (56.7)

Abbreviations: Adalimumab-EU adalimumab sourced from the European Union, *CCP* cyclic citrullinated peptide, *DAS28–4(CRP)* Disease Activity Score-28: four components based on high-sensitivity C-reactive protein, *DMARD* disease-modifying anti-rheumatic drug, *HAQ-DI* Health Assessment Questionnaire Disability Index, *hs-CRP* high-sensitivity C-reactive protein, *ITT* intention-to-treat, *MTX* methotrexate, *n* number of patients in each category, *RA* rheumatoid arthritis, *RF* rheumatoid factor, *SD* standard deviation

[a]Randomization stratified by geographic region (North America and Western Europe; Japan; Republic of Korea and Taiwan; Latin America; rest of world)

observed data in the ITT population, 204 (68.7%) out of 297 patients in the PF-06410293 arm and 218 (72.7%) out of 300 in the adalimumab-EU arm achieved an ACR20 response at week 12, and treatment difference was −3.98%. For the ITT population, response was imputed as non-responder in 19 patients, the treatment difference was −2.98%, based on ACR20 response in 203 (68.4%) out of 297 patients in the PF-06410293 arm and 214 (71.3%) out of 300 in the adalimumab-EU arm, and the 95% CI (−10.38%, 4.44%) was entirely contained within the symmetric margin (Fig. 2a) and 90% CI (−9.25%, 3.28%) was entirely contained within the asymmetric margin (Fig. 2b).

For the PP population sensitivity analysis, 189 (71.1%) out of 266 patients in the PF-06410293 arm and 191 (75.2%) out of 254 in the adalimumab-EU arm achieved an ACR20 response at week 12. The treatment difference was −4.14%, and the corresponding 95% (−11.79%, 3.61%) and 90% (−10.60%, 2.38%) CIs were entirely contained within the symmetric (±14%) and asymmetric (−12%, 15%) equivalence margins, respectively. Other sensitivity analyses of the primary endpoint, including

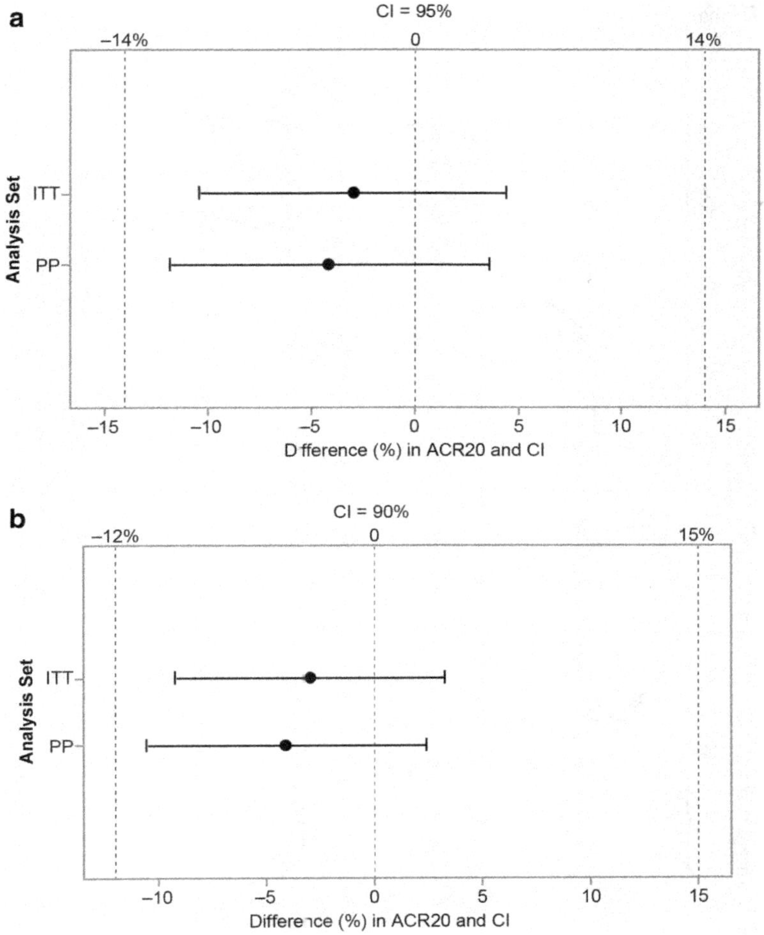

Fig. 2 Primary efficacy endpoint of ACR20 at week 12 (with non-responder imputation). **a** Difference (95% CI) between PF-06410293 and adalimumab-EU using a symmetric equivalence margin. **b** Difference (90% CI) between PF-06410293 and adalimumab-EU using an asymmetric equivalence margin. Abbreviations: *ACR20* American College of Rheumatology 20% improvement, *Adalimumab-EU* adalimumab sourced from the European Union, *CI* confidence interval, *ITT* intention-to-treat, *PP* per protocol

an analysis adjusting for the stratification variable of geographic region and a multiple imputation-based tipping point analysis for missing data, were consistent with the primary result of therapeutic equivalence between PF-06410293 and adalimumab-EU (Additional file 4).

The ACR20 rates at week 12 for subgroups were numerically higher in ADA-negative (70.9% and 77.2%) compared with ADA-positive (63.7% and 65.7%) patients for the PF-06410293 and adalimumab-EU arms, respectively, defined as subjects with a positive ADA test in the first 26 weeks. ACR20 rates for NAb-negative patients were also numerically higher (70.9% and 74.0%) as compared with NAb-positive patients (50.0% and 64.0%) for the PF-06410293 and adalimumab-EU arms, respectively.

Secondary endpoints

The ACR20/50/70 response rates through week 26 were similar between the PF-06410293 and adalimumab-EU arms (Fig. 3a). Mean changes from baseline in DAS28–4(CRP) were similar between treatment arms at each study visit, and the changes from baseline at week 26 were −2.7 for the PF-06410293 arm and −2.8 for the adalimumab-EU arm (Fig. 3b). At week 26, 162 (54.5%) out of 297 and 147 (49.0%) out of 300 of patients had a good EULAR response in the PF-06410293 and adalimumab-EU arms, respectively (Additional file 5). In the PF-06410293 arm, 87 (29.3%) out of 297 patients achieved DAS28–4(CRP) of less than 2.6 at week 26 compared with 99 (33.0%) out of 300 in the adalimumab-EU arm (Additional file 6). A total of 38 (12.8%) out of 297 patients in the PF-06410293 arm and 44 (14.7%) out of 300 in the adalimumab-EU arm achieved ACR/EULAR remission at week 26, including 26 (8.8%) out of 297 and 27 (9.0%) out of 300 using only the Boolean definition (Additional file 6). At week 26, mean HAQ-DI decreased from baseline by 0.654 in the

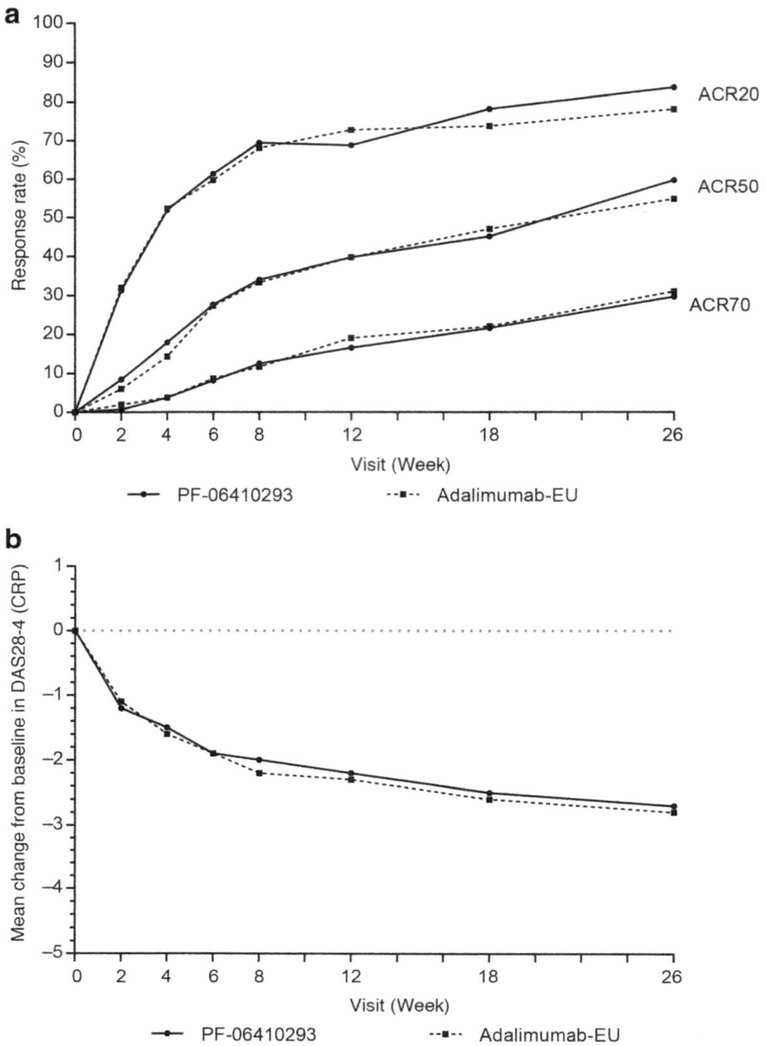

Fig. 3 Secondary efficacy endpoints (intention-to-treat population). **a** ACR20/50/70 response rates by study visit. **b** Mean change from baseline in DAS28–4(CRP) by study visit. Abbreviations: *Adalimumab-EU* adalimumab sourced from the European Union, *ACR20/50/70* American College of Rheumatology 20%/50%/70% improvement, *DAS28–4(CRP)* Disease Activity Score-28: four components based on high-sensitivity C-reactive protein

PF-06410293 arm and by 0.674 in the adalimumab-EU arm (Additional file 7).

Safety

A total of 143 (48.1%) out of 297 patients in the PF-06410293 arm and 143 (47.8%) out of 299 in the adalimumab-EU arm reported one or more TEAEs. The System Organ Classes (SOCs) with the highest proportion of patients with AEs were infections and infestations in 24.9% and 25.1%, musculoskeletal and connective tissue disorders in 10.4% and 8.7%, and investigations in 8.8% and 7.7% for the PF-06410293 and adalimumab-EU patients, respectively. The number of patients who permanently discontinued treatment because of TEAEs was 11 (3.7%) versus 14 (4.7%) and the number of patients who temporarily discontinued treatment because of TEAEs was 17 (5.7%) versus 29 (9.7%) in the PF-06410293 and adalimumab-EU arms, respectively.

Serious adverse events (SAEs) were reported by 4.0% (PF-06410293) and 4.3% (adalimumab-EU) of patients (Table 2). This included one death due to myocardial infarction in the adalimumab-EU arm. The SOC with the highest proportion of patients with SAEs was infections and infestations, occurring in three patients in each treatment arm.

In total, 5.7% of patients in the PF-06410293 arm and 7.0% in the adalimumab-EU arm reported TEAEs of grade 3 or higher. All-causality grade 4 TEAEs were reported in two patients in the PF-06410293 arm (intentional self-injury, and hemorrhoids with rectal hemorrhage and resulting anemia) and four patients in

Table 2 All-causality treatment-emergent adverse events (safety population)

	PF-06410293 *n* = 297	Adalimumab-EU *n* = 299
Number of AEs	343	379
Patients with events, n (%)		
AEs	143 (48.1)	143 (47.8)
SAEs	12 (4.0)	13 (4.3)
Grade 3 AEs	15 (5.1)	16 (5.4)[a]
Grade 4 AEs	2 (0.7)	4 (1.3)
Grade 5 AEs	0	1 (0.3)
Patients with temporary treatment discontinuation due to AEs, n (%)	17 (5.7)	29 (9.7)
Patients discontinued from treatment due to AEs[c], n (%)	11 (3.7)[b]	14 (4.7)
Patients discontinued from the study due to AEs, n (%)	8 (2.7)	9 (3.0)

AEs were graded in accordance with National Cancer Institute Common Terminology Criteria for Adverse Events version 4.03. Grade 1–5 AEs are defined as mild, moderate, severe, life-threatening AEs, and death related to AE, respectively.
Abbreviations: Adalimumab-EU adalimumab sourced from the European Union, *AE* adverse event, *SAE* serious adverse event
[a]One patient had an AE of neutropenia incorrectly recorded as grade 2; the correct severity was grade 3 (not corrected in this table)
[b]One patient was incorrectly recorded as treatment discontinuation due to an AE; the correct reason was insufficient clinical response (not corrected in this table)
[c]The System Organ Class with the highest proportion of subjects who had AEs leading to permanent treatment discontinuation was infections and infestations (8 [2.7%] subjects on PF-06410293 and 3 [1.0%] subjects on adalimumab-EU)

the adalimumab-EU arm (atrial fibrillation, ileus secondary to colon cancer, gastroenteritis, and papillary thyroid cancer).

The most frequently reported TEAEs occurring in at least 2% of patients in any treatment arm were viral upper respiratory tract infections, increased alanine aminotransferase, hypertension, and headaches (Additional file 8).

Of the TEAEs of special interest, ISRs were reported by five (1.7%) and six (2.0%) patients in the PF-06410293 and adalimumab-EU arms, respectively (Table 3). The primary symptom was redness (three patients in the PF-06410293 arm and two in the adalimumab-EU arm). In addition, one patient in each arm reported pain and swelling. No patients discontinued treatment because of an ISR. For one patient in the PF-06410293 arm and two patients in the adalimumab-EU arm, the ISR occurred on or after the date the patient first tested positive for ADA.

Overall infection rates were similar at 24.9% and 25.1% for the PF-06410293 and adalimumab-EU arms, respectively. Opportunistic infections (predefined in the study as including latent TB) were reported by seven (2.4%) in the PF-06410293 arm and five (1.7%) patients in the adalimumab-EU arm (Table 3). One case of herpes zoster was reported in the PF-06410293 arm and three cases in the adalimumab-EU arm. Five and one cases of seroconversion with a subsequent diagnosis of latent TB (based on specialist consultation following a positive week-26 QuantiFERON-TB Gold test result) were reported in the PF-06410293 and adalimumab-EU arms, respectively. The RD for latent TB (1.35, 95% CI −0.35, 3.59) was not statistically significant. In total, 5.6% of patients in the PF-06410293 arm and 4.9% in the adalimumab-EU arm had a negative QuantiFERON-TB test at screening and a positive test at week 26. There were

Table 3 All-causality treatment-emergent adverse events of special interest with risk difference (safety population)

Event of special interest	PF-06410293 *n* = 297 n (%)	Adalimumab-EU *n* = 299 n (%)	Risk difference (95% CI) (%)
Injection-site reactions	5 (1.7)	6 (2.0)	−0.32 (−2.84, 2.12)
Opportunistic infections	7 (2.4)	5 (1.7)	0.69 (−1.80, 3.32)
Herpes zoster	1 (0.3)	3 (1.0)	−0.67 (−2.61, 0.97)
Latent tuberculosis	5 (1.7)	1 (0.3)	1.35 (−0.35, 3.59)
Confirmed active tuberculosis	0	0	0 (NA)
Oral candidiasis	0	1 (0.3)	−0.33 (−1.87, 0.95)
Pneumocystis jirovecii pneumonia	1 (0.3)	0	0.34 (−0.94, 1.88)
Urticaria, angioedema, anaphylactic reaction[a]	0	2 (0.7)	−0.67 (−2.41, 0.61)

Abbreviations: Adalimumab-EU adalimumab sourced from the European Union, *CI* confidence interval, *NA* not applicable
[a]Only urticaria reported

no cases of active TB in any patient in either treatment arm. One case of oral candidiasis (adalimumab-EU) and one case of *Pneumocystis jirovecii* pneumonia (PF-06410293) were reported. Overall, pneumonia was reported by 0.7% and 2.0% of the PF-06410293 and adalimumab-EU arms, respectively. There were no cases of anaphylaxis or angioedema in either treatment arm; two cases of urticaria were reported in the adalimumab-EU arm.

A total of 39.1% of patients in each arm reported 183 (PF-06410293) and 202 (adalimumab-EU) AEs in one or more prespecified TEAE categories of interest (Table 4). Hypersensitivity TEAEs were reported in 13 (4.4%) out of 297 patients in the PF-06410293 arm compared with 25 (8.4%) out of 299 in the adalimumab-EU arm (RD −3.98, 95% CI −8.15, −0.06). The most frequently reported hypersensitivity TEAEs were cough (5 versus 3), erythema (4 versus 1), and rash (1 versus 3) in the PF-06410293 and adalimumab-EU arms, respectively. Hypersensitivity TEAEs occurring on or after the date a patient first tested positive for ADA included six AEs reported by five patients in the PF-06410293 arm and nine AEs reported by seven patients in the adalimumab-EU arm. Two patients in the PF-06410293 arm reported grade 3 hypersensitivity SAEs, including interstitial lung disease and toxic skin eruption. The rate of blood and lymphatic system events was numerically higher in the PF-06410293 versus adalimumab-EU arms—22 (7.4%) out of 297 versus 14 (4.7%) out of 299—but this was not statistically significant (RD 2.73, 95% CI −1.15, 6.79). The reported malignancies included one (basal cell carcinoma) and two (adenocarcinoma of the colon and papillary thyroid cancer) patients in the PF-06410293 and adalimumab-EU arms, respectively.

Immunogenicity, PK, and PD

Overall, 44.4% and 50.5% of patients in the PF-06410293 and adalimumab-EU treatment arms, respectively, had at least one post-dose sample that tested positive for ADA (Fig. 4; Additional file 9). ADAs were transient in 11.4% of patients in the PF-06410293 arm and in 6.0% in the adalimumab-EU arm. Of the ADA-positive patients, 31.1% in the PF-06410293 and 27.8% in the adalimumab-EU treatment arms tested positive for NAb.

The mean serum drug trough concentrations at week 26 were 8244 and 7190 ng/mL in the PF-06410293 and adalimumab-EU arms, respectively. Mean serum concentrations of both drugs were lower in ADA-positive patients (4683 and 4041 ng/mL) compared with ADA-negative patients (11,090 and 10,460 ng/mL) for the PF-06410293 and adalimumab-EU arms, respectively. The mean hs-CRP concentrations (prespecified PD marker) were decreased at week 26 in both arms (ITT population); the changes from baseline to week 26 were −11.1 (PF-06410293) and −13.6 mg/L (adalimumab-EU).

Discussion

This comparative clinical study was conducted to evaluate the biosimilarity of PF-06410293 and adalimumab-EU. The primary goal of the study was met by demonstrating therapeutic equivalence of PF-06410293 and adalimumab-EU using the symmetric and asymmetric margins for the week-12 ACR20 primary endpoint comparison. Sensitivity analyses of the primary endpoint supported a conclusion of therapeutic equivalence. As expected, ACR20 response rates at week 12 were numerically higher in ADA-negative patients compared with ADA-positive in both treatment arms. Secondary endpoints reported up to week 26, including ACR50, ACR70,

Table 4 Prespecified treatment-emergent adverse event categories of interest with risk difference (safety population)

Category	PF-06410293 *n* = 297 n (%)	Adalimumab-EU *n* = 299 n (%)	Risk difference (95% CI) (%)
Blood and lymphatic system events	22 (7.4)	14 (4.7)	2.73 (−1.15, 6.79)
Cardiovascular events	9 (3.0)	16 (5.4)	−2.32 (−5.84, 0.96)
Demyelinating conditions	0	0	0 (NA)
Gastric/hepatic events	11 (3.7)	14 (4.7)	−0.98 (−4.44, 2.39)
Hypersensitivity[a]	13 (4.4)	25 (8.4)	−3.98 (−8.15, −0.06)
Infections and infestations	74 (24.9)	75 (25.1)	−0.17 (−7.13, 6.80)
Neoplasms	5 (1.7)	5 (1.7)	0.01 (−2.38, 2.42)
Other[b]	11 (3.7)	10 (3.3)	0.36 (−2.80, 3.57)

Abbreviations: Adalimumab-EU adalimumab sourced from the European Union, *CI* confidence interval, *MedDRA* Medical Dictionary for Regulatory Activities, *NA* not applicable

[a]Hypersensitivity events identified by Hypersensitivity Standardized MedDRA Query (broad and narrow), Anaphylactic reactions Standardized MedDRA Query (broad and narrow), and High-Level Group Terms Immunology and allergy investigations

[b]Other events identified by High-Level Group Terms Skin Vascular Abnormalities, Central Nervous System Vascular Abnormalities and Medication Errors; Higher Level Terms Connective Tissue Disorders, Vasculitides (not elsewhere classified), Rashes, Eruptions and Exanthems (not elsewhere classified); Lower Level Teams Seizure and Convulsions; and Preferred Terms Lupus-like Syndrome, Headache and Migraine

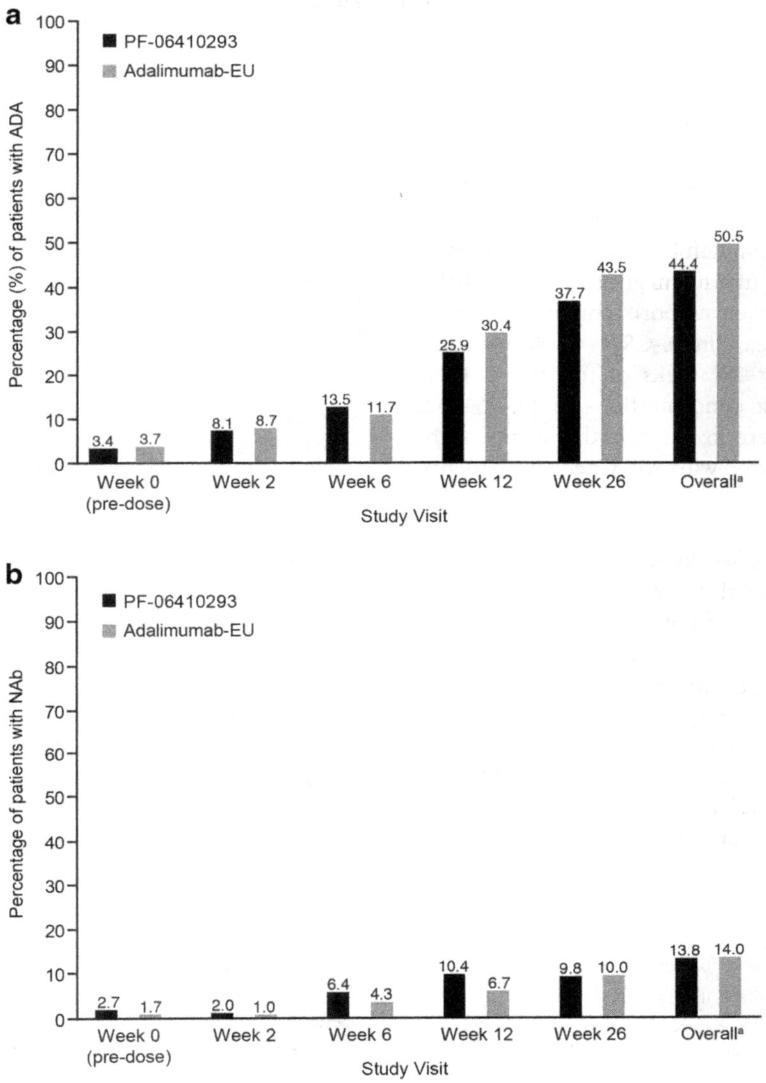

Fig. 4 ADA and NAb incidence by study visit (safety population). **a** ADA incidence. **b** NAb incidence. The percentage of NAb-positive patients is based on the total number of patients in each treatment group. [a]"Overall" includes data from week 2, week 6, week 12, week 26, end-of-treatment/early termination, follow-up, and unplanned visits in treatment period 1. Abbreviations: *ADA* anti-drug antibody, *Adalimumab-EU* adalimumab sourced from the European Union, *NAb* neutralizing antibody

change from baseline in DAS28–4(CRP), EULAR response, DAS28–4(CRP) of less than 2.6, ACR/EULAR remission, and HAQ-DI all supported therapeutic equivalence.

The safety profiles of PF-06410293 and adalimumab-EU to week 26 were comparable, including similar findings with respect to the number of AEs, SAEs, and prespecified TEAEs and TEAE categories of special interest. The only statistically significant safety difference was a lower rate of hypersensitivity events observed in the PF-06410293 arm compared with the adalimumab-EU arm; however, no correction for multiplicity was performed in this study. As might be expected in a single clinical trial, numerical differences were observed between the treatment arms, including an imbalance in the development of latent TB (more common in the PF-06410293 group) and hypersensitivity events (more common in the adalimumab-EU group). Of note, the diagnosis of latent TB was based on investigator judgment, local practice, and consultation with a pulmonary or infectious disease specialist and after a protocol-mandated QuantiFERON-TB test was performed. The percentage of patients who converted to a QuantiFERON-TB test positive at week 26 was balanced between the treatment arms, suggesting that there was no clinically meaningful difference in the rate of QuantiFERON-TB test conversion between PF-06410293 and adalimumab-EU. The safety profile for both study drugs appears to be consistent with the known safety profile of reference adalimumab-EU.

The immunogenicity profiles observed during the first 26 weeks of treatment were similar for the two treatment arms, and there was a somewhat lower incidence of patients testing positive for ADA in the PF-06410293 arm. Serum drug concentrations were numerically higher in the PF-06410293 arm; however, these differences were not considered clinically meaningful, as the clinical response was similar in the two treatment arms. The hs-CRP response as a PD biomarker supports this lack of clinical significance, as the decrease in hs-CRP was similar for the two arms over the first 26 weeks of treatment. As expected, the serum drug concentrations of PF-06410293 and adalimumab-EU were lower in both treatment arms for ADA-positive compared with ADA-negative patients.

Conclusions

Results from the first 26 weeks of dosing demonstrated no clinically meaningful differences in efficacy, safety, immunogenicity, PK, or PD between PF-06410293 and adalimumab-EU in patients with active RA. Upcoming data from the subsequent 6 months of the trial will provide additional efficacy, safety, and immunogenicity information, including data on patients after a blinded transition from adalimumab-EU to PF-06410293 and those who receive a total of 1 year of treatment with either PF-06410293 or adalimumab-EU.

Additional files

Additional file 1: Inclusion criteria for study enrollment. (DOCX 48 kb)

Additional file 2: Exclusion criteria. (DOCX 53 kb)

Additional file 3: Consolidated Standards of Reporting Trials (CONSORT) flow diagram of patient progress in the two treatment arms. [a]Patients may screen fail for more than one reason. [b]Patients may be excluded from the per-protocol population for more than one reason. Abbreviation: *Adalimumab-EU* adalimumab sourced from the European Union. (PNG 171 kb)

Additional file 4: Multiple imputation-based tipping-point analysis. (DOCX 48 kb)

Additional file 5: EULAR response by study visit (ITT population). Abbreviations: *EULAR* European League Against Rheumatism, *ITT* intention-to-treat. (DOCX 48 kb)

Additional file 6: DAS28–4(CRP) of less than 2.6 and ACR/EULAR remission by study visit (ITT population). Abbreviations: *ACR/EULAR* American College of Rheumatology/European League Against Rheumatism, *DAS28–4(CRP)* Disease Activity Score 28 joints: four components based on high-sensitivity C-reactive protein, *ITT* intention-to-treat. (DOCX 50 kb)

Additional file 7: Mean change from baseline in HAQ-DI by visit (ITT population). Abbreviations: *Adalimumab-EU* adalimumab sourced from the European Union, *HAQ-DI* health assessment questionnaire disability index, *ITT* intention-to-treat (PNG 84 kb)

Additional file 8: All-causality treatment-emergent adverse events in at least 2% of patients in any treatment arm (safety population). (DOCX 49 kb)

Additional file 9: ADA and NAb incidence by study visit (safety population). Abbreviations: *ADA* anti-drug antibody, *NAb* neutralizing antibody. (DOCX 52 kb)

Abbreviations

ACR: American College of Rheumatology; ACR20: American College of Rheumatology 20% improvement; ADA: Anti-drug antibody; Adalimumab-EU: Adalimumab sourced from the European Union; AE: Adverse event; bDMARD: Biologic disease-modifying anti-rheumatic drug; CI: Confidence interval; DAS28–4(CRP): Disease Activity Score 28 joints: four components based on high-sensitivity C-reactive protein; DMARD: Disease-modifying anti-rheumatic drug; ESR: Erythrocyte sedimentation rate; EULAR: European League Against Rheumatism; FDA: US Food and Drug Administration; HAQ-DI: Health Assessment Questionnaire Disability Index; hs-CRP: High-sensitivity C-reactive protein; ISR: Injection-site reaction; ITT: Intention-to-treat; MTX: Methotrexate; NAb: Neutralizing antibody; PD: Pharmacodynamics; PK: Pharmacokinetics; PP: Per protocol; RA: Rheumatoid arthritis; RD: Risk difference; SAE: Serious adverse event; SOC: System Organ Class; TB: Tuberculosis; TEAE: Treatment-emergent adverse event; TNF: Tumor necrosis factor

Acknowledgments

Medical writing support was provided by Jacqui Oliver and Neel Misra of Engage Scientific Solutions and was funded by Pfizer Inc.

Funding

This study was sponsored by Pfizer Inc.

Availability of data and materials

The policies of Pfizer Inc. on the provision of clinical trial data are set out in http://www.pfizer.com/research/clinical_trials/trial_data_and_results. In addition to posting clinical trial results on the ClinicalTrials.gov registry, Pfizer will provide access to anonymized patient-level data in response to scientifically valid research protocols. Data from Pfizer-sponsored global interventional clinical studies are available from trials conducted for medicines, vaccines, and medical devices for indications that have been approved in the US or the European Union or both and from trials conducted for medicines, vaccines, and medical devices that have been terminated (that is, development for all indications has been discontinued). Data from these trials will be made available 24 months after study completion. Pfizer will make reasonable efforts to fulfill all data requests for legitimate research purposes, but there may be instances in which retrieval or delivery of data is not feasible (for example, if Pfizer does not have legal authority to provide the data or if costs of retrieval of older or pre-electronic data are prohibitive; see page 5 at the following link: https://www.pfizer.com/files/research/research_clinical_trials/A_Guide_to_Requesting_Pfizer_Patient-Level_Clinical_Trial_Data_2017.pdf). Further detail can be found at http://www.pfizer.com/research/clinical_trials/trial_data_and_results/data_requests. Pfizer's practices adhere to the principles for responsible data sharing laid out by the European Federation of Pharmaceutical Industries and Associations (EFPIA) and the Pharmaceutical Research and Manufacturers of America (PhRMA): http://phrma.org/sites/default/files/pdf/PhRMAPrinciplesForResponsibleClinicalTrialDataSharing.pdf.

Authors' contributions

KLS, DA, and AEB made substantial contributions to study conception and design. SYH, CC, KLS, and AEB analyzed the data and SYH provided statistical support. RMF, RA, and MP contributed to the acquisition of data. RMF reviewed for investigator approval all study data in the clinical study report written by KLS. All authors made substantial contributions to the interpretation of data, were involved in drafting the manuscript or revising it critically for important intellectual content or both, and read and approved the final manuscript for submission.

Competing interests

RMF has received research grants and consulting fees from Pfizer Inc. and AbbVie. RA has received research grants and honoraria from Pfizer Inc. MP declares that she has no competing interests. SYH was an employee of and held stock holdings or stock options (or both) from Pfizer Inc. at the time of the study. KL, CC, DA, AEB, and KLS are full-time employees of and declare stock holdings or stock options (or both) from Pfizer Inc.

Author details

[1]Southwestern Medical Center, Metroplex Clinical Research Center, University of Texas, 8144 Walnut Hill Lane, Suite 810, Dallas, TX 75231, USA. [2]Schlosspark-Klinik, University Medicine Berlin, Heubnerweg 2, Berlin 14059, Germany. [3]Department of Rheumatology, Hospital of Lithuanian University of Health Sciences, Eiveniu str.2, Kaunas, LT 50161, Lithuania. [4]Pfizer Inc., 500 Arcola Road Collegeville, Collegeville, PA 19426, USA. [5]Pfizer Inc., 10777 Science Center Drive, CB1/2103, San Diego, CA 92121, USA. [6]Pfizer Inc., 300 Technology Square, Cambridge, MA 02139, USA.

References

1. Curtis JR, Singh JA. Use of biologics in rheumatoid arthritis: current and emerging paradigms of care. Clin Ther. 2011;33:679–707. https://doi.org/10.1016/j.clinthera.2011.05.044.
2. Weinblatt ME, Keystone EC, Furst DE, Moreland LW, Weisman MH, Birbara CA, et al. Adalimumab, a fully human anti-tumor necrosis factor alpha monoclonal antibody, for the treatment of rheumatoid arthritis in patients taking concomitant methotrexate: the ARMADA trial. Arthritis Rheum. 2003;48:35–45. https://doi.org/10.1002/art.10697.
3. Keystone EC, Kavanaugh AF, Sharp JT, Tannenbaum H, Hua Y, Teoh LS, et al. Radiographic, clinical, and functional outcomes of treatment with adalimumab (a human anti-tumor necrosis factor monoclonal antibody) in patients with active rheumatoid arthritis receiving concomitant methotrexate therapy: a randomized, placebo-controlled, 52-week trial. Arthritis Rheum. 2004;50:1400–11. https://doi.org/10.1002/art.20217.
4. Breedveld FC, Weisman MH, Kavanaugh AF, Cohen SB, Pavelka K, van Vollenhoven R, et al. The PREMIER study: a multicenter, randomized, double-blind clinical trial of combination therapy with adalimumab plus methotrexate versus methotrexate alone or adalimumab alone in patients with early, aggressive rheumatoid arthritis who had not had previous methotrexate treatment. Arthritis Rheum. 2006;54:26–37. https://doi.org/10.1002/art.21519.
5. European Medicines Agency. HUMIRA (adalimumab) summary of product characteristics. 2017 (last update: 10 May 2017). http://www.ema.europa.eu/docs/en_GB/document_library/EPAR_-_Product_Information/human/000481/WC500050870.pdf. Accessed 19 Feb. 2018.
6. Abbott Laboratories. HUMIRA (adalimumab) package insert. 2003 (last update: 26 September 2003). https://www.accessdata.fda.gov/drugsatfda_docs/label/2002/adalabb123102LB.htm. Accessed 19 Feb. 2018.
7. US Food and Drug Administration. Scientific considerations in demonstrating biosimilarity to a reference product. Guidance for industry. 2015 (last update: April 2015). https://www.fda.gov/downloads/drugs/guidances/ucm291128.pdf. Accessed 19 Feb. 2018.
8. European Medicines Agency. Guideline on similar biological medicinal products. 2014 (last update: July 2014). http://www.ema.europa.eu/docs/en_GB/document_library/Scientific_guideline/2014/10/WC500176768.pdf. Accessed 19 Feb. 2018.
9. QuintilesIMS. The impact of biosimilar competition in Europe. 2017 (last update: May 2017). http://www.medicinesforeurope.com/wp-content/uploads/2017/05/IMS-Biosimilar-2017_V9.pdf. Accessed 19 Feb. 2018.
10. Mulcahy A, Predmore Z, Soeren M. The cost savings potential of biosimilar drugs in the United States. 2014. https://www.rand.org/content/dam/rand/pubs/perspectives/PE100/PE127/RAND_PE127.pdf. Accessed 19 Feb. 2018.
11. Crespi-Lofton J, Skelton JB. The growing role of biologics and biosimilars in the United States: Perspectives from the APhA Biologics and Biosimilars Stakeholder Conference. J Am Pharm Assoc (2003). 2017;57:e15–27. https://doi.org/10.1016/j.japh.2017.05.014.
12. Derzi D, Ripp S, Ng C, Shoieb A, Finch G, Lorello L, et al. Comparative nonclinical assessments of the potential biosimilar PF-06410293 and adalimumab [abstract no. 276]. In: Society of Toxicology 53rd Annual Meeting and ToxExpo 2014; Phoenix, Arizona; 2014.
13. ClinicalTrials.gov. A study of PF-06410293 (adalimumab-Pfizer) and adalimumab (Humira) In healthy subjects (REFLECTIONS B538–07)) (B538–07). 2014 (last update: 13 April 2015). https://clinicaltrials.gov/ct2/show/NCT02237729. Accessed 19 Feb. 2018.
14. Aletaha D, Neogi T, Silman AJ, Funovits J, Felson DT, Bingham CO 3rd, et al. 2010 rheumatoid arthritis classification criteria: an American College of Rheumatology/European league against rheumatism collaborative initiative. Arthritis Rheum. 2010;62:2569–81. https://doi.org/10.1002/art.27584.
15. Felson DT, Anderson JJ, Boers M, Bombardier C, Furst D, Goldsmith C, et al. American College of Rheumatology. Preliminary definition of improvement in rheumatoid arthritis. Arthritis Rheum. 1995;38:727–35.
16. Fleischmann R, van der Heijde D, Koenig AS, Pedersen R, Szumski A, Marshall L, et al. How much does disease activity score in 28 joints ESR and CRP calculations underestimate disease activity compared with the simplified disease activity index? Ann Rheum Dis. 2015;74:1132–7. https://doi.org/10.1136/annrheumdis-2013-204920.
17. Kim HY, Lee SK, Song YW, Yoo DH, Koh EM, Yoo B, et al. A randomized, double-blind, placebo-controlled, phase III study of the human anti-tumor necrosis factor antibody adalimumab administered as subcutaneous injections in Korean rheumatoid arthritis patients treated with methotrexate. APLAR J Rheumatol. 2007;10:9–16. https://doi.org/10.1111/j.1479-8077.2007.00248.x.
18. Chen DY, Chou SJ, Hsieh TY, Chen YH, Chen HH, Hsieh CW, et al. Randomized, double-blind, placebo-controlled, comparative study of human anti-TNF antibody adalimumab in combination with methotrexate and methotrexate alone in Taiwanese patients with active rheumatoid arthritis. J Formos Med Assoc. 2009;108:310–9. https://doi.org/10.1016/S0929-6646(09)60071-1.
19. Miettinen O, Nurminen M. Comparative analysis of two rates. Stat Med. 1985;4:213–26.
20. Shankar G, Arkin S, Cocea L, Devanarayan V, Kirshner S, Kromminga A, et al. Assessment and reporting of the clinical immunogenicity of therapeutic proteins and peptides-harmonized terminology and tactical recommendations. AAPS J. 2014;16:658–73. https://doi.org/10.1208/s12248-014-9599-2.

19

Tophus resolution in patients with chronic refractory gout who have persistent urate-lowering responses to pegloticase

Brian F. Mandell[1], Anthony E. Yeo[2] and Peter E. Lipsky[3*]

Abstract

Background: Pegloticase is a recombinant mammalian uricase conjugated to polyethylene glycol approved in the United States for treatment of chronic refractory gout. It can profoundly decrease serum urate to < 1 mg/dl. In patients receiving pegloticase who did not generate high-titer antidrug antibodies (responders), the serum urate remained low for the duration of therapy, 6 months in the phase III clinical trials plus the open-label extension. The objective of this study was to assess the velocity of tophus resolution in subjects treated with pegloticase.

Methods: Data from two randomized controlled trials of pegloticase in chronic refractory gout were analyzed. Tophi were assessed by computer-assisted measurements of standardized digital photographs. Subjects were designated as responders and nonresponders based on maintenance of serum urate < 6 mg/dl at months 3 and 6 of treatment. The projected time of complete resolution of all tophi was determined by linear regression analysis.

Results: The mean total tophus area at baseline was 585.8 mm^2 for responders, 661.5 mm^2 for nonresponders, and 674.4 mm^2 for placebo-treated patients. Complete resolution at 6 months of at least one tophus was achieved by 69.6% of 23 responders, 27.9% of 43 nonresponders, and 14.3% of 21 patients who received placebo. Complete resolution of all photographed tophi was achieved by 34.8% of biochemical responders, 11.6% of nonresponders, and 0% of placebo-treated patients. The mean velocity of resolution of all tophi was 60.1 mm^2/month in responders with a mean projected time of complete resolution of 9.9 months (4.6–32.6 months). There was a significant inverse correlation between serum urate AUC and tophus resolution velocity ($r = -0.40$, $P = 0.0002$), although considerable heterogeneity in the velocity of resolution was noted. The only patient characteristic that correlated with the velocity of tophus resolution was the baseline tophus area.

Conclusions: Pegloticase treatment caused a rapid resolution of tophi in responders that correlated with the serum urate lowering associated with this therapy.

Keywords: Gout, Serum urate, Tophus, Pegloticase

Background

The tophus, a cardinal feature of gout, is a complex mass comprised of monosodium urate (MSU) crystals, a variety of immune and inflammatory cells, and a fibrous capsule [1, 2]. Tissue deposition of urate crystals initiates tophus formation with a local inflammatory and subsequent fibrotic tissue response. Clinically, it is difficult to dissect the various components of a tophus, and these may vary between different anatomical sites and different patients. Stimulation of immune/inflammatory system cells by MSU crystals may lead to chronic inflammation, pain, and tissue remodeling, including bone erosions [3, 4]. Much of the inflammatory capacity of urate crystals results from their capacity to stimulate the NLRP3 inflammasome with resultant production of IL-1β. The presence of tophi in patients with gout is associated with significantly decreased quality of life [5–12]. It has also been shown that clinically evident foot or ankle tophi are associated with muscle force deficits that may contribute to reduced muscular activation and consequent disuse muscle atrophy

* Correspondence: peterlipsky@comcast.net
[3]AMPEL BioSolutions, LLC, 250 West Main Street, Charlottesville, VA 22902, USA
Full list of author information is available at the end of the article

[13]. Tophaceous disease strongly predicts decreased hand function in patients with gout [14], because flexor or extensor tendon sheath deposition of urate can markedly reduce the ability to grasp and make a fist. The presence of tophi in patients with gout has also been associated with elevated mortality risk [15].

The most recent guidelines for treatment of gout from the American College of Rheumatology recognize the impact of tophi on patients and recommend that "the target serum urate should be lowered sufficiently to durably improve signs and symptoms of gout, including palpable and visible tophi detected by physical examination, and that this may involve therapeutic serum urate-lowering to below 5 mg/dl" [16].

Multiple studies have demonstrated the ability of urate-lowering therapy to reduce or resolve tophi [17–25]. However, results from most clinical trials indicate only modest decreases in tophi, perhaps owing to their relatively short duration [17, 21, 22]. Although there appears to be a significant correlation between the magnitude of serum urate reduction and resolution of tophi [26, 27], and although oral urate-lowering therapies are capable of decreasing serum urate from baseline by 50–60%, resulting in levels that are between 4 and 6 mg/dl [17, 20, 22], this may be insufficient for rapid tophus resolution.

Pegloticase is a recombinant mammalian uricase conjugated to polyethylene glycol approved in the United States for treatment of patients with chronic refractory gout. It profoundly decreases serum urate in biochemical responders to < 1 mg/dl [28]. The results of the pegloticase randomized clinical trials (RCTs) [18] provided the opportunity to determine the impact of persistent and markedly low levels of serum urate on the velocity of tophus resolution. Case reports and small-scale studies have indicated that treatment with pegloticase can produce rapid decreases in tophus mass in patients with gout [29–31]. Tophus reductions with pegloticase were also evaluated in the RCTs of this agent [19], but this analysis combined results from patients who responded to this treatment with sustained reductions in serum urate and those who did not. The present analysis focuses on tophus reduction in patients who responded with persistent urate lowering to pegloticase and compares results from this group with those from patients who did not have a persistent response (nonresponders) and those who received placebo.

Methods

Design of pegloticase clinical trials

Results from two identical RCTs of pegloticase were analyzed (NCT00325195, NCT01356498) [18, 28]. The methods for these studies have been described in detail elsewhere [18, 28] and are summarized only briefly herein. These studies received institutional review board approval at each site. Written informed consent and Health Insurance Portability and Accountability Act assurances were completed for each participant before enrollment. The design and conduct of the study complied with the Declaration of Helsinki.

Patients

Patients were ≥ 18 years of age with chronic refractory gout, defined as baseline serum urate ≥ 0.476 mmol/L (8 mg/dl), and at least one of the following: (1) at least three self-reported gout flares during the previous 18 months, (2) at least one tophus, and/or (3) gouty arthropathy, defined clinically or radiographically as joint damage caused by gout, and (4) contraindication to treatment with allopurinol or history of failure to normalize urate despite ≥ 3 months of treatment with the maximum medically appropriate allopurinol dose. Patients were randomized to 6 months of treatment with intravenous infusions of either pegloticase 8 mg at each infusion (8 mg q2w), pegloticase 8 mg alternating with placebo (q4w), or placebo [28].

Tophus assessment

Tophus assessment was carried out using Computer-Assisted Photographic Evaluation in Rheumatology methodology [32]. Each study site was supplied with a calibrated digital camera, digital media storage cards, preprinted templates for hand and foot photography, and a light stand. A designated individual was trained and took all photographs at each site.

Photographs of the hands and feet were taken for each patient at baseline and repeated at weeks 13, 19, and 25 of the RCTs using the same views of the tophus sites identified at baseline. Serial photographs of up to two additional regions were taken at the discretion of the investigator, based on other tophi identified at baseline. Digital media cards containing the photographs were sent to RadPharm (Princeton, NJ, USA), where central readers, who were blinded to treatment assignment, evaluated the photographs prospectively and identified sites of tophi present at the start of treatment as well as response to therapy.

Endpoints

Biochemical responder analysis

A responder (primary endpoint for the RCTs) was defined as a patient with plasma UA < 0.36 mmol/L (6 mg/dl) for ≥ 80% of the 15 measurements taken during periods of intensive monitoring from the week 9 infusion to just before the week 13 infusion (bracketing 3 months after the initiation of infusions) and from the week 21 infusion to the week 25 final study visit (bracketing 6 months after the initiation of infusions).

Tophus resolution

Two measures were used to assess the effects of pegloticase treatment on the photographed tophi. The first was the complete resolution of at least one tophus without development of new tophi or progressive enlargement of any other tophus. This was the definition employed in an earlier evaluation of the effects of pegloticase on tophi [19]. The second measure was based on the total number of photographically identified tophi at baseline and assessed as total area of all tophi combined. In this analysis, a response was defined as complete resolution of all of these tophi.

Serum urate exposure

AUCs of serum urate during the 6-month study were calculated according to the equation:

$$AUC = \int_a^b F(X)dX,$$

where a and b are points on the x-axis and F(X) is the integral of function using SAS software (SAS Institute, Cary, NC, USA). Because the curves were not always continuous functions, the trapezoidal rule was employed to approximate the definitive integral.

Analysis populations

Results from three groups were evaluated: (1) patients treated with pegloticase q2w who were responders (defined above), (2) patients who received pegloticase the entire 6 months but did not meet the criteria for a response (nonresponders), and (3) patients who received placebo.

Results for responders were also subdivided on the basis of baseline tophus burden into tertiles as low (total baseline tophus area < 668 mm^2), medium (baseline tophus burden 688–1690 mm^2), and high (baseline tophus burden > 1690 mm^2), and the velocity of tophus resolution was determined for each of these groups.

Data analysis

Kaplan-Meier analysis was used for evaluation of time to events. Because the number of subjects in each group was small, nonparametric tests were used. Unpaired two-sample Wilcoxon tests were used when comparing groups. One-way analyses of variance were employed to derive group means for all variables. Between-group differences for categorical variables were determined by Fisher's exact tests. The projected time of complete resolution of all tophi was determined by linear regression using SAS software. The relationship between serum urate exposure and velocity of tophus reduction was evaluated with a Pearson product-moment correlation, and significance was determined with a t test. $P < 0.05$ was the accepted level of significance for all significance tests.

Results

Patients

The analysis included results from 66 patients who received pegloticase every 2 weeks (q2w) (23 responders, 43 nonresponders, and 21 patients who received placebo). The baseline demographic and clinical characteristics of these patients are summarized in Table 1. Except for age, there were no significant differences among the three groups for any demographic or clinical variable.

Tophus resolution

The mean total tophus area (mean [SD]) at baseline was 585.8 mm^2 (795.0) for responders, 661.5 mm^2 (1298.7) for nonresponders, and 674.4 mm^2 (1011.6) for placebo patients ($p = 0.32$). Complete resolution of at least one tophus without development of new tophi or progressive enlargement of any other

Table 1 Baseline demographic characteristics of the three groups of patients included in the analysis

Characteristic	Responders ($n = 23$)	Nonresponders ($n = 43$)	Placebo ($n = 21$)	P value
Age, years, mean (SD)	63.0 (14.1)	53.5 (14.0)	56.8 (10.5)	0.043
Sex, n	17 M, 6F	37 M, 6F	17 M, 4F	0.48
Disease duration, years, mean (SD)	17.0 (17.2)	15.1 (9.8)	14.9 (9.9)	0.97
sUA, mg/dl, mean (SD)	10.22 (1.76)	10.50 (1.62)	10.19 (1.82)	0.68
Number of tophi assessed	93	98	68	NC
Total tophus area, mm^2, mean (SD)	585.8 (795.0)	661.5 (1298.7)	674.4 (1011.6)	0.32
Comorbidities, n				
Hypertension	16	30	17	0.60
Dyslipidemia	14	17	10	0.25
Diabetes mellitus	4	7	4	0.96
Coronary artery disease	4	3	2	0.41

Abbreviations: M Male, *F* Female, *NC* Not computed

P value is for comparison of responders, nonresponders, and placebo tophus was achieved by 69.6% of responders, and the median time to resolution for this subgroup of patients was 132 days. This goal was achieved by 27.9% of nonresponders with a median time to resolution of 162 days; 14.3% of patients who received placebo achieved this outcome, and the median time to resolution was 171 days (Fig. 1a). The percentage of responders who achieved this criterion was significantly higher than for nonresponders ($P = 0.001$) or patients treated with placebo ($P = 0.0006$). The response rate for nonresponders was not significantly different from that for patients who received placebo ($P = 0.24$).

Complete resolution of all tophi photographed was achieved by 34.8% of responders (93 tophi assessed) in the 6 months of the RCT, 11.6% of nonresponders (98 tophi assessed), and 0% of placebo-treated patients (69 tophi assessed) (Fig. 1b). The percentage of

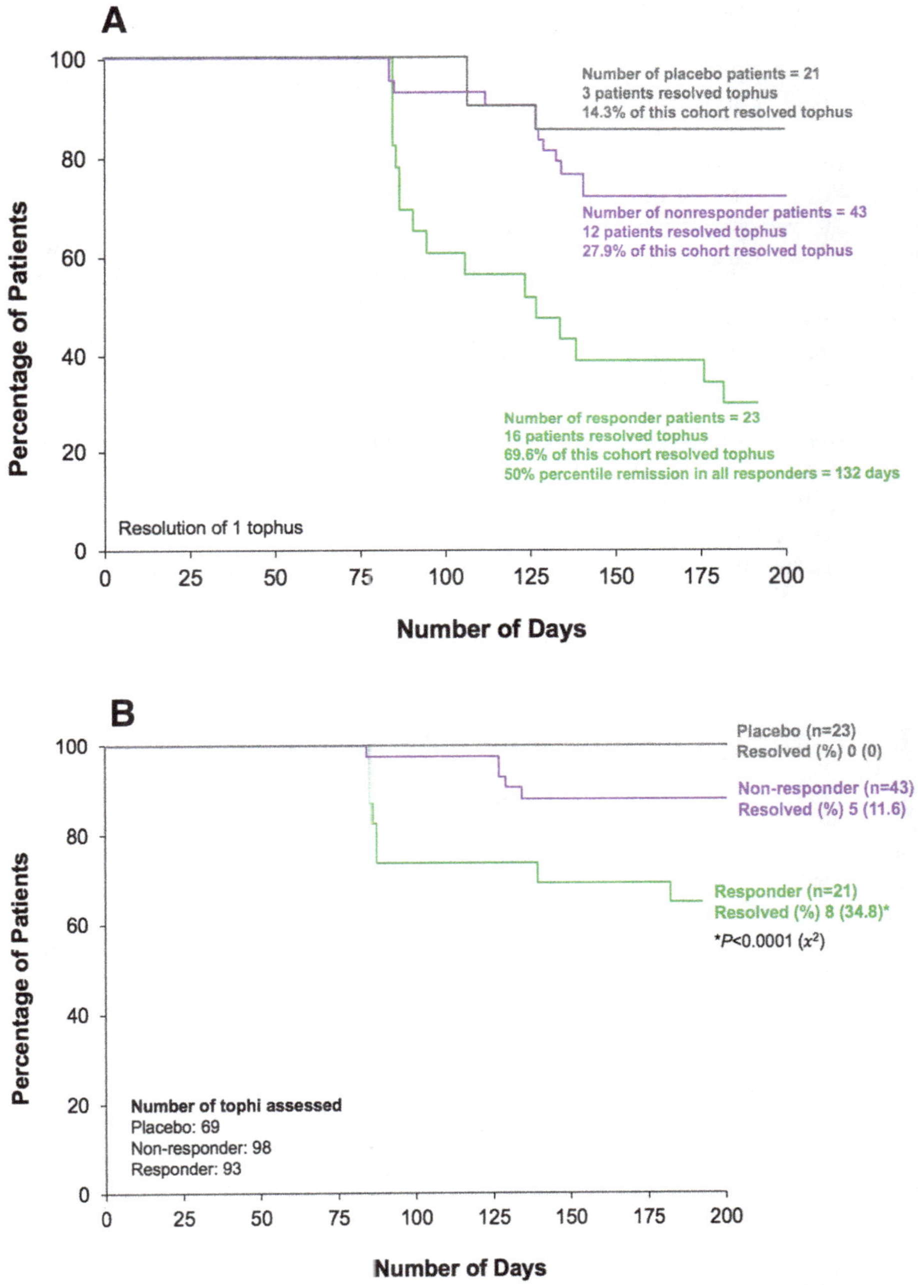

Fig. 1 **a** Kaplan-Meier analysis of time to complete resolution of at least one tophus without development of new tophi or progressive enlargement of any other tophus. **b** Kaplan-Meier analysis of time to complete resolution of all tophi

responders who achieved this criterion was significantly higher than for nonresponders and patients treated with placebo ($P < 0.001$). The frequency of subjects who completely resolved tophi for nonresponders was not significantly different from that for patients who received placebo ($P = 0.16$).

Velocity of tophus resolution

Comparison of results for responders, nonresponders, and patients who received placebo indicated significant differences among groups for tophus area at all postbaseline assessments (Fig. 2) (all $P \leq 0.01$). Reductions from baseline to the end of 6 months were significant for responders and nonresponders ($P < 0.0001$ and $P = 0.0005$, respectively), but not for those who received placebo ($P = 0.32$). The velocity of tophus resolution for the responders was 60.1 mm^2 per month, with a projected time of full resolution of 9.9 months. The velocity of tophus resolution was statistically different from that for the nonresponders (22.3 mm^2 per month, $P = 0.053$) and for patients treated with placebo (28.4 mm^2 per month, $P = 0.0034$). The projected time to complete tophus resolution in biochemical responders was 9.9 months.

Exposure to different serum urate treatment groups

The mean (SD) serum urate values at the end of treatment were 0.49 mg/dl (01.41) (0.029 mmol/L) for the biochemical responders, 8.47 mg/dl (3.61) (0.504 mmol/L) for the nonresponders, and 10.25 mg/dl (1.23) (0.610 mmol/L) for the patients who received placebo ($P < 0.0001$ for responders vs the other two groups). The most unbiased approach for determining serum urate exposure over the course of the RCTs was determination of the AUC for all of the measurements made during the study (Fig. 3a). The mean (SD) value for this measure for biochemical responders was 2907.0 mg/dl·h (1834.3), and it was significantly lower than values for either nonresponders (31,615.6 [10,814.9]) ($P < 0.0001$) or patients treated with placebo (42,442.6 [6234.1]) ($P < 0.0001$) (Fig. 3b).

Relationship between serum urate exposure and velocity of tophus reduction

Combined analysis of results from all three groups of patients included in this analysis indicated a significant inverse correlation between serum urate AUC and tophus resolution velocity ($r = -0.40$, $P = 0.0002$) (Fig. 4). The mean time to resolution of all tophi for biochemical responders was 9.9 months (range, 4.6 to 32.6 months). Clinical features, including age, body mass index, gender, race, and tophus location, did not significantly influence velocity of tophus resolution.

Baseline tophus burden and tophus reduction

In responders, the mean (SD) baseline tophus areas at baseline were 419.4 mm^2 (202.4) for patients with low baseline tophus burden, 1176.9 mm^2 (238.7) for those with moderate tophus burden, and 4260.4 mm^2 (2784.9) for those with high baseline tophus burden (Fig. 5a).

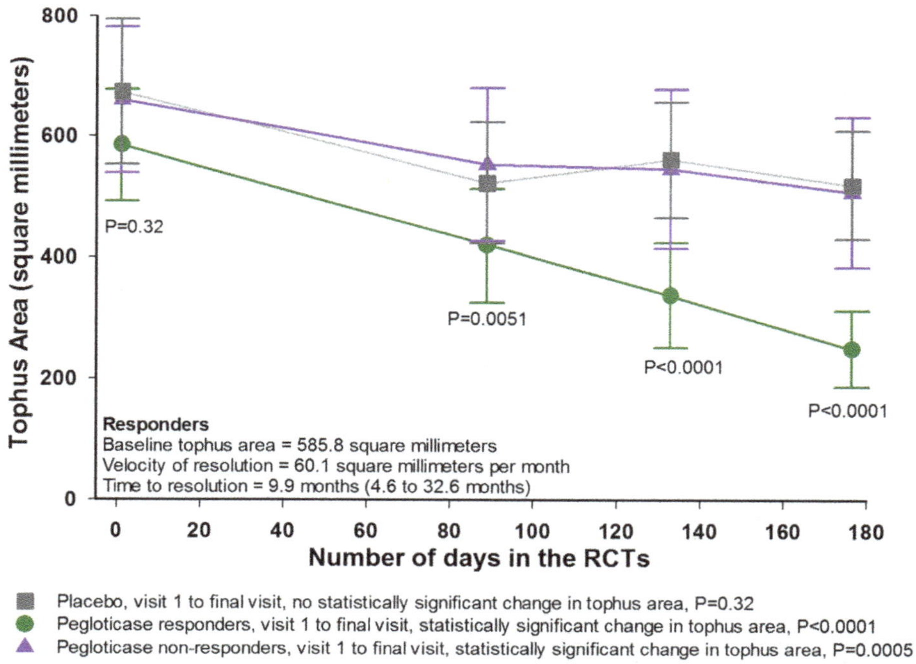

Fig. 2 Mean (±SD) tophus area over time for the three groups of patients evaluated

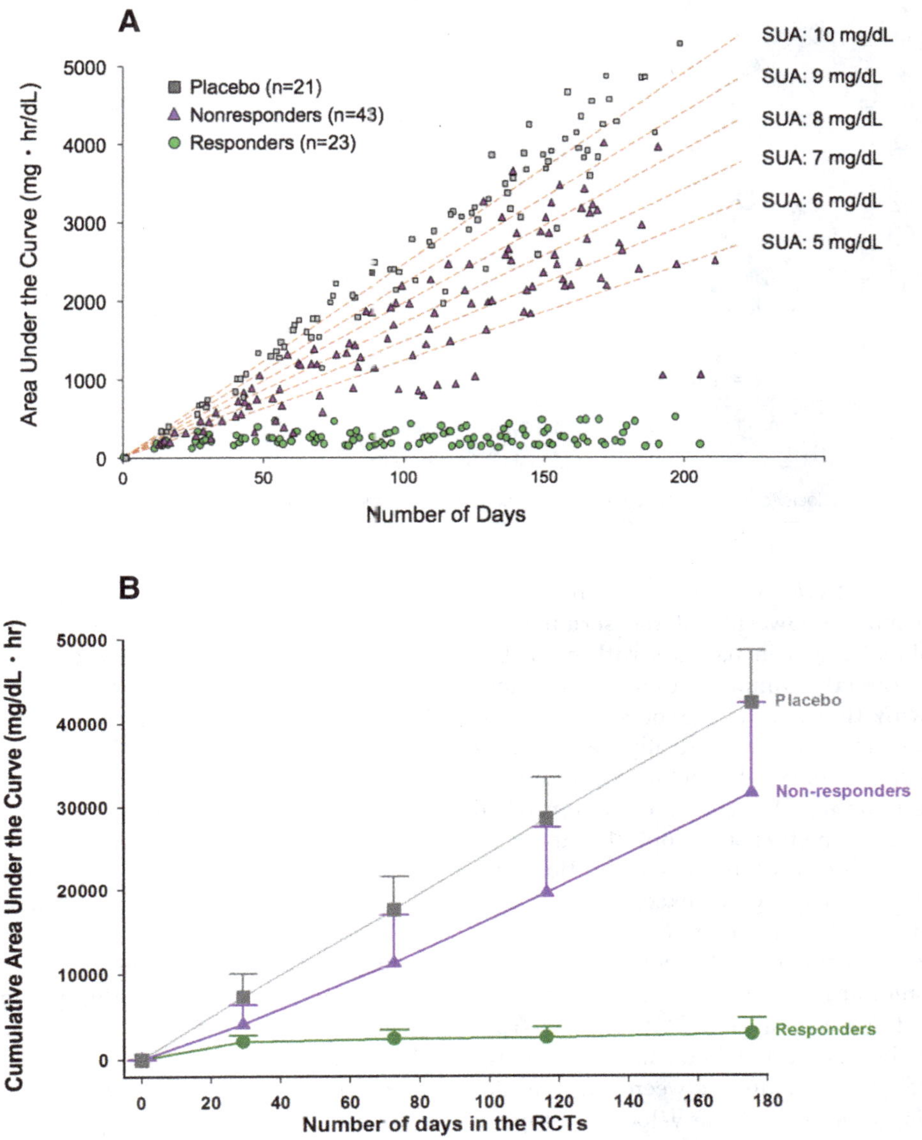

Fig. 3 **a** Cumulative serum urate AUC values for individual patients at different time points and projected cumulative serum urate AUCs for different mean serum urate values over the course of the study. **b** Mean AUC [±SD] for serum urate in the three groups included in the analysis

The mean (SD) velocity of tophus resolution was 28.7 (13.6) mm^2/month, and the mean time to tophus resolution was 6.98 months (range, 5.02 to 10.0 months) for patients with low baseline tophus burden ($P < 0.0001$ compared with those with high tophus burden). For those with moderate baseline tophus burden, these values were 60.2 (53.5) mm^2/month and 7.14 months (range, 5.21 to 10.1 months) ($P < 0.0001$ compared with those with high tophus burden), and for those with high baseline tophus burden, they were 89.5 (38.7) mm^2/month and 12.02 months (range, 6.73 to 27.91 months) ($P = 0.0477$) (Fig. 5b and c).

Discussion

This analysis demonstrates that about one-third of patients who responded biochemically to pegloticase as defined in the RCTs achieved resolution of all tophi within the 6 months of the RCTs. This goal was also achieved by 11.6% of pegloticase-treated patients who did not have sustained reductions in sUA to < 6 mg/dl for the duration of the study, but in none of those receiving placebo. Correlational analysis showed further that reduction in exposure to serum urate achieved with pegloticase was correlated with the velocity of tophus resolution.

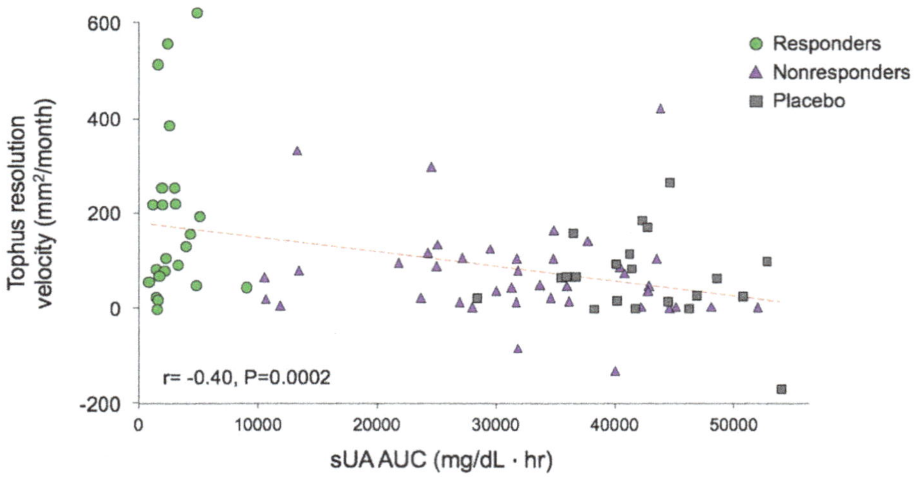

Fig. 4 Serum urate AUC vs velocity of tophus reduction in responders, nonresponders, and placebo-treated patients

Previous studies have shown that treatments achieving more modest lowering of the serum urate can reduce tophus burden in patients with gout, but it is difficult to directly compare results from those clinical trials with those from the present analysis. In other studies, results are generally reported as the percentage of patients who achieved resolution of a single target tophus [17, 20] or reduction of all tophi [22]. However, neither the tophus burden at baseline nor the velocity of tophus resolution was reported in these trials. One exception to this generalization is a trial in which 63 patients with microscopically confirmed tophaceous gout were treated with allopurinol, benzbromarone, or the combination of these two agents [23]. Results from that study, like those reported here, indicated a significant inverse relationship between the serum urate level during therapy and the velocity of tophus reduction. The mean time from onset of urate-lowering therapy to the disappearance of the target tophus for all patients was 20.8 months (range, 6–64 months). This is much longer than that reported in our analysis, and it is almost certainly related to the fact that the average on-treatment serum urate for the patients evaluated ranged from 3.97 to 5.37 mg/dl in different treatment arms of the trial reported by Perez-Ruiz vs an end-of-treatment value of 0.49 mg/dl for the biochemical responders in the present analysis. The highest velocity of tophus reduction (decrease in diameter) was 1.53 mm per month, and the initial tophus diameter for patients in the Perez-Ruiz study was 14.5 mm. Assuming that the tophi were approximately circular, this equates to a reduction in area of 33.2 mm^2 per month, which is approximately one-half of that for the responders in this analysis and only slightly higher than that for the nonresponders.

Nonresponders to pegloticase typically have an initial profound reduction in serum urate that is followed by a gradual increase in serum urate over approximately 6 weeks. This loss of response is strongly associated with development of high titer of antibodies to pegloticase [28, 33]. The results of the present analysis suggest that these patients may have received some benefit from pegloticase with respect to tophus reduction, because complete resolution of at least one tophus without development of new tophi or progressive enlargement of any other tophus was achieved by 27.9% of this group, and resolution of all photographed tophi was achieved by 11.6%. This is consistent with previous observations in patients treated with pegloticase and the suggestion that even transient lowering of serum urate levels may decrease tophus volume because they are dynamic structures and begin to decline in size as soon as serum urate levels are decreased [30].

A final point worth noting is that the incomplete tophus resolution in any study employing photographs for this determination may underestimate the benefit of serum urate-lowering treatment. A typical tophus consists of a mostly acellular crystalline core surrounded by a corona zone with multiple cell types, including macrophages, mast cells, and lymphocytes, and an outer, loose fibrovascular zone [3, 34]. The reductions in tophus size reported here probably reflect decreases in the mass of MSU crystals, which might be complete but still leave chronic inflammation and a fibrotic "shell," which may take various periods of time to resolve. The heterogeneous composition of tophi along with interindividual variations in urate solubilization likely contributed to the

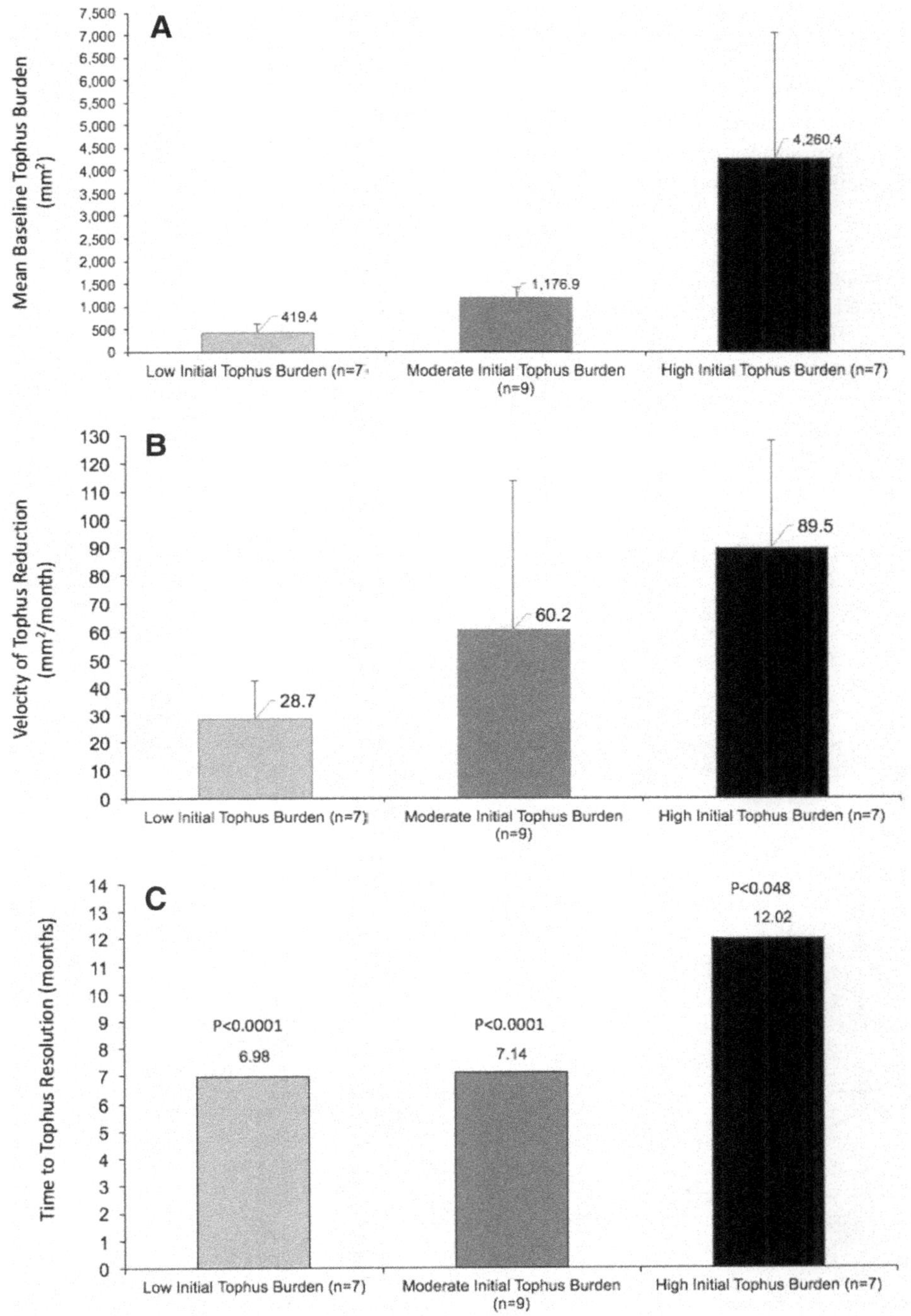

Fig. 5 **a** Baseline tophus areas for biochemical responders with low, medium, and high tophus burden at baseline. **b** Velocity of tophus resolution for patients the three groups. **c** Mean time to tophus resolution for patients with low, medium, and high tophus burden at baseline. Error bars are SDs

high interpatient variability in velocity of tophus resolution. Subject characteristics, including age, body mass index, sex, race, and tophus location were not correlated with velocity of tophus resolution. However, there was a significant positive correlation between initial tophus area and velocity of resolution. Presumably, larger tophi may have a greater relative component of urate crystals that can be mobilized rapidly by pegloticase treatment.

The limitations of this study include the post hoc nature of the analysis, the assessment of only subcutaneous tophi, and the use of photographic rather than clinical measures of tophus area. It is possible that deeper tophi respond with a different velocity than subcutaneous ones and that clinical evaluation of tophi might have been more effective by allowing assessment of the consistency of the lesion as well as its dimensions. Despite these caveats, the data contribute to understanding of the relationship between serum urate burden and tophus resolution and also indicate the heterogeneity in tophus resolution.

Conclusions

Pegloticase treatment causes a rapid resolution of tophi in responders, as predicted from the profound and persistent serum urate lowering associated with this therapy. Even transient reductions in serum urate observed in nonresponders may result in complete resolution of tophi in some patients over the course of 6 months or less.

Abbreviations

MSU: Monosodium urate crystals; q2w: Every 2 weeks; q4w: Every 4 weeks; RCT: Randomized clinical trial; sUA: Serum uric acid; UA: Uric acid

Acknowledgements

Not applicable.

Funding

This analysis was supported by Horizon Pharma, which did not influence the analysis or the conclusions reported in this article.

Authors' contributions

All authors had full access to the study data, contributed to the writing and review of the manuscript, and read and approved the final version for publication.

Competing interests

BFM reports being a clinical investigator for and receiving consulting fees from Horizon Pharma. PEL reports receiving consulting fees from Celgene, Horizon Pharma, Janssen, Medimmune, and Sanofi. AEY reports receiving fees as a contractor from Horizon Pharma.

Author details

[1]Department of Rheumatologic and Immunologic Disease, Cleveland Clinic, Cleveland, OH, USA. [2]Horizon Pharma, Lake Forest, IL, USA. [3]AMPEL BioSolutions, LLC, 250 West Main Street, Charlottesville, VA 22902, USA.

References

1. Ruoff G, Edwards NL. Overview of serum uric acid treatment targets in gout: why less than 6 mg/dL? Postgrad Med. 2016;128:706–15.
2. Sapsford M, Gamble GD, Aati O, Knight J, Horne A, Doyle AJ, et al. Relationship of bone erosion with the urate and soft tissue components of the tophus in gout: a dual energy computed tomography study. Rheumatology (Oxford). 2017;56:129–33.
3. Dalbeth N, Pool B, Gamble GD, Smith T, Callon KE, McQueen FM, et al. Cellular characterization of the gouty tophus: a quantitative analysis. Arthritis Rheum. 2010;62:1549–56.
4. Franklin BS, Mangan MS, Latz E. Crystal formation in inflammation. Annu Rev Immunol. 2016;34:173–202.
5. Roddy E, Zhang W, Doherty M. Is gout associated with reduced quality of life? A case-control study. Rheumatology (Oxford). 2007;46:1441–4.
6. Chandratre P, Roddy E, Clarson L, Richardson J, Hider SL, Mallen CD. Health-related quality of life in gout: a systematic review. Rheumatology (Oxford). 2013;52:2031–40.
7. Becker MA, Schumacher HR, Benjamin KL, Gorevic P, Greenwald M, Fessel J, et al. Quality of life and disability in patients with treatment-failure gout. J Rheumatol. 2009;36:1041–8.
8. Khanna P, Persselin J, Hays R, Furst D, Paulus H, Maranian P, et al. Health related quality of life (HRQOL) in tophaceous vs. non-tophaceous gout. Arthritis Rheum. 2010;62((Suppl 10)):Abstract:1365.
9. Khanna PP, Perez-Ruiz F, Maranian P, Khanna D. Long-term therapy for chronic gout results in clinically important improvements in the health-related quality of life: short form-36 is responsive to change in chronic gout. Rheumatology (Oxford). 2011;50:740–5.
10. Khanna PP, Nuki G, Bardin T, Tausche AK, Forsythe A, Goren A, et al. Tophi and frequent gout flares are associated with impairments to quality of life, productivity, and increased healthcare resource use: results from a cross-sectional survey. Health Qual Life Outcomes. 2012;10:117.
11. Khanna P, Tafesse E, Baumgartner S, Walker A, Morlock R. Comparing the burden of illness of patients with tophaceous and non-tophaceous gout in France, Germany, Italy, Spain, UK, and USA [abstract]. Arthritis Rheumatol. 2016;68(Suppl 10):Abstract: 223 Available at: http://acrabstracts.org/abstract/comparing-the-burden-of-illness-of-patients-with-tophaceousand-non-tophaceous-gout-in-france-germany-italy-spain-uk-and-usa/. Accessed 11 Jul 2017.
12. Mandell BF, Baraf HSB, Yeo A, Lipsky PE. Rapid tophus resolution in chronic refractory gout patients treated with pegloticase [abstract]. Arthritis Rheumatol. 2017;69(suppl 10) http://acrabstracts.org/abstract/rapid-tophus-resolution-in-chronic-refractory-gout-patients-treated-with-pegloticase/. Accessed 2 Jan 2018.
13. Stewart S, Dalbeth N, Otter S, Gow P, Kumar S, Rome K. Clinically-evident tophi are associated with reduced muscle force in the foot and ankle in people with gout: a cross-sectional study. J Foot Ankle Res. 2017;10:25.
14. Dalbeth N, Collis J, Gregory K, Clark B, Robinson E, McQueen FM. Tophaceous joint disease strongly predicts hand function in patients with gout. Rheumatology (Oxford). 2007;46:1804–7.
15. Vincent Z, Gamble G, House M, Knight J, Horne A, Taylor WJ, et al. Predictors of mortality in people with recent onset of gout: a prospective observational study. J Rheumatol. 2017 Mar;44(3):368–73.
16. Khanna D, Fitzgerald JD, Khanna PP, Sangmee B, Singh M, Neogi T, et al. American College of Rheumatology guidelines for management of gout. Part 1: systematic nonpharmacologic and pharmacologic therapeutic approaches to hyperuricemia. Arthritis Care Res (Hoboken). 2012;64:1431–46.
17. Saag KG, Fitz-Patrick D, Kopicko J, Fung M, Bhakta N, Adler S, et al. Lesinurad combined with allopurinol: a randomized, double-blind, placebo-controlled study in gout patients with an inadequate response to standard-of-care allopurinol (a US-based study). Arthritis Rheumatol. 2017;69:203–12.
18. Becker MA, Baraf HS, Yood RA, Dillon A, Vazquez-Mellado J, Ottery FD, et al. Long-term safety of pegloticase in chronic gout refractory to conventional treatment. Ann Rheum Dis. 2013;72:1469–74.
19. Baraf HS, Becker MA, Gutierrez-Urena SR, Treadwell EL, Vazquez-Mellado J, Rehrig CD, et al. Tophus burden reduction with pegloticase: results from phase 3 randomized trials and open-label extension in patients with chronic gout refractory to conventional therapy. Arthritis Res Ther. 2013;15:R137.
20. Schumacher HR Jr, Becker MA, Lloyd E, MacDonald PA, Lademacher C. Febuxostat in the treatment of gout: 5-yr findings of the FOCUS efficacy and safety study. Rheumatology (Oxford). 2009;48:188–94.
21. Schumacher HR Jr, Becker MA, Wortmann RL, Macdonald PA, Hunt B, Streit J, et al. Effects of febuxostat versus allopurinol and placebo in reducing serum urate in subjects with hyperuricemia and gout: a 28-week, phase III, randomized, double-blind, parallel-group trial. Arthritis Rheum. 2008;59:1540–8.
22. Becker MA, Schumacher HR Jr, Wortmann RL, MacDonald PA, Eustace D, Palo WA, et al. Febuxostat compared with allopurinol in patients with hyperuricemia and gout. N Engl J Med. 2005;353:2450–61.
23. Perez-Ruiz F, Calabozo M, Pijoan JI, Herrero-Beites AM, Ruibal A. Effect of urate-lowering therapy on the velocity of size reduction of tophi in chronic gout. Arthritis Rheum. 2002;47:356–60.
24. McCarthy GM, Barthelemy CR, Veum JA, Wortmann RL. Influence of antihyperuricemic therapy on the clinical and radiographic progression of gout. Arthritis Rheum. 1991;34:1489–94.
25. Goldfarb E, Smyth CJ. Effects of allopurinol, a xanthine oxidase inhibitor, and sulfinpyrazone upon the urinary and serum urate concentrations in eight

patients with tophaceous gout. Arthritis Rheum. 1966;9:414–23.
26. Peiteado D, Villalba A, Martín-Mola E, Balsa A, De Miguel E. Ultrasound sensitivity to changes in gout: a longitudinal study after two years of treatment. Clin Exp Rheumatol. 2017;35(5):746–51.
27. Perez-Ruiz F, Martin I, Canteli B. Ultrasonographic measurement of tophi as an outcome measure for chronic gout. J Rheumatol. 2007;34:1888–93.
28. Sundy JS, Baraf HS, Yood RA, Edwards NL, Gutierrez-Urena SR, Treadwell EL, et al. Efficacy and tolerability of pegloticase for the treatment of chronic gout in patients refractory to conventional treatment: two randomized controlled trials. JAMA. 2011;306:711–20.
29. Modjinou DV, Krasnokutsky S, Gyftopoulos S, Pike VC, Karis E, Keenan RT, et al. Comparison of dual-energy CT, ultrasound and surface measurement for assessing tophus dissolution during rapid urate debulking. Clin Rheumatol. 2017;36(9):2101–7.
30. Araujo EG, Bayat S, Petsch C, Englbrecht M, Faustini F, Kleyer A, et al. Tophus resolution with pegloticase: a prospective dual-energy CT study. RMD Open. 2015;1:e000075.
31. Dalbeth N, Doyle AJ, McQueen FM, Sundy J, Baraf HS. Exploratory study of radiographic change in patients with tophaceous gout treated with intensive urate-lowering therapy. Arthritis Care Res (Hoboken). 2014;66:82–5.
32. Maroli AN, Waltrip R, Alton M, Baraf HSB, Huang B, Rehrig C, et al. First application of computer-assisted analysis of digital photographs for assessing tophus response: phase 3 studies of pegloticase in treatment failure gout [abstract]. Arthritis Rheum. 2009;60:1111.
33. Lipsky PE, Calabrese LH, Kavanaugh A, Sundy JS, Wright D, Wolfson M, et al. Pegloticase immunogenicity: the relationship between efficacy and antibody development in patients treated for refractory chronic gout. Arthritis Res Ther. 2014;16:R60.
34. Palmer DG, Hogg N, Denholm I, Allen CA, Highton J, Hessian PA. Comparison of phenotype expression by mononuclear phagocytes within subcutaneous gouty tophi and rheumatoid nodules. Rheumatol Int. 1987;7:187–93.

Baseline JAK phosphorylation profile of peripheral blood leukocytes, studied by whole blood phosphospecific flow cytometry, is associated with 1-year treatment response in early rheumatoid arthritis

Krista Kuuliala[1*], Antti Kuuliala[1], Riitta Koivuniemi[2], Hannu Kautiainen[3,4,5], Heikki Repo[1] and Marjatta Leirisalo-Repo[2]

Abstract

Background: We found recently that baseline signal transducer and activator of transcription 3 phosphorylation in peripheral blood CD4$^+$ T cells of patients with early rheumatoid arthritis (RA) is associated with treatment response to synthetic disease-modifying antirheumatic drugs (DMARDs). This prompted us to study the baseline phosphorylation profiles of Janus kinases (JAKs) in blood leukocytes with respect to treatment response in early RA.

Methods: Thirty-five DMARD-naïve patients with early RA provided blood samples for whole blood flow cytometric determination of phosphorylation of JAKs in CD4$^+$ and CD8$^+$ T cells, CD19$^+$ B cells, and CD14$^+$ monocytes. Treatment response was determined after 1 year of treatment with synthetic DMARDs, with remission defined as absence of tender and swollen joints and normal erythrocyte sedimentation rate. Exact logistic regression was used to investigate the association of baseline variables with treatment response. Ninety-five percent CIs of means were estimated by bias-corrected bootstrapping.

Results: High JAK3 phosphorylation in CD4$^+$ and CD8$^+$ T cells, CD19$^+$ B cells, and CD14$^+$ monocytes and low JAK2 phosphorylation in CD14$^+$ monocytes were significantly associated with remission following treatment with synthetic DMARDs.

Conclusions: Baseline JAK phosphorylation profile in peripheral blood leukocytes may provide a means to predict treatment response achieved by synthetic DMARDs among patients with early RA.

Keywords: Rheumatoid arthritis, Disease-modifying antirheumatic drug, Janus kinases, Phosphorylation, Blood, Leukocyte, Biomarker

* Correspondence: krista.kuuliala@helsinki.fi
[1]Bacteriology and Immunology, Helsinki University Hospital and University of Helsinki, Helsinki, Finland
Full list of author information is available at the end of the article

Background

Rheumatoid arthritis (RA) is a chronic autoimmune disease characterized by inflammatory synovitis; articular destruction; extra-articular manifestations; and, when not responding to treatment satisfactorily, progressive disability and increased mortality. The disease is heterogeneous, and its pathogenetic mechanisms are not clear, but they are known to involve both genetic and environmental factors as well as innate and adaptive immunity [1]. Synthetic disease-modifying antirheumatic drugs (sDMARDs) are the first treatment option in untreated RA, used either as monotherapy or in various combinations [2–4]. Recently, highly selective immunological agents have been developed for the treatment of RA, including biological disease-modifying antirheumatic drugs (DMARDs), especially blockers of inflammatory cytokines and immune cell surface receptors [5], and agents inhibiting intracellular signal transduction pathway members. As to the latter, Janus kinases (JAKs) are tempting targets because they are required for classical immune cytokine receptor signal transduction and consequently are involved in the pathophysiology of several inflammatory and immune disorders [6, 7]. Despite the multiple drug options for treatment of RA, the lack of reliable predictive biomarkers poses a challenge to finding the most effective and suitable treatment for each individual rapidly, preferably within 3–4 months from the onset of symptoms [8].

A few years ago, we started to study the phosphorylation of the signal transducer and activator of transcription (STAT) transcription factors as biomarkers of disease activity and treatment response in RA [9]. We found that baseline phosphorylation of STAT3 in whole blood leukocytes is associated with the treatment response achieved by use of sDMARDs [10]. In the present study, we made progress in studying the JAK-STAT pathway and aimed at elucidating if JAK phosphorylation levels are able to distinguish DMARD-naïve patients with RA who will respond well to sDMARDs from those who will require still other treatment options. Using a phosphospecific whole blood flow cytometric method, we measured the baseline phosphorylation levels of all known JAKs (i.e., JAK1, JAK2, JAK3, and tyrosine kinase 2 [Tyk2]) in whole blood T cells, B cells, and monocytes of patients with early untreated RA.

Methods

Subjects

The study included 35 patients diagnosed with early RA at the Division of Rheumatology, Helsinki University Central Hospital, Helsinki, Finland, between April 2012 and April 2013. The patients fulfilled the American College of Rheumatology/European League Against Rheumatism 2010 classification criteria [11]. At study entry, the patients had received no DMARDs or oral glucocorticoids. Twenty-one healthy volunteers (62% women; mean age 47 years [SD 13 years]) with no infectious symptoms or history of autoimmune disease and derived from hospital and laboratory staff served as reference subjects. All subjects were white Finnish persons residing in the Helsinki metropolitan area. The study protocol was approved by the ethical review board of the Joint Authority for the Hospital District of Helsinki and Uusimaa, and written informed consent was obtained from each patient.

Clinical evaluation

A comprehensive clinical and laboratory evaluation was undertaken at entry concomitant to blood sampling. Joints were evaluated for swelling and pain (66 and 68 joints, respectively). Patient global assessment of disease activity was recorded on a 100-mm visual analogue scale. Laboratory measurements, including white blood cell count, erythrocyte sedimentation rate (ESR), and plasma C-reactive protein (CRP) level, were logged. The 28-joint Disease Activity Score (DAS28) was calculated [12]. After a mean 12-month follow-up, the patients were reexamined. Patients with no tender or swollen joints (68 and 66 joints, respectively) and normal ESR were considered to be in remission.

Blood samples

At study entry, an 8-ml blood sample was taken by venipuncture from the antecubital vein into a Falcon polypropylene tube (BD Biosciences, Bedford, MA, USA) supplemented with 800 μl of pyrogen-free acid citrate dextrose solution A (ACD-A; Baxter Healthcare Ltd, Thetford, UK). Cells were prepared for flow cytometry within 3 h of blood sampling.

Antibodies

The following antibodies were purchased from BD Biosciences (San Jose, CA, USA): fluorescein isothiocyanate (FITC)-conjugated anti-CD14 (MφP9), anti-CD4 (SK3), and anti-CD19 (SJ25C1); phycoerythrin (PE)-conjugated anti-CD3 (SP34-2); peridinin chlorophyll protein complex (PerCP)-conjugated anti-CD3 (SK7); Alexa Fluor 647-conjugated anti-CD8 (RPA-T8) mouse anti-human monoclonal antibodies; and PE-conjugated anti-rabbit secondary antibody. Anti-phosphorylated (anti-p)-JAK1 (PhosphoDetect Tyr1022/1023) rabbit anti-human antibody was purchased from EMD Millipore (Darmstadt, Germany). The following antibodies were purchased from Santa Cruz Biotechnology (Dallas, TX, USA): anti-pJAK2 (Tyr1007/Tyr1008), anti-pJAK3 (Tyr980), anti-pTyk2 (Tyr1054) rabbit anti-human antibodies, and PerCP-conjugated anti-rabbit secondary antibody. The amounts of the antibodies were optimized, and their compatibility was assured in preliminary examinations.

Preparing leukocytes for flow cytometry

Blood leukocytes were prepared for flow cytometry using a protocol and buffers by BD Biosciences [13]. Aliquots (50 µl) of blood were deposited into 12 polystyrene tubes (BD Biosciences). Four tubes were supplemented with anti-CD14-FITC, four with anti-CD4-FITC and anti-CD8-Alexa Fluor 647, and four with anti-CD19-FITC for surface marker staining of monocytes, $CD4^+/CD8^+$ T cells, and B cells, respectively. Following a 15-minute incubation at 37 °C, leukocytes were fixed and erythrocytes lysed by adding 1× Lyse/Fix Buffer (BD Biosciences). After being pelleted, leukocytes were permeabilized and washed by incubating them twice in 1× Perm/Wash Buffer (BD Biosciences) at room temperature protected from light for 15 minutes. Cells were pelleted and resuspended in Perm/Wash Buffer. One tube each containing anti-CD14, anti-CD4 and anti-CD8, and anti-CD19 were supplemented with either anti-pJAK1, anti-pJAK2, anti-pJAK3, or anti-pTyk2. The tubes were incubated at room temperature protected from light for 1 h, and then cells were pelleted and resuspended in Perm/Wash Buffer. Tubes containing the anti-pJAK1, anti-pJAK2, or anti-pTyk2 were supplemented with PE-conjugated secondary antibody, and tubes containing anti-pJAK3 were supplemented with PerCP-conjugated secondary antibody. The anti-CD4- and anti-CD8-containing tubes, as well as the anti-CD19-containing tubes, were also supplemented with the T-cell marker antibody anti-CD3-PerCP (for anti-pJAK1, anti-pJAK2, and anti-pTyk2 tubes) or anti-CD3-PE (for anti-pJAK3 tubes). Following incubation at room temperature protected from light for 40 minutes, cells were washed in Perm/Wash Buffer and suspended in Stain Buffer (BD Biosciences). The samples were kept on ice for a maximum of 3 h until flow cytometric acquisition.

Flow cytometry

Flow cytometric data were acquired using a BD FACSCanto II flow cytometer and analyzed with BD FACSDiva software (BD Biosciences), as described previously [14]. $CD3^+CD4^+$ and $CD3^+CD8^+$ T lymphocytes, $CD19^+$ B lymphocytes, and $CD14^+$ monocytes were identified, and pJAK1-PE, pJAK2-PE, pJAK3-PerCP, and pTyk2-PE fluorescence intensities of the respective cell populations were determined as relative fluorescence units (RFU).

Statistical analysis

The data are presented as means with SDs and numbers of patients with percentages, and groups were compared using a permutation test or chi-square test. Exact logistic regression was used to investigate crude and adjusted relationships of the study entry variables to remission at 12 months. The 95% CIs of means were estimated by bias-corrected bootstrapping (5000 replications). pJAK1-PE, pJAK2-PE, pTyk2-PE, and pJAK3-PerCP fluorescence intensities are presented as standardized fluorescence intensities (mean 0, SD 1) of RFU. Correlation coefficients were calculated by the Spearman method using Šidák-adjusted probabilities. The Stata 14.1 statistical software package (StataCorp, College Station, TX, USA) was used for the analyses.

Results

Treatment and outcome

The study included 35 DMARD-naïve patients with recent-onset RA (Table 1). After blood sampling, 33 patients started sDMARD therapy (methotrexate, sulfasalazine, hydroxychloroquine) according to the Finnish national care guidelines [4] (Table 1). In addition, 16 patients (46%) started a course of low-dose (≤10 mg/day) oral prednisone. Intra-articular glucocorticoid injections were also applied to treat swollen joints according to the Finnish national guidelines [4].

During follow-up (mean duration 12 months, SD 3.6 months), the drug treatment was modified when appropriate, targeting remission. After follow-up, 33 patients (91%) were on sDMARDs, including 3 patients (9%) on oral prednisone. Twenty patients (57%) were in remission (no swollen or tender joints, and normal ESR). No patients were on biological DMARDs. The patients in remission started with a lower DAS28 score, lower number of tender joints, and lower patient global assessment at study entry (Table 1).

Phosphorylation levels of JAKs

Baseline phosphorylation of levels of JAKs were compared between the patients who subsequently were in remission after 12-month follow-up and the patients who were not (Fig. 1). JAK3 phosphorylation in $CD8^+$ and $CD4^+$ T cells and $CD19^+$ B cells was found to be higher in the patients who achieved remission than in those who did not (p values of 0.015, 0.024, and 0.038, respectively). No correlations were found between baseline JAK phosphorylation levels and plasma ESR or plasma CRP levels (data not shown).

In order to further elucidate the predictive value of JAK phosphorylation in each cell population, crude and adjusted exact logistic regression models of the baseline phosphorylation levels of JAK1, JAK2, JAK, and Tyk2 were constructed (Table 2). In the models adjusted for anti-cyclic citrullinated peptide, number of DMARDs started at entry, smoking, and white blood cell count, high phosphorylation level of JAK3 was associated with remission in all leukocyte types studied. In addition, low

Table 1 Baseline characteristics of the patients categorized according to remission at 12-month follow-up

Variable	All patients ($n = 35$)	Remission at follow-up		p Value[a]
		No ($n = 15$)	Yes ($n = 20$)	
Age, years, mean (SD)	55 (14)	57 (15)	53 (14)	0.43
Female sex, n (%)	28 (80%)	15 (75%)	13 (87%)	0.39
Rheumatoid factor-positive, n (%)	26 (74%)	10 (67%)	16 (80%)	0.37
Anti-citrullinated protein antibody-positive, n (%)	27 (77%)	10 (67%)	17 (85%)	0.20
Smokers, n (%)	8 (23%)	5 (33%)	3 (15%)	0.20
Duration of symptoms, months, mean (SD)	6 (7)	6 (10)	6 (4)	0.89
Number of tender joints, 0–68, mean (SD)	7 (6)	10 (7)	6 (5)	0.040
Number of swollen joints, 0–66, mean (SD)	6 (5)	6 (4)	7 (6)	0.78
Erythrocyte sedimentation rate, mm/h, mean (SD)	19 (15)	22 (18)	16 (13)	0.32
Plasma C-reactive protein, mg/L, mean (SD)	7 (7)	6 (3)	8 (9)	0.41
White blood cell count, $\times 10^9$/L, mean (SD)	6.9 (2.4)	7.5 (3.1)	6.5 (1.6)	0.23
Patient global assessment, 0–100-mm VAS, mean (SD)	40 (25)	54 (24)	31 (21)	0.0073
DAS28 score, mean (SD)	3.63 (1.14)	4.08 (1.19)	3.29 (1.01)	0.040
Number of DMARDs started, mean (range)	2.2 (0–3)	2.1 (1–3)	2.3 (0–3)	0.72
Single DMARD, n	4	2	2	
Combination of two DMARDs, n	13	9	4	
Combination of three DMARDs, n	16	4	12	
None, n	2	0	2	

Abbreviations: VAS Visual analogue scale, *DAS28* 28-Joint Disease Activity Score, *DMARD* Disease-modifying antirheumatic drug
[a] Significance of difference between No and Yes groups calculated using permutation test or chi-square test

JAK2 phosphorylation level in CD14$^+$ monocytes at baseline emerged to be associated with remission.

Tyk2 phosphorylation level was higher in patients than in healthy reference subjects in all leukocyte types studied (Table 3): CD4$^+$ T cells ($p = 0.0014$), CD8$^+$ T cells ($p = 0.037$), CD19$^+$ B cells ($p = 0.049$), and CD14$^+$ monocytes ($p < 0.001$). This indicated constitutive activation of Tyk2 in the patients' circulating leukocytes. Also, JAK2 phosphorylation of CD14$^+$ monocytes was higher in patients than in healthy reference subjects ($p = 0.011$) (Table 3).

Discussion

The results of the present study show that high baseline JAK3 phosphorylation in all peripheral blood leukocyte subtypes studied (i.e., CD4$^+$ and CD8$^+$ T cells, B cells, and monocytes) is associated with remission achieved by sDMARDs among patients with early untreated RA. The JAK signaling profile of the patients who turned out as good sDMARD responders also included low JAK2 phosphorylation in CD14$^+$ monocytes. Although there is evidence of JAK activation within inflamed joints observed in a few studies using animal models [15] or synovial cells from patients with RA [16–18], there are no prior studies, to the best of our knowledge, on the phosphorylation of JAKs in peripheral blood leukocytes of patients with RA. Consequently, the potential of the JAK phosphorylation profile in leukocytes as a predictor of treatment response in RA has not been studied before.

There are a number of possible explanations for the association we found between baseline JAK3 phosphorylation level and treatment response. First, the sDMARDs used can be effective in downregulating JAK3-involving inflammatory pathways, although the detailed mechanisms remain to be elucidated. In this context, it may be noteworthy that JAK3 cannot be replaced by other JAKs in transducing signals from the receptors of interleukin (IL)-2, IL-4, IL-7, IL-9, IL-15, and IL-21 (γc receptors) [7]. These cytokines are among those whose levels in peripheral blood are affected by DMARDs [19–22], which may represent a disease-modifying mechanism involving JAK3 signaling. Second, the anti-inflammatory or regulatory processes that are also triggered by JAK3 can possibly facilitate the amelioration of RA. It has been observed that JAK3 signaling limits T-helper cell type 17 differentiation in CD4$^+$ T cells [23], maintains circulating quiescent T cells [24], and negatively regulates the production of inflammatory cytokines in innate immune cells [25, 26]. In fact, in developing kinase inhibitor therapies for the treatment of RA, the challenge is to halt the pathogenic effects while preserving the homeostatic and advantageous effects of the kinases [27].

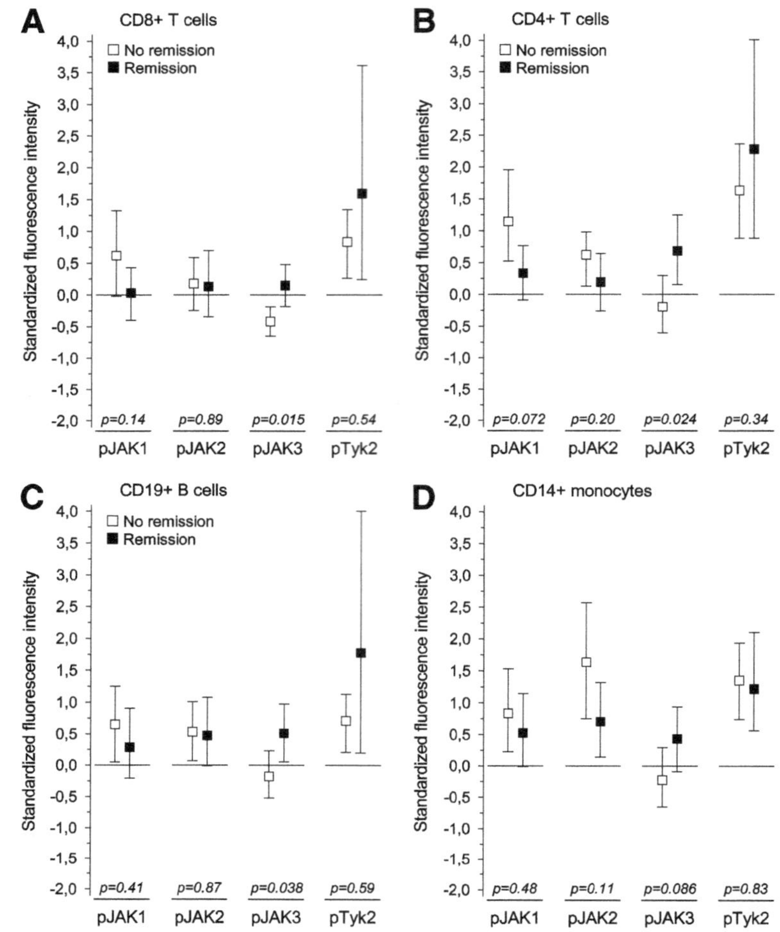

Fig. 1 Baseline Janus kinase phosphorylation (pJAK) profiles of peripheral blood **a** CD8+ T cells, **b** CD4+ T cells, **c** CD19+ B cells, and **d** CD14+ monocytes according to remission at 12-month follow-up. *Squares* indicate group means, and *whiskers* indicate group 95% CIs. The fluorescence intensities are standardized to controls (mean 0 and SD 1). *Horizontal lines* show controls' means. Remission groups are compared using a permutation test

Table 2 ORs for remission after 1 year of follow-up

Model	Variable	$CD8^+$ T cells		$CD4^+$ T cells		$CD19^+$ B cells		$CD14^+$ monocytes	
		OR (95% CI)	*p* Value	OR (95% CI)	*p* Value	OR (95% CI)	*p* Value	OR (95% CI)	*p* Value
Unadjusted	pJAK1	0.57 (0.25–1.18)	0.14	0.47 (0.18–1.03)	0.053	0.75 (0.36–1.49)	0.42	0.78 (0.38–1.56)	0.49
	pJAK2	0.96 (0.48–1.89)	0.90	0.63 (0.30–1.26)	0.20	0.95 (0.48–1.88)	0.88	0.55 (0.25–1.10)	0.092
	pJAK3	3.01 (1.20–9.55)	0.017	2.40 (1.08–6.11)	0.032	2.19 (1.03–5.32)	0.044	1.84 (0.91–4.00)	0.094
	pTyk2	1.34 (0.64–3.24)	0.49	1.23 (0.61–2.84)	0.61	1.46 (0.65–3.78)	0.44	0.92 (0.46–1.82)	0.80
Adjusted[a]	pJAK1	0.42 (0.13–1.14)	0.083	0.46 (0.16–1.09)	0.077	0.68 (0.30–1.49)	0.32	0.84 (0.36–1.94)	0.70
	pJAK2	0.97 (0.46–2.1)	0.94	0.53 (0.25–1.20)	0.14	0.66 (0.29–1.42)	0.29	0.42 (0.16–0.96)	0.034
	pJAK3	3.87 (1.33–16.65)	0.009	2.73 (1.16–7.90)	0.017	2.87 (1.11–8.87)	0.029	2.22 (1.01–5.31)	0.045
	pTyk2	1.40 (0.64–3.25)	0.45	1.32 (0.62–3.05)	0.52	1.47 (0.63–3.47)	0.44	0.92 (0.45–1.93)	0.83

pJAK Phosphorylated Janus kinase, *Tyk* Tyrosine kinase

[a] The models are adjusted for anti-citrullinated protein antibody, number of disease-modifying antirheumatic drugs at entry, smoking, and white blood cell count. ORs are calculated per 1 SD

Table 3 Baseline phosphorylatad Janus kinase fluorescence intensities in peripheral blood leukocytes of patients and healthy reference subjects

Fluorescence	Cell type	Patients (*n* = 35)	Healthy control subjects (*n* = 17)	*p* Value
pJAK1-PE	$CD4^+$ T	385 (32)	335 (75)	0.054
	$CD8^+$ T	387 (39)	365 (79)	0.41
	$CD19^+$ B	549 (151)	497 (121)	0.23
	$CD14^+$ Mo	863 (240)	737 (193)	0.06
pJAK2-PE	$CD4^+$ T	4443 (1446)	3885 (1484)	0.20
	$CD8^+$ T	4282 (1792)	4016 (1761)	0.62
	$CD19^+$ B	7675 (3026)	6340 (2680)	0.12
	$CD14^+$ Mo	6571 (2703)	4727 (1674)	0.011
pJAK3-PerCP	$CD4^+$ T	823 (197)	773 (163)	0.37
	$CD8^+$ T	1350 (283)	1388 (396)	0.69
	$CD19^+$ B	1040 (214)	994 (213)	0.47
	$CD14^+$ Mo	2035 (442)	1976 (385)	0.65
pTyk2-PE	$CD4^+$ T	380 (144)	297 (41)	0.001
	$CD8^+$ T	342 (128)	287 (43)	0.037
	$CD19^+$ B	361 (177)	295 (51)	0.049
	$CD14^+$ Mo	1118 (342)	827 (228)	<0.001

Abbreviations: pJAK Phosphorylated Janus kinase, *Mo* Monocyte, *PE* Phycoerythrin, *PerCP* Peridinin chlorophyll protein complex, *Tyk* Tyrosine kinase
The fluorescence intensities are shown as means (SDs) in relative fluorescence units, with *p* values calculated using a permutation test

The association between low JAK2 phosphorylation in monocytes and good treatment response may reflect the critical roles of JAK2 in innate immune responses. It has been demonstrated in monocytic cells that JAK2 inhibition blunts the production of both early and late inflammatory mediators [28], and that the prolonged effect of interferon-γ on lipopolysaccharide-induced tumor necrosis factor production is apparently mediated by JAK2 [29]. It is noteworthy that the JAK inhibitor tofacitinib has high affinity for JAK3, but it also inhibits JAK1 and, to a lesser extent, JAK2, and also STAT1 and STAT3 [6]. Thus, the efficacy of tofacitinib in treating RA [6, 7, 30] may actually be due to its effects on target molecules other than JAK3. It has also been reported on the basis of in vitro studies on rheumatoid synovial fibroblasts that JAK3-selective inhibition is insufficient to control the proinflammatory cascade, and inhibition of JAK1 and JAK2 may be needed instead [31].

It should be noted that because the patients' JAK3 phosphorylation levels overlapped with those of healthy reference subjects, they cannot serve as diagnostic markers for RA. The phenomenon in which levels of a marker distinguish patients with RA according to divergent outcomes while not distinguishing patients from healthy control subjects has recently been described for other potential markers, including microRNAs [32]. Hence, JAK3 phosphorylation may serve as a surrogate marker, and the possibility remains that markers that discriminate patients with RA from healthy individuals will be discovered along the same signaling pathway.

We also observed that, in contrast to the other JAKs, Tyk2 phosphorylation in lymphocytes and monocytes of patients with RA was significantly higher than in those of healthy reference subjects. Because this phosphorylation was not associated with measures of disease activity or treatment response, the context of the finding remains elusive. Tyk2, for its part, promotes interferon-γ production [33] and can be activated by IL-13 [34]. Methotrexate treatment (which was an essential sDMARD in our study) reduces the levels of both of these cytokines in patients with RA [19]. So, it is possible that Tyk2 phosphorylation increases along with the inflammatory processes during the development of RA and decreases along with the amelioration achieved by sDMARDs, but its effects are not directly related to clinical manifestations of RA. Interestingly, genetic variants of *Tyk2* have been reported to protect against RA, systemic lupus erythematosus, and possibly other autoimmune diseases, such as inflammatory bowel disease [35]. Accordingly, Tyk2 phosphorylation in patients with early RA (as a consequence of either genetic factors or pathogenetic processes) may be associated with increased risk for development of RA, though not directly correlating to disease activity.

The quite low number of subjects is a limitation of the present study. The strengths of the study include the advantages of the phosphospecific whole blood flow cytometric method we used. Blood samples were easily obtained, and only a small volume of blood (a couple of milliliters) was required. Also, ex vivo phosphorylation due to sample handling was minimized, and the procedure was quick (within hours) and has been evaluated as being applicable for rapid immune status determination before starting immunomodulatory therapy in inflammatory diseases [36]. If our results are confirmed in larger studies, it is possible that JAK3 phosphorylation, either alone or with other markers from, for example, the JAK-STAT pathway, is able to serve as treatment response marker in RA.

Conclusions

Baseline JAK phosphorylation profile in circulating leukocytes of patients with early untreated RA is associated with treatment response achieved with sDMARDs. High JAK3 phosphorylation level in both $CD4^+$ and $CD8^+$ T cells, in $CD19^+$ B cells, and in $CD14^+$ monocytes is a promising predictor of good treatment response to sDMARDs in RA.

Abbreviations

CRP: C-reactive protein; DAS28: 28-joint Disease Activity Score; DMARD: Disease-modifying antirheumatic drug; ESR: Erythrocyte sedimentation rate; FITC: Fluorescein isothiocyanate; IL: Interleukin; JAK: Janus kinase; Mo: Monocyte; PE: Phycoerythrin; PerCP: Peridinin chlorophyll protein complex; RA: Rheumatoid arthritis; RFU: Relative fluorescence unit; sDMARD: Synthetic disease-modifying antirheumatic drug; STAT: Signal transducer and activator of transcription; Tyk: Tyrosine kinase; VAS: Visual analogue scale

Acknowledgements

The authors thank Maija-Leena Peltoperä for excellent technical assistance.

Funding

The study was supported by Paulo Foundation and Finnish Cultural Foundation (to KK), and by Helsinki University Central Hospital Research Funds and Finska Läkaresällskapet (to MLR and HR).

Authors' contributions

KK, AK, HR, and MLR conceived of and designed the study, analyzed and interpreted the data, and drafted the manuscript. KK and AK carried out the laboratory work. RK and MLR recruited and examined the patients. HK carried out the statistical analysis. All authors helped to critically revise the manuscript for intellectual content. All authors read and approved the final manuscript.

Competing interests

The authors declare that they have no competing interests.

Author details

[1]Bacteriology and Immunology, Helsinki University Hospital and University of Helsinki, Helsinki, Finland. [2]Rheumatology, Helsinki University Hospital and University of Helsinki, Helsinki, Finland. [3]Primary Health Care, Helsinki University Hospital and University of Helsinki, Helsinki, Finland. [4]General Practice, Helsinki University Hospital and University of Helsinki, Helsinki, Finland. [5]Unit of Primary Health Care, Kuopio University Hospital, Kuopio, Finland.

References

1. McInnes IB, Schett G. The pathogenesis of rheumatoid arthritis. N Engl J Med. 2011;365:2205–19.
2. Smolen JS, Landewé R, Breedveld FC, Dougados M, Emery P, Gaujoux-Viala C, et al. EULAR recommendations for the management of rheumatoid arthritis with synthetic and biological disease-modifying antirheumatic drugs. Ann Rheum Dis. 2010;69:964–75.
3. Singh JA, Saag KG, Bridges Jr SL, Akl EA, Bannuru RR, Sullivan MC, et al. 2015 American College of Rheumatology Guideline for the Treatment of Rheumatoid Arthritis. Arthritis Care Res (Hoboken). 2016;68:1–25.
4. Working group appointed by the Finnish Medical Society Duodecim and the Finnish Society for Rheumatology. Rheumatoid arthritis [in Finnish]. In: Current Care Guidelines. The Finnish Medical Society Duodecim. 2015. http://www.kaypahoito.fi/web/kh/suositukset/suositus?id=hoi21010. Accessed 22 Aug 2016.
5. Tak P, Kalden JR. Advances in rheumatology: new targeted therapeutics. Arthritis Res Ther. 2011;13 Suppl 1:S5.
6. Ghoreschi K, Laurence A, O'Shea J. Janus kinases in immune cell signaling. Immunol Rev. 2009;228:273–87.
7. Laurence A, Pesu M, Silvennoinen O, O'Shea J. JAK kinases in health and disease: an update. Open Rheumatol J. 2012;6:232–44.
8. van Nies JA, Tsonaka R, Gaujoux-Viala C, Fautrel B, van der Helm-van Mil AH. Evaluating relationships between symptom duration and persistence of rheumatoid arthritis: does a window of opportunity exist? Results on the Leiden early arthritis clinic and ESPOIR cohorts. Ann Rheum Dis. 2015;74:806–12.
9. Kuuliala K, Kuuliala A, Aittomäki S, Oksanen S, Siitonen S, Kautiainen H, et al. STAT3 phosphorylation of circulating leukocytes correlates with disease activity in early untreated rheumatoid arthritis. Arthritis Rheum. 2011;63 Suppl 10:S1008.
10. Kuuliala K, Kuuliala A, Koivuniemi R, Oksanen S, Hämäläinen M, Moilanen E, et al. Constitutive STAT3 phosphorylation in circulating $CD4^+$ T lymphocytes associates with disease activity and treatment response in recent-onset rheumatoid arthritis. PLoS One. 2015;10:e0137385.
11. Aletaha D, Neogi T, Silman AJ, Funovits J, Felson DT, Bingham 3rd CO, et al. 2010 rheumatoid arthritis classification criteria: an American College of Rheumatology/European League Against Rheumatism collaborative initiative. Ann Rheum Dis. 2010;69:1580–8.
12. Prevoo ML, van 't Hof MA, Kuper HH, van Leeuwen MA, van de Putte LB, van Riel PL. Modified disease activity scores that include twenty-eight-joint counts: development and validation in a prospective longitudinal study of patients with rheumatoid arthritis. Arthritis Rheum. 1995;38:44–8.
13. BD Biosciences. Technical data sheet: BD Perm/Wash Buffer. http://www.bdbiosciences.com/ds/pm/tds/554723.pdf. Accessed 22 Aug 2016.
14. Oiva J, Mustonen H, Kylänpää ML, Kyhälä L, Kuuliala K, Alanärä T, et al. Acute pancreatitis with organ dysfunction associates with abnormal blood lymphocyte signaling: controlled laboratory study. Crit Care. 2010;14:R207.
15. Shahrara S, Amin MA, Woods JM, Haines GK, Kock AE. Chemokine receptor expression and in vivo signaling pathways in the joints of rats with adjuvant-induced arthritis. Arthritis Rheum. 2003;48:3568–83.
16. Walker JG, Ahern MJ, Coleman M, Weedon H, Papangelis V, Beroukas D, et al. Changes in synovial tissue Jak-STAT expression in rheumatoid arthritis in response to successful DMARD treatment. Ann Rheum Dis. 2006;65:1558–64.
17. Carrión M, Juarranz Y, Martinez C, González-Àlvaro I, Pablos JL, Gutiérrez-Canas I, et al. IL-22/IL-22R1 axis and S100A8/A9 alarmins in human osteoarthritic and rheumatoid arthritis synovial fibroblasts. Rheumatology (Oxford). 2013;52:2177–86.
18. Li CH, Xu LL, Zhao JX, Sun L, Yao ZQ, Deng XL, et al. CXCL16 upregulates RANKL expression in rheumatoid arthritis synovial fibroblasts through the JAK2/STAT3 and p38/MAPK signaling pathway. Inflamm Res. 2016;65:193–202.
19. Gerards AH, de Lathouder S, de Groot ER, Dijkmans BAC, Aarden LA. Inhibition of cytokine production by methotrexate: studies in healthy volunteers and patients with rheumatoid arthritis. Rheumatology. 2003;42:1189–96.
20. van Roon JA, Jacobs K, Verstappen S, Bijlsma J, Lafeber F. Reduction of serum interleukin 7 levels upon methotrexate therapy in early rheumatoid arthritis correlates with disease suppression. Ann Rheum Dis. 2008;67:1054–5.

21. Ally MM, Hodkinson B, Meyer PW, Musenge E, Tintinger GR, Tikly M, et al. Circulating anti-citrullinated peptide antibodies, cytokines and genotype as biomarkers of response to disease-modifying antirheumatic drug therapy in early rheumatoid arthritis. BMC Musculoskelet Disord. 2015;16:130.
22. Kremer JM, Lawrence DA, Hamilton R, McInnes IB. Long-term study of the impact of methotrexate on serum cytokines and lymphocyte subsets in patients with active rheumatoid arthritis: correlation with pharmacokinetic measures. RMD Open. 2016;2:e000287.
23. Martín P, Gómez M, Lamana A, Cruz-Adalia A, Ramírez-Huesca M, Ursa MA, et al. CD69 association with Jak3/Stat5 proteins regulates Th17 cell differentiation. Mol Cell Biol. 2010;30:4877–89.
24. Sohn SJ, Forbush KA, Nguyen N, Witthuhn B, Nosaka T, Ihle JN, et al Requirement for Jak3 in mature T cells: its role in regulation of T cell homeostasis. J Immunol. 1998;160:2130–8.
25. Wang H, Brown J, Gao S, Liang S, Jotwani R, Zhou H, et al. The role of JAK-3 in regulating TLR-mediated inflammatory cytokine production in innate immune cells. J Immunol. 2013;191:1164–74.
26. Kim HJ, Hart J, Knatz N, Hall MW, Wewers MD. Janus kinase 3 down-regulates lipopolysaccharide-induced IL-1β-converting enzyme activation by autocrine IL-10. J Immunol. 2004;172:4948–55.
27. Chakravarty SD, Poulikakos PI, Ivashkiv LB, Salmon JE, Kalliolas GD. Kinase inhibitors: a new tool for the treatment of rheumatoid arthritis. Clin Immunol. 2013;148:66–78.
28. Pena G, Cai B, Deitch EA, Ulloa L. JAK2 inhibition prevents innate immune responses and rescues animals from sepsis. J Mol Med. 2010;88:851–9.
29. Lee JY, Sullivan KE. Gamma interferon and lipopolysaccharide interact at the level of transcription to induce tumor necrosis factor alpha expression. Infect Immun. 2001;69:2847–52.
30. Schwartz DM, Bonelli M, Gadina M, O'Shea JJ. Type I/II cytokines, JAKs, and new strategies for treating autoimmune diseases. Nat Rev Rheumatol. 2016; 12:25–36.
31. Migita K, Izumi Y, Torigoshi T, Satomura K, Izumi M, Nishino Y, et al. Inhibition of Janus kinase/signal transducer and activator of transcription (JAK/STAT) signalling pathway in rheumatoid synovial fibroblasts using small molecule compounds. Clin Exp Immunol. 2013;174:356–63.
32. Filková M, Aradi B, Senolt L, Ospelt C, Vettori S, Mann H, et al. Association of circulating miR-223 and miR-16 with disease activity in patients with early rheumatoid arthritis. Ann Rheum Dis. 2014;73:1898–904.
33. Karaghiosoff M, Steinborn R, Kovarik P, Kriegshäuser G, Baccarini M, Donabauer B, et al. Central role for type I interferons and Tyk2 in lipopolysaccharide-induced endotoxin shock. Nat Immunol. 2003;4:471–7.
34. Roy B, Bhattacharjee A, Xu B, Ford D, Maizel AL, Cathcart MK. IL-13 signal transduction in human monocytes: phosphorylation of receptor components, association with Jaks, and phosphorylation/activation of Stats. J Leukoc Biol. 2002;72:580–9.
35. Diogo D, Bastarache L, Liao KP, Graham RR, Fulton RS, Greenberg JD, et al. TYK2 protein-coding variants protect against rheumatoid arthritis and autoimmunity, with no evidence of major pleiotropic effects on non-autoimmune complex traits. PLoS One. 2015;10:e0122271.
36. Caldwell CC, Hotchkiss RS. The first step in utilizing immune-modulating therapies: immune status determination. Crit Care. 2011;15:108.

Risk factors for flare and treatment of disease flares during pregnancy in rheumatoid arthritis and axial spondyloarthritis patients

Stephanie van den Brandt[1,2], Astrid Zbinden[1], Dominique Baeten[2], Peter M. Villiger[1], Monika Østensen[1] and Frauke Förger[1*]

Abstract

Background: During pregnancy, patients with rheumatoid arthritis (RA) and axial spondyloarthritis (axSpA) can experience active disease, which might be influenced by adjustment of treatment around conception. The aim of this study was to identify possible risk factors of disease flares during pregnancy and to evaluate the effect of treatment in pregnant patients experiencing a flare.

Methods: Pregnant patients with RA and axSpA were prospectively followed before, during, and after pregnancy. Disease activity and flares of disease activity were analyzed in regard to medication.

Results: Among 136 pregnant patients, disease flares during pregnancy occurred in 29% of patients with RA and in 25% of patients with axSpA. In both diseases, active disease and tumor necrosis factor inhibitor (TNFi) discontinuation in early pregnancy were identified as risk factors for disease flares during pregnancy. Of 75 patients with RA, 15 patients were on TNFi and discontinued the treatment at the time of the positive pregnancy test. After stopping TNFi, disease activity increased, which was reflected by peaking C-reactive protein levels at the first trimester. The relative risk of flare in patients with RA stopping TNFi was 3.33 (95% CI 1.8–6.1). Initiation of TNFi or glucocorticosteroid (GC) treatment in 60% of these patients resulted in disease improvement at the second and third trimesters. In comparison, patients with RA without TNFi in the preconception period, most of whom had used pregnancy-compatible antirheumatic drugs, showed mild and stable disease activity before and during pregnancy. Of 61 patients with axSpA, 24 patients were on TNFi and discontinued the treatment at the time of the positive pregnancy test. In patients with axSpA stopping TNFi, a disease aggravation at the second trimester could be observed. The relative risk of flare in this group was 3.08 (95% CI 1.2–7.9). In spite of initiated TNFi or GC treatment in 62.5% of these patients, disease activity remained elevated throughout pregnancy. Patients with axSpA without TNFi in the preconception period showed persistent high disease activity from prepregnancy until the postpartum period.

Conclusions: On the basis of a risk-benefit analysis, to stabilize disease activity and to prevent a flare during pregnancy in patients with RA and axSpA, tailored medication including TNF inhibitors should be considered beyond conception.

Keywords: Rheumatoid arthritis, Axial spondyloarthritis, Tumor necrosis factor inhibitors, Treatment, Pregnancy

* Correspondence: frauke.foerger@insel.ch
[1]Department of Rheumatology, Immunology and Allergology, University Hospital, University of Bern, Freiburgstrasse 8, 3010 Bern, Switzerland
Full list of author information is available at the end of the article

Background

Rheumatoid arthritis (RA) and axial spondyloarthritis (axSpA) often affect women of childbearing age. In patients wishing for children, pregnancy represents a challenge in the management of the disease because current disease activity, the influence of pregnancy on the disease, and the safety of antirheumatic drugs in pregnancy have to be taken into account [1]. During pregnancy, active disease can be found in about 35% to 52% of patients with RA and in 60% to 80% of patients with axSpA [2–5].

In RA, the positivity for or elevated level of rheumatoid factor or anticitrullinated antibodies is associated with more active disease during pregnancy [6, 7]. Disease activity before conception seems to be an additional factor that influences the disease course during pregnancy in patients with RA because quiescent disease often remains stable throughout pregnancy [3]. Active disease or flares during pregnancy in patients with rheumatic disease can harm maternal and fetal health and should therefore be avoided.

Up to now, it is unknown whether changes of treatment before conception or early in pregnancy have an influence on the disease course during pregnancy in patients with RA and axSpA. This information would be of clinical importance, however, in the management of patients with RA and axSpA before and during pregnancy.

The aim of this study was to analyze the frequency of flares during pregnancy in patients with RA and axSpA and to delineate risk factors for flares. In addition, we analyzed the response to therapy in controlling disease activity after the occurrence of a flare in both diseases during pregnancy.

Methods

Patients and medications

In total, 136 pregnant patients with RA or axSpA were prospectively followed between 2000 and 2015 at the Center for Pregnancy in Rheumatic Diseases at the Department of Rheumatology of the Inselspital Bern, Switzerland. Patients with RA had to fulfill the revised 1987 American College of Rheumatology classification criteria for RA [8]. Patients with spondyloarthritis (SpA) fulfilled the European Spondylarthropathy Study Group criteria for SpA [9]. All patients with SpA also fulfilled the Assessment of SpondyloArthritis international Society (ASAS) criteria for axSpA; for patients recruited before 2009, the ASAS criteria were applied in retrospect [10]. The study was approved by the ethics committee of the Canton of Bern, Switzerland, and patients were included after they provided written informed consent. Patients were examined within 6 months before conception, at each trimester (gestational weeks 10–12, 20–22, and 30–32) and 6–8 weeks postpartum. At each visit, detailed information on medication, disease activity, and pregnancy were recorded. Flare was analyzed at each visit during pregnancy and postpartum. If demanded by maternal disease, tumor necrosis factor inhibitor (TNFi) or glucocorticosteroid (GC) treatment was initiated during pregnancy, based on a risk-benefit analysis as well as informed and shared decision making.

Assessments and definitions

In patients with RA, disease activity states were assessed by the three-variable Disease Activity Score in 28 joints based on C-reactive protein (DAS28-CRP) [11]. DAS28-CRP scores below 2.6 were defined as clinical remission, DAS28-CRP scores from 2.7 to 3.2 as low disease activity, DAS28-CRP scores from 3.3 to 5.1 as intermediate disease activity, and DAS28-CRP scores above 5.1 as high disease activity [11]. Flare was defined by an increase of DAS28-CRP greater than 0.6 [12] in combination with an elevated C-reactive protein (CRP) level. Active disease was defined by DAS28-CRP scores higher than 3.2. In patients with axSpA, disease activity states were measured by the patient global assessment, the Bath Ankylosing Spondylitis Disease Activity Index, and the Ankylosing Spondylitis Disease Activity Score based on C-reactive protein (ASDAS-CRP). In patients with axSpA recruited before the development of the ASDAS-CRP in 2009 [13], the ASDAS-CRP scores were calculated retrospectively. Categories of the ASDAS-CRP were defined as inactive disease for scores below 1.3, moderate disease activity for scores from 1.3 to 2.0, high disease activity for scores from 2.1 to 3.5, and very high disease activity for scores above 3.5 [14]. Active disease was defined by ASDAS-CRP scores higher than 2.1. Flare of disease activity was defined by an increase of ASDAS-CRP greater than 0.6 in combination with an elevated CRP level. A flare during pregnancy was defined as a flare observed during the first, second, or third trimester.

Statistical analysis

For longitudinal comparisons of paired samples, the Wilcoxon signed-rank test was used. The Mann-Whitney *U* test was performed to analyze unpaired data as well as in groupwise comparisons. To analyze categorical data, Fisher's exact test was performed. A significant difference was considered in case of P values less than 0.05.

Results

Flare rates during pregnancy in patients with RA and axSpA are associated with active disease and TNFi discontinuation in early pregnancy

A total of 136 pregnant patients were identified, comprising 75 patients with RA and 61 patients with axSpA. Patients' characteristics and medical treatment at baseline are displayed in Table 1.

Table 1 Patients' characteristics and treatments before conception

	RA ($n = 75$)	axSpA ($n = 61$)
Age at conception, years (median)	31 (21–40)	31 (22–41)
Age at diagnosis, years (median)	27 (20–38)	24 (17–33)
Rheumatoid factor-positive	50 (66)	–
HLA-B27-positive	–	43 (70.5)
axSpA with peripheral arthritis	–	27 (44.3)
Medication within 3 months before conception		
Methotrexate[a]	2 (2.7)	–
NSAIDs	8 (10.7)	18 (29.5)
TNFi[b]	15 (20.0)	24 (39.3)
Glucocorticosteroids[c]	25 (33.3)	5 (8.2)
DMARDs	29 (38.7)	5 (8.2)
SSZ	18 (24.0)	5 (8.2)
HCQ	8 (10.7)	
SSZ and HCQ	3 (4.0)	

Abbreviations: axSpA Axial spondyloarthritis, *DMARD* Disease-modifying antirheumatic drug, *HCQ* Hydrochloroquine, *HLA* Human leukocyte antigen, *NSAID* Nonsteroidal anti-inflammatory drug, *RA* Rheumatoid arthritis, *SSZ* Sulfasalazine, *TNFi* Tumor necrosis factor inhibitor
[a]Methotrexate, discontinued 1 month before the planned conception
[b]TNFi, discontinued at the time of the positive pregnancy test
[c]Prednisone or prednisolone

Before pregnancy, 61 patients with RA had low disease activity, and 8.6% had active disease with DAS28-CRP scores greater than or equal to 3.2. However, during pregnancy, a flare of disease activity occurred in 29% of patients with RA. Most flares emerged in the first trimester (Table 2). No patient with RA experienced more than one episode of flare during pregnancy. Comparing patients with flares with those without them, the discontinuation of TNFi in early pregnancy correlated with the risk of flares ($P = 0.001$) (Table 3). Flares during the course of pregnancy were also associated with elevated disease activity and CRP at early pregnancy ($P = 0.038$ and $P = 0.008$, respectively) (Table 3 and Additional file 1: Table S1).

During the prepregnancy period, patients with RA treated with TNFi showed disease activity comparable to that of patients without TNFi treatment during the same period. Among the 15 patients treated with TNFi during at least 20 weeks before conception, all discontinued the treatment at the positive pregnancy test; the median time point of discontinuation was gestational week 3. After the discontinuation of TNFi, the relative risk of a flare during pregnancy was 3.33 (95% CI 1.8–6.1). Patients with RA who discontinued TNFi showed active disease at the first trimester and peaking CRP levels ($P = 0.04$ prepregnancy to first trimester, $P = 0.03$ first trimester to second trimester) (Fig. 1). The aggravation of disease activity led to a treatment adjustment in 60% of the patients. In most patients with RA without TNFi treatment, disease activity remained stable throughout pregnancy, with DAS28-CRP scores ranging from 2.6 to 3.1 and low CRP levels (Fig. 1a, b). The therapies received by patients with RA with and without TNFi are shown in Table 2. Among patients without TNFi, a higher proportion received pregnancy-compatible drugs such as sulfasalazine, hydroxychloroquine, GCs, and nonsteroidal anti-inflammatory drugs before and during pregnancy than those treated with TNFi.

Among patients with axSpA, 24.6% showed active disease with ASDAS scores greater than or equal to 2.1 before pregnancy. Flares of disease activity during pregnancy occurred in 25% of patients with axSpA and were most often seen in the second half of pregnancy (Table 2). The discontinuation of TNFi treatment at the positive pregnancy test ($P = 0.017$), elevated CRP levels ($P = 0.006$), and active disease at early pregnancy were associate with flares during pregnancy in these women (Table 3, Additional file 1: Table S1).

Among the 61 patients with axSpA, 24 patients received TNFi treatment before pregnancy and had a median ASDAS-CRP of 1.95 preconceptionally. After discontinuation of TNFi treatment at the positive pregnancy test (median time point of discontinuation was gestational week 3), the relative risk of flare was 3.08 (95% CI 1.2–7.9) (Table 3). Patients with axSpA who discontinued TNFi treatment experienced high disease activity throughout pregnancy, with ASDAS-CRP scores ranging between 2.4 and 2.8 and CRP peaking at the second trimester (Fig. 1c, d). There was no patient with more than one flare episode during pregnancy. Among patients with axSpA discontinuing TNFi, an initiation or restart of medication was required in 62.5% during gestation. In patients with axSpA without TNFi treatment, ASDAS-CRP scores ranged from 2.2 to 2.7 throughout pregnancy, and stable low CRP levels were measured. Of these patients, 10.8% required a start of new medication during pregnancy (Table 2). Comparing patients without TNFi treatment and patients discontinuing TNFi treatment at the positive pregnancy test, higher CRP values were found in the latter group throughout pregnancy ($P = 0.04$ for first trimester, $P = 0.03$ for second trimester, $P = 0.01$ for third trimester) (Fig. 1d).

Response to initiation of TNFi or GC treatment during pregnancy

During pregnancy, 25 patients with RA (flare in $n = 22$, increase of disease activity in $n = 3$) and 19 patients with axSpA (flare in $n = 15$, increase of disease activity in $n = 4$) experienced a disease aggravation with the need to step up medication. Among patients with RA, 9 patients started TNFi treatment and 16 started GC treatment during pregnancy (Table 2). Upon TNFi treatment, median

Table 2 Flares and medical treatments during pregnancy in patients with and without tumor necrosis factor inhibitor use until early pregnancy

	RA		axSpA	
	TNFi until positive pregnancy test[a] ($n = 15$)	TNFi-negative ($n = 60$)	TNFi until positive pregnancy test ($n = 24$)	TNFi-negative ($n = 37$)
Patients (n) with flare at				
First trimester	6	4	1	2
Second trimester	3	4	5	1
Third trimester	1	4	4	2
Medication at conception				
TNFi	15 (100)	0 (0)	24 (100)	0 (0)
NSAIDs	1 (6.7)	13 (21.7)	11 (45.8)	23 (61.2)
Glucocorticosteroids[b]	1 (6.7)	23 (38.3)	2 (8.3)	1(3.7)
DMARDs	2 (13.3)	27 (45)	3 (12.5)	2 (5.4)
SSZ	1 (6.7)	17(28.3)	3 (12.5)	2 (5.4)
HCQ	1 (6.7)	7 (11.7)		
SSZ and HCQ		3 (5)		
Medication during pregnancy				
TNFi	4 (26.7)	5 (8.3)	10 (41.7)	1 (2.7)
NSAIDs	5 (33.3)	23 (38.3)	15 (62.5)	27 (73)
Glucocorticosteroids[b]	7 (46.7)	29 (48.3)	12 (50.0)	3 (8.1)
DMARDs	7 (46.7)	38 (63.3)	3 (12.5)	2 (5.4)
SSZ	1 (6.7)	23 (38.3)	3 (12.5)	2 (5.4)
HCQ	1 (6.7)	9 (15)		
SSZ and HCQ	5 (33.3)	6 (10)		
Initiation of medication during pregnancy	9 (60)	16 (26.7)	15 (62.5)	4 (10.8)
TNFi[c]	4 (26.7)	5 (8.3)	10 (41.7)	1 (2.7)
Start at visit 1 T-2 T-3 T	2-2-0	1-3-1	4-4-2	0-0-1
Glucocorticosteroids[b]	5 (33.3)	11(18.6)	12 (50)	3 (8.1)
Start at visit 1 T-2 T-3 T	0-4-1	3-6-2	4-5-3	0-2-1

Abbreviations: axSpA Axial spondyloarthritis, *DMARD* Disease-modifying antirheumatic drug, *HCQ* Hydrochloroquine, *NSAID* Nonsteroidal anti-inflammatory drug, *RA* Rheumatoid arthritis, *SSZ* Sulfasalazine, *TNFi* Tumor necrosis factor inhibitor, *1 T* First trimester, *2 T* Second trimester, *3 T* Third trimester

Numbers are count or count (percent); the percentages are calculated for each column

[a]NSAIDs used until gestational week 32

[b]Prednisone or prednisolone

[c]TNFi initiated during pregnancy: 11 certolizumab, 8 etanercept, 1 adalimumab

CRP values decreased significantly from 26 mg/L to 3 mg/L ($P = 0.03$) (Fig. 2a), and median DAS28-CRP scores decreased from 4.25 to 2.60. Upon initiation of GC treatment in pregnant patients with RA, median CRP values of 13 mg/L decreased to normal levels ($P = 0.04$) (Fig. 2b), and DAS28-CRP dropped from 3.95 to 2.45, indicating inactive disease.

Among patients with axSpA, TNFi treatment was initiated in 11 and GC treatment in 15 during pregnancy (Table 2). Upon initiation of TNFi, pregnant patients with axSpA showed a significant decrease of median CRP levels from 18.5 mg/L to 12 mg/L ($P = 0.04$) (Fig. 2c). In spite of the improved CRP levels, disease activity remained high, with slightly elevated CRP levels and median ASDAS-CRP scores of 4.0 before and 3.7 after initiation of TNFi therapy (not shown). Upon GC treatment, elevated CRP values persisted, with a median CRP level of 12 mg/L (Fig. 2d) and a median ASDAS-CRP score of 3.14.

Discussion

For the management of patients with RA and axSpA who are planning a pregnancy, both disease activity and therapeutic regimens have to be considered with regard to maternal and fetal health. Any beneficial effect of pregnancy on diseases such as RA could buffer a reduction of the antirheumatic therapy [2, 3, 7]. However, the adjustment of therapy around conception might also be

Table 3 Risk factors for flare during the course of pregnancy

	Patients with RA ($n = 75$)					Patients with axSpA ($n = 61$)				
	Flare	No flare	RR	95% CI	*P* value	Flare	No flare	RR	95% CI	*P* value
Treatment										
TNFi before pregnancy[a] and discontinued at positive pregnancy test	10 of 22 (45.5)	5 of 53 (9.4)	3.333	(1.8–6.1)	0.001*	10 of 15 (66.7)	14 of 46 (30.4)	3.083	(1.2–7.9)	0.017*
TNFi during first trimester	3 of 22 (13.6)	5 of 53 (9.4)	1.322	(0.5–3.5)	0.686	6 of 15 (40)	12 of 46 (26.1)	1.593	(0.7–3.8)	0.340
GCs before pregnancy	8 of 22 (36.4)	17 of 53 (32.1)	1.143	(0.6–2.4)	0.790	1 of 15 (6.7)	4 of 46 (8.7)	0.800	(0.1–4.9)	0.642
GCs during first trimester	8 of 22 (36.4)	17 of 53 (32.1)	1.143	(0.6–2.4)	0.790	1 of 15 (6.7)	6 of 46 (13)	0.551	(0.1–3.6)	0.178
DMARDs before pregnancy	10 of 22 (45.5)	22 of 53 (41.5)	1.120	(0.6–2.3)	0.801	3 of 15 (20)	5 of 46 (10.9)	1.656	(0.6–4.6)	0.589
DMARDs during first trimester	8 of 22 (36.4)	22 of 53 (42.5)	0.860	(0.4–1.8)	0.798	2 of 15 (13.3)	3 of 46 (6.5)	1.723	(0.5–5.6)	0.589
NSAIDs before pregnancy	2 of 22 (9.1)	6 of 53 (11.3)	0.838	(0.2–2.9)	0.568	3 of 15 (20)	15 of 46 (32.6)	0.597	(0.2–1.9)	0.518
NSAIDs during first trimester	3 of 22 (13.6)	6 of 53 (11.3)	1.158	(0.4–3.1)	0.716	3 of 15 (20)	15 of 46 (32.6)	0.597	(0.2–1.9)	0.518
Disease activity										
Active disease before pregnancy[a]	5 of 22 (22.7)	9 of 53 (17.0)	1.282	(0.6–2.9)	0.536	2 of 15 (13.3)	4 of 46 (8.7)	1.410	(0.4–4.8)	0.630
Active disease during first trimester	8 of 22 (36.4)	10 of 53 (18.9)	0.456	(0.2–0.9)	0.038*	5 of 15 (33.3)	11 of 46 (23.9)	0.717	(0.3–1.7)	0.510
Elevated CRP before pregnancy[a]	3 of 22 (13.6)	8 of 53 (15.1)	0.584	(0.3–1.3)	0.282	1 of 15 (6.7)	2 of 46 (4.3)	0.724	(0.1–3.8)	0.718
Elevated CRP during first trimester	9 of 22 (40.9)	12 of 53 (22.6)	0.553	(0.2–0.7)	0.008*	7 of 15 (46.7)	6 of 46 (13)	0.280	(0.1–0.7)	0.006*

Abbreviations: axSpA Axial spondyloarthritis, *CRP* C-reactive protein, *DMARD* Disease-modifying antirheumatic drug, *GC* Glucocorticosteroid, *NSAID* Nonsteroidal anti-inflammatory drug, *RA* Rheumatoid arthritis, *RR* Relative risk, *SpA* Spondyloarthritis, *TNFi* Tumor necrosis factor inhibitor

[a] "Before pregnancy" refers to period from 20 weeks prior to conception until the positive pregnancy test

* $p < 0.05$

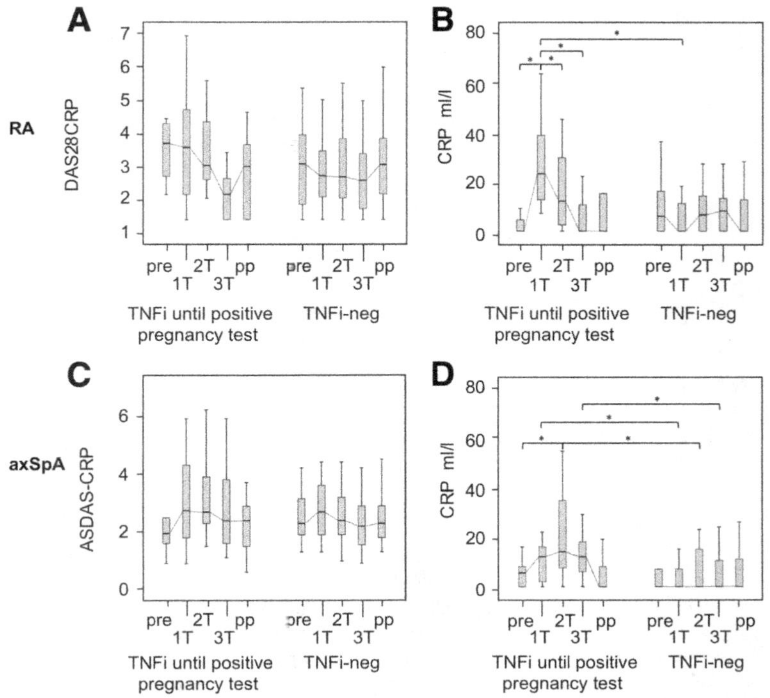

Fig. 1 Disease activity over the course of pregnancy in patients with rheumatoid arthritis (RA) and axial spondyloarthritis (axSpA) treated with and without tumor necrosis factor inhibitors (TNFi) until early pregnancy. Disease activity is compared between patients who received TNFi until the positive pregnancy test and patients without TNFi treatment (TNFi-neg). The *upper panels* show Disease Activity Score in 28 joints based on C-reactive protein (DAS28-CRP) levels (**a**) and C-reactive protein (CRP) levels (**b**) in patients with RA (prepregnancy [pre]: number of patients [n] = 54, first trimester [1 T]: $n = 59$, second trimester [2 T]: $n = 66$, third trimester [3 T]: $n = 64$, postpartum [pp]: $n = 53$). The *lower panels* display Ankylosing Spondylitis Disease Activity Score based on C-reactive protein (ASDAS-CRP) levels (**c**) and CRP levels (**d**) in patients with axSpA (pre: $n = 44$, 1 T: $n = 46$, 2 T: $n = 58$, 3 T: $n = 54$, pp: $n = 46$). Box plots present the medians and the interquartile ranges. *$P < 0.051$

associated with disease reactivation during gestation, especially in diseases such as axSpA, in which no major beneficial effect has been observed during pregnancy [15]. In the present study, disease flares during pregnancy were observed in 29% of patients with RA and 25% of patients with axSpA. Interestingly, our study shows that, in the subgroup of patients with RA and axSpA treated with TNFi for at least 5 months before conception, the discontinuation of TNFi early in pregnancy could be a risk factor for disease flares during pregnancy. Both groups of patients experienced an aggravation of disease several weeks after withdrawal of TNFi. Disease-specific characteristics as well as disease activity at the time of TNFi withdrawal might play a role in this respect because elevated disease activity in early pregnancy is another risk factor for a flare during the course of pregnancy. In nonpregnant patients with axSpA, the discontinuation of TNFi leads to disease flares in 76% to 100% [16]. In nonpregnant patients with RA, the results vary with regard to whether the withdrawal of TNFi may lead to a deterioration of disease activity [17, 18]. Factors predictive of maintaining low disease activity in RA include low disease activity at the time of TNFi discontinuation [17]. However, others report immediate disease deterioration in patients with early RA in whom TNFi were withdrawn after they achieved remission while receiving TNFi and methotrexate [18]. Presumably, the time in remission is a prerequisite in patients with RA for persisting clinical benefits after TNFi discontinuation [17]. Accordingly, withdrawing TNFi later in pregnancy in patients with sustained inactive disease did not result in a flare in patients with inflammatory bowel disease [19].

In patients with RA without TNFi, 63.3% of whom were on pregnancy-compatible disease-modifying drugs, both the DAS28-CRP scores as well as CRP levels showed low disease activity during the course of pregnancy, and only 26.7% of patients required initiation of therapy. This confirms that patients with RA with low disease activity at the first trimester mostly continue with stable and low disease activity throughout gestation [3]. By contrast, the possible pregnancy-ameliorating effect in RA was not strong enough to compensate the disease aggravation that occurred after TNFi discontinuation around conception. In addition, the subpopulation of patients treated with TNFi in the period before

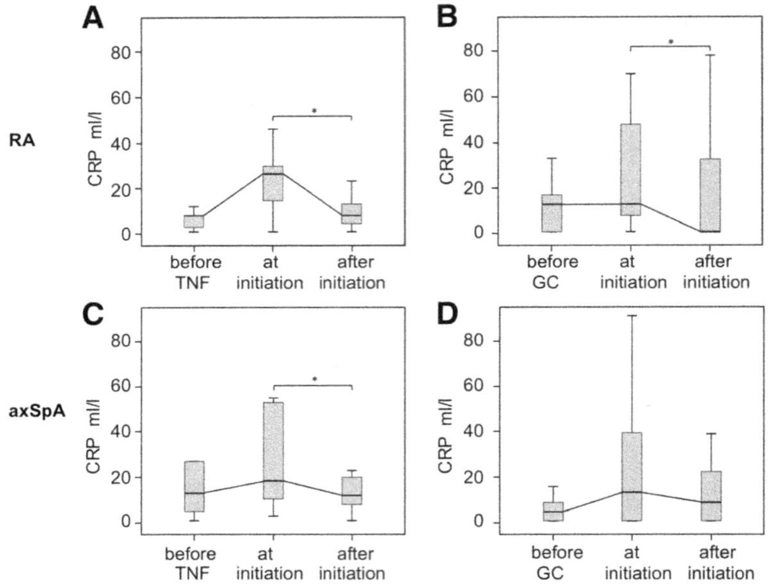

Fig. 2 Response to treatment of flares with tumor necrosis factor inhibitor (TNFi) or glucocorticosteroid (GC) treatment in patients with rheumatoid arthritis (RA) and axial spondyloarthritis (axSpA) during pregnancy. The *upper panels* show the time course of C-reactive protein (CRP) levels in patients with RA in whom TNFi treatment (**a**) or GC treatment (**b**) was initiated during pregnancy. The *lower panels* show the time course of CRP levels in patients with axSpA in whom TNFi treatment (**c**) or GC treatment (**d**) was initiated during pregnancy. Box plots present the medians and the interquartile ranges. *$P < 0.05$

pregnancy represents patients with more severe disease because symptoms were not sufficiently controlled with disease-modifying antirheumatic drugs alone. In the latter patient group, smoldering disease activity might erupt to disease flares after TNFi discontinuation even under the tolerance-inducing condition of pregnancy. Sixty-three percent of patients with axSpA who discontinued TNFi around conception had increased CRP levels at the second trimester. Disease flares in this group occurred around gestational week 20, which corresponds to the median time to flare of 16 weeks after discontinuation of TNFi in nonpregnant patients with axSpA [16]. Patients with axSpA not treated with TNFi before conception showed stable and low CRP levels but high ASDAS-CRP scores throughout gestation. The discrepancy could be explained by the composition of the ASDAS-CRP, which consists of the objective CRP as well as the subjective parameters [11]. A previous study comparing clinical scores and the Medical Outcomes Study 36-item Short Form Health Survey also confirmed the importance of subjective symptoms resulting in high disease activity measured in patients with axSpA throughout pregnancy [20].

The success of new initiation or reintroduction of therapy for the treatment of flares differed significantly in pregnant patients with RA and axSpA. In RA, the start of TNFi because of flare in pregnancy resulted in improvement and in achievement of disease remission in the majority of patients. The median CRP levels decreased by 69% after the start of therapy and normalized during the third trimester. By contrast, in patients with axSpA in whom TNFi treatment was initiated, median CRP levels decreased by only 35%, and CRP levels remained elevated during pregnancy. Thus, high disease activity in axSpA could be ameliorated but not controlled by restart or initiation of TNFi in pregnancy. Our results for patients with RA and axSpA suggest that the initiation of TNFi during pregnancy may be more effective in patients with active RA than in patients with active axSpA.

GC therapy has been accepted for treating flares of rheumatic disease during pregnancy [21]. Our study showed that the response of CRP values to GC treatment differed in patients with RA and patients with axSpA. Patients with RA responded with a significant decrease of disease activity and CRP levels after the start of GC treatment during pregnancy, whereas patients with axSpA showed a minimal decrease of CRP. This weak response in patients with axSpA is consistent with the lack of effect of GC treatment in nonpregnant patients with axSpA [22].

The strength of our study is the prospective design and the inclusion of two rheumatic diseases with different responses to pregnancy. It is the first report on the effect of discontinuing TNFi in early pregnancy, and on the response to the restart or the initiation of medication at a flare in pregnant patients with RA and axSpA. A limitation is the number of TNFi-treated patients, which did not allow more detailed statistical analysis.

Conclusions

Elevated disease activity and TNFi discontinuation in early pregnancy may cause a relapse of disease activity in patients with RA and axSpA. Restart of medication controls disease activity in pregnant patients with RA but shows insufficient effect in pregnant patients with axSpA. The data indicate that tailored medication should be considered beyond conception to stabilize low disease activity and to prevent a flare during pregnancy.

Abbreviations

ASAS: Assessment of SpondyloArthritis international Society; ASDAS-CRP: Ankylosing Spondylitis Disease Activity Score based on C-reactive protein; axSpA: Axial spondyloarthritis; CRP: C-reactive protein; DAS28-CRP: Disease Activity Score in 28 joints based on C-reactive protein; DMARD: Disease-modifying antirheumatic drug; GC: Glucocorticosteroid; HCQ: Hydrochloroquine; HLA: Human leukocyte antigen; NSAID: Nonsteroidal anti-inflammatory drug; RA: Rheumatoid arthritis; RR: Relative risk; SpA: Spondyloarthritis; SSZ: Sulfasalazine; TNFi: Tumor necrosis factor inhibitor

Acknowledgements

We would like to thank Dr. Lukas Bütkofer from the Clincal Trials Unit Bern for his statistical guidance.

Funding

Not applicable.

Authors' contributions

SvdB made substantial contributions to acquisition of data, analysis and interpretation of data using SPSS software, the drafting and revision of the manuscript. AZ carried out acquisition of data and was involved in the revision of the manuscript. FF and MØ were involved in conception and design as well as drafting and revision of the manuscript. DB and FMV contributed to conception and design and were involved in the critical revision of the manuscript. All authors gave final approval of the version to be published and agreed to be accountable for all aspects of the work in ensuring that questions related to the accuracy or integrity of any part of the work are appropriately investigated and resolved. All authors read and approved the final manuscript.

Competing interests

The authors declare that they have no competing interests.

Author details

[1]Department of Rheumatology, Immunology and Allergology, University Hospital, University of Bern, Freiburgstrasse 8, 3010 Bern, Switzerland. [2]Clinical Immunology and Rheumatology, Academic Medical Center/University of Amsterdam, Meibergdreef 9, 1105, AZ, Amsterdam, The Netherlands.

References

1. Ostensen M, Förger F. How safe are anti-rheumatic drugs during pregnancy? Curr Opin Pharmacol. 2013;13(3):470–5.
2. Barrett JH, Brennan P, Fiddler M, Silman AJ. Does rheumatoid arthritis remit during pregnancy and relapse postpartum? Results from a nationwide study in the United Kingdom performed prospectively from late pregnancy. Arthritis Rheum. 1999;42(6):1219–27.
3. de Man YA, Dolhain RJ, van de Geijn FE, Willemsen SP, Hazes JM. Disease activity of rheumatoid arthritis during pregnancy: results from a nationwide prospective study. Arthritis Rheum. 2008;59(9):1241–8.
4. Ostensen M, Ostensen H. Ankylosing spondylitis—the female aspect. J Rheumatol. 1998;25(1):120–4.
5. Ostensen M, Fuhrer L, Mathieu R, Seitz M, Villiger PM. A prospective study of pregnant patients with rheumatoid arthritis and ankylosing spondylitis using validated clinical instruments. Ann Rheum Dis. 2004;63(10):1212–7.
6. Förger F, Vallbracht I, Helmke K, Villiger PM, Ostensen M. Pregnancy mediated improvement of rheumatoid arthritis. Swiss Med Wkly. 2012;142:w13644.
7. de Man YA, Bakker-Jonges LE, Goorbergh CM, Tillemans SP, Hooijkaas H, Hazes JM, et al. Women with rheumatoid arthritis negative for anti-cyclic citrullinated peptide and rheumatoid factor are more likely to improve during pregnancy, whereas in autoantibody-positive women autoantibody levels are not influenced by pregnancy. Ann Rheum Dis. 2010;69(2):420–3.
8. Verstappen SM, King Y, Watson KD, Symmons DP, Hyrich KL, BSRBR Control Centre Consortium, BSR Biologics Register. Anti-TNF therapies and pregnancy: outcome of 130 pregnancies in the British Society for Rheumatology Biologics Register. Ann Rheum Dis. 2011;70(5):823–6.
9. Dougados M, van der Linden S, Juhlin R, Huitfeldt B, Amor B, Calin A, et al. The European Spondylarthropathy Study Group preliminary criteria for the classification of spondylarthropathy. Arthritis Rheum. 1991;34(10):1218–27.
10. Rudwaleit M, van der Heijde D, Landewé R, Listing J, Akkoc N, Brandt J, et al. The development of Assessment of SpondyloArthritis international Society classification criteria for axial spondyloarthritis (part II): validation and final selection. Ann Rheum Dis. 2009;68(6):777–83.
11. de Man YA, Hazes JM, van de Geijn FE, Krommenhoek C, Dolhain RJ. Measuring disease activity and functionality during pregnancy in patients with rheumatoid arthritis. Arthritis Rheum. 2007;57(5):716–22.
12. Smolen JS, Keystone EC, Emery P, Breedveld FC, Betteridge N, Burmester GR, et al. Consensus statement on the use of rituximab in patients with rheumatoid arthritis. Ann Rheum Dis. 2007;66(2):143–50.
13. Lukas C, Landewé R, Sieper J, Dougados M, Davis J, Braun J, et al. Development of an ASAS-endorsed disease activity score (ASDAS) in patients with ankylosing spondylitis. Ann Rheum Dis. 2009;68(1):18–24.
14. Machado P, Landewé R, Lie E, Kvien TK, Braun J, Baker D, et al. Ankylosing Spondylitis Disease Activity Score (ASDAS): defining cut-off values for disease activity states and improvement scores. Ann Rheum Dis. 2011;70(1):47–53.
15. Østensen M, Villiger PM, Förger F. Interaction of pregnancy and autoimmune rheumatic disease. Autoimmun Rev. 2012;11(6-7):A437–46.
16. Navarro-Compan V, Plasencia-Rodriguez C, de Miguel E, Balsa A, Martin-Mola E, Seoane-Mato D, et al. Anti-TNF discontinuation and tapering strategies in patients with axial spondyloarthritis: a systematic literature review. Rheumatology. 2016;55(7):1188–94.
17. Kavanaugh A, Lee SJ, Curtis JR, Greenberg JD, Kremer JM, Soto L, et al. Discontinuation of tumour necrosis factor inhibitors in patients with rheumatoid arthritis in low-disease activity: persistent benefits. Data from the Corrona registry. Ann Rheum Dis. 2015;74(6):1150–5.
18. Wiland P, Dudler J, Veale D, Tahir H, Pedersen R, Bukowski J, et al. The effect of reduced or withdrawn etanercept-methotrexate therapy on patient-reported outcomes in patients with early rheumatoid arthritis. J Rheumatol. 2016;43(7):1268–77.
19. Zelinkova Z, van der Ent C, Bruin KF, van Baalen O, Vermeulen HG, Smalbraak HJ, et al. Effects of discontinuing anti-tumor necrosis factor therapy during pregnancy on the course of inflammatory bowel disease and neonatal exposure. Clin Gastroenterol Hepatol. 2013;11(3):318–21.
20. Förger F, Ostensen M, Schumacher A, Villiger PM. Impact of pregnancy on health related quality of life evaluated prospectively in pregnant women with rheumatic diseases by the SF-36 Health Survey. Ann Rheum Dis. 2005;64(10):1494–9.
21. Götestam Skorpen C, Hoeltzenbein M, Tincani A, Fischer-Betz R, Elefant E, Chambers C, et al. The EULAR points to consider for use of antirheumatic drugs before pregnancy, and during pregnancy and lactation. Ann Rheum Dis. 2016;75(5):795–810.
22. Braun J, van den Berg R, Baraliakos X, Boehm H, Burgos-Vargas R, Collantes-Estevez E, et al. 2010 update of the ASAS/EULAR recommendations for the management of ankylosing spondylitis. Ann Rheum Dis. 2011;70(6):896–904.
23. van der Maas A, Lie E, Christensen R, Choy E, de Man YA, van Riel P, Woodworth T, den Broeder AA. Construct and criterion validity of several proposed DAS28-based rheumatoid arthritis flare criteria: an OMERACT cohort validation study. Ann Rheum Dis. 2013;72(11):1800–5.
24. Gossec L, Portier A, Landewe R, Etcheto A, Navarro-Compan V, Kroon F, van der Heijde D, Dougados M. Preliminary definitions of 'flare' in axial spondyloarthritis, based on pain, BASDAI and ASDAS-CRP: an ASAS initiative. Ann Rheum Dis. 2016;75(6):991–6.

22

Discovery of new candidate genes for rheumatoid arthritis through integration of genetic association data with expression pathway analysis

Klementy Shchetynsky*, Lina-Marcella Diaz-Gallo, Lasse Folkersen, Aase Haj Hensvold, Anca Irinel Catrina, Louise Berg, Lars Klareskog and Leonid Padyukov

Abstract

Background: Here we integrate verified signals from previous genetic association studies with gene expression and pathway analysis for discovery of new candidate genes and signaling networks, relevant for rheumatoid arthritis (RA).

Method: RNA-sequencing-(RNA-seq)-based expression analysis of 377 genes from previously verified RA-associated loci was performed in blood cells from 5 newly diagnosed, non-treated patients with RA, 7 patients with treated RA and 12 healthy controls. Differentially expressed genes sharing a similar expression pattern in treated and untreated RA sub-groups were selected for pathway analysis. A set of "connector" genes derived from pathway analysis was tested for differential expression in the initial discovery cohort and validated in blood cells from 73 patients with RA and in 35 healthy controls.

Results: There were 11 qualifying genes selected for pathway analysis and these were grouped into two evidence-based functional networks, containing 29 and 27 additional connector molecules. The expression of genes, corresponding to connector molecules was then tested in the initial RNA-seq data. Differences in the expression of *ERBB2*, *TP53* and *THOP1* were similar in both treated and non-treated patients with RA and an additional nine genes were differentially expressed in at least one group of patients compared to healthy controls. The *ERBB2*, *TP53*. *THOP1* expression profile was successfully replicated in RNA-seq data from peripheral blood mononuclear cells from healthy controls and non-treated patients with RA, in an independent collection of samples.

Conclusion: Integration of RNA-seq data with findings from association studies, and consequent pathway analysis implicate new candidate genes, *ERBB2*, *TP53* and *THOP1* in the pathogenesis of RA.

Keywords: Rheumatoid arthritis, Molecular genetics, Immunology, Genome-wide, RNA-seq

Background

Implementation of next-generation sequencing (NGS) to analyse RNA expression has revolutionized our capacity to approach different cell functions. However, the precise functional interpretation of whole-transcriptome expression data is still challenging [1]. Currently, there are multiple approaches to analysing the output of RNA-sequencing (RNA-seq), but there is little consensus on the algorithms used to process and interpret the data. Integration of multiple RNA-seq data sets with extensive amounts of data from genome-wide association studies (GWAS) and protein interaction databases may improve the interpretation of data and contribute to the discovery of new molecular targets that are supported by experimental evidence on multiple levels [2].

Here we attempted to incorporate previous knowledge from genome-wide association studies and pathway analyses into the framework of an RNA-seq-based study of differential gene expression in rheumatoid arthritis (RA). RA is a common autoimmune disease, manifesting

* Correspondence: klementy.shchetynsky@ki.se
Rheumatology Unit, Department of Medicine Centre of Molecular Medicine, CMM:L8:04, Karolinska Institutet/Karolinska University Hospital Solna, 171 61 Stockholm, Sweden

as chronic inflammation of the joints, and characterized by a significant genetic contribution [3–5] and gender bias (1.8–3.6 female-to-male ratio) [6, 7].

Refinement and meta-analysis of large-scale GWAS have found associations between risk of RA and more than a hundred variants in non-human leukocyte antigen (HLA) loci [8–11]. A comprehensive review by Okada et al. summarises a multitude of verified genetic variants playing a role in RA susceptibility, suggesting 377 genes for prospective study, based on their proximity to verified RA-associated single nucleotide polymorphisms (SNPs) [12]. Multiple previous studies suggest enrichment for cis-acting variants, located in close proximity to coding genes [13].

Focusing on previously validated genetic variants associated with RA (with genome-wide significant association), we used RNA-seq to address the expression of the genes proximal to these SNPs, in whole-blood samples from patients with RA and from healthy individuals. We differentiated between treated and non-treated patients with (early) RA to identify common expression signals in these two groups, and controlled for the effects of treatment when comparing them to healthy controls. We applied pathway analysis to differentially expressed genes from RNA-seq data, which correspond to previously validated genetic variants associated with RA, with the goal of identifying new functionally meaningful candidate genes and gene networks playing a role in the disease. A new gene set derived from interconnections in pathway analysis, was analyzed for differential expression and validated in a larger independent collection of samples, sharing a similar structure with our discovery cohort.

Methods

Cohorts of patients and controls

We studied 12 female patients from Karolinska University Hospital, Solna, Sweden, who had RA that corresponded to the American College of Rheumatology (ACR) 1987 criteria and the European League Against Rheumatism (EULAR)/ACR 2010 criteria for RA, according to assessment by trained rheumatologists. Of the 12 patients with RA, 5 were non-treated and had not previously used anti-rheumatic drugs (patients with early RA with symptom duration less than 1 year), and 7 of the patients were receiving anti-rheumatic treatment (either methotrexate or biological agents). Patients with early RA, not yet receiving anti-rheumatic treatment, could still receive non-steroid anti-inflammatory drugs (NSAIDs). The study also included 12 matched healthy female individuals as a control group. An additional non-overlapping validation cohort (COMBINE) consisted of 46 non-treated female patients with RA, 27 female patients with RA treated with methotrexate and 34 healthy female controls. Additional clinical information for the studied groups, including age range, disease activity score in 28 joints (DAS28) and anti-citrullinated peptide antibody (ACPA) status is presented in Additional file 1: Table S1.

RNA extraction and sequencing

Whole blood from all patients and healthy controls was collected in PAXgene Blood RNA Tubes according to the manufacturer's protocol and saved at -20 °C. RNA was extracted using PAXgene Blood miRNA kit (PreAnalytiX, Switzerland). Sample quality was assessed using Agilent Technologies Bioanalyzer with Agilent RNA 6000 Nano Kit (Agilent Technologies, Sweden). RNA-seq was based on the Illumina HiSeq 2000 platform and TruSeq library construction, with 20-m pair-end reads per sample (Illumina, CA, USA). For the RNA-seq data from the initial discovery cohort and the COMBINE validation cohort, TopHat-Cufflinks 2.0 software package was used for RNA-seq data alignment and analysis, as described previously [14], against an hg19 USCS human genome reference. Cufflinks 2.0 was used for abundance estimation and quantification of transcripts. These data have been deposited in the NCBI Gene Expression Omnibus repository [GEO:GSE90081] [15]. The PBMC samples for the COMBINE validation cohort were collected as citrated blood and isolated using Ficoll-Paque (GE Healthcare, Sweden). A detailed description of the validation cohort has been published previously [16].

Pathway analysis

RA-associated loci were chosen based on the selection reported previously by Okada et al. [17], and corresponding proximal genes were defined as being either 2 kbp away or in linkage disequilibrium of $r2 > 0.50$ with any of the 100 verified non-HLA RA risk loci from this study. The workflow is presented schematically in Additional file 2: Figure S1. The network construction was based on the Ingenuity Pathway Analysis (IPA) (QIAGEN, CA, USA) experimental evidence database (human, mouse and rat). The IPA score of 5 and above was used to assign a credible interaction network, requiring that the latter contains at least five of the input genes. The same input dataset was used for analysis with no restrictions on tissue type and a separate analysis, restricted to experimental data from immune primary cells and immune cell lines.

Statistics

A significance cutoff of 0.05 was used for Cuffdiff results of comparison of either of the RA patient groups to controls, and followed by visualisation with R-based cummeRbund software [14]. The Cuffdiff approach to calculate differential gene expression is based on the beta negative binomial model to estimate the variance of the RNA-seq data by *t*-like statistics from fragments per kilobase of transcript per million mapped reads (FPKM) values [18].

The Cuffdiff-derived *p* values of genes with similarly directed fold changes from the separate analyses of treated and non-treated patients with RA were meta-analysed, using Fisher's combined probability test. The results were adjusted for the number of tests performed, using Benjamini and Hochberg false discovery rate (FDR) correction with the adjusted *p* value threshold of 0.05 [19].

Quantitative expression data in the COMBINE validation cohort was analysed by the non-parametric Kruskal-Wallis H test. The threshold for significance was $p = 0.05$. For multiple tests, a false discovery rate threshold *q* value of 0.05 was used. Simple linear regression was used to assess the effect of gene expression on DAS28 score.

Results

Genes proximal to RA associated variants are differentially expressed

Candidate genes were chosen based on proximity to validated genetic variants from previous GWAS and meta-analyses, summarized in the publication by Okada et al. as shown in Additional file 3: Data sheet [17]. Out of 377 genes from RA-associated loci, 22 genes were differentially expressed (DE) based on comparison of RNA-seq data between any of the two groups (with non-treated RA or treated RA) with controls after correction for multiple testing, as shown in (Additional file 4: Figure S2). However, the expression difference was significant only for 11 genes and was unidirectional in both non-treated and treated RA compared to healthy controls (Fig. 1a). As expected, clustering based on the expression pattern of these 11 genes resulted in a reasonably good separation of healthy controls and patients with RA, with group mismatches for only a single patient with RA and two control individuals (Fig. 1b). Predictably, there was no clear distinction between the groups with different treatment status.

Pathway-based analysis of differentially expressed genes reveals new candidate genes for RA

As an outcome of the pathway analysis, corresponding molecules for 6 out of 11 DE genes were interconnected in a reasonably sized functional molecular network, involving 29 additional interacting molecules (Fig. 2a), based on the database for immune cells and cell-lines within Ingenuity Pathway Analysis (IPA). These networks included genes functionally attributed to cellular development, cellular growth and proliferation, and haematological system development and function. An additional inclusive analysis was carried out without restrictions on tissue specificity (Fig. 2b). The resulting network contained corresponding molecules for 8 out of 11 DE genes and 27 additional "connectors". TNF and molecules corresponding to 6 out of 11 input genes were present in both networks.

We used the set of connector molecules produced by pathway analysis to re-interrogate the initial RNA-seq data: 24 IPA-derived connector molecules had quantifiable expression values in our RNA-seq data, and 11 were DE (Additional file 1: Table S2). The meta-analysis approach was used for genes that were DE in a unilateral fashion in both RA groups, when compared to healthy controls. These new candidate genes were selected for further validation.

Replication of expression of differentially expressed genes confirms three new candidates

To replicate our findings we employed analysis of RNA-seq data from the independent COMBINE validation cohort of 46 non-treated female patients with RA, 27 methotrexate-treated female patients with RA and 34 healthy female controls. On the discovery stage we noticed that *ERBB2* RNA expression in whole blood from both non-treated and treated patients with RA was significantly lower than in healthy controls (Kruskal-Wallis test $p = 0.04$).

A similar pattern was observed for *ERBB2* in the COMBINE validation cohort (Fig. 3a), with a significant difference in ERBB2 expression between healthy controls and non-treated patients (Kruskal-Wallis test $p = 0.03$). We also observed significantly lower *TP53* mRNA in non-treated and treated patients with RA compared to healthy controls in the discovery cohort (Kruskal-Wallis test $p = 0.02$) and subsequently demonstrated a similar expression profile in the COMBINE validation cohort (Kruskal-Wallis test $p = 0.05$) (Fig. 3b).

Finally, we discovered a difference in whole blood in the RNA expression of *THOP1*, which was significantly lower in both treated and non-treated patients with RA, compared to healthy controls (Kruskal-Wallis test $p = 0.001$) and was confirmed in the COMBINE validation cohort (Kruskal-Wallis test $p = 0.02$), although there was only a trend towards a difference between the control group and non-treated patients (Fig. 3c). *THOP1* expression was also negatively correlated to DAS28-C-reactive protein (CRP) score with a *p* value of 0.03 and an adjusted R^2 of 0.09 in PBMCs from 43 untreated female patients with RA (data not shown). Additionally, we also used RNA-seq data from the COMBINE validation cohort to assess the expression of 349 genes out of 377 reported by Okada et al. Only one gene - *DNase gamma* (*DNASE1L3*) - was DE in this analysis after correction for multiple testing (data not shown).

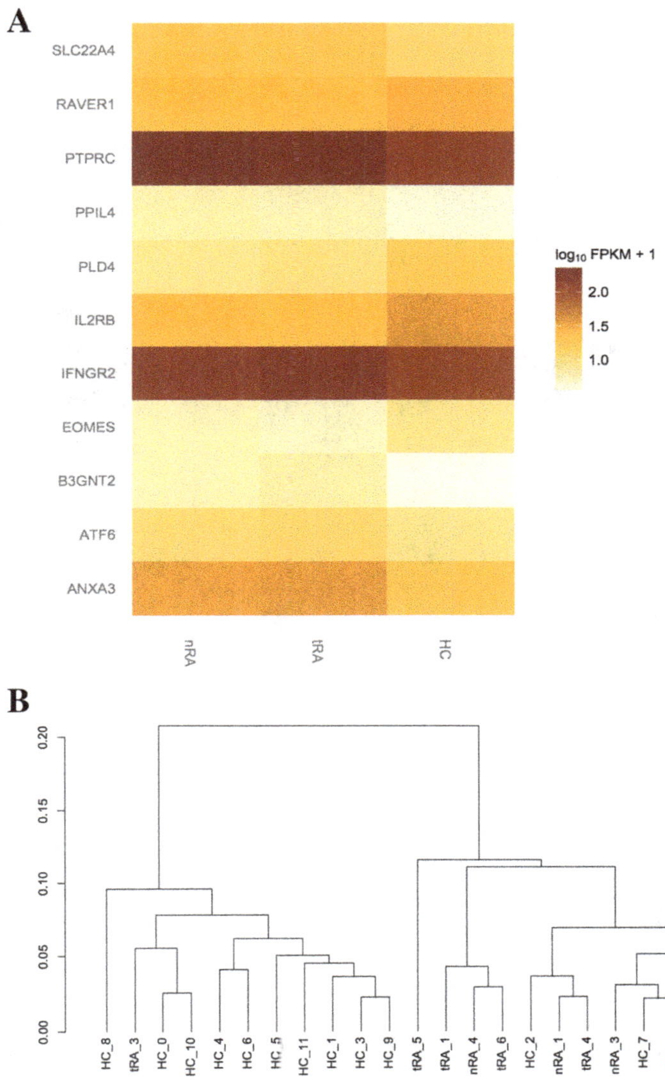

Fig. 1 a Of the 377 genes associated with rheumatoid arthritis (RA) that were reported by Okada et al., 11 were uni-directionally differentially expressed in whole blood from both treated patients (*tRA*) and untreated patients (*nRA*) with RA, when compared to 12 healthy controls (*HC*). The *p* values from both analyses were combined by Fisher's method. A significance threshold of $p = 0.05$ after correction for false discovery rate was applied. *FPKM* fragments per kilobase of transcript per million mapped reads. **b** Clustering on the 11-gene expression profile for grouping of individual samples using Jensen-Shannon distance (shown on axis Y)

Discussion

Our data suggest at least three new candidate genes involved in the development of RA: *ERBB2*, *TP53* and *THOP1*. This finding is based on the integration of previous knowledge from RA association studies, our own RNA-seq expression data and comprehensive pathway analysis with replication in the COMBINE validation cohort.

Initially we hypothesised that genes close to previously found genetic association hits might influence disease-related phenotypes through regulation of RNA expression. This type of association may point to other genes important in RA development, which are part of the same disease-related pathway but do not exhibit a significant change in allelic frequencies defined in conventional GWAS.

The selection of genes proximal to associated loci was based on the criteria previously utilized by Okada et al. [12]. By using this approach we first identified that 11 genes, proximal to validated RA-associated genetic variations, were indeed differentially expressed in whole blood from patients with RA in comparison to healthy controls. Notably, samples could be reasonably grouped into RA and non-RA based on this expression profile alone. This particular gene set, however, did not provide a distinctive clustering between treated and non-treated

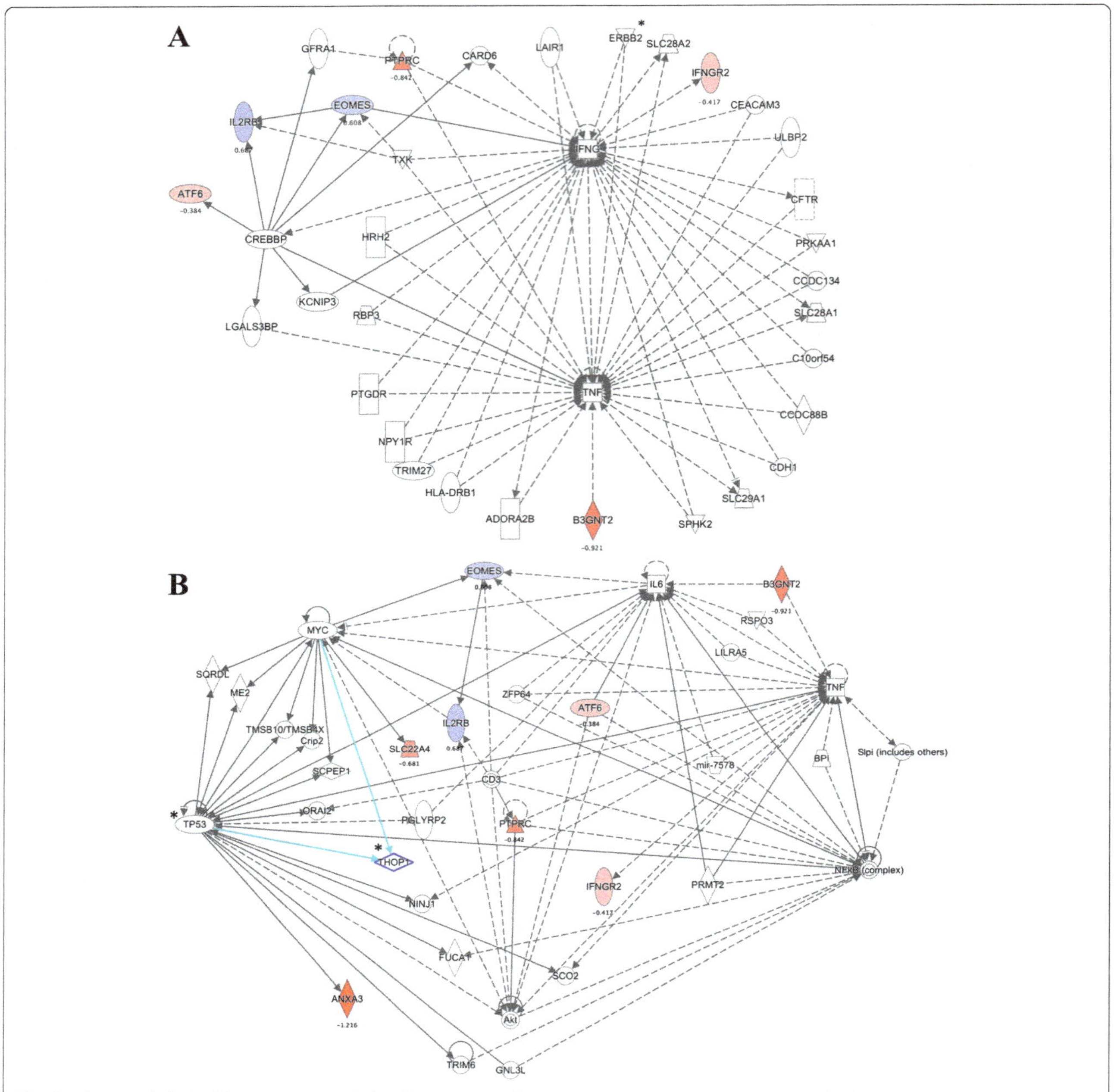

Fig. 2 a A network derived from experimental data for immune cells containing corresponding input molecules for six genes, which were differentially expressed in whole blood RNA-sequencing (RNA-seq) data (Ingenuity Pathway Analysis (IPA)). **b** A network derived from experimental data with no tissue filter applied, containing corresponding input molecules for eight genes, which were differentially expressed in whole blood according to RNA-seq data. *Coloured shapes* represent genes previously associated with RA, which were also DE in RNA-seq data (input data) - expression log2 fold change is represented with colour intensity (*red* increased expression in patients with RA; *blue* decreased expression in patients with RA) and a corresponding value (RA patients versus healthy controls); *white shapes* represent interaction molecules; *solid lines* direct interaction evidence; *broken lines* indirect interaction evidence; *verified differentially expressed connector molecules, IPA

patients with RA. This circumstance aligns with our intention to avoid genes, displaying heterogeneity of gene expression depending on response to treatment among patients with RA.

Using the IPA service in the second part of the discovery stage, we obtained information about the functional relations between the DE genes from RA-associated loci. As a result, 6 out of 11 input genes were grouped into a single network, where *IFNG* and *TNF* served as connecting hubs. Importantly, this network also contained *HLA-DRB1*. It is notable that shared epitope alleles of this gene are well established as the strongest genetic risk

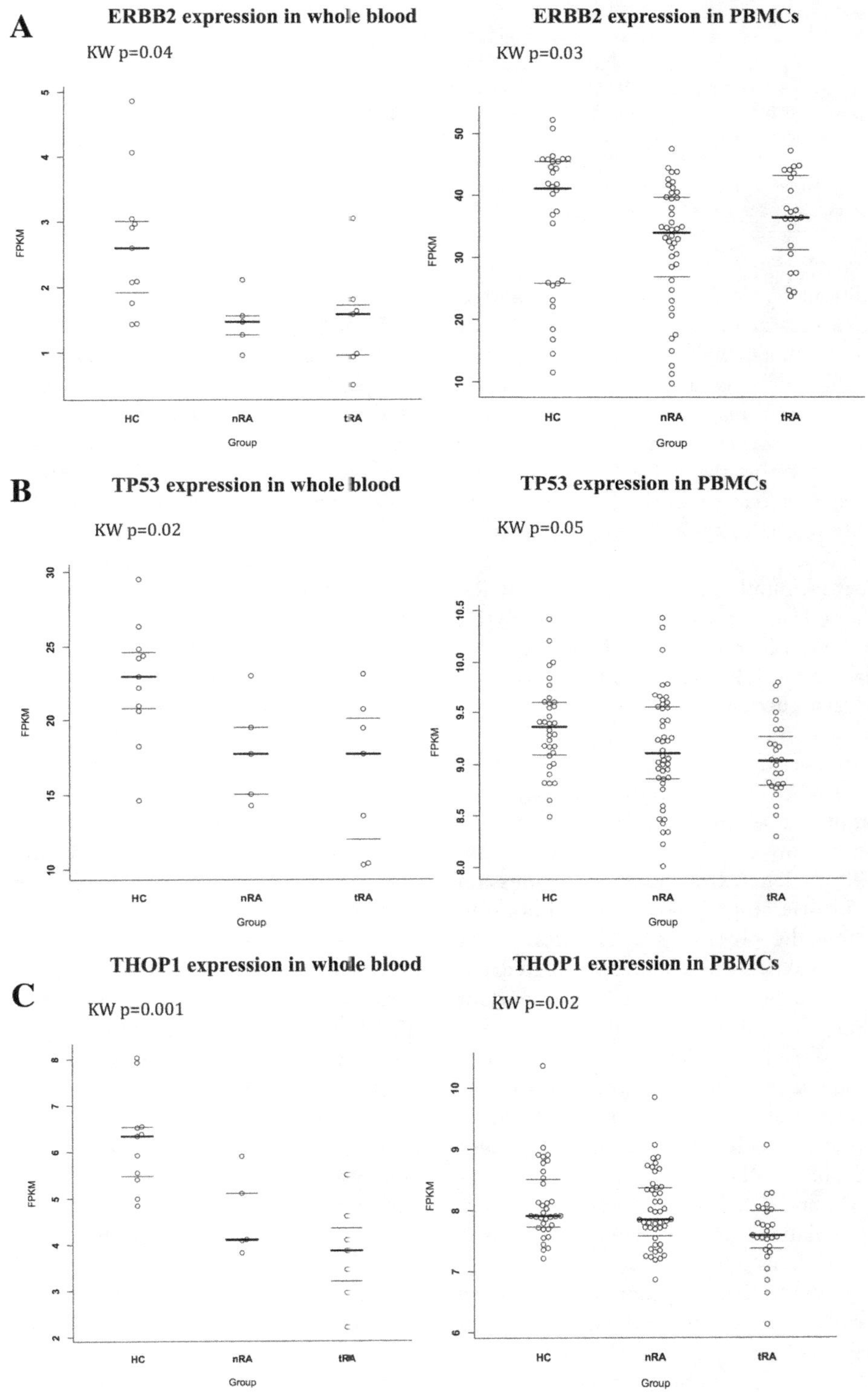

Fig. 3 (See legend on next page.)

(See figure on previous page.)

Fig. 3 a *ERBB2* was significantly differentially expressed (DE) in whole blood from 5 non-treated patients with rheumatoid arthritis (*nRA*) and 12 healthy controls (HC) and for 7 treated patients with RA (*tRA*) versus 12 healthy controls ($p = 0.04$). The expression difference between nRA and HC was replicated in peripheral blood mononuclear cell (*PBMC*) samples from an independent cohort of 46 nRA, 27 methotrexate-treated patients with RA and 34 HC ($p = 0.033$). **b** *TP53* was differentially expressed in whole blood from 5 nRA and 7 tRA versus 12 HC ($p = 0.02$). There was a similar TP53 expression profile in PBMC samples from an independent cohort of 46 nRA, 27 methotrexate-treated patients with RA versus 34 HC ($p = 0.05$). **c** *THOP1* was differentially expressed in whole blood from 5 nRA and 7 tRA versus 12 healthy controls (p = 0.001); there was a significant difference in expression between 27 tRA and 34 HC in PBMC samples ($p = 0.02$). A *p* value of 0.05 was used as the significance threshold for the Kruskal-Wallis (*KW*) non-parametric test. *FPKM* fragments per kilobase of transcript per million mapped reads

factor of RA. Additionally, TNF was earlier identified as one of the most successful drug targets and currently significant number of patients with RA are receiving anti-TNF treatment [20]. IFNγ is also a well-established contributor to autoimmune reactions during RA course; anti-IFNγ treatment, however, show significant side effects [21]. Thus, discovering that HLA-DRB1, TNF and IFNγ are components in our networks is reassuring in terms of the validity of the integrative approach used in this study.

An important feature of all current treatments for RA is the absence of long lasting post-treatment effect: joint destruction, pain and inflammation reoccur after the cancellation of medication [22]. Based on these observations, we assumed that currently available treatments for RA (including most common methotrexate treatment, anti-TNF treatment and other disease modifying anti-rheumatic drugs, DMARDs) are only palliative and influence the symptoms of inflammation rather than disease-developing pathways. Although we cannot exclude the possibility of DMARDs modifying expression of genes involved in disease pathways, it is tempting to hypothesise that only the physiological changes in RA that are common between treated and non-treated patients in comparison to healthy controls are important for the fundamental mechanisms of the disease. Following this hypothesis, we were prompted to compare non-treated and treated patients versus controls without pooling RA samples into a single group, but rather focusing on common effects in independent patient groups. We used Fisher method for combining p-values as an established approach to distinguish common effects in similar populations with an expected degree of heterogeneity [23, 24]. This approach may be helpful in pointing to gene products that may not be affected by current anti-rheumatic treatments, and has been used previously in expression data analyses [25].

Addressing the expression of the "connector" genes, suggested by the pathway analysis, revealed that some of them were DE in whole blood. Although not previously connected to RA, several of these genes were recently shown to be implicated in autoimmunity (e.g. CARD6 in psoriasis [26], PTGDR in asthma [27], BPI in cystic fibrosis [27]) and immune-related processes [28, 29].

However, with the exception of *HLA-DRB1, ERBB2, TP53* and *THOP1,* DE was limited to the comparison of healthy individuals to either treated or non-treated RA groups, but not both. This could be potentially attributed to the heterogeneity introduced by treatment. The study design involving both early and established RA was intended to favour genes contributing to disease development, rather then those connected to the acute manifestation of inflammatory symptoms. Therefore, the validation of *ERBB2, TP53* and *THOP1* expression in a similarly-structured independent material may point at the importance of these genes in the pathogenesis of RA.

Multiple studies have previously implicated *TP53* in RA pathogenesis, showing that decreased expression on both mRNA and protein level contributes to severe defects in apoptosis, potentially enhancing the severity of autoimmune processes in patients with RA (reviewed in [30, 31]). However, genetic association studies never recognised this gene as associated with RA. Our findings of lower *TP53* expression in patients with RA fall in line with the results of previously published studies.

Our data also indicate lower expression of ERBB2 in whole blood and PBMCs of both treated and non-treated Patients with RA compared to controls. *ERBB2* (HER2/neu) is a receptor tyrosine-protein kinase erbB-2, previously implicated in promoting hyperproliferative growth in arthritic synovial tissue [32]. Notably, it is known that ERBB2 protein plays an important role in the regulation of the NFkB pathway and, potentially, TNF signalling [33, 34], which are both implicated in RA.

THOP1 (Thimet Oligopeptidase 1, also known as TOP) was implicated in RA for the first time in this study. Interestingly, *THOP1* has been found to promote rapid degradation of the antigenic peptides, and could affect antigen presentation in vivo [35]. One could speculate that lower expression of *THOP1* observed in whole blood and PBMCs from patients with RA could result in abnormal antigen presentation, which might contribute to the pathogenesis of RA. In this context, it is tempting to investigate a possible functional relationship between *THOP1* and *HLA-DRB1* - the major genetic risk factor for RA.

It is important to mention the limitations of the current study. The discovery cohort is relatively small. Combined with the heterogeneity of gene expression measurements in clinical samples this could lead to insufficient power to detect of some of the genes. Indeed, on testing for DE in the COMBINE validation cohort independently from the discovery cohort, we observed discrepancies that may be indicative of multiple alternative mechanisms leading to differences in regulation of gene expression, different cell composition or more complex timing in this regulation.

Additionally, the RNA in the initial analysis was derived from whole blood, whereas the data from the COMBINE validation cohort is based on RNA from PBMCs. This may explain the discrepant DE results from the two materials on the same gene set, proposed by Okada et al. While useful for verifying and generalizing more consistent signals, this approach does not directly replicate results derived from whole blood. Therefore, it is possible that some of the existing signals could be missed by the current study. The search for pathways underlying RA-associated genes will benefit from larger studies with more stringent replication conditions.

Conclusion

Integration of RNA-seq data with prior data from association studies and pathway analysis, allowed us to infer new candidate genes and molecular pathways that are potentially involved in RA pathogenesis and could be tested as drug targets. Pathway analysis implies that *ERBB2*, *TP53* and *THOP1* could play a role in a signalling network that could contribute to better understanding of the pathological mechanisms behind RA.

Additional files

Additional file 1: Table S1. Clinical features of studied groups of patients with RA and healthy controls. **Table S2** The expression and replication status of genes, which were grouped in common functional networks with genes previously associated with RA. (XLSX 55 kb)

Additional file 2: Figure S1. Schematic representation of the study workflow. Out of the initial set of genes in direct proximity to reported RA variants, those DE in our RNA-seq data were assessed using Ingenuity Pathway Analysis software. Interaction molecules suggested by IPA were again compared to the RNA-seq DE results. (TIFF 966 kb)

Additional file 3: Data sheet. RA-associated variants and corresponding proximal genes as defined in the study by Okada et al. (XLS 62 kb)

Additional file 4: Figure S2. Out of the 377 RA-associated genes reported by Okada et al., 22 were differentially expressed in whole blood from either of the RA patient groups, when compared to 12 healthy controls. (TIFF 772 kb)

Abbreviations

ACPA: anti-citrullinated peptide antibody; ACR: American College of Rheumatology; DAS28: disease activity score (assessment of 28 joints); DE: differentially expressed; DMARDs: disease-modifying anti-rheumatic drugs; ERBB2: Erb-B2 receptor tyrosine kinase 2; EULAR: European League Against Rheumatism; FDR: false discovery rate; FPKM: fragments per kilobase of transcript per million mapped reads; GWAS: genome-wide association studies; HLA: human leukocyte antigen; IFN: interferon; IPA: Ingenuity Pathway Analysis; NFkB: nuclear factor kappa B; NGS: next-generation sequencing; NSAIDs: non-steroid anti-inflammatory drugs; PBMCs: peripheral blood mononuclear cells; RA: rheumatoid arthritis; SNP: single nucleotide polymorphism; THOP1: thimet oligopeptidase 1; TNF: tumor necrosis factor; TP53: tumor protein P53

Acknowledgements

We would like to thank Barbro Larsson for help in performing this study. We would like to thank The National Genomics Infrastructure (NGI) Sweden for access to UPPMAX and the Science for Life Laboratory for the help with RNA-sequencing.

Funding

This study was supported by The Swedish Research Council (Vetenskaprådet) and Be The Cure consortium.

Authors' contributions

KS provided the study design, executed data analysis and interpretation and drafted the manuscript. LMDG provided quality control for RNA samples and edited the manuscript. LF assisted with management and analysis of data from the COMBINE validation cohort and revised the manuscript. AHH and AIC collected clinical material, performed management and analysis of clinical data and revised the manuscript. LB coordinated sharing and management of genetic and clinical data for the COMBINE validation cohort and edited the manuscript. LK and LP have contributed to the study design, drafting and editing of the manuscript. All authors read and approved the final manuscript.

Competing interests

The authors declare that they have no competing interests.

References

1. de Klerk E, t Hoen PA. Alternative mRNA transcription, processing, and translation: insights from RNA sequencing. Trends Genet. 2015;31:128–39.
2. Finotello F, Di Camillo B. Measuring differential gene expression with RNA-seq: challenges and strategies for data analysis. Brief Funct Genomics. 2015; 14:130–42.
3. Raychaudhuri S, Sandor C, Stahl EA, Freudenberg J, Lee HS, Jia X, et al. Five amino acids in three HLA proteins explain most of the association between MHC and seropositive rheumatoid arthritis. Nat Genet. 2012;44:291–6.
4. Padyukov L, Silva C, Stolt P, Alfredsson L, Klareskog L. A gene-environment interaction between smoking and shared epitope genes in HLA-DR provides a high risk of seropositive rheumatoid arthritis. Arthritis Rheum. 2004;50:3085–92.
5. Klareskog L, Stolt P, Lundberg K, Kallberg H, Bengtsson C, Grunewald J, et al. A new model for an etiology of rheumatoid arthritis: smoking may trigger HLA-DR (shared epitope)-restricted immune reactions to autoantigens modified by citrullination. Arthritis Rheum. 2006;54:38–46.
6. Tedeschi SK, Bermas B, Costenbader KH. Sexual disparities in the incidence and course of SLE and RA. Clin Immunol. 2013;149:211–8.
7. Barragan-Martinez C, Amaya-Amaya J, Pineda-Tamayo R, Mantilla RD, Castellanos-dela Hoz J, Bernal-Macias S, et al. Gender differences in Latin-American patients with rheumatoid arthritis. Gend Med. 2012;9:490–510. e5.
8. Freudenberg J, Lee HS, Han BG, Shin HD, Kang YM, Sung YK, et al. Genome-wide association study of rheumatoid arthritis in Koreans: population-specific loci as well as overlap with European susceptibility loci. Arthritis Rheum. 2011;63:884–93.
9. Okada Y, Terao C, Ikari K, Kochi Y, Ohmura K, Suzuki A, et al. Meta-analysis identifies nine new loci associated with rheumatoid arthritis in the Japanese population. Nat Genet. 2012;44:511–6.
10. Stahl EA, Raychaudhuri S, Remmers EF, Xie G, Eyre S, Thomson BP, et al. Genome-wide association study meta-analysis identifies seven new rheumatoid arthritis risk loci. Nat Genet. 2010;42:508–14.

11. Eyre S, Bowes J, Diogo D, Lee A, Barton A, Martin P, et al. High-density genetic mapping identifies new susceptibility loci for rheumatoid arthritis. Nat Genet. 2012;44:1336–40.
12. Okada Y, Wu D, Trynka G, Raj T, Terao C, Ikari K, et al. Genetics of rheumatoid arthritis contributes to biology and drug discovery. Nature. 2014;506:376–81.
13. Sahlen P, Abdullayev I, Ramskold D, Matskova L, Rilakovic N, Lotstedt B, et al. Genome-wide mapping of promoter-anchored interactions with close to single-enhancer resolution. Genome Biol. 2015;16:156.
14. Trapnell C, Roberts A, Goff L, Pertea G, Kim D, Kelley DR, et al. Differential gene and transcript expression analysis of RNA-seq experiments with TopHat and Cufflinks. Nat Protoc. 2012;7:562–78.
15. NCBI Gene Expression Omnibus, project number: GSE90081. http://www.ncbi.nlm.nih.gov/geo/query/acc.cgi?acc=GSE90081. Accessed 24 Nov 2016.
16. Folkersen L, Brynedal B, Diaz-Gallo LM, Ramskold D, Shchetynsky K, Westerlind H, et al. Integration of known DNA, RNA and protein biomarkers provides prediction of anti-TNF response in rheumatoid arthritis: results from the COMBINE study. Mol Med. 2016;22:322–8.
17. Chen J, Weiss WA. Alternative splicing in cancer: implications for biology and therapy. Oncogene. 2015;34:1–14.
18. Trapnell C, Williams BA, Pertea G, Mortazavi A, Kwan G, van Baren MJ, et al. Transcript assembly and quantification by RNA-Seq reveals unannotated transcripts and isoform switching during cell differentiation. Nat Biotechnol. 2010;28:511–5.
19. Yosef BYH. Controlling the false discovery rate: a practical and powerful approach to multiple testing. J Roy Statist Soc Ser. 1995;B 57:289–300.
20. Abe T, Takeuchi T. Rheumatoid arthritis and tumor necrosis factor alpha. Autoimmunity. 2001;34:291–303.
21. Raanani P, Ben-Bassat I. Immune-mediated complications during interferon therapy in hematological patients. Acta Haematol. 2002;107:133–44.
22. Moots RJ, Naisbett-Groet B. The efficacy of biologic agents in patients with rheumatoid arthritis and an inadequate response to tumour necrosis factor inhibitors: a systematic review. Rheumatology. 2012;51:2252–61.
23. Li Q, Hu J, Ding J, Zheng G. Fisher's method of combining dependent statistics using generalizations of the gamma distribution with applications to genetic pleiotropic associations. Biostatistics. 2014;15:284–95.
24. Infante-Rivard C, Mirea L, Bull SB. Combining case-control and case-trio data from the same population in genetic association analyses: overview of approaches and illustration with a candidate gene study. Am J Epidemiol. 2009;170:657–64.
25. Hess A, Iyer H. Fisher's combined p-value for detecting differentially expressed genes using Affymetrix expression arrays. BMC Genomics. 2007;8:96.
26. Tervaniemi MH, Katayama S, Skoog T, Siitonen HA, Vuola J, Nuutila K, et al. NOD-like receptor signaling and inflammasome-related pathways are highlighted in psoriatic epidermis. Sci Rep. 2016;6:22745.
27. Skopelja S, Hamilton BJ, Jones JD, Yang ML, Mamula M, Ashare A, et al. The role for neutrophil extracellular traps in cystic fibrosis autoimmunity. JCI Insight. 2016;1:e88912.
28. Cheung AK, Ko JM, Lung HL, Chan KW, Stanbridge EJ, Zabarovsky E, et al. Cysteine-rich intestinal protein 2 (CRIP2) acts as a repressor of NF-kappaB-mediated proangiogenic cytokine transcription to suppress tumorigenesis and angiogenesis. Proc Natl Acad Sci U S A. 2011;108:8390–5.
29. Kennedy JM, Fodil N, Torre S, Bongfen SE, Olivier JF, Leung V, et al. CCDC88B is a novel regulator of maturation and effector functions of T cells during pathological inflammation. J Exp Med. 2014;211:2519–35.
30. Sun Y, Cheung HS. p53, proto-oncogene and rheumatoid arthritis. Semin Arthritis Rheum. 2002;31:299–310.
31. Maas K, Westfall M, Pietenpol J, Olsen NJ, Aune T. Reduced p53 in peripheral blood mononuclear cells from patients with rheumatoid arthritis is associated with loss of radiation-induced apoptosis. Arthritis Rheum. 2005;52:1047–57.
32. Kitamura T, Sekimata M, Kikuchi S, Homma Y. Involvement of poly(ADP-ribose) polymerase 1 in ERBB2 expression in rheumatoid synovial cells. Am J Physiol Cell Physiol. 2005;289:C82–8.
33. Yamaoka T, Yan F, Cao H, Hobbs SS, Dise RS, Tong W, et al. Transactivation of EGF receptor and ErbB2 protects intestinal epithelial cells from TNF-induced apoptosis. Proc Natl Acad Sci U S A. 2008;105:11772–7.
34. Omenn GS, Guan Y, Menon R. A new class of protein cancer biomarker candidates: differentially expressed splice variants of ERBB2 (HER2/neu) and ERBB1 (EGFR) in breast cancer cell lines. J Proteomics. 2014;107:103–12.
35. Saric T, Beninga J, Graef CI, Akopian TN, Rock KL, Goldberg AL. Major histocompatibility complex class I-presented antigenic peptides are degraded in cytosolic extracts primarily by thimet oligopeptidase. J Biol Chem. 2001;276:36474–81.

23

Semaphorin 7A as a potential immune regulator and promising therapeutic target in rheumatoid arthritis

Jianmin Xie[1*] and Hao Wang[2]

Abstract

Background: Semaphorin 7A (Sema7A) is expressed by several different classes of lymphoid and myeloid cells and is a potent immunomodulator. We examined the role of Sema7A in modulating cellular immune responses and to provide experimental data validating the therapeutic potential of Sema7A in rheumatoid arthritis (RA).

Methods: Soluble Sema7A (sSema7A) levels in the serum and synovial fluid from patients with RA or osteoarthritis, as well as cytokine secretions, were analyzed with an enzyme-linked immunosorbent assay. The cell surface levels and transcripts of Sema7A were evaluated in T cells and monocytes from patients with RA. The effect of Sema7A on the functions of primary T cells isolated from the peripheral blood of healthy donors was observed. Detection of the activation of the signal mediator focal adhesion kinase was performed by Western blotting. Shedding of sSema7A was evaluated in monocytes. The introduction of anti-Sema7A antibody to mice with collagen-induced arthritis (CIA) was observed in vivo.

Results: Upregulation of sSema7A levels in both the serum and synovial fluid of patients with RA was correlated with disease activity markers. sSema7A markedly increased Th1/Th17 cytokine secretion and induced evident upregulation of T-bet and retinoic acid receptor-related orphan nuclear receptor γt levels in T cells. Cell surface Sema7A was cleaved by a disintegrin and metalloprotease 17 (ADAM17) in monocytes. Interleukin-6 and tumor necrosis factor-α stimulated ADAM17 secretion in synovial macrophages. Blocking of β1-integrin abrogated the Sema7A-mediated cytokine secretion. Treatment with an anti-Sema7A antibody significantly attenuated CIA.

Conclusions: These findings indicate that Sema7A as a potent activator of T cells and monocytes in the immune response contributes to the inflammation and progression of RA, suggesting its therapeutic potential in the treatment of RA.

Keywords: Rheumatoid arthritis, Semaphorin 7A, ADAM17, Cytokine, T cell

Background

Rheumatoid arthritis (RA) is an autoimmune and systemic inflammatory disorder characterized by synovial inflammation, destruction of cartilage and bone, and systemic manifestations [1, 2]. RA synovial inflammation evokes arthritis symptoms and causes articular bone and cartilage destruction. In RA joints, the immune cells infiltrating the synovium include T cells, macrophages, B cells, and dendritic cells [3]. Activated synovial T cells and macrophages secrete various types of proinflammatory cytokines, including interleukin-6 (IL-6), tumor necrosis factor-α (TNF-α), and IL-17 [4, 5]. Among the different inflammatory cells, T-helper cell type 1 (Th1) cells, as potent cytokine producers, are considered to be crucial effector cells in RA [6]. Recently, considerable evidence has been presented, both in humans and in mice, for the importance of Th 17 cells as the main source of IL-17 in the development and progression of autoimmune diseases. However, the role of inflammatory cells in RA has remained elusive.

Semaphorins comprise a large family of transmembrane proteins and secreted proteins that have been described as axon guidance molecules during neuronal development.

* Correspondence: xiejmdoc@163.com
[1]Department of Rheumatology, Second Affiliated Hospital of Nanjing Medical University, Nanjing, People's Republic of China
Full list of author information is available at the end of the article

They are divided into eight classes based on sequence similarities and distinct structural features [7, 8]. Of the eight classes of semaphorins, classes 1 and 2 semaphorins are found in invertebrates, whereas classes 3–7 semaphorins are found in vertebrates and class 8 semaphorins are viral. Plexin-semaphorin-integrin domains, immunoglobulin-like domains, PDZ domains, and/or thrombospondin domains have also been shown to be part of the semaphorin protein structure. Semaphorins were initially described for their role in axon guidance during neurogenesis [9]. It has since been found that semaphorins branch beyond the nervous system to cover an ample overlap of molecular repertoires. Semaphorins are also involved in physiological processes such as organogenesis, immune cell regulation, and vascular growth [10].

Semaphorin 7A (Sema7A) is the only class 7 semaphorin, also known as CD108, with a membrane-associated, glycosylphosphatidylinositol (GPI)-linked semaphorin protein that contains arginine-glycine-aspartate [11], a well-conserved, integrin-binding motif, in its Sema domain. Sema7A has an immune function in both the innate and adaptive immune systems [12]. Previous studies have shown that semaphorins have important roles in immunologic disorders, such as multiple sclerosis, contact hypersensitivity, experimental autoimmune encephalomyelitis, granulomatosis with polyangiitis (Wegener's), and RA [13, 14]. Recently, on one hand, several studies have shown that Sema7A is a potent stimulator of monocytes inducing the production of proinflammatory cytokines [15]. On the other hand, Sema7A has been shown to function as a regulator of the T-cell immune response by its effects on T-cell proliferation [16]. Notably, Sema7A has been demonstrated to have a clear effect on the migration processes of osteoblasts and osteoclasts in bone remodeling and a distinct role in tumor angiogenesis [17, 18]. Neovascularization, immunologic abnormality, and bone erosion all have crucial roles in the progression of RA [19, 20], suggesting that Sema7A may aggravate RA. However, the pathologic significance of Sema7A in RA remains unclear.

On the basis of these observations, we analyzed the role of secreted Sema7A in the modulation of cellular immunological functions and the pathogenesis of RA. Our findings identified that Sema7A is an attractive activator of T cells and monocytes in the synovial lesions of patients with RA. Furthermore, the elevated levels of soluble semaphorin 7A (sSema7A) were proteolytically shed from the cell surface, and the resultant sSema7A contributed to inflammation, suggesting that an inflammatory activation loop exists in RA synovium. Moreover, we demonstrate that Sema7A mediates its intracellular effects via interactions with β1-integrins and the activation of focal adhesion kinase (FAK). The inhibition of Sema7A attenuated the development of collagen-induced arthritis (CIA). In the present study, we explored the key role of Sema7A in immunoregulation, and we provide experimental data validating the therapeutic potential of Sema7A in RA.

Methods

Subjects

Blood samples were collected from 55 patients with RA and 12 with osteoarthritis (OA). Blood samples were also obtained from healthy donors. Synovial tissue and fluid samples were collected during knee joint replacement surgery from patients with RA (n =15) and patients with OA (n = 10). These patients presented with high levels of C-reactive protein (CRP) (29–138 mg/L, mean 66 mg/L) and rheumatoid factor (RF) (63–432 U/ml, mean 214.8 U/ml). Thirty-three of the 55 patients with RA had a Disease Activity Score in 28 joints (DAS28) ≥3.2 [21]. All patients with RA fulfilled the revised American College of Rheumatology criteria [22]. All cases of OA were classified as grade IV on the basis of clinical and radiological criteria according to the Kellgren-Lawrence grading scale [23]. All of the patients provided written informed consent to participate in this study. The ethics committee of Nanjing Medical University approved this study.

Cell isolation and culture

Isolation of human peripheral blood mononuclear cells (PBMCs) was performed as described previously [20]. PBMCs were analyzed on a fluorescence-activated cell-sorting (FACS) flow cytometer (BD Biosciences, San Jose, CA, USA) using FlowJo software (FlowJo, Ashland, OR, USA). $CD4^+$ T cells and $CD14^+$ monocytes were purified from PBMCs by incubating cells with anti-CD4 and anti-CD14 monoclonal antibody (mAb). The following antibodies were used: anti-human CD4 phycoerythrin (PE) (BD Biosciences) and anti-human CD14 PE (BD Biosciences). The purity of isolated $CD4^+$ T cells and $CD14^+$ monocytes was >95% in all experiments. The cell surface expression of Sema7A in peripheral blood $CD4^+$ and $CD14^+$ cells was detected by flow cytometric analyses using PE-conjugated anti-human Sema7A (BioLegend, San Diego, CA, USA). THP-1 cells were cultured in RPMI 1640 medium supplemented with 10% heat-inactivated FBS and penicillin-streptomycin.

Synovial macrophage isolation

After synovial tissues were digested, the samples were filtered using a cell strainer (BioLegend). The adherent synovial cells were harvested. After overnight culture, primary synovial cells were employed for synovial macrophage isolation using a magnetic-activated cell sorting separation column system (Miltenyi Biotec, Bergisch Gladbach, Germany) as previously described [23]. Adherent cells were incubated with CD14-labeled microbeads for 30 minutes at 4 °C, and this mixture was then applied to a magnetic column. The positive fraction ($CD14^+$) was used as the synovial macrophage. CD14$^+$ cells were incubated for 24 h with 1 mg/ml of IL-6 and 0.1 mg/ml of TNF-α (PeproTech, Rocky Hill, NJ, USA) in Dulbecco's modified Eagle's medium containing 10% fetal calf serum. The concentrations of a disintegrin and metalloprotease 17 (ADAM17) and Sema7A in the culture supernatants were also measured by enzyme-linked immunosorbent assay (ELISA).

Cytokine production assay

For the analysis of cytokine secretions, freshly isolated CD4$^+$ T and CD14$^+$ cells (2×10^5) from patients with RA were incubated in the presence of Sema7A-Fc fusion protein (10 ng/ml) at the indicated concentrations for 48 h. Cells cultured in the absence of Sema7A (negative control [NC]) or in the presence of heat-denatured Sema7A (DSema7A) were used as an NC or an additional control. DSema7A was produced by incubating Sema7A at 95 °C for 20 minutes. Supernatants from T-cell cultures were then collected and analyzed for cytokine secretion. The concentrations of human TNF-α, IL-6, interferon-γ (IFN-γ), IL-22, and IL-17 in the culture supernatants were determined using ELISA kits for each cytokine (R&D Systems, Minneapolis, MN, USA). For the blocking experiments, the CD14$^+$ cells were cocultured with 10 ng/ml of Sema7A and 10 ng/ml of anti-Sema7A antibody, anti-β1-integrin antibody, or anti-plexin C1 antibody (BioLegend), or with immunoglobulin G (IgG) as a control, for 36 h. The levels of IL-6 and TNF-α in the supernatants were evaluated by ELISA.

sSema7A levels in patients' serum and synovial fluid samples from and in the cell culture supernatants were detected using an ELISA kit (R&D Systems). The levels of ADAM17 in the serum and synovial fluid samples were also determined using an ELISA kit (MyBioSource, San Diego, CA, USA).

Human Sema7A-Fc fusion proteins were produced as previously described [11, 16], and recombinant human IgG1-Fc (R&D Systems) was used as a control. Naturally cleaved sSema7A was affinity-purified, performed as previously described [16].

Reverse transcription-quantitative polymerase chain reaction

PBMCs or CD4$^+$ or CD14$^+$ cells (2×10^5) were isolated using a FACS flow cytometer (BD Biosciences). The total RNA was extracted from the cells using TRIzol reagent (Invitrogen, Carlsbad, CA, USA) according to the manufacturer's instructions. The complementary DNA was synthesized using SuperScript III reverse transcriptase (Invitrogen) according to the manufacturer's protocol. A LightCycler (Roche, Basel, Switzerland) and a SYBR reverse transcription-polymerase chain reaction (RT-PCR) kit (Toyobo, Osaka, Japan) were used for the quantitative real-time RT-PCR analysis in accordance with the manufacturer's instructions. The sequences of the primer sets for Sema7A, β1-integrin, and plexin C1, as well as the target sites on the messenger RNA (mRNA) and the PCR product sizes, are shown in Table 1. β-actin was used to normalize the samples. The relative quantification of each gene was determined using LightCycler 480SW software (Roche).

Western blot analysis

Cultured CD4$^+$ T cells from healthy control subjects were stimulated with Sema7A for 3 h. Unstimulated cells or T cells treated with DSema7A were used as controls. The cells were washed twice with ice-cold PBS and lysed in lysis buffer consisting of 25 mM Tris-HCl, pH 7.5, 150 mM NaCl, 1% Triton X-100, 0.1% SDS, and cOmplete Mini protease inhibitor cocktail (Roche). For phosphorylation-specific immunoblot analysis, phosphatase inhibitors (10 mM NaF, 12.5 mM β-glycerophosphate, and 1 mM Na_3VO_4) were added to the lysis buffer. Whole-cell lysates were subjected to SDS-PAGE under reducing conditions. Immunoblotting was performed using antibodies specific to retinoic acid receptor-related orphan nuclear receptor γt (RORγt; BioLegend) and T-bet (BD Biosciences).

The CD14$^+$ cells from patients with RA were stimulated with 10 ng/ml of recombinant Sema7A or DSema7A for 15 minutes. CD14$^+$ cells stimulated with DSema7A were used as negative controls. The activation of FAK was evaluated by immunoblotting using antibodies specific to FAK (Santa Cruz Biotechnology, Dallas, TX, USA), phospho-FAK (Tyr397) (BD Biosciences), and glyceraldehyde 3-phosphate dehydrogenase (Abcam, Cambridge, UK).

Shedding of sSema7A

The THP-1 cell line and CD14$^+$ cells from patients with RA were cultured in RPMI 1640 medium containing 1 μM of BMS-561392 (Bristol-Myers Squibb, New York, NY, USA) or 100 μM of GM6001 (Calbiochem, San Diego, CA, USA) for 7 minutes at room temperature before the THP-1 and CD14$^+$ cells were incubated for 12 h with 0.1 mg/ml of TNF-α and 1.0 mg/ml of IL-6. sSema7A concentrations were measured by Western blotting.

Table 1 Primers for human semaphorin 7A, β1-integrin, and plexin C1

Transcript	Forward primer	Reverse primer	Length
Semaphorin7A	TCATCAAAGC CACCATCG	AGCTCACATAC AGCTTCCTCC	771
β1-integrin	CAAAGGAAC AGCAGAGAAGC	GTGGAAAACA CCAGCAGC	537
Plexin C1	AACCATTGCA CTGCAAACC	GATTCCATCTTC AAGAATCACG	557

Small interfering RNA experiments

HEK293T cells were transduced with a pcDNA3.1 vector containing the Sema7A sequence. HEK293T cells stably expressing Sema7A (HEK293T_Sema7A) were infected with a lentiviral vector containing short-hairpin RNA (shRNA) specific for *ADAM17* (5′-GCTTGATTCTTTGCTCTCA-3′) or a nonspecific shRNA. The preparation of the lentiviral vector and cell transduction were performed according to previously described protocols [24]. ADAM17 mRNA expression was assayed by RT-PCR 48 h after cell transduction. sSema7A levels in the cell supernatant were determined by Western blot analysis 5 days after the silencing of ADAM-17 expression.

Induction and assessment of CIA

The CIA model was induced in the mice as previously described [25, 26]. Briefly, DBA/1 mice were obtained from the Shanghai Animal Center (Shanghai, China). Eight-week-old DBA/1 mice were given intradermal injections of 100 μg/mouse of bovine collagen type II (CII) (Cosmo Bio, Tokyo, Japan) emulsified in complete Freund's adjuvant containing 250 μg/mouse of heat-killed *Mycobacterium tuberculosis* H37Ra (BD Biosciences). Twenty-one days after immunization, the mice were given a booster injection at the base of the tail with 100 μg/mouse of bovine CII. Mice with CIA were given intraperitoneal injections of 12 μg/mouse of anti-Sema7A antibody (AF1835, goat IgG; R&D Systems) ($n = 8$), 9 μg/mouse of anti-Sema7A antibody ($n = 8$), or isotype control antibodies (R&D Systems) on days 1, 10, 20, 30, and 40. Serum was collected on day 50. Serum levels of TNF-α, IL-6, and IL-17 were evaluated by ELISA (R&D Systems).

To evaluate the incidence and severity of arthritis, arthritis was scored by two calibrated examiners via a visual assessment scoring system using a scale of 0–4 per limb as previously described [25, 27]. The severity scores were defined as follows: 0 = no evidence of erythema and swelling; 1 = erythema and mild swelling confined to the midfoot (tarsals) or ankle joint; 2 = erythema and mild swelling extending from the ankle to the foot; 3 = erythema and moderate swelling extending from the ankle to the metatarsal joints; and 4 = erythema and severe swelling encompassing the ankle, foot, and digits. The paws of mice stimulated with anti-Sema7A antibody ($n = 8$), the control antibody ($n = 8$), or no antibody ($n = 6$) were fixed and decalcified. Histologic scoring and the histomorphometric analysis of the paws were performed by an investigator blinded to treatment status.

Statistical analysis

Statistical analysis of the data was performed using SPSS version 16 software (SPSS, Chicago, IL, USA). Nonparametric Mann-Whitney *U* tests were used to compare two groups, and comparisons between three groups were performed using the Kruskal-Wallis test followed by the Mann-Whitney *U* test. *P* values less than or equal to 0.05 were considered significant. Correlations between clinical parameters and Sema7A were determined using Spearman's correlation. The data are presented as SDs.

Results

Significantly increased levels of sSema7A in patients with RA and correlation with disease activity

Several members of the semaphorin family have been characterized with respect to their function in immunity. To explore the pathologic role of Sema7A in RA, we first detected the serum levels of Sema7A in patients with immunologic and joint-destructive diseases. The serum levels of secreted Sema7A were determined by ELISA in a large cohort of patients with RA ($n = 55$) and patients with OA ($n = 12$) in comparison with healthy individuals ($n = 60$).

Interestingly, the levels of serum sSema7A were remarkably increased in patients with RA compared with healthy subjects (mean ± SD 13.6 ± 3.7 ng/ml versus 5.7 ± 2.8 ng/ml; $P < 0.01$). In contrast, serum sSema7A levels were not elevated in patients with OA. We next performed ELISA to determine the Sema7A levels in the synovial fluid of patients with RA and OA. A significantly increased level of Sema7A was detected in fluid from patients with RA (12.3 ± 6.5 ng/ml) compared with that from patients with OA (3.1 ± 2.4 ng/ml) ($P < 0.01$) (Fig. 1a). To investigate the clinical significance of sSema7A, we analyzed the correlations between clinical features and levels of serum sSema7A. Importantly, there was a positive correlation between sSema7A and disease activity markers such as the DAS28 ($r^2 = 0.817$, $P < 0.01$), the CRP level ($r^2 = 0.760$, $P < 0.01$), and the RF titer ($r^2 = 0.621$, $P < 0.01$) (Fig. 1b). In contrast, no relationship between serum sSema7A levels and disease duration, age, or sex were observed (data not shown).

Serum levels of sSema7A were examined before and 6 months after the beginning of biologic disease-modifying antirheumatic drug (DMARD) therapy (31 patients were treated with TNF inhibitors). A significant reduction in serum sSema7A levels after biologic DMARD treatment was observed (mean ± SD 12.6 ± 4.3 ng/ml versus 6.7 ± 2.6 ng/ml; $P < 0.01$) in patients who were good responders according to the European League Against Rheumatism response criteria [28] (Fig. 1c), suggesting the involvement of Sema7A in determining the clinical status of RA.

Expression of Sema7A and its upregulation of secretion of proinflammatory cytokines in T cells and monocytes/macrophages

Studies suggest that members of the semaphoring family are important players during the immune response because they regulate interactions between T cells and antigen-presenting cells during the primary immune response [29, 30]. To

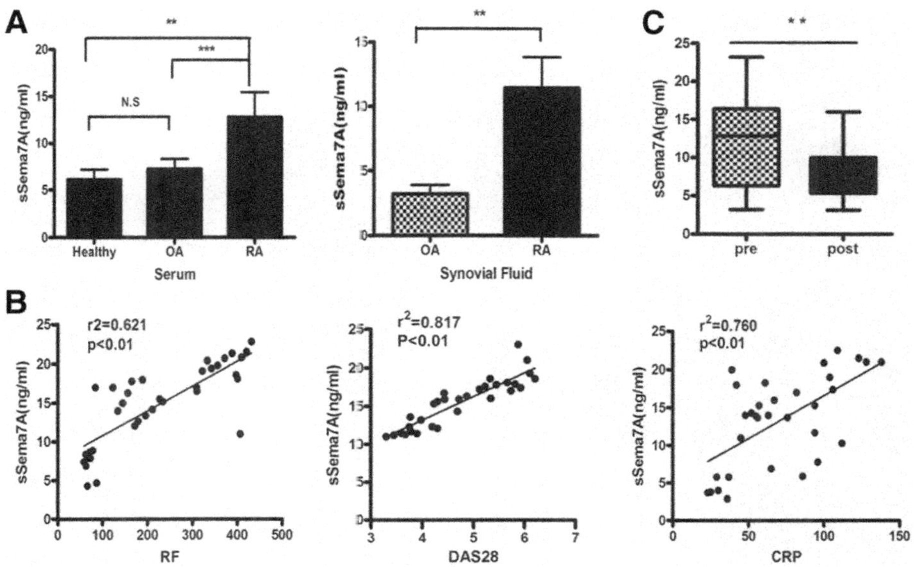

Fig. 1 Levels of soluble semaphorin 7A (sSema7A) and correlation with markers of rheumatoid arthritis (RA) disease activity. **a** sSema7A levels in serum and synovial fluid samples from patients with RA and patients with osteoarthritis (OA). **b** Serum sSema7A levels before and after biologic disease-modifying antirheumatic drug treatment in good responders according to the European League Against Rheumatism response criteria. Values in **a** and **b** are mean ± SD. $^{**}P < 0.01$; $^{***}P < 0.001$. *N.S* Not significant. **c** Correlation between serum sSema7A levels with rheumatoid factor (RF) titer, Disease Activity Score in 28 joints (DAS28), and C-reactive protein (CRP) level ($n = 31$ samples)

explore whether Sema7A expression by T cells and monocytes differed in patients with RA compared with control subjects, we isolated $CD4^+$ cells and $CD14^+$ cells and performed flow cytometry. Notably, cell surface Sema7A expression was downregulated on all cells from patients with RA (Fig. 2a). Furthermore, cell surface Sema7A was expressed richly on $CD14^+$ and $CD4^+$ cells in healthy individuals. In contrast, the expression of the Sema7A transcript was not reduced in $CD4^+$ and $CD14^+$ cells from patients with RA compared with healthy donors (Fig. 2b), suggesting that the reduction in cell surface Sema7A was due to shedding of Sema7A from the cell surface.

Next, we assessed the effect of Sema7A on the cytokine production of PBMCs from healthy subjects. Culture supernatants were collected after 48 h of incubation and analyzed for secreted cytokines by ELISA. The secretions of IL-6, TNF-α, and IL-17 were significantly increased after stimulation with Sema7A (Fig. 2c). Notably, the in vitro stimulation of $CD4^+$ cells with Sema7A led to a significant increase in the secretion of Th17/Tc17 cytokines, including IL-17, IFN-γ, and IL-22, compared with unstimulated cells or cells stimulated with DSema7A (Fig. 2d). These data indicate that sSema7A can strongly increase the production of inflammatory cytokines, in particular Th17/Tc17 and Th1/Tc1, by T cells in vitro.

Previous studies have shown that Sema7A is a potent stimulator of monocytes and induces the production of proinflammatory cytokines. Monocytes and macrophages are critical effector cells of the inflammatory immune response in RA [30, 31]. Next, to examine whether Sema7A serves a crucial role by affecting inflammatory immune functions in RA, we assessed the effect of sSema7A on monocyte IL-6 and TNF-α production among patients with RA in vitro. Treatment with cleaved sSema7A or sSema7A-Fc increased the production of TNF-α and IL-6 by $CD14^+$ monocytes/macrophages. Moreover, the anti-Sema7A antibody suppressed IL-6 and TNF-α secretion stimulated by sSema7A (Fig. 2e). These results showed that sSema7A can induce inflammatory cytokine production by monocytes/macrophages, suggesting that Sema7A might have a pathogenic role in RA.

Role of Sema7A in the expression of T-bet and RORγt by T cells

Increasing data indicate that the latter types of $CD4^+$ cells, such as Th1 and Th17 cells, are key players in the development of RA [6, 31, 32]. Th1 cells are characterized by their expression of the transcription factor T-bet [33]. Th17 cells are a subgroup of helper T cells with the capability to produce high levels of IL-17, which is their main characteristic, along with the expression of the transcription factor RORγt [34]. As mentioned above, T cells stimulated with Sema7A induced the production of cytokines that were relevant to Th1/Tc1 and Th17/Tc17 subclasses. Next, we evaluated the effect of Sema7A stimulation on RORγt and T-bet expression in T cells. After the induction of $CD4^+$ cells by Sema7A, we found that Sema7A caused a significant elevation in the expression of both RORγt

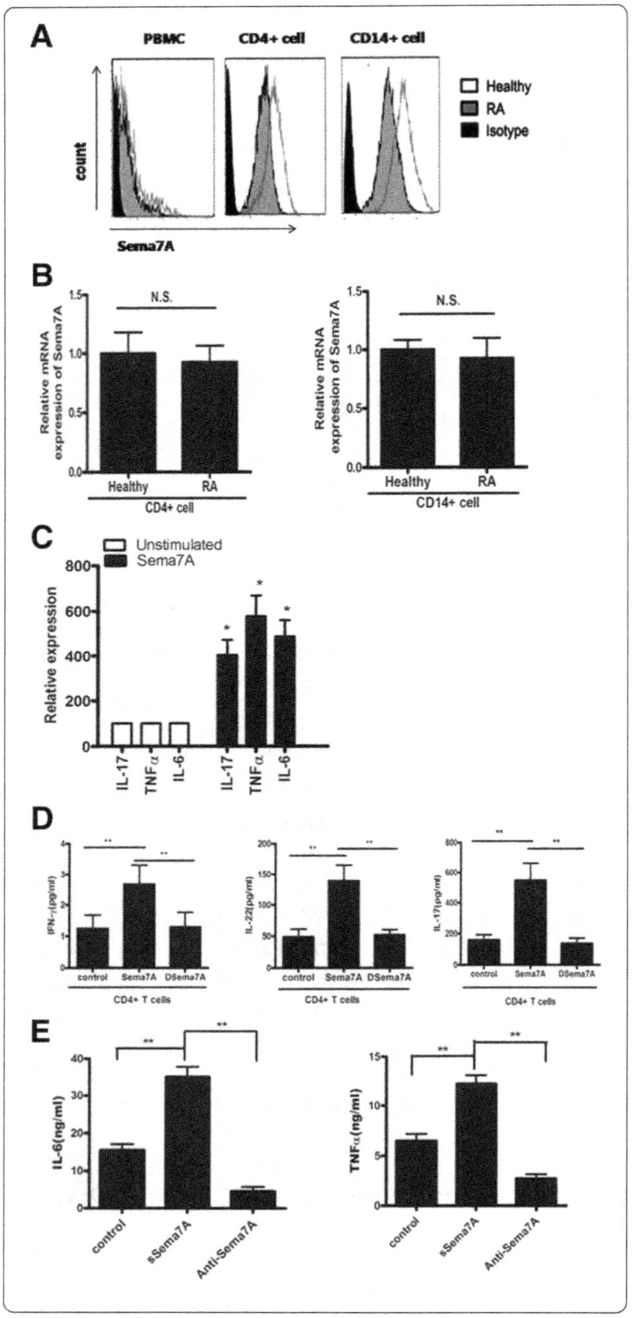

Fig. 2 Semaphorin 7A (Sema7A) expression, and inflammatory cytokine synthesis induced by Sema7A in primary human cells. **a** Cell surface expression of Sema7A in peripheral blood $CD4^+$ and $CD14^+$ cells and peripheral blood mononuclear cells (PBMCs) from patients with rheumatoid arthritis (RA) and healthy volunteer donors. Results shown are representative of findings from nine patients with RA and eight healthy volunteer donors. **b** Expression of messenger RNA (mRNA) for Sema7A in peripheral blood $CD4^+$ and $CD14^+$ cells. Results shown are from nine patients with RA and eight healthy individuals. *N.S.* Not significant. **c** Cytokine production by PBMCs from healthy donors ($n = 6$ percytokine) after treatment with or without Sema7A (10 ng/ml) for 24 h. Supernatants were analyzed for expression of IL-17, TNF-α, and IL-6 by enzyme-linked immunosorbent assay. Results are shown as the mean of triplicate values ± SD from one of three representative experiments. *$P<0.05$ versus unstimulated controls. **d** Interferon-γ (IFN-γ), IL-17, and IL-22 synthesis by primary human $CD4^+$ T cells from patients with RA after treatment with either Sema7A or heat-denatured Sema7A (DSema7A) (both at 10 ng/ml) for 24 h. Data are shown as the mean of triplicate values ± SD as compared with DSema7A (10 ng/ml) or unstimulated $CD4^+$ T cells. **$P < 0.01$. **e** Tumor necrosis factor-α (TNF-α) and interleukin-6 (IL-6) production by primary human $CD14^+$ monocytes from patients with RA after stimulation with naturally cleaved soluble Sema7A (sSema7A) for 48 h with or without anti-Sema7A antibody. Results shown are representative of three independent experiments

and T-bet compared with unstimulated cells or cells stimulated with DSema7A (Fig. 3a and b). These data suggested that Sema7A induced $CD4^+$ cells to differentiate into Tc1/Tc17 and Th1/Th17 subclasses, respectively.

Effect of Sema7A receptors on cytokine production

The effects of Sema7A are believed to be mediated via two receptors: plexin C1 and the β1-integrin subunit [35, 36]. To investigate whether β1-integrin and/or plexin C1 is implicated in the stimulatory effect of Sema7A observed in monocytes, we first evaluated the mRNA levels of β1-integrin and plexin C1 by quantitative RT-PCR in $CD14^+$ monocytes derived from patients with RA and healthy subjects. We found that the mRNA levels of β1-integrin and plexin C1 were significantly upregulated in patients with RA compared with healthy subjects. Interestingly, the mRNA levels of β1-integrin were significantly higher than the levels of plexin C1 in RA $CD14^+$ monocytes (Fig. 4a).

Next, blocking assays were performed with anti-plexin C1 or anti-β1-integrin antibody. The monocytes were stimulated with Sema7A or anti-plexin C1 or anti-β1-integrin antibody, and cytokine secretion was analyzed. Sema7A-induced cytokine secretion was significantly inhibited in the presence of the anti-β1-integrin antibody compared with control cells stimulated with Sema7A in the absence of the anti-β1-integrin antibody. Notably, cytokine secretion by Sema7A was barely inhibited in the presence of the anti-plexin C1 antibody compared with the presence of the anti-β1-integrin antibody (Fig. 4b). These data indicate that Sema7A may induce cytokine secretion from $CD14^+$ cells via interactions with β1-integrin.

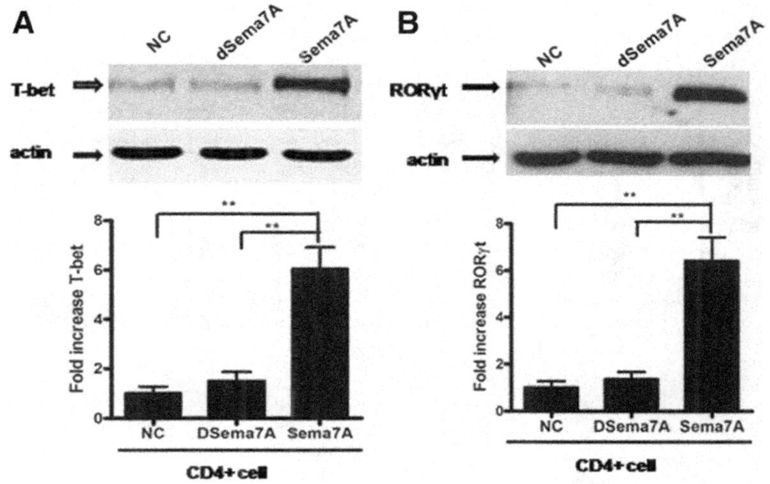

Fig. 3 Semaphorin 7A (Sema7A) enhances expression of retinoic acid receptor-related orphan nuclear receptor γt (RORγt) and T-bet transcription factor in CD4$^+$ T cells from healthy donors. Freshly isolated T cells (CD4$^+$) were stimulated with 10 ng/ml of Sema7A or heat-denatured Sema7A (DSema7A) for 2 h. The expression of (**a**) T-bet and (**b**) RORγt was detected by immunoblotting. Bars show the mean ± SD of three independent experiments. **$P < 0.01$ versus unstimulated control or DSema7A. *NC* Negative control cells cultured in the absence of Sema7A

Although it has been proposed that plexin C1 is a Sema7A receptor, the effect of Sema7A on monocytes is independent of plexin C1. These observations further reinforce that β1-integrin may be the major receptor for Sema7A in monocytes from patients with RA.

Sema7A signaling through β1-integrin activates FAK

Sema7A has been reported to promote axon outgrowth through the activation of non-receptor tyrosine kinase FAK during the embryonic development of neuronal progenitor cells [37]. FAK is a pivotal signal transducer downstream of integrins [38, 39]. Moreover, it is known that signaling through integrins such as β1-integrin activates FAK [39]. To determine whether Sema7A elicits integrin-dependent signaling responses in CD14$^+$ monocytes from patients with RA, we measured the level of FAK phosphorylation by performing immunoblot analysis in CD14$^+$ monocytes and THP-1 cells stimulated with Sema7A or DSema7A for 1 h. As shown in Fig. 4c, the phosphorylation of FAK was detected after stimulation with Sema7A. In contrast, DSema7A was used as a negative control and did not cause FAK phosphorylation. These data indicate the role of integrin-associated signal transduction machinery in propagating Sema7A signals.

Cleavage of Sema7A from cell surface

Previous studies established that Sema7A as a transmembrane protein can produce a soluble form by shedding from the cell surface [40]. The mechanism by which Sema7A is cleaved from the cell surface is not well understood. It is now clear that metalloproteinases are involved in the ectodomain shedding of many important cell surface proteins [41]. Previous studies have established that the cleavage of GPIbα and Sema4D is mediated by ADAM17 [42, 43]. Sema7A is a GPI-anchored member of the semaphorin family [44]. Thus, we determined whether ADAM17 was implicated in the shedding of Sema7A from the monocyte membrane. We incubated Sema7A-expressing cells (THP-1 cells and CD14$^+$ cells) with BMS-561392, a potent and selective inhibitor of ADAM17, or GM6001, a general inhibitor of metalloproteinases [45]. GM6001 inhibits Sema7A cleavage by 72% when CD14$^+$ cells are activated by IL-6 and TNF-α. The corresponding proportion for BMS-561392 is 65% (Fig. 5a). Thus, the results validated the detection of sSema7A in the shedding analysis and suggest that ADAM17 is probably the shedddase. Consistent with this finding, we measured the enhanced levels of ADAM17 in the serum and synovial fluid of patients with RA (Fig. 5b and c), and we found that TNF-α and IL-6 stimulated the secretion of ADAM17 by monocytes/macrophages detected in the patients with RA in this study (Fig. 5d).

To further investigate the role of ADAM17 in the shedding of Sema7A, we established stable HEK293T cell lines overexpressing ADAM17 or Sema7A. sSema7A was detected in the cell culture supernatants with nonspecific shRNA expression. ADAM17 expression was silenced using a vector encoding for ADAM17-specific shRNA in HEK293T cell lines overexpressing ADAM17 or Sema7A. ADAM17 shRNA resulted in a significant decrease in the levels of sSema7A in the cell culture supernatant of HEK293T cells overexpressing ADAM17 or Sema7A (Fig. 5e). Thus, these results validate the detection of Sema7A in the shedding analysis and suggest that ADAM17 is probably shed in patients with RA.

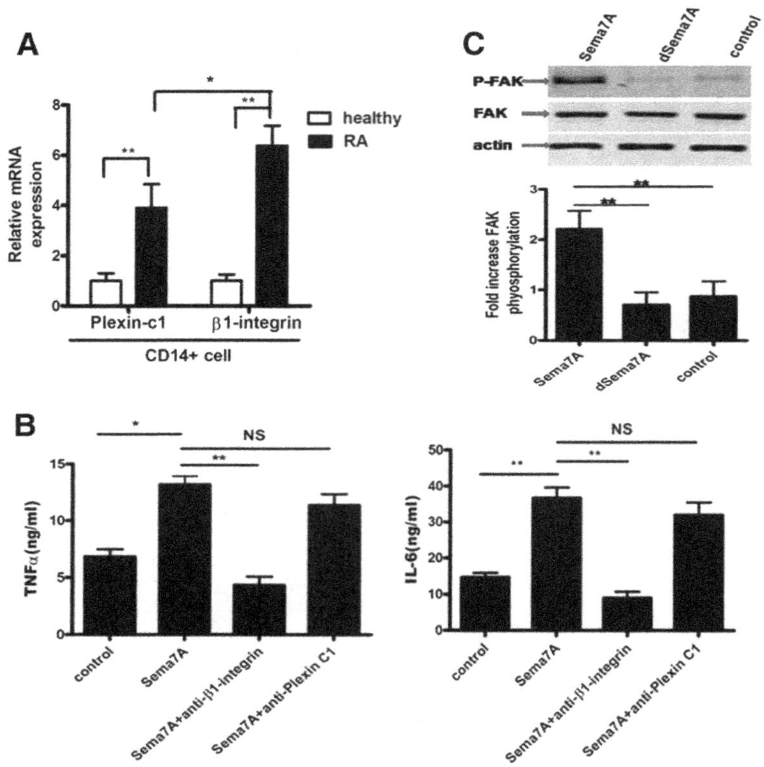

Fig. 4 Blocking β1-integrin abrogates semaphorin 7A (Sema7A)-induced cytokine production from $CD14^+$ cells in rheumatoid arthritis (RA). **a** Expression of messenger RNA (mRNA) for Sema7A receptors (plexin C1 and β1-integrin) in peripheral blood $CD14^+$ cells from patients with RA and from healthy individuals. Results shown are from 14 patients with RA and 12 healthy individuals. Values in a–c are mean ± SEM. *$P < 0.05$, **$P < 0.01$. **b** RA $CD14^+$ cells were incubated with the anti-β1-integrin monoclonal antibody (mAb) or anti-plexin C1 mAb in the presence of soluble Sema7A. After 48-h cultivation, supernatants were collected for expression of TNF-α and IL-6 by enzyme-linked immunosorbent assay. Results shown are representative of findings from eight patients with RA and six healthy volunteer donors. **c** Phosphorylation of focal adhesion kinase (FAK) in THP-1 and $CD14^+$ cells upon exposure to Sema7A. Isolated $CD14^+$ cells were exposed to 10 ng/ml of recombinant Sema7A. Cells exposed to heat-inactivated Sema7A (DSema7A) were used as negative controls. Phosphorylation of FAK was evaluated by immunoblot analysis. Activation of FAK was detected after 3 min of incubation with Sema7A. Results shown are representative of three independent experiments. *NS* Not significant

Blocking of Sema7A attenuates CIA

Next, we investigated whether the blocking of Sema7A using an anti-Sema7A antibody has the ability to prevent and treat the development of CIA in DBA/1 mice, a surrogate model of human RA. For the CIA treatment studies, mice with established clinical arthritis (an average score of 4) were randomized and given an injection with anti-Sema7A antibody or a control antibody. In the prevention model, blocking Sema7A demonstrated that treatment with anti-Sema7A antibody significantly reduced the development of CIA. Indeed, we observed that the arthritis scores and paw swelling in mice treated with anti-Sema7A antibody were significantly reduced compared with those in control mice (Fig. 6b), and the reduction in the arthritis scores was attenuated in mice treated with half a dose of the antibody. Histologic examination revealed that blocking Sema7A in mice with CIA also reduced disease severity and was accompanied by reduced bone erosion, synovial hyperplasia, and inflammatory infiltration into the joint compartment (Fig. 6a). The histologic scores in the joints of mice treated with anti-Sema7A antibody were significantly decreased (Fig. 6d). Moreover, serum TNF-α, IL-17, and IL-6 levels on day 50 were significantly decreased in mice treated with anti-Sema7A antibody (Fig. 6c).

Discussion

Although Sema7A has been involved in immunologic disorders, there are few reports regarding its expression and immunological function in RA. The present study is the first, to our knowledge, to show that sSema7A is significantly increased in the synovial fluid and serum of patients with the inflammatory autoimmune disease RA compared with OA. Furthermore, we demonstrate that the levels of sSema7A strongly stimulated inflammatory T-cell and monocyte/macrophage responses in vitro. Second, we demonstrated that Sema7A is involved in the inflammatory response in RA and is also correlated with disease activity.

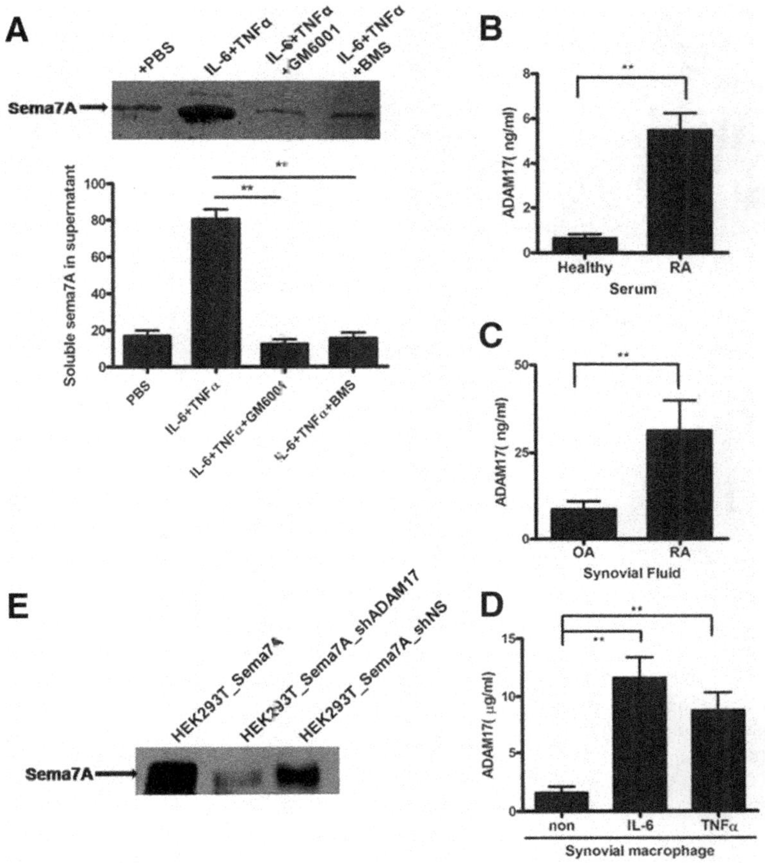

Fig. 5 A disintegrin and metalloprotease 17 (ADAM17) contributes to the shedding of semaphorin 7A (Sema7A). **a** Shedding of Sema7A is inhibited by metalloproteinase inhibitors. Western blots show Sema7A in the supernatant of THP-1 and $CD14^{+}$ cells stimulated with tumor necrosis factor-α (TNF-α) and interleukin-6 (IL-6) in the presence of the metalloprotease inhibitor GM6001 or the ADAM17-selective inhibitor BMS-561392 (BMS). Results shown are representative of three independent experiments. **b** Elevated serum ADAM17 levels in 26 patients with rheumatoid arthritis (RA) and 23 healthy donors. **d** Synovial fluid levels of ADAM17 in 11 patients with RA and 8 patients with osteoarthritis (OA). **c** Synovial fluid levels of ADAM17 in 11 patients with RA and 8 patients with osteoarthritis (OA). **d** ADAM17 protein levels in primary cultures of TNF-α- and IL-6-stimulated synovial macrophages from patients with RA. Data were compiled from three independent experiments. Values are mean ± SEM. $^{**}P < 0.01$. **e** HEK293T cells stably expressing transmembrane Sema7A (HEK293T_Sema7A) were transduced with vectors encoding an ADAM17-specific short-hairpin RNA (shADAM17) or a nonspecific short-hairpin RNA (shNS). Levels of secreted Sema7A in the cell culture supernatant were analyzed by Western blotting. Results shown are representative of three independent experiments

We assessed the relationship between serum sSema7A levels and known clinical and biologic markers usually used in the diagnosis and prediction of RA. Interestingly, a significant correlation between serum sSema7A levels and the levels of DAS28, CRP, and RF in patients with RA was observed. Furthermore, successful treatment with biologic DMARDs in patients with RA decreased serum sSema7A levels. In general, these data indicate that sSema7A is a potentially useful biomarker for RA disease activity, further supporting its role in the progression of RA.

An increasing amount of data shows that Sema7A is an important player during the immune response because it regulates the interactions between T cells and monocytes during the primary immune response [29]. The immunogenetics of RA suggest the key role for abnormal pathways of T-cell and monocyte activation in the perpetuation of disease [46]. Thus, we decided to investigate the role of Sema7A in RA. Recombinant sSema7A was performed to evaluate its effects on T cells and monocytes. Our data reveal that sSema7A regulated cytokine secretion by T cells and monocytes. An analysis of T-cell and monocyte cytokine production showed that stimulation with Sema7A led to strongly enhanced production of proinflammatory cytokines, such as TNF-α and IL-6. Interestingly, it has been shown that these cytokines play central roles in RA disease progression and recruit inflammatory cells to erode the joints of patients with RA [46]. It thus appears that Sema7A is involved in the pathogenesis of RA.

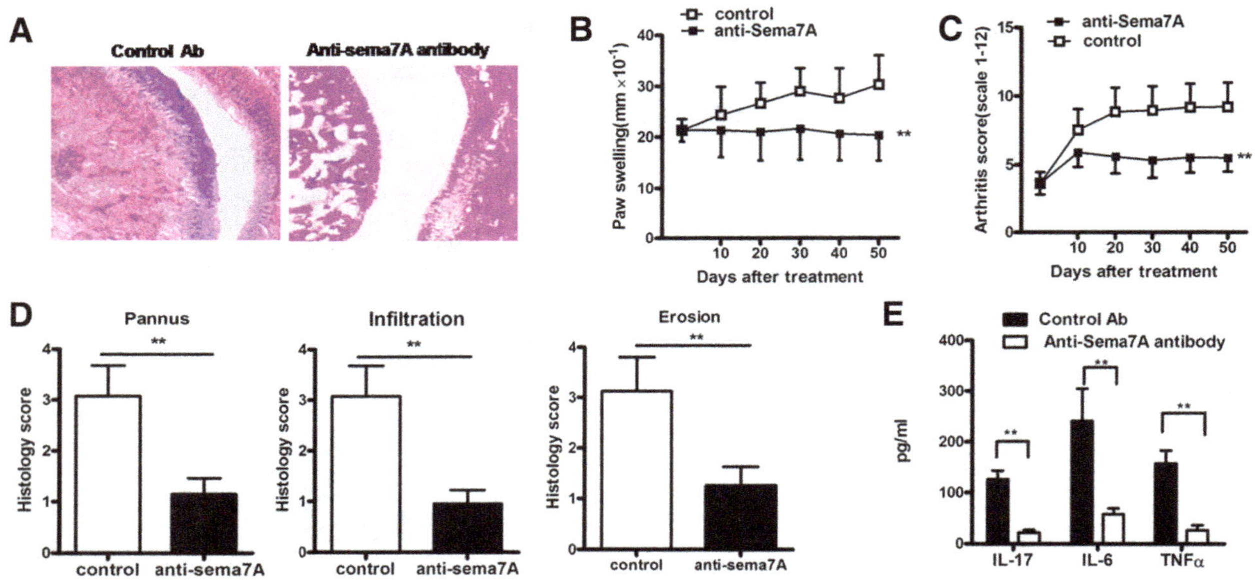

Fig. 6 Blocking of semaphorin 7A (Sema7A) attenuates severity of collagen-induced arthritis (CIA) in mice. **a** Histological examination of a mouse ankle joint on day 50 after treatment with anti-Sema7A antibody. Sections were stained with hematoxylin and eosin. Original magnification × 400. **b** and **c** Average arthritis scores and paw swelling of mice with CIA. Mice ($n = 8$ per group) were immunized with collagen type II, randomized, and, at onset of disease (clinical score of 4), anti-Sema7A or control antibody (Ab) (12 μg/mouse) was administered intraperitoneally on days 1, 10, 20, 30, and 40 ($n = 8$ mice per group). Data are representative of three independent experiments. **d** Average histologic scores of paw sections on day 50 ($n = 8$ mice per group). **e** Serum samples were collected for expression of tumor necrosis factor-α (TNF-α), interleukin-17 (IL-17), and IL-6 by enzyme-linked immunosorbent assay on day 50 ($n = 8$ mice per group). Data were compiled from three independent experiments. Values are mean ± SEM. $^{**}P < 0.01$

In this study, we also demonstrated that the production of the inflammatory cytokines IFN-γ (formally attributed to Th1 response) and IL-17 (the well-known Th17-derived cytokine) was significantly increased in T-cell culture supernatant induced by sSema7A. These results were also confirmed by the significant upregulation of the expression of transcription factor T-bet and RORγt in $CD4^+$ T cells following stimulation with Sema7A. A previous report suggested that T-bet and RORγt promote the differentiation of T cells into Th1/Tc1 and Th17/Tc17 subsets, respectively [47]. Recently, it has become clear that both Th1 and Th17 cytokines are key players in the development of RA [48]. Furthermore, we observed that Sema7A significantly enhanced the production of Th17/Tc17 cytokines, including IFN-γ, IL-22, and IL-17, in comparison with cells treated with DSema7A. Collectively, these findings demonstrate that Sema7A can strongly elevate the production of inflammatory cytokines, particularly Th17/Tc17 and Th1/Tc1, which is strongly similar to the characteristic cytokine profile of patients with RA displayed by T cells in vitro.

To further determine the possible mechanism of action of Sema7A, we explored intracellular signal transduction pathways. Plexin C1 and β1-integrin molecules were shown to serve as Sema7A receptors. To determine whether both receptors may play roles in the stimulatory effect of Sema7A observed in T cells and monocytes, we evaluated the plexin C1 and β1-integrin mRNA levels in T cells and monocytes isolated from patients with RA and healthy subjects. Both receptor mRNA levels were significantly upregulated in patients with RA compared with healthy subjects. Next, we tested whether Sema7A mediates its intracellular effects via interactions with plexin C1 and β1-integrin. Blocking assays were performed in $CD14^+$ cells with anti-β1-integrin antibody or anti-plexin C1 antibody in the presence or absence of Sema7A. Interestingly, Sema7A-induced cytokine secretion was attenuated by the blockage of β1-integrin but not plexin C1 in $CD14^+$ cells, suggesting that β1-integrin is a binding partner for Sema7A in monocytes. As previously reported, our results showed that the Sema7A-induced cytokine secretion from monocytes was also significantly inhibited by an anti-β1-integrin mAb alone. In the present study, we observed that Sema7A induces the activation of FAK in $CD14^+$ cells. These results suggest that Sema7A signaling occurs through the engagement of β1-integrin in monocytes, given that signaling through integrins commonly leads to FAK activation.

In the present study, the expression of Sema7A mRNA was stable in $CD4^+$ cells, and $CD14^+$ cells. However, the expression levels of Sema7A at the cell surface were actually decreased in T cells and monocytes from the peripheral blood of patients with RA. Thus, we speculated that the relative decrease in cellular Sema7A levels may be attributable to the shedding of Sema7A from the cell surface. In support of this notion, other studies established that the transmembrane semaphorins can be proteolytically cleaved to produce soluble proteins, and the proteinase responsible for cleavage has been identified: It is a member of the ADAM family [49]. It has been shown that the cleavage of GPIbα is mediated by ADAM17. On the basis of our analysis of the results described above, we speculated that Sema7A, a GPI-anchored member of the semaphorin family, might be one of the proteins cleaved by ADAM17. Consistent with this finding, our results validated the detection of Sema7A in the shedding analysis and suggest that ADAM17 was probably the sheddase. In addition, our results indicated that sSema7A induced TNF-α and IL-6 production and that both TNF-α and IL-6 induced the production of ADAM17. The levels of ADAM17 were increased in synovial fluid and serum from patients with RA. Hence, we propose that Sema7A functions as an autocrine stimulator of the IL-6/TNF-α inflammatory axis in patients with RA.

To further confirm that Sema7A has a distinct role in the pathogenesis of RA in vivo, we introduced anti-Sema7A antibody into a T-cell- and monocyte-dependent animal model of RA, namely, CIA. Blocking Sema7A in CIA exerted favorable therapeutic effects and achieved a dramatic arrest in disease progression, as confirmed by the clinical, histopathological, and immunological manifestations of arthritis. These observations extend our findings demonstrating that Sema7A has a distinct role in regulating inflammatory responses in vivo, suggesting that Sema7A might be a possible therapeutic target for RA. Furthermore, sSema7A has been reported to promote angiogenesis. Angiogenesis is thought to have an important role in the progression of arthritic lesions in RA. Therefore, it is attractive to speculate that Sema7A may be further involved in the pathogenesis of RA by promoting the angiogenesis of joint tissue, which would recruit the inflammatory cells into the synovium.

Conclusions

Taken together, our results show that the levels of secreted Sema7A were significantly high in the serum and synovial fluid of patients with RA and that Sema7A is a promising biomarker for RA disease. The crucial roles of Sema7A in the pathogenesis of RA suggest that Sema7A is a potential therapeutic target for RA. Therefore, our results provide a further rationale for prospective clinical studies designed to evaluate whether Sema7A provides effective therapeutic activities in RA and other autoimmune diseases.

Abbreviations

ADAM: A disintegrin and metalloprotease; CIA: Collagen-induced arthritis; CII: Collagen type II; CRP: C-reactive protein; DAS28: Disease Activity Score in 28 joints; DMARD: Disease-modifying antirheumatic drug; DSema7A: Heat-denatured Sema7A; ELISA: Enzyme-linked immunosorbent assay; FACS: Fluorescence-activated cell-sorting; FAK: Focal adhesion kinase; GPI: glycosylphosphatidylinositol; IFN-γ: Interferon-gamma; IgG: Immunoglobulin G; IL-17: Interleukin-17; mAb: Monoclonal antibody; mRNA: Messenger RNA; OA: Osteoarthritis; PBMC: Peripheral blood mononuclear cell; PE: phycoerythrin; PFAK: Phosphorylated focal adhesion kinase; RA: Rheumatoid arthritis; RF: Rheumatoid factor; RORγt: Retinoic acid receptor-related orphan nuclear receptor γt; RT-PCR: Reverse transcription-polymerase chain reaction; Sema7A: Semaphorin 7A; shRNA: Short-hairpin RNA; sSema7A: Soluble semaphorin 7A; Th17: T-helper cell type 17; TNF-α: Tumor necrosis factor-α

Acknowledgements

The authors thank the study participants as well as the staff involved in the collection of blood samples.

Funding

This work was supported by grants from the National Natural Science Foundation of China (30600560), a project funded by the Peak Foundation Six Talent Peaks Program of Jiangsu Province of China. The funders had no role in study design, data collection and analysis, the decision to publish, or the preparation of the manuscript.

Authors' contributions

JX carried out the animal experiments as well as the histological and immunological analyses, conceived of the study, participated in its design and coordination, and drafted the manuscript. HW carried out the animal experiments and helped to revise the manuscript. Both authors read and approved the final manuscript.

Authors' information

Not applicable.

Competing interests

The authors declare that they have no competing interests.

Author details

[1]Department of Rheumatology, Second Affiliated Hospital of Nanjing Medical University, Nanjing, People's Republic of China. [2]Experimental Center of Basic Medicine, Shanghai Medical College, Fudan University, Shanghai, People's Republic of China.

References

1. Holmdahl R, Malmström V, Burkhardt H. Autoimmune priming, tissue attack and chronic inflammation—the three stages of rheumatoid arthritis. Eur J Immunol. 2014;44(6):1593–9.
2. McInnes IB, Schett G. Cytokines in the pathogenesis of rheumatoid arthritis. Nat Rev Immunol. 2007;7(6):429–42.
3. Firestein GS. Evolving concepts of rheumatoid arthritis. Nature. 2003; 423(6937):356–61.
4. Hot A, Miossec P. Effects of interleukin (IL)-17A and IL-17 F in human rheumatoid arthritis synoviocytes. Ann Rheum Dis. 2011;70(5):727–32.
5. Chomarat P, Kjeldsen-Kragh J, Quayle AJ, Natvig JB, Miossec P. Different cytokine production profiles of γδ T cell clones: relation to inflammatory arthritis. Eur J Immunol. 1994;24(9):2087–91.
6. Miltenburg AM, van Laar JM, de Kuiper R, Daha MR, Breedveld FC. T cells cloned from human rheumatoid synovial membrane functionally represent the Th1 subset. Scand J Immunol. 1992;35(5):603–10.

7. Worzfeld T, Offermanns S. Semaphorins and plexins as therapeutic targets. Nat Rev Drug Discov. 2014;13(8):603–21.
8. Nogi T, Yasui N, Mihara E, Matsunaga Y, Noda M, Yamashita N, et al. Structural basis for semaphorin signalling through the plexin receptor. Nature. 2010;467(7319):1123–7.
9. Pasterkamp RJ, Giger RJ. Semaphorin function in neural plasticity and disease. Curr Opin Neurobiol. 2009;19(3):263–74.
10. Kang S, Kumanogoh A. Semaphorins in bone development, homeostasis, and disease. Semin Cell Dev Biol. 2012;24(3):163–71.
11. Czopik AK, Bynoe MS, Palm N, Raine CS, Medzhitov R. Semaphorin 7A is a negative regulator of T cell responses. Immunity. 2006;24(5):591–600.
12. Kang HR, Lee CG, Homer RJ, Elias JA. Semaphorin 7A plays a critical role in TGF-β1-induced pulmonary fibrosis. J Exp Med. 2007;204(5):1083–93.
13. Costa C, Martínez-Sáez E, Gutiérrez-Franco A, Eixarch H, Castro Z, Ortega-Aznar A, et al. Expression of semaphorin 3A, semaphorin 7A and their receptors in multiple sclerosis lesions. Mult Scler. 2015;21(13):1632–43.
14. Kim CW, Cho EH, Lee YJ, Kim YH, Hah YS, Kim DR. Disease-specific proteins from rheumatoid arthritis patients. J Korean Med Sci. 2006;21(3):478–84.
15. Kang S, Okuno T, Takegahara N, Takamatsu H, Nojima S, Kimura T, et al. Intestinal epithelial cell-derived semaphorin 7A negatively regulates development of colitis via $\alpha_v\beta_1$ integrin. J Immunol. 2011;188(3):1108–16.
16. Holmes S, Downs AM, Fosberry A, Hayes PD, Michalovich D, Murdoch P, et al. Sema7A is a potent monocyte stimulator. Scand J Immunol. 2002;56(3):270–5.
17. Ghanem RC, Han KY, Rojas J, Ozturk O, Kim DJ, Jain S, et al. Semaphorin 7A promotes angiogenesis in an experimental corneal neovascularization model. Curr Eye Res. 2011;36(11):989–96.
18. Garcia-Areas R, Libreros S, Amat S, Keating P, Carrio R, Robinson P, et al. Semaphorin 7A promotes tumor growth and exerts a pro-angiogenic effect in macrophages of mammary tumor-bearing mice. Front Physiol. 2014;5:17.
19. Onuora S. Targeting myostatin could prevent bone destruction in inflammatory arthritis. Nat Rev Rheumatol. 2015;11(9):504.
20. Bodolay E, Koch AE, Kim J, Szegedi G, Szekanecz Z. Angiogenesis and chemokines in rheumatoid arthritis and other systemic inflammatory rheumatic diseases. J Cell Mol Med. 2002;6(3):357–76.
21. Prevoo ML, Hof MA v 't, Kuper HH, van Leeuwen MA, van de Putte LB, van Riel PL. Modified disease activity scores that include twenty-eight-joint counts: development and validation in a prospective longitudinal study of patients with rheumatoid arthritis. Arthritis Rheum. 1995;38(1):44–8.
22. Arnett FC, Edworthy SM, Bloch DA, McShane DJ, Fries JF, Cooper NS, et al. The American Rheumatism Association 1987 revised criteria for the classification of rheumatoid arthritis. Arthritis Rheum. 1988;31(3):315–24.
23. The MARS Group. Osteoarthritis classification scales: interobserver reliability and arthroscopic correlation. J Bone Joint Surg Am. 2014;96(14):1145–51.
24. Figueiredo C, Goudeva L, Horn PA, Eiz-Vesper B, Blasczyk R, Seltsam A. Generation of HLA-deficient platelets from hematopoietic progenitor cells. Transfusion. 2010;50(8):1690–701.
25. Rabinovich GA, Daly G, Dreja H, Tailor H, Riera CM, Hirabayashi J, et al. Recombinant galectin-1 and its genetic delivery suppress collagen-induced arthritis via T cell apoptosis. J Exp Med. 1999;190(3):385–98.
26. Sarkar S, Cooney LA, White P, Dunlop DB, Endres J, Jorns JM, et al. Regulation of pathogenic IL-17 responses in collagen-induced arthritis: roles of endogenous interferon-gamma and IL-4. Arthritis Res Ther. 2009;11(5):R158.
27. Marchesan JT, Gerow EA, Schaff R, Taut AD, Shin SY, Sugai J, et al. *Porphyromonas gingivalis* oral infection exacerbates the development and severity of collagen-induced arthritis. Arthritis Res Ther. 2013;15(6):R186.
28. van Gestel AM, Prevoo ML, Hof MA v 't, van Rijswijk MH, van de Putte LB, van Riel PL. Development and validation of the European League Against Rheumatism response criteria for rheumatoid arthritis: comparison with the preliminary American College of Rheumatology and the World Health Organization/International League Against Rheumatism Criteria. Arthritis Rheum. 1996;39(1):34–40.
29. Kumanogoh A, Kikutani H. Immune semaphorins: a new area of semaphorin research. J Cell Sci. 2003;116(Pt 17):3463–70.
30. Gras C, Eiz-Vesper B, Seltsam A, Immenschuh S, Blasczyk R, Figueiredo C. Semaphorin 7A protein variants differentially regulate T-cell activity. Transfusion. 2012;53(2):270–83.
31. Li J, Yang P, Wu Q, Li H, Ding Y, Hsu HC, et al. Death receptor 5-targeted depletion of interleukin-23-producing macrophages, Th17, and Th1/17 associated with defective tyrosine phosphatase in mice and patients with rheumatoid arthritis. Arthritis Rheum. 2013;65(10):2594–605.
32. Lee J, Choi J, Lee W, Ko K, Kim S. Dehydrodiconiferyl alcohol (DHCA) modulates the differentiation of Th17 and Th1 cells and suppresses experimental autoimmune encephalomyelitis. Mol Immunol. 2015;68(2 Pt B):434–44.
33. Szabo SJ, Kim ST, Costa GL, Zhang X, Fathman CG, Glimcher LH. A novel transcription factor, T-bet, directs Th1 lineage commitment. Cell. 2000; 100(6):655–69.
34. Unutmaz D. RORC2: the master of human Th17 cell programming. Eur J Immunol. 2009;39(6):1452–5.
35. Scott GA, McClelland LA, Fricke AF, Fender A. Plexin C1, a receptor for semaphorin 7a, inactivates cofilin and is a potential tumor suppressor for melanoma progression. J Invest Dermatol. 2009;129(4):954–63.
36. Scott GA, McClelland LA, Fricke AF. Semaphorin 7a promotes spreading and dendricity in human melanocytes through β1-integrins. J Invest Dermatol. 2008;128(1):151–61.
37. Pasterkamp RJ, Peschon JJ, Spriggs MK, Kolodkin AL. Semaphorin 7A promotes axon outgrowth through integrins and MAPKs. Nature. 2003; 424(6947):398–405.
38. Mitra SK, Hanson DA, Schlaepfer DD. Focal adhesion kinase: in command and control of cell motility. Nat Rev Mol Cell Biol. 2005;6(1):56–68.
39. Schlaepfer DD, Hunter T. Integrin signalling and tyrosine phosphorylation: just the FAKs? Trends Cell Biol. 1998;8(4):151–7.
40. Althoff K, Müllberg J, Aasland D, Voltz N, Kallen K, Grötzinger J, et al. Recognition sequences and structural elements contribute to shedding susceptibility of membrane proteins. Biochem J. 2001;353(Pt 3):663–72.
41. Ito N, Nomura S, Iwase A, Ito T, Kikkawa F, Tsujimoto M, et al. ADAMs, a disintegrin and metalloproteinases, mediate shedding of oxytocinase. Biochem Biophys Res Commun. 2004;314(4):1008–13.
42. Zhu L, Bergmeier W, Wu J, Jiang H, Stalker TJ, Cieslak M, et al. Regulated surface expression and shedding support a dual role for semaphorin 4D in platelet responses to vascular injury. Proc Natl Acad Sci U S A. 2007;104(5):1621–6.
43. Bergmeier W, Piffath CL, Cheng G, Dole VS, Zhang Y, von Andrian UH, et al. Tumor necrosis factor-α-converting enzyme (ADAM17) mediates GPIbα shedding from platelets in vitro and in vivo. Circ Res. 2004;95(7):677–83.
44. Gardiner EE, Karunakaran D, Shen Y, Arthur JF, Andrews RK, Berndt MC. Controlled shedding of platelet glycoprotein (GP)VI and GPIb-IX-V by ADAM family metalloproteinases. J Thromb Haemost. 2007;5(7):1530–7.
45. Moss ML, Sklair-Tavron L, Nudelman R. Drug insight: tumor necrosis factor-converting enzyme as a pharmaceutical target for rheumatoid arthritis. Nat Clin Pract Rheumatol. 2008;4(6):300–9.
46. Wei ST, Sun YH, Zong SH, Xiang YB. Serum levels of IL-6 and TNF-alpha may correlate with activity and severity of rheumatoid arthritis. Med Sci Monit. 2015;21:4030–8.
47. McGuire DJ, Rowse AL, Li H, Peng BJ, Sestero CM, Cashman KS, et al. CD5 enhances Th17-cell differentiation by regulating IFN-gamma response and RORγt localization. Eur J Immunol. 2013;44(4):1137–42.
48. Barros-Martins J, Schmolka N, Fontinha D, Pires De Miranda M, Simas JP, Brok I, et al. Effector γδ T cell differentiation relies on master but not auxiliary Th cell transcription factors. J Immunol. 2016;196(9):3642–52.
49. Koenen RR, Pruessmeyer J, Soehnlein O, Fraemohs L, Zernecke A, Schwarz N, et al. Regulated release and functional modulation of junctional adhesion molecule A by disintegrin metalloproteinases. Blood. 2009;113(19):4799–809.

Permissions

All chapters in this book were first published in AR&T, by BioMed Central; hereby published with permission under the Creative Commons Attribution License or equivalent. Every chapter published in this book has been scrutinized by our experts. Their significance has been extensively debated. The topics covered herein carry significant findings which will fuel the growth of the discipline. They may even be implemented as practical applications or may be referred to as a beginning point for another development.

The contributors of this book come from diverse backgrounds, making this book a truly international effort. This book will bring forth new frontiers with its revolutionizing research information and detailed analysis of the nascent developments around the world.

We would like to thank all the contributing authors for lending their expertise to make the book truly unique. They have played a crucial role in the development of this book. Without their invaluable contributions this book wouldn't have been possible. They have made vital efforts to compile up to date information on the varied aspects of this subject to make this book a valuable addition to the collection of many professionals and students.

This book was conceptualized with the vision of imparting up-to-date information and advanced data in this field. To ensure the same, a matchless editorial board was set up. Every individual on the board went through rigorous rounds of assessment to prove their worth. After which they invested a large part of their time researching and compiling the most relevant data for our readers.

The editorial board has been involved in producing this book since its inception. They have spent rigorous hours researching and exploring the diverse topics which have resulted in the successful publishing of this book. They have passed on their knowledge of decades through this book. To expedite this challenging task, the publisher supported the team at every step. A small team of assistant editors was also appointed to further simplify the editing procedure and attain best results for the readers.

Apart from the editorial board, the designing team has also invested a significant amount of their time in understanding the subject and creating the most relevant covers. They scrutinized every image to scout for the most suitable representation of the subject and create an appropriate cover for the book.

The publishing team has been an ardent support to the editorial, designing and production team. Their endless efforts to recruit the best for this project, has resulted in the accomplishment of this book. They are a veteran in the field of academics and their pool of knowledge is as vast as their experience in printing. Their expertise and guidance has proved useful at every step. Their uncompromising quality standards have made this book an exceptional effort. Their encouragement from time to time has been an inspiration for everyone.

The publisher and the editorial board hope that this book will prove to be a valuable piece of knowledge for researchers, students, practitioners and scholars across the globe.

List of Contributors

Panagiota Drivelegka, Lennart T. H. Jacobsson and Mats Dehlin
Department of Rheumatology and Inflammation Research, Sahlgrenska Academy, University of Gothenburg, Grona Straket 12, Sahlgrenska University Hospital, 413 45 Gothenburg, Sweden

Valgerdur Sigurdardottir
Department of Rheumatology and Inflammation Research, Sahlgrenska Academy, University of Gothenburg, Grona Straket 12, Sahlgrenska University Hospital, 413 45 Gothenburg, Sweden
Centre of Clinical Research Dalarna, Falun, Sweden

Anna Svärd
Centre of Clinical Research Dalarna, Falun, Sweden

Durga M. S. H. Chandrupatla, Gerrit Jansen and Conny J. van der Laken
Amsterdam Rheumatology and Immunology Center, VU University Medical Center, De Boelelaan 1117, 1081 HV Amsterdam, The Netherlands

Ricardo Vos, Mariska Verlaan, Albert D. Windhorst, Adriaan A. Lammertsma and Carla F. M. Molthoff
Department of Radiology & Nuclear Medicine, VU University Medical Center, De Boelelaan 1117, 1081 HV Amsterdam, The Netherlands

Qingshou Chen and Philip S. Low
Department of Chemistry, Purdue University, 720 Clinic Drive, West Lafayette, IN 47907-2084, USA

Michael Ziegelasch, Thomas Skogh and Alf Kastbom
Department of Rheumatology, Department of Clinical and Experimental Medicine, Linköping University, Linköping, Sweden

Kristina Forslind
Section of Rheumatology, Department of Medicine, Helsingborg Hospital, Helsingborg, Sweden
Department of Clinical Sciences, Section of Rheumatology, Lund University, Helsingborg, Sweden

Katrine Riklund
Department of Diagnostic radiology, Umeå university Hospital, Umeå, Sweden

Ewa Berglin
Department of Public Health and Clinical Medicine/ Rheumatology, Umeå university Hospital, Umeå, Sweden

Michael Schiff
University of Colorado School of Medicine, Denver, CO 80045, USA

Tsutomu Takeuchi
Keio University, Tokyo, Japan

Roy Fleischmann
Metroplex Clinical Research Center, University of Texas Southwestern Medical Center, Dallas, TX 75231, USA

Ji-Eon Won
Eli Lilly and Company, Seoul, Republic of Korea

Jeffrey R. Curtis
Division of Clinical Immunology and Rheumatology, University of Alabama at Birmingham, FOT 802, 510 20th Street South, Birmingham, AL 35294, USA

Christopher Herrem
Mylan, 1000 Mylan Blvd, Canonsburg, PA 15317, USA

Matladi N. Ndlovu and Cathy O'Brien
UCB Pharma, Allée de la Recherche 60, 1070 Brussels, Belgium

Yusuf Yazici
NYU Hospital for Joint Diseases, New York University School of Medicine, 301 East 17th Street, New York, NY 10003, USA

Dena D'Souza
Department of Molecular Medicine and Pathology, Faculty of Medical and Health Sciences, The University of Auckland, Private Bag 92019, Auckland, New Zealand

Fiona M. McQueen
Department of Molecular Medicine and Pathology, Faculty of Medical and Health Sciences, The University of Auckland, Auckland, New Zealand
Department of Rheumatology, Greenlane Clinical Centre, Auckland District Health Board, 214 Green Lane West, Epsom, Auckland 1051, New Zealand

Terina Pollock and Anthony Doyle
Department of Radiology, Auckland City Hospital, 2 Park Rd, Grafton, Auckland 1023, New Zealand

Arier C. Lee
Section of Epidemiology & Biostatistics, School of Population Health (Tamaki Campus), University of Auckland, Auckland 1142, New Zealand

Nicola Dalbeth
Bone & Joint Research Group, Department of Medicine, The University of Auckland, Auckland, New Zealand
Department of Rheumatology, Greenlane Clinical Centre, Auckland District Health Board, 214 Green Lane West, Epsom, Auckland 1051, New Zealand

Karen Lindsay
Department of Rheumatology, Greenlane Clinical Centre, Auckland District Health Board, 214 Green Lane West, Epsom, Auckland 1051, New Zealand

Peter Chapman
Department of Rheumatology, Immunology & Allergy, Christchurch Hospital, Christchurch 8140, New Zealand

Lisa Stamp
Department of Medicine, University of Otago, Christchurch 8140, New Zealand

Josef S. Smolen
Division of Rheumatology, Department of Medicine 3, Medical University of Vienna, Waehringer Guertel 18-20, 1090 Vienna, Austria
Hietzing Hospital, Vienna, Austria

Annette Szumski
inVentiv Health, Princeton, NJ, USA

Andrew S. Koenig, Thomas V. Jones and Lisa Marshall
Pfizer, Collegeville, PA, USA

Uta Kiltz, Christine von Zabern, Xenofon Baraliakos, Bernd Mintrop, Michael Sarholz and Jürgen Braun
Rheumazentrum Ruhrgebiet, Claudiusstraße 45, 44649 Herne, Germany

Frank Heldmann
Zeisigwaldklinik Bethanien Chemnitz, Zeisigwaldstraße 101, 09130 Chemnitz, Germany

Dietmar Krause
Rheumatology private office in Gladbeck, Friedrich-Ebert-Straße 2, 45964 Gladbeck, Germany

Friedrich Dybowski
Rheumatology private office in Herne, Claudiusstraße 45, 44649 Herne, Germany

Ludwig Kalthoff
Rheumatology private office in Bochum, Gudrunstrasse 56, 44791 Bochum, Germany

Deborah R. Winter
Department of Medicine, Division of Rheumatology, Northwestern University Feinberg School of Medicine, Chicago, IL 60611, USA

T. Martijn Kuijper, Riëtte Folmer, Johanna M. W. Hazes and Jolanda J. Luime
Department of Rheumatology, Erasmus Medical Center, Room Na-609, CA Rotterdam, The Netherlands

Elly A. Stolk
Institute for Medical Technology Assessment, Erasmus University, Rotterdam, The Netherlands

George W. Reed
University of Massachusetts Medical School, 55 Lake Ave North, Worcester, MA 01605, USA
Corrona LLC, Southborough, MA, USA

David H. Collier
Amgen Inc., Thousand Oaks, CA, USA

Andrew S. Koenig and Sameer Kotak
Pfizer Inc., Collegeville, PA, USA

Katherine C. Saunders and Heather J. Litman
Corrona LLC, Southborough, MA, USA

Dimitrios A. Pappas
Corrona LLC, Southborough, MA, USA
Columbia University College of Physicians and Surgeons, New York, NY, USA

Joel M. Kremer
Corrona LLC, Southborough, MA, USA
Albany Medical College and The Center for Rheumatology, Albany, NY, USA

Hirofumi Shoda, Yasuo Nagafuchi, Yumi Tsuchida, Keiichi Sakurai, Shuji Sumitomo, Keishi Fujio and Kazuhiko Yamamoto
Department of Allergy and Rheumatology, Graduate School of Medicine, the University of Tokyo, 7-3-1 Hongo, Bunkyo-ku, Tokyo, Japan

Shinichiro Nakachi, Shuji Sumitomo, Yumi Tsuchida, Haruka Tsuchiya, Masanori Kono, Rika Kato, Keiichi Sakurai, Norio Hanata, Yasuo Nagafuchi, Kazuhiko Yamamoto and Keishi Fujio
Department of Allergy and Rheumatology, Graduate School of Medicine, the University of Tokyo, 7-3-1 Hongo, Bunkyo-ku, Tokyo 113-8655, Japan

Shoko Tateishi and Hiroko Kanda
Department of Allergy and Rheumatology, Graduate School of Medicine, the University of Tokyo, 7-3-1 Hongo, Bunkyo-ku, Tokyo 113-8655, Japan
Department of Immunotherapy Management, Graduate School of Medicine, the University of Tokyo, 7-3-1 Hongo, Bunkyo-ku, Tokyo 113-8655, Japan

Tomohisa Okamura
Department of Allergy and Rheumatology, Graduate School of Medicine, the University of Tokyo, 7-3-1 Hongo, Bunkyo-ku, Tokyo 113-8655, Japan
Max Planck-The University of Tokyo Center for Integrative Inflammology, The University of Tokyo, 4-6-1 Komaba, Meguro-ku, Tokyo 153-8505, Japan

Florent Garrigues
Radiology Department, Cavale Blanche Hospital and Brest Occidentale University, Brest, France

Anaïs Huwart
Radiology Department, Cavale Blanche Hospital and Brest Occidentale University, Brest, France
Radiology Unit, Hôpital de Cornouaille, 14 avenue Yves Thépot, F 29000 Quimper, France

Thierry Marhadour, Dewi Guellec and Divi Cornec
Rheumatology Department, Cavale Blanche Hospital and Brest Occidentale University, Brest, France

Sandrine Jousse-Joulin, Alain Saraux and Valérie Devauchelle-Pensec
Rheumatology Department, Cavale Blanche Hospital and Brest Occidentale University, Brest, France
INSERM UMR 1227, Laboratoire d'Immunothérapie et Pathologies lymphocytaires B, Labex "Immunotherapy, Graft, Oncology", Brest Occidentale University, 29609 Brest Cedex, France

Maelenn Gouillou
Clinical Investigation Centre (CIC) 1412, Institut National de la Santé et de la Recherche Médicale (INSERM), Brest, France

Mark Genovese
Division of Immunology and Rheumatology, Stanford School of Medicine, Stanford, CA, USA
Division of Immunology and Rheumatology, Stanford School of Medicine, 1000 Welch RD #203, Palo Alto, CA 94304, USA

Rene Westhovens
Department of Development and Regeneration KU Leuven, Skeletal Biology and Engineering Research Center; Rheumatology, University Hospitals Leuven, Leuven, Belgium

Luc Meuleners, Annegret Van der Aa, Pille Harrison and Chantal Tasset
Galapagos NV, Mechelen, Belgium

Arthur Kavanaugh
University of California San Diego, La Jolla, CA, USA

L. E. Burgers and D. M. Boeters
Department of Rheumatology, Leiden University Medical Center, C-01-046, 2300 RC Leiden, The Netherlands

A. H. M. van der Helm-van Mil
Department of Rheumatology, Leiden University Medical Center, C-01-046, 2300 RC Leiden, The Netherlands
Department of Rheumatology, Erasmus Medical Center, Rotterdam, the Netherlands

M. Reijnierse
Department of Radiology, Leiden University Medical Center, Leiden, the Netherlands

Katie L. Druce
Arthritis Research UK Centre for Epidemiology, Faculty of Biology Medicine and Health, the University of Manchester, Manchester M13 9PT, UK

Laraine Aikman and Piotr Szczypa
Medical Affairs, Pfizer, Sandwich, UK

Maria Dilleen
Statistics, Global Product Development, Pfizer, Sandwich, UK

Annie Burden
Quanticate, Hitchin, UK

Neil Basu
Epidemiology Group, School of Medicine, Medical Sciences and Nutrition, University of Aberdeen, Aberdeen, UK
Aberdeen Centre for Arthritis and Musculoskeletal Health, University of Aberdeen, Aberdeen, UK
Arthritis Research UK/MRC Centre for Musculoskeletal Health and Work, University of Aberdeen, Aberdeen, UK

Roy M. Fleischmann
Southwestern Medical Center, Metroplex Clinical Research Center, University of Texas, 8144 Walnut Hill Lane, Suite 810, Dallas, TX 75231, USA

Rieke Alten
Schlosspark-Klinik, University Medicine Berlin, Heubnerweg 2, Berlin 14059, Germany

Margarita Pileckyte
Department of Rheumatology, Hospital of Lithuanian University of Health Sciences, Eiveniu str.2, Kaunas, LT 50161, Lithuania

Kasia Lobello, Carol Cronenberger and Daniel Alvarez
Pfizer Inc., 500 Arcola Road Collegeville, Collegeville, PA 19426, USA

Steven Y. Hua
Pfizer Inc., 10777 Science Center Drive, CB1/2103, San Diego, CA 92121, USA

Amy E. Bock and K. Lea Sewell
Pfizer Inc., 300 Technology Square, Cambridge, MA 02139, USA

Brian F. Mandell
Department of Rheumatologic and Immunologic Disease, Cleveland Clinic, Cleveland, OH, USA

Anthony E. Yeo
Horizon Pharma, Lake Forest, IL, USA

Peter E. Lipsky
AMPEL BioSolutions, LLC, 250 West Main Street, Charlottesville, VA 22902, USA

Krista Kuuliala, Antti Kuuliala and Heikki Repo
Bacteriology and Immunology, Helsinki University Hospital and University of Helsinki, Helsinki, Finland

Riitta Koivuniemi and Marjatta Leirisalo-Repo
Rheumatology, Helsinki University Hospital and University of Helsinki, Helsinki, Finland

Hannu Kautiainen
Primary Health Care, Helsinki University Hospital and University of Helsinki, Helsinki, Finland
General Practice, Helsinki University Hospital and University of Helsinki, Helsinki, Finland
Unit of Primary Health Care, Kuopio University Hospital, Kuopio, Finland

Astrid Zbinden, Peter M. Villiger, Monika Østensen and Frauke Förger
Department of Rheumatology, Immunology and Allergology, University Hospital, University of Bern, Freiburgstrasse 8, 3010 Bern, Switzerland

Stephanie van den Brandt
Department of Rheumatology, Immunology and Allergology, University Hospital, University of Bern, Freiburgstrasse 8, 3010 Bern, Switzerland
Clinical Immunology and Rheumatology, Academic Medical Center/University of Amsterdam, Meibergdreef 9, 1105, AZ, Amsterdam, The Netherlands

Dominique Baeten
Clinical Immunology and Rheumatology, Academic Medical Center/University of Amsterdam, Meibergdreef 9, 1105, AZ, Amsterdam, The Netherlands

Klementy Shchetynsky, Lina-Marcella Diaz-Gallo, Lasse Folkersen, Aase Haj Hensvold, Anca Irinel Catrina, Louise Berg, Lars Klareskog and Leonid Padyukov
Rheumatology Unit, Department of Medicine Centre of Molecular Medicine, CMM:L8:04, Karolinska Institutet/Karolinska University Hospital Solna, 171 61 Stockholm, Sweden

Jianmin Xie
Department of Rheumatology, Second Affiliated Hospital of Nanjing Medical University, Nanjing, People's Republic of China

Hao Wang
Experimental Center of Basic Medicine, Shanghai Medical College, Fudan University, Shanghai, People's Republic of China

Index

CPSIA information can be obtained
at www.ICGtesting.com
Printed in the USA
LVHW061314290122
709673LV00007B/652

9 781639 274741